Pediatric
Neuro-
Ophthalmogy

Springer
New York
Berlin
Heidelberg
Barcelona
Budapest
Hong Kong
London
Milan
Paris
Santa Clara
Singapore
Tokyo

Pediatric
Neuro-
Ophthalmology

Michael C. Brodsky, MD

Associate Professor of Ophthalmology and Pediatrics
University of Arkansas for Medical Sciences, Jones Eye Institute
Chief of Pediatric Ophthalmology
Arkansas Children's Hospital
Little Rock, Arkansas

Robert S. Baker, MD

Chairman and Professor of Ophthalmology
Professor of Pediatrics, Neurosurgery, and Neurology
University of Kentucky Medical Center
Lexington, Kentucky

Latif M. Hamed, MD, FACS

Associate Professor of Ophthalmology and Pediatrics
Chief, Section of Pediatric Ophthalmology
University of Florida College of Medicine
Gainesville, Florida

Foreword by John Flynn, MD

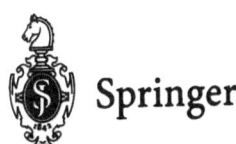 Springer

Michael C. Brodsky, MD
University of Arkansas for Medical Sciences
Little Rock, AR 72202-3591
USA

Robert S. Baker, MD
University of Kentucky
Lexington, KY 40536-0284
USA

Latif M. Hamed, MD
University of Florida College of Medicine
Gainesville, FL 32610
USA

With 229 illustrations, 82 in full color

Library of Congress Cataloging-in-Publication Data
Brodsky, Michael C.,
    Pediatric neuro-ophthalmology / Michael C. Brodsky, Robert S.
Baker, Latif M. Hamed.
        p.   cm.
    Includes bibliographical references and index.
    ISBN 0-387-94464-8 (alk. paper)
    1. Pediatric neuro-ophthalmology.   I. Baker, Robert S.   II. Hamed,
Latif M.   III. Title
    [DNLM: 1. Eye Diseases—in infancy & childhood. 2. Eye Diseases—
etiology 3. Nervous System Diseases—in infancy & childhood.
4. Nervous System Diseases—complications.   WW   600   B864p   1995]
RE725.B76   1995
618.92'0977—dc20   95-16249

Printed on acid-free paper.

© 1996 Springer-Verlag New York, Inc.
Softcover reprint of the hardcover 1st edition 1996

Production coordinated by Impressions, a division of Edwards Brothers, Inc. and managed
by Bill Imbornoni; manufacturing supervised by Joe Quatela.
Typeset by Impressions, a division of Edwards Brothers, Inc., Madison, WI.

9 8 7 6 5 4 3 2 1

ISBN-13: 978-1-4613-8459-5   e-ISBN-13: 978-1-4613-8457-1
DOI: 10.1007/978-1-4613-8457-1

Foreword

In today's world, an increasing number of voices ask, in at times querulous tones, where is medicine going and why? Perhaps no more succinct statement of the goal of our art and science can be found than words spoken in 1952 by Nobel laureate MacFarlane Burnet:

> The aim of medicine in the broadest sense is to provide for every human being, from conception to death, the greatest fullness of health and length of life that is allowed by his genetic constitution and by the accidents of life.

From the standpoint of the reader, this book documents progress in a field of medical research that indeed fulfills that goal in the sense of Burnet's thoughtful analysis. Progress in our understanding of the basic mechanisms of human nervous system development in its broadest context and its derangements—as well as our ability to use this information clinically—has been little short of astounding. This is nowhere more apparent than in the development of the visual system on its sensory and motor side. Though this has not always resulted in immediate therapeutic successes in the treatment of the many maladies that affect the visual system, particularly during its protean developmental phase, it has provided the ample infrastructure of basic knowledge that necessarily precedes such treatment breakthroughs. An apt analogy might be that of our understanding of human cancer, where huge advances are coming in avalanche fashion today. The groundwork for this progress was laid by painstaking and careful research in such disparate fields as cell biology and energetics, molecular genetics, pharmacology, epidemiology and the like, begun decades ago. Today we witness the coming together of the hard-won knowledge in all these disciplines in a coherent story and an enhanced understanding of cancer biology that is revolutionary. And we are indeed its benefactors. In like fashion, the many fields encompassed by the generic term neurosciences, from developmental embryology to neural imaging and neuropharmacology, are laying the groundwork for the breakthroughs in understanding, treatment, and, most importantly, prevention sure to come in the subject areas of this text.

In this work, the authors have more than filled a void long empty at the interface between pediatric and neuro-ophthalmology. They have created a new sense of the essential unity shared by the two disciplines as concerns the visual development of the child. This book is an expression of esteem, dedication, and, yes, love for their specialty on the part of the authors. This is not a book for the beginner. It takes no shortcuts, makes no sacrifices of rigor for simplicity, and spares us no detail that will illuminate our understanding of the nuance and variety of the entities it covers in its 11 chapters. In contrast to the multiauthored compendia that comprise today's encyclopedic texts in medicine, the work clearly reflects the distinctive approaches of the three authors to their subject. This does produce a bit of redundancy but leaves one with the sense of having viewed the topic from many different perspectives, thereby deepening and expanding one's appreciation of its many sides. It was a delight for this reader to encounter the many facets of optic nerve development and disease in Chapters 2, 3, and 4 and hear again echoes of these discussions in Chapter 1 and again in Chapter 5. The redundancy I find not at all boring, but enriching. Nor do they slight the basic sciences and their clinical contributions to our current understanding of, for example, the metabolic derangements leading to the spectrum of the storage diseases. On still another level, each author provides for the reader the algorithms that constitute his clinical approach to a given problem, say visual loss or nystagmus. For the physician, whatever his/her level of skill and expertise, trainee to consultant, this too is an asset. One may differ with the authors' approach, but it is there, clearly spelled out in the text together with the reasons behind their choices. I may not always agree with the intensity of the workup that they propose for an entity such as a hypoplastic optic nerve in an otherwise healthy infant, based on my experience with it over the decades, yet the text makes me fully aware of what I may be overlooking in so choosing.

It is not within the purview of my task to play the role of a reviewer and dissect the text chapter by chapter. Others much more astute and knowledgeable than I will do this. Rather, I see it as my responsibility to put the work in perspective for the reader-to-be. One can approach this book "cover to cover," as the small cadre of physicians with the special interest and expertise in the area will probably do. They will be rewarded for the effort with a truly encyclopedic coverage of their subject, likely to remain the reference standard for the coming years. For the physician with a more general background and specific need, the approach will likely be patient and problem oriented, and the volume serves this use as well. The bibliography is selective and remarkably up-to-date, reaching back to cite seminal works from the past as well as current citations in fast changing fields as neurochemistry and molecular genetics.

In closing, it is both a joy and a privilege to provide a foreword to this book. I have learned immensely from it.

John T. Flynn, MD
Miami, Florida
February 1995

Preface

The developing brain is at once inherently vulnerable and uniquely resilient in its response and adaptation to neurological injury. It is for this reason that neurological diseases in children differ in their clinical presentation, natural history, prognosis, and treatment response from similar injuries to the mature brain. This book was borne out of the recognition that ophthalmologists, neurologists, neurosurgeons, pediatricians, and orthoptists frequently encounter children with complex neuro-ophthalmologic disorders and would be well-served by a book covering various aspects of the discipline. Readers with an interest in pediatric neuro-ophthalmology must currently consult an array of textbooks in order to piece together answers to complex clinical questions. In this book, we have tried to accomplish the somewhat contradictory task of providing a clinical manual that is readily applicable to the child who is sitting in the examining chair, while offering a thoughtful analysis of each condition in light of current information. In so doing, we hope to provide the clinician with the insight needed to offer an accurate prognosis and treatment and thereby empower the clinician to provide appropriate support and guidance to the families of these children.

The evolution of pediatric neuro-ophthalmology as a discipline represents the confluence of a number of rapidly evolving fields, including neuroimaging, neurology, neurosurgery, neuropharmacology, genetics, and pediatrics. The unspoken goal of researchers in pediatric neuro-ophthalmology is to someday unite strabismus, amblyopia, and congenital nystagmus with the myriad other neuro-ophthalmologic disorders discusses in this book into one conceptual framework. Rapid advances in our understanding of the neuroanatomical and neurocellular substrates of strabismus and amblyopia will hopefully enable future editions of this book to accomplish this goal.

In this decade, which has been dubbed the decade of the brain, many of the disorders discusses in this book that have heretofore been untreatable may become treatable as advances occur in genetic therapy, neuron rescue, and preventative medicine. Twenty years from now, the analysis contained herein may be considered as merely an attempt to define the problem.

Michael C. Brodsky, MD
Robert S. Baker, MD
Latif M. Hamed, MD

Acknowledgments

The authors express their deep gratitude to the following individuals for their help and guidance in the preparation of this book: Frederick A. Boop, MD, Edward G. Buckley, MD, James C. Corbett, MD, Lou Dell'Osso, PhD, Gerald M. Fenichel, MD, Kathleen M. Fitzgerald, PhD, Katherine J. Fritz, CO, Charles M. Glasier, MD, May Griebel, MD, William V. Good, MD, Creig S. Hoyt, MD, William F. Hoyt, MD, James E. Jan, MD, Stephen P. Kraft, MD, Mark J. Kupersmith, MD, Burton J. Kushner, MD, Scott R. Lambert, MD, Patrick J. Lavin, MD, Nancy J. Newman, MD, Stephen C. Pollock, MD, Valerie Purvin, MD, Gregory B. Sharp, MD, Richard A. Saunders, MD, Charles Teo, MD, and Russell Walker, MD.

Contents

1

The Apparently Blind Infant

Introduction

Visual unresponsiveness in an otherwise healthy infant is an alarming finding. Parents are understandably anxious and inquisitive about the cause, severity, and prognosis of the condition. Depending upon the underlying cause, the visual outcome may range from normal vision to complete blindness. The importance of establishing an accurate diagnosis in this setting is obvious.

Decreased vision in infancy is generally due to developmental malformations or acquired lesions of the eyes, anterior visual pathways, or posterior visual pathways. Some causes involving ocular structures will be readily identifiable on careful eye examination (e.g., cataracts, corneal opacities, refractive errors). However, most congenital retinal dystrophies (e.g., Leber congenital amaurosis (LCA), congenital stationary night blindness (CSNB), achromatopsia) lack conspicuous ophthalmoscopic signs in early infancy and necessitate electroretinography to establish the diagnosis. Neurological visual impairment (e.g., cortical visual impairment (CVI)) can also be suspected clinically but requires neuroimaging to confirm.

Mentally retarded or autistic children may appear visually unresponsive despite intact visual pathways. However, physically or mentally disabled children may also have occult ophthalmologic disorders that are difficult to diagnose because of their disability.[62] The diagnosis of disorders causing visual disability in infants and children depends first and foremost on a pertinent clinical history and a thorough examination. The information thus obtained should enable a clinician with a thorough grasp of the various clinical entities that may cause an infant to act blind to formulate a list of differential diagnoses. The correct diagnosis may then be reached using a thoughtful diagnostic paradigm to work up such patients (Figure 1.1).

Important clues to the cause of blindness in an infant may be derived from various aspects of the ophthalmologic evaluation. Congenital nystagmus is absent in children with cortical visual loss but is a common feature in those with congenital ocular or anterior visual pathway disorders. It is now well established that the majority of patients with congenital nystagmus have underlying visual sensory disorders,[71,72] even when the eyes appear to be structurally normal.[228] It should be emphasized that the clinical appearance and the electro-oculographic waveforms of congenital nystagmus are identical whether or not a sensory deficit is detectable. The term "congenital" nystagmus is a misnomer, since the nystagmus is usually first noted between 8 and 12 weeks of age.[112] If damage to ocular or anterior visual pathway structures occurs postnatally, the nystagmus appears about 1 month after visual loss and only develops when the visual loss occurs prior to 2 years of age. During the first 2 months of life, the absence of nystagmus (in infants who will subsequently acquire it) eliminates an important diagnostic clue in differentiating an anterior visual pathway disorder from lesions of the posterior pathway. This distinction becomes especially important when dealing with ocular conditions that show minimal ophthalmoscopic signs in early infancy (e.g., LCA) or at any age (e.g., achromatopsia, CSNB).

Infants with nystagmus due to anterior visual pathway abnormalities typically have certain

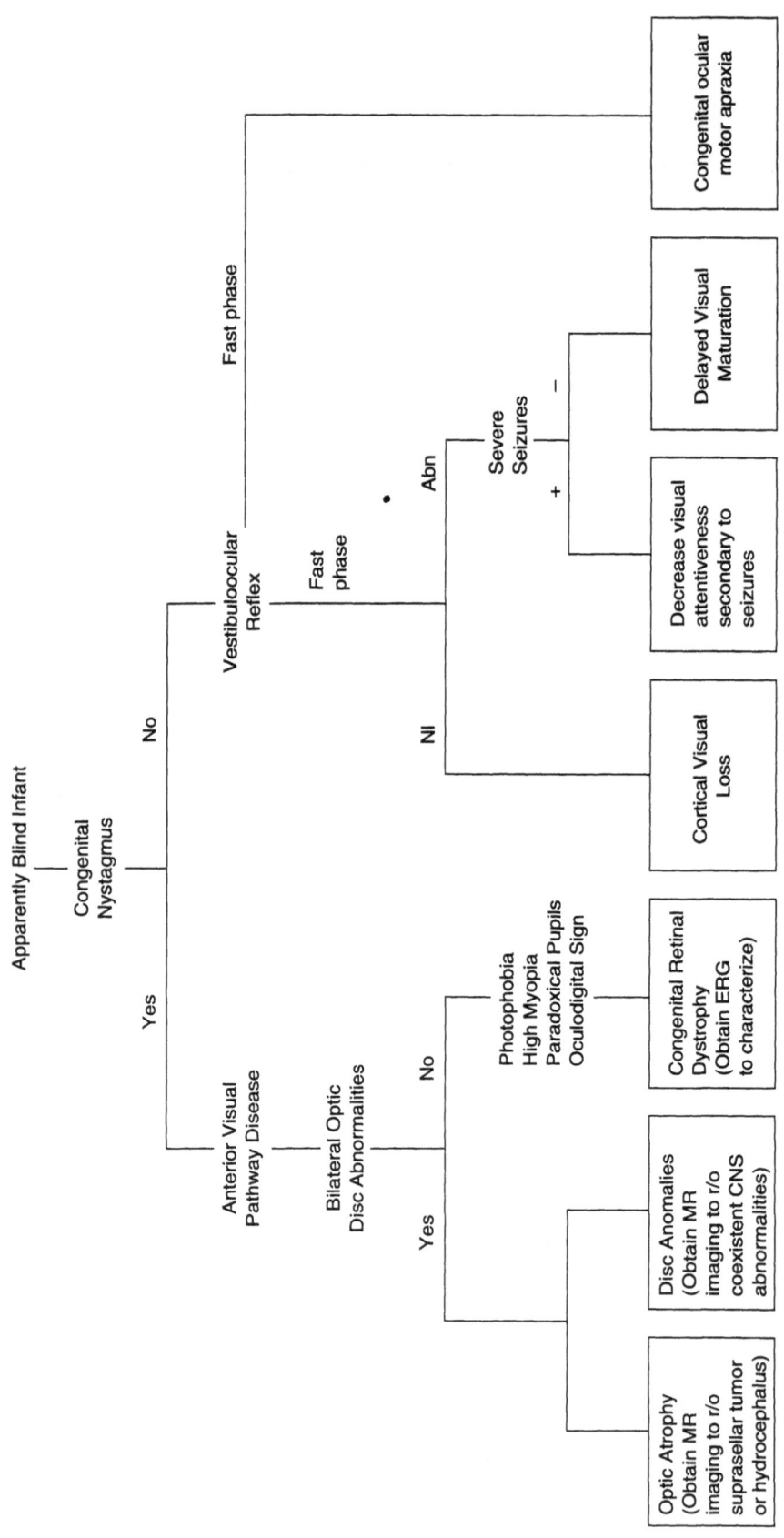

ONH = optic nerve hypoplasia
DVM = delayed visual maturation

FIGURE 1.1. This flow chart depicts a simplified diagnostic algorithm that may be used in the evaluation of the apparently blind infant.

directions of gaze in which the nystagmus is less intense and the vision is better (null points or null zones). Such children may hold their heads at eccentric angles when fixating an object. The presence of such a preferential head posture usually implies the presence of fixation and functional vision. Unlike head nodding observed in patients with spasmus nutans, the head shaking seen in some patients with congenital nystagmus and poor vision presumably does not prolong foveation time and would not, therefore, be expected to improve vision. However, this is a controversial issue, with some authorities maintaining that the head shaking is a learned, voluntary neurovisual adaptation to improve vision.[115a] This is supported by the observation that the head shaking is noted during intense visual fixation.[115a]

Congenital nystagmus due to sensory visual dysfunction should be distinguished from "roving" or "drifting" eye movements, the latter implying worse visual function. Roving eye movements are often seen in affixational patients with ocular or anterior visual pathway lesions whose vision is worse than 20/400. They are not seen in patients with pure cortical visual impairment. They consist of slow, aimless drifting of the eyes back and forth, usually horizontally.[112] Jan et al[112] likened fixation to an "anchor" without which the eyes "rove" back and forth. Nystagmus may be seen in some patients with roving eye movements when an object is held close enough to allow some fixation or may replace roving altogether in those whose vision improves.[112] Jan et al observed that some characteristics of congenital nystagmus due to anterior visual pathway abnormalities correspond with the age of the onset of visual loss and level of vision. Thus, nystagmus associated with extremely poor vision and/or vision loss before 6 months of age showed slow velocity and large amplitudes. Roving eye movements may represent one extreme in this continuum.

To summarize, nystagmus in an apparently blind infant is a valuable clinical marker for anterior visual pathway disease. Patients with bilateral disorders of the eye or anterior visual pathways may display roving eye movements, if the vision is extremely poor with absent fixation; horizontal nystagmus, if the vision is less than 20/70 in the better eye but fixation is present; or neither, if the vision is better than 20/70. The 20/70 cutoff is somewhat arbitrary, and variations on this are common. It is not unusual to see patients with CSNB, albinism, or blue-cone monochromatism with visual acuity as good as 20/40 who display nystagmus. It is therefore probably an oversimplification to suggest that the nystagmus is a result of the visual deficit in such patients. The finding of ocular movement abnormalities, including nystagmus, in obligate carriers of blue-cone monochromatism who had visual acuity of 20/20 or better suggests that the nystagmus is intrinsic to the disease and can appear independent of the visual impairment.[78] Theoretically, the two traits (the cone disorder and the associated nystagmus) may be inherited through linked genes rather than a single gene.

The pupillary examination may provide valuable clues to the diagnosis in this setting to the extent that it can be reliably performed in small, uncooperative infants. Infants with blindness due to congenital retinal disorders show sluggishly reactive pupils, whereas the pupillary light reaction is usually spared in patients with pure CVI. A "paradoxical" pupillary response (initial constriction of the pupil to darkness) may be present in certain retinal disorders, such as CSNB and congenital achromatopsia.[11,64,178] It is not specific to these disorders, however, as it may also be present in some patients with optic nerve abnormalities (e.g., developmental optic nerve disorders, bilateral optic neuritis, dominant optic atrophy), patients with strabismus and amblyopia or nystagmus but without apparent retinal or optic nerve disease, or even those patients with normal eyes.[68] Paradoxical pupillary responses are often difficult to detect in infants but become more apparent over the first few years of life.

Certain congenital retinal disorders are characteristically associated with high refractive errors: high hyperopia in LCA[8,67] and high myopia in patients with CSNB and other congenital retinal dystrophies.[136] Albinos may have high hyperopia or high myopia. These associations are not constant but are sufficiently frequent to warrant consideration of retinal disorders in a blind infant with nystagmus.

The funduscopic appearance of the infant eye differs sufficiently from that of the adult eye in ways that may cause a diagnostic problem to the clinician. The optic discs of young infants often appear pale, even when undue pressure on the globe is avoided while opening the eyelids. In equivocal cases, the presence of asymmetric disc appearance or peripapillary nerve fiber layer dropout may serve to corroborate the impression of genuine disc pallor. The fundus of young infants often has a pale, speckled appearance that may be difficult to distinguish from an abnormal fundus with ophthalmoscopy. Foveal hypoplasia is one of the more difficult causes of decreased vision to diagnose. Although a common feature of ocular albinism and aniridia, it may occasionally occur as an isolated familial disorder.[173]

Some congenital retinal disorders are associated with various degrees of photophobia (intolerance to light). Most notably, children with congenital achromatopsia display an extreme aversion to light. Marked photophobia may also be seen in cone–rod dystrophy and LCA. Children with optic nerve hypoplasia and dominant optic atrophy are often mildly photophobic. Photophobia and glare arising from corneal or lenticular opacities can be readily classified as such on ocular examination. Even when other ocular disorders (e.g., media opacities, iritis, albinism, aniridia) are excluded, photophobia is not invariably of retinal origin. A variety of neurological disorders are associated with photophobia, including meningitis, subarachnoid hemorrhage, migraine, trigeminal neuralgia, thalamic infarct, head injuries, and tumors compressing the anterior visual pathways.

It has been recently demonstrated that CVI can also be associated with photophobia (approximately one-third of patients in the study by Jan et al[115]), presumably a result of associated thalamic damage or the cortical lesion itself. The photophobia in most patients is mild, with a tendency to resolve or diminish along with visual and other symptomatic improvement. Jan et al[115] did not find a close relationship between the photophobia and the severity of the visual loss or the peripheral field defects. It should be noted that some patients with CVI show a compulsive tendency to gaze at room lights, especially fluorescent lights, or other bright objects, including the sun (light gazing).[116] Photophobia and light gazing in patients with CVI are not mutually exclusive, with many children, paradoxically, exhibiting both.[115] Jan et al[115] feel that "light-gazing is such a compulsive behavior that even the presence of photophobia is not a deterrent." The presence of mild photophobia cannot, therefore, be used to distinguish a primary

retinal disease from cortical visual loss. However, the marked photophobia is highly suggestive of congenital retinal dystrophy.

Some children with very poor vision habitually press on their eyes with a finger or a fist. This "oculodigital sign" appears to be specific for bilateral congenital or very early-onset blindness due to retinal disease (e.g., LCA, retinopathy of prematurity, congenital retinal infections, retinal dysplasia, congenital cone–rod dystrophy).[113] It does not occur in children with only one blind eye irrespective of cause and is not seen in children with cortical blindness, media opacities, or optic nerve disease. Children who engage in frequent eye poking often exhibit sunken eyes due to orbital fat atrophy. Jan et al[113] speculated that eye pressing stimulates the visual cortex by mechanically triggering ganglion cell action potentials (phosphenes). Absence of eye pressing in children with blockage of the visual pathways due to optic nerve or cortical damage supports his speculation. This probably explains the observation that children with CVI do not show deep-set orbits.[114] Eye pressing should be distinguished from eye rubbing and eye poking.[113a] For example, children who are sleepy tend to rub their eyes, those with blinding ocular disorders tend to press their eyes, whereas severely mentally disabled children with self-injurious behavior may poke their eyes or even rub their corneas, sometimes with disasterous results.[113a] We have seen vigorous eye poking in children with Down syndrome lead to dislocation of the crystalline lens. In addition to eye pressing, children with retinal blindness may wave their fingers between their eyes and a bright light (finger waving). Finger waving may also be seen in photoconvulsive epilepsy and autism.

Some children with bilaterally poor vision display a phenomenon termed "overlooking" (Figure 1.2). Instead of looking at the object of regard directly, affected children look above the object. Initially attributed to relative preservation of the inferior visual field in patients with certain retinal disorders,[210] it was later reported not to be disease specific but rather to represent a sign of bilateral central scotomas (and vision of 20/200 or worse) in children from a variety of causes.[73] Nevertheless, the majority of patients who display this sign will be found to have congenital retinal disorders. Overlooking may initially be mistaken for either

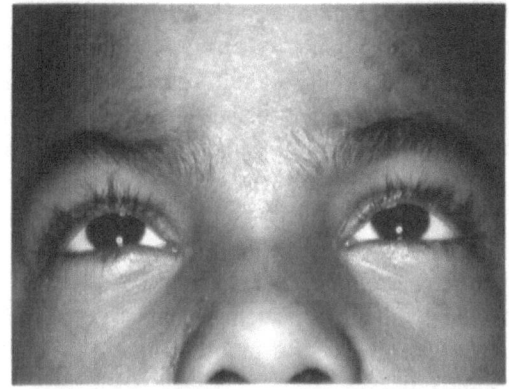

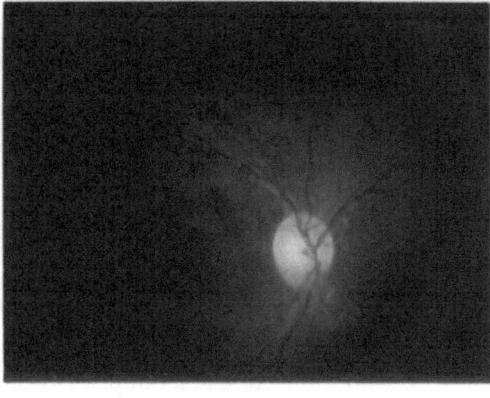

FIGURE 1.2. Overlooking. This 8-year-old boy habitually views objects by looking above them. (**A**) Patient attempting to view a target attached to the camera's lens. (**B** and **C**) The fundus pictures depict arteriolar narrowing and mottling of the retinal pigment epithelium. He was diagnosed as having rod–cone dystrophy.

lack of cooperation or comprehension on the part of the patient or may be misinterpreted as a primary ocular motor disorder.

Blind patients at various ages may experience formed and/or unformed hallucinations. These have been considered, in the absence of epilepsy, to represent a release phenomenon.[141] Release phenomena refer to neurological disorders resulting from maladaptive activity of disinhibited neurons following damage to their source of inhibition.

The fixation pattern of children with congenital visual defects follows a general pattern based on the extent of the vision loss: Children with vision better than 20/200 follow mostly with their eyes, those with 20/200 follow with both their eyes and head, and those with severe vision loss follow mostly with their head.[112] Those with severe, congenital loss of vision have difficulty with producing willful saccades into any suggested direction, with upward gaze being most markedly limited.[112] The suggestion that this limitation in upgaze results because the superior fields are relatively unimportant (and thus infrequently uti-

lized)[112] may be valid, although this would appear to be more applicable to adults than to children, in whom (because of short stature) much of the world resides in the superior fields.

A preference to view objects of regard at very close range may be seen occasionally in normal children, reflecting a transient behavioral pattern. Children with poor vision often do so consistently to produce linear magnification (by shortening the focal length), to dampen an existing nystagmus to improve vision, or in the case of uncorrected aphakic children, to induce a miotic response to increase depth of focus and create a pinhole effect.[75]

Assessment of vision in children with severe visual deficits requires the utilization of specialized techniques or specific adaptations of techniques commonly used in children. The usual qualitative subjective methods of assessing the ability of the child to fix and follow, the steadiness of fixation, and the ability to maintain fixation are not as helpful since most such children are affixational. It is practically more relevant to obtain a measure of overall visual function than to simply attempt measurement of distance visual acuity, which is difficult or impossible with severe visual impairment. Snellen acuity charts and similar tests are often useless. Parental accounts of the child's visual behavior are usually good starting points. Patiently playing with affected children using a variety of toys of different colors and sizes provides useful information. Can the child recognize various objects in the environment, navigate effectively, and interact visually with other people? How does the child respond to the examiner's face, larger objects, or movement of the parent nearby? How does the child react to penlight or to flickering of room lights on and off? A widening of the palpebral fissures when room lights are extinguished indicates the presence of at least light perception.

A measure of vision can be achieved with the dynamic vestibulo-ocular reflex. This is evoked by holding the infant face-to-face with the examiner at about arm's length and spinning the infant around. The infant develops nystagmus as the eyes move counter to the direction of rotation and, at the limit of their excursion, make a quick movement in the opposite direction before the cycle is repeated. When the spinning stops, the inertia of the endolymph in the semicircular canal evokes nystagmus in the opposite direction that is dampened within 5 seconds in a child with good vision; the nystagmus lasts longer in a blind infant due to poor fixation. Visual function may also be qualitatively evaluated with the optokinetic reflex. When the visual field moves with respect to the eyes, as with a rotating optokinetic drum, the eyes track the moving field to the limit of their excursion and then make a recovery saccade in the opposite direction and so on, producing optokinetic nystagmus. Totally blind infants cannot generate optokinetic nystagmus. It has been estimated that visually impaired patients with horizontal nystagmus who are able to generate an optokinetic nystagmus to a vertically rotating drum should be able to achieve a significant measure of visual independence (i.e., they probably will not be required to be in a school for the blind).

Generally, the vision of infants and children with various neurological diseases (e.g., cerebral palsy, mental retardation) is more difficult to evaluate irrespective of its level. Numerous studies have demonstrated a higher prevalence of subnor-

mal acuity in children with cerebral palsy than in age-matched controls.[149] Hertz and Rosenberg[91] found that the more severe the physical and neurological disability in children with cerebral palsy, the worse the visual performance on the acuity cards. They reasoned that poorer visual performance may reflect a combination of genuine poor visual function and difficulty in test administration and interpretation in this group of patients. The poorer vision in more severely affected children with cerebral palsy is not surprising given the diffuse nature of the encephalopathic process.

The vision of infants and children with cerebral palsy and mental retardation, with or without severe visual impairment, may be quantitatively evaluated with preferential looking techniques (e.g., Teller acuity cards).[46,58,91] These techniques are also useful to document the visual improvement that occurs in some of these patients, especially those with CVI or delayed visual maturation.[80] However, the results of Teller acuity card testing and similar tests of grating acuity should be interpreted with caution.[131a] Hoyt[99] suggested that Teller acuity card methods have low sensitivity in detecting significant visual dysfunction during infancy. Infants who score entirely within the normal range with Teller acuity cards may later be found to have significantly reduced acuity with recognition visual acuity testing (e.g., Snellen acuity). Droste et al[47] presented evidence that visual function in visually impaired children is more accurately evaluated by a combination of Teller acuity cards and a battery of other visual function behavioral tests than by the Teller cards alone. Citing these and other potential pitfalls, Kushner[130] presented a cogent argument against using the results of grating acuity to classify children as legally blind for social service purposes. Doing so, he cautioned, may overestimate their visual function, which would unjustifiably deny financial benefits to qualified children.

Unfortunately, visual evoked potential (VEP) is not a reliable method of quantitative visual evaluation in patients with cerebral palsy, mental retardation, or severe neurological disease (see below). In children with poor vision and nystagmus due to anterior visual pathway disorders, Jan et al[117] proposed the performance of the "unequal nystagmus test" to determine which eye, if any, has better vision. The test is performed by noting the degree of nystagmus while the child views an attractive toy at a distance with both eyes open and then with alternate eyes covered. The nystagmus is similar in patients with similar acuity in both eyes. When the acuities are different, wider and slower excursions of nystagmus are noted in the worse eye, and faster and smaller-amplitude nystagmus is noted in the better eye. Other batteries of tests with the stated purpose of evaluating vision in children with severe visual deficits have been recently reported.[47]

Much valuable clinical information about visual impairment in children has been gleaned from the collaborative efforts of various subspecialists working as multidisciplinary diagnostic teams. The collaborative efforts of pediatric ophthalmologists, pediatric neurologists, electrophysiologists, behavioral psychologists, and developmental specialists, among others, will be needed to further enhance our understanding of the various disorders discussed within.

Besides rendering accurate diagnoses and treating the remediable causes of blindness, the clinician should be acquainted with the mental, psychological, neuroendocrinologic, developmental, and educational needs of visually impaired children. Knowledge of the various available programs that may act as resources to affected children and their families is essential, especially since, unfortunately, definitive treatment of many of the underlying conditions remains elusive.

This chapter will address causes of blindness that are neurological in origin or that have features that warrant including them in the differential diagnoses of neurologic causes of blindness. Emphasis will be placed on CVI and related disorders. Causes of blindness due to congenital ocular disorders associated with obvious structural ocular abnormalities (e.g., albinism, congenital cataracts, chorioretinal colobomas, retinopathy of prematurity) will be discussed elsewhere.

Hereditary Retinal Disorders

Causes of blindness in infancy due to opacities of the optical media or to refractive errors are usually discovered during a thorough ophthalmologic evaluation. Optic nerve hypoplasia may be poten-

tially overlooked if the examiner mistakes the border of the outside ring in the classic double-ring sign with the border of the disc.[135] Generally, hereditary diseases of the retina should be suspected in children who present with bilateral decrease in vision, light sensitivity, color deficiency, visual impairment confined to either daytime or nighttime, and a tendency to bump into objects and to hold objects very close to the face. A family history of similarly affected members may be elicited, and a history of consanguinity is highly suggestive since many of these disorders are recessively inherited.

Many patients with congenital retinal dystrophies have characteristic features that are highly suggestive, if not virtually diagnostic, of a specific underlying disorder. For instance, profound photophobia and nystagmus in a blind child with generally normal-appearing eyes otherwise highly suggest rod monochromatism, whereas blindness and nystagmus in the presence of diffuse pigmentary retinal changes suggest LCA. Unfortunately, not all patients can be pigeonholed into these classic presentations; some require further investigation, for instance, the young blind infant with an ostensibly normal fundus appearance who has LCA. Many congenital retinal dystrophies are distinguishable on the electrophysiological level but remain otherwise poorly defined as simply cone dystrophies, cone–rod dystrophies, or rod–cone dystrophies, although diagnosis at the molecular level is rapidly becoming available.

Leber Congenital Amaurosis

Leber congenital amaurosis is a recessively inherited, severe retinal dystrophy involving both rods and cones. It is characterized by the onset of blindness at birth, a variable fundus picture, and an absent or extremely attenuated electroretinogram (ERG). Photophobia is seldom present and is never of the degree found in congenital achromatopsia. Patients show nystagmus, poorly reactive or unreactive pupils, and a positive oculodigital sign of Franceschetti (pushing on the eyes or rubbing them with a finger or fist) to create phosphenes. The fundus picture may appear normal at birth or shortly thereafter. However, a variety of pigmentary changes may develop over months to years (Figure 1.3). These include salt and pepper pigmentation, yellowish flecks, a mosaic pattern, periarteriolar distribution of yellow lesions, a retinitis pigmentosa-like fundus, or macular coloboma. The abnormal retinal appearance may be progressive, leading to a variable picture of chorioretinal degenerative changes, vascular narrowing, and optic disc pallor. The vascular narrowing is probably present at birth but is easily overlooked. Patients have a higher-than-normal risk for developing keratoconus and cataracts later on in life.

The pattern VEP is absent, as is the flash VEP in most cases. It is estimated that LCA accounts for 10% to 18% of childhood blindness. This disorder may comprise a number of genetically heterogeneous conditions.[88] The visual acuity ranges from 20/200 (rare) to no light perception.[136,138] Parents can be reassured that the visual impairment is usually nonprogressive, despite the visible progression of the fundus findings.[88] Exceptional cases showing further visual deterioration with time belong either to the subgroup of LCA with macular colobomas or to harbor cataracts or keratoconus.[88] Conversely, some patients with Leber amaurosis may show some visual improvement within the first several years of life, enough to have visually guided behavior and measurable grating acuity. A similar phenomenon occurs in some albinos and some children with optic nerve hypoplasia. It is attributed to a secondary delay in maturation of the posterior visual pathways.[58,59]

As many as half of the patients with LCA examined before 1 year of age may show a normal retinal appearance,[88] although careful examination using direct ophthalmoscopy shows marked arteriolar narrowing. Since nystagmus may not be present during the first few months of life, the normal retinal appearance in many infants with LCA may pose a diagnostic dilemma, raising the specter of CVI or delayed visual maturation, among others. The ERG is the definitive test in establishing the diagnosis of LCA. The range of refractive errors associated with LCA is wide, ranging from high hyperopia to high myopia, with high hyperopia being far more common. Some studies have suggested that associated high hyperopia differentiates a distinct subset of the disorder, uncomplicated by neurologic or systemic disease. Subsequent studies disproved this distinction, showing that high hyperopia does not differentiate complicated from uncomplicated cases.[36] A careful consideration of neurologic, systemic, or biochemical disorders should be offered to patients with LCA, regardless of refractive error.[136]

The optic discs appear normal early on, but may later develop pallor (Figure 1.3). Sullivan et al[208] retrospectively reviewed the optic disc findings in 77 patients with LCA. Sixty-nine percent showed normal discs, 23% showed varying degrees of optic atrophy, 3% showed pseudopapilledema, and 1% showed gray discs. They concluded that the optic discs are frequently normal, even in older patients with LCA. They suggested that the find-

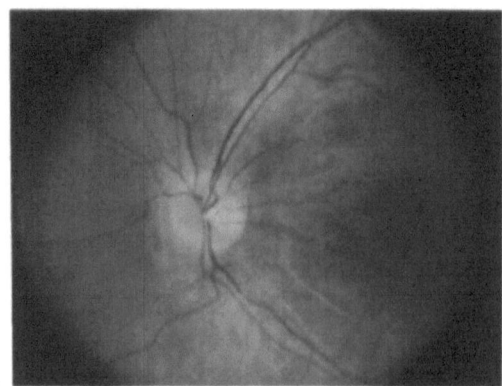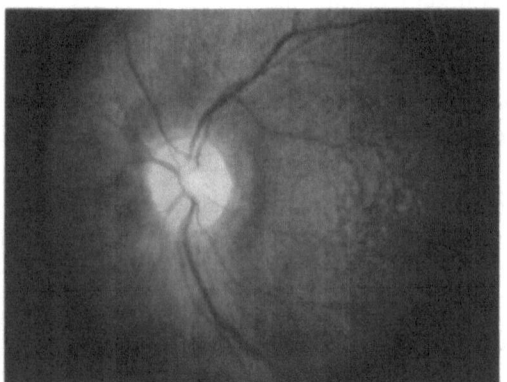

FIGURE 1.3. (A) Fundus appearance of an infant with LCA shows somewhat attenuated retinal arterioles but little, if any, pigmentary changes. (B) Fundus appearance in a 5-year-old boy with LCA shows pallor of the optic disc, retinal arteriolar attenuation, and diffuse mottling of the retinal pigment epithelium.

ing of significant optic atrophy in an infant suspected to have LCA may suggest one of the systemic, metabolic disorders associated with infantile retinal dystrophies (e.g., peroxisomal disorders).

A number of disorders manifesting a congenital retinal dystrophy in association with other neurologic or systemic disorders have been previously grouped with LCA. These include medullary cystic kidney disease or nephronophtisis (Senior–Loken syndrome), cone-shaped epiphyses of the hand and cerebellar ataxia (Saldino–Mainzer syndrome), vermis hypoplasia, ocular motor disturbances and neonatal respiratory problems (Joubert syndrome), psychomotor retardation, mental retardation, autistic behavior, hydrocephalus, deafness, epilepsy, or cardiomyopathy. The ever-increasing identification of distinct disorders once grouped with LCA and the heterogeneity of the findings associated with LCA support the idea that LCA is not a single nosologic entity but rather a group of genetically heterogeneous disorders awaiting further characterization.[2] For example, many children with peroxisomal disorders and blindness get classified as LCA until their underlying metabolic disturbance becomes evident.[82] It should be noted that the various disorders of congenital retinal dystrophy described earlier do not have identical clinical presentations. For instance, most patients with the Senior–Loken syndrome show better (some even normal) visual acuity in early infancy than the typical case of LCA.

A number of oculocerebral disorders associated with peroxisomal dysfunction and a high blood level of very long-chain fatty acids[66,176] may simulate LCA. The peroxisome is a single-membrane subcellular organelle that mediates the catabolism of very long-chain fatty acids, phytanic acid, and pipecolic acid, as well as the biosynthesis of some types of membrane lipids. Cerebro-hepato-renal syndrome (Zellweger syndrome), neonatal adrenoleukodystrophy, and infantile Refsum disease are associated with peroxisomal dysfunction and progressive deterioration of rod and cone function.[234] All three conditions show rapidly progressive neurological deterioration, but the initial manifestation before this deterioration occurs may resemble LCA both clinically and electrophysiologically. In fact, it is felt that some patients described in the older literature (before the advent of advanced metabolic testing) with LCA and neurological disease might have belonged to this group of disorders. In an infant with poor vision and nystagmus, the findings of seizures, failure to thrive, developmental delay, neurosensory deafness, neurological deterioration, or dysmyelination on magnetic resonance imaging (MRI) of the brain should suggest a peroxisomal disorder and prompt a metabolic workup. Therefore, infants or young children suspected to harbor LCA, especially if other neurodevelopmental abnormalities exist, should not only have a thorough ophthalmologic examination but should also be seen by a pediatrician or pediatric neurologist experienced in metabolic disorders.[38]

A minority of patients with Leber amaurosis may show associated neuroimaging abnormalities, such as ventriculomegaly, dysmyelination, or cerebellar vermis hypoplasia.[202] The finding of vermis hypoplasia should suggest a diagnosis of Joubert syndrome (Figure 1.4).

Does early-onset blindness due to ocular disorders such as Leber amaurosis affect myelination and maturation of the posterior visual pathway? Steinlin et al[203] performed MRI in seven children (aged 5 months to 16 years) with LCA. The

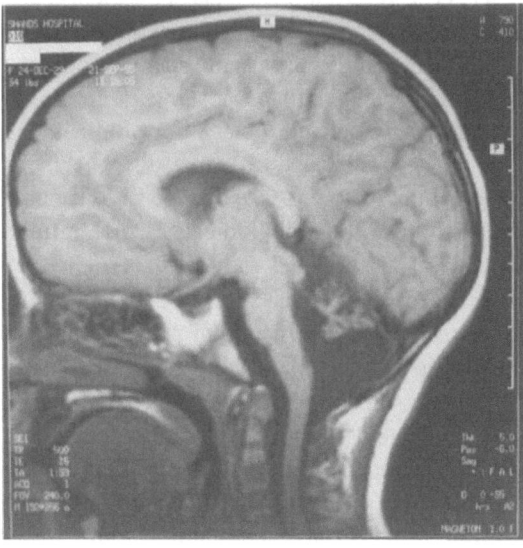

FIGURE 1.4. Joubert syndrome. MRI scan shows severe vermis hypoplasia with a large fourth ventricle.

posterior visual pathway showed grossly normal myelination on MRI, leading the authors to conclude that myelination of the optic radiation is not interrupted by greatly diminished visual sensory input in patients with LCA. Curless et al[35] described two brothers with Leber amaurosis and dysmyelination detected by MRI who had no peroxisomal defect. Both patients had delayed psychomotor development, and one had autistic features. On the basis of the study by Steinlin et al,[203] these two patients probably represent a heretofore undetermined disorder, probably of metabolic origin.

Leber congenital amaurosis should be differentiated from non-ocular causes of blindness like cortical blindness or delayed visual maturation. Infants with LCA may be thought to have CVI within the first few weeks of life, before the nystagmus appears. Conditions that are commonly mistaken for LCA include CSNB, achromatopsia, infantile-onset retinitis pigmentosa, peroxisomal disorders, Joubert syndrome, and neuronal ceroid lipofuscinosis.[136]

Electroretinography is particularly helpful in distinguishing between the various disorders in infants with poor vision, nystagmus, and a seemingly normal ocular examination. The three most common such disorders are LCA, CSNB, and congenital achromatopsia. Leber congenital amaurosis is characterized by extinguished or markedly attenuated ERG. Achromatopsia shows markedly attenuated or nonremarkable cone-mediated ERG; the rod-mediated ERG is usually spared. Congenital stationary night blindness shows a normal a wave but an attenuated b wave on rod-mediated ERG; the cone-mediated ERG may also be abnormal. It is important to realize that the ERG is not a prognostic test. It simply indicates which retinal components are affected and to what extent, but the test needs to be repeated if one is to determine whether or not a disorder is progressive and at what rate in a given individual.

Our understanding of the genetic retinal disorders is undergoing tremendous changes due to advances in molecular biology. The precise gene defects have been uncovered for conditions such as gyrate atrophy, blue-cone monochromacy, X-linked cone degeneration, dominant retinitis pigmentosa, and choroideremia.[143] Knowledge of the gene defects that may eventuate in LCA will un-

doubtedly cast further light on the pathophysiology of LCA and provide potential new avenues for treatment.

Joubert Syndrome

Joubert syndrome was first described in 1969.[120] It is characterized by a variable combination of the following features: episodic neonatal tachypnea and apnea, rhythmic protrusion of the tongue, ataxia, hypotonia, and variable degree of psychomotor retardation.[134] The episodic tachypnea presents in the neonatal period and alternates with periods of apnea, resembles the panting of a dog, and usually resolves or improves. Notable associated eye findings may include congenital retinal dystrophy, nystagmus, abnormal supranuclear eye movements, colobomas, or congenital ocular fibrosis and other forms of strabismus. A congenital retinal dystrophy is seen in approximately 50% of patients with Joubert syndrome.[107,123] This retinal dystrophy was at first labeled as a variant of LCA. It was subsequently considered different from LCA in that the visual loss is usually not as profound (20/60 to 20/200, as compared with count fingers or worse), and the VEPs are relatively spared (mild to moderate reduction in amplitudes, as compared with absent or highly attenuated signals). Both conditions show flat or highly attenuated ERGs. Ocular motor disorders described in Joubert syndrome include slow, hypometric saccades, ocular motor apraxia, periodic alternating gaze deviation, pendular torsional nystagmus, seesaw nystagmus, skew deviation, and defective smooth pursuit as well as optokinetic and vestibular responses.[134]

Dysgenesis or hypoplasia of the cerebellar vermis is a typical and a highly characteristic morphological feature of Joubert syndrome[122] (Figure 1.4). Complete agenesis of the cerebellar vermis may also occur, but this is readily distinguishable from the vermian agenesis that occurs with the Dandy–Walker variant by the associated findings. For instance, hydrocephalus and cystic dilatation of the fourth ventricle do not occur with the Joubert syndrome. Additional sporadic structural defects reported in association with the Joubert syndrome include other cerebellar midline defects, a dilated fourth ventricle, short neck, occipital meningoencephalocele, microcephaly, unsegmented midbrain tectum, absence of the corpus callosum and brainstem, multicystic kidneys, congenital ocular fibrosis, and bilateral retinal colobomas. The condition may be sporadic, but familial cases are inherited in an autosomal recessive pattern.

The Joubert syndrome has some overlapping features with the Arima syndrome (cerebro-oculo-hepato-renal syndrome). The Arima syndrome exhibits pigmentary degeneration suggestive of LCA, severe psychomotor retardation, hypotonia, characteristic facies, polycystic kidneys, and absent cerebellar vermis. Joubert and Arima syndromes may be distinguished by such clinical features as neonatal tachypnea, which is one of the cardinal features of Joubert.

Congenital Stationary Night Blindness

This condition may be classified into two subtypes: one with a normal fundus appearance and another with abnormal fundus.[161] Subtypes of congenital stationary night blindness with abnormal fundi include Oguchi disease and fundus albipunctatus. Vision of affected children ranges from 20/20 to 20/200 and does not deteriorate with time. Those with reduced vision often have a myopic refractive error and typically show nystagmus. The disorder is inherited as an X-linked trait (most common) or as an autosomal recessive or dominant trait (less common). Typically, the ERG shows a normal *a* wave and an attenuated *b* wave under scotopic conditions. The dark adaptation curve is usually 2 to 3 log units higher than normal. The various types of CSNB are detailed in chapter 9.

Achromatopsia

This is a congenital, nonprogressive defect of the cone photoreceptors. Affected children present with nystagmus, decreased vision, defective or absent color discrimination, photophobia, and paradoxical pupils (initial constriction upon dimming ambient light). The fundus appears normal. Achromatopsia has been subdivided into two categories: complete (autosomal recessive), in which cone function is absent and vision ranges from 20/200 to 20/400, and incomplete (autosomal recessive or X-linked), in which residual cone function is present and vision may range from 20/40 to

20/400. The incomplete variety may be further subdivided on the basis of residual sensitivity to one or a combination of red, green, or blue light stimuli. The associated nystagmus in some incomplete cases may improve with time or may disappear altogether. The ERG is characterized by diminished or absent cone response and a normal rod response.

Congenital Optic Nerve Disorders

Some congenital disorders of the optic nerves should be mentioned in the context of infant blindness, although these disorders are discussed at length in other chapters. The most relevant for this discussion is bilateral optic nerve hypoplasia (Chapter 2) and congenital or early-onset optic atrophy (Chapter 4). Neuroimaging studies are generally required in patients with optic nerve hypoplasia as a part of both a neuroendocrinologic workup (i.e., the presence of posterior pituitary ectopia on MRI is a useful marker for associated pituitary gland dysfunction) and a neurodevelopmental evaluation (i.e., the presence of hemispheric abnormalities on computed tomography (CT) or MRI scanning is a clinical marker for associated developmental abnormalities.[25,26,198] Congenital or early-onset bilateral optic atrophy always warrants neuroimaging to look for suprasellar tumors (craniopharyngioma, glioma) or hydrocephalus.[183]

Cortical Visual Impairment

Introduction

At the outset, clarification of certain aspects of related terminology may be useful. Cortical blindness refers to complete loss of vision resulting from disorders of the geniculostriate pathway. Some investigators prefer to more accurately refer to the visual deficit as cerebral rather than cortical, because damage either to the optic radiations, to the occipital cortex, or to both diminishes vision. The term cortical continues to be the one in common use and will be employed by us in this discussion. Furthermore, since the degree of vision loss resulting from a cortical insult is highly variable, rarely complete, and often shows a degree of recovery, many investigators prefer the term cortical visual impairment (CVI) over cortical blindness to avoid the dismal prognostic implications suggested by the term blindness.[114,229] We also discourage the term cortical blindness, since affected children usually have residual vision.

Cortical visual impairment is one of the major forms of visual loss in children in the developed world. The proportion of blindness in children attributable to this disorder has increased as a result of two major factors: (1) Advancement in neonatal medicine has resulted in saving the lives of an increasing number of premature infants and children with severe brain damage. (2) Advancement of ophthalmologic techniques to treat other causes of blindness in children, such as cataracts, has reduced the proportion of such children in schools for the blind. Medical advances to prevent and treat CVI have lagged behind.

The most common definition of CVI found in the literature is derived almost entirely from experience with adult patients who have acquired cortical lesions. In this context, the diagnosis of CVI requires very poor vision, normal pupillary light reflexes, no nystagmus, and an otherwise normal eye examination. However, congenital or early-acquired cortical visual loss in children may be quite different from the acquired variety in adult life. The immature, extremely adaptable infantile brain may react differently to injury than the adult brain. As the entity of CVI in infants and children is explored further in this chapter, the reader should keep in mind that some qualifying remarks are necessary for each of the classic features included in the above definition. First, the visual loss need not be severe; CVI represents a spectrum of disability. Second, contrary to classic teaching, the pupillary reaction to light may not be completely normal. This finding may be due to coexisting disorders of the anterior visual pathway, the sympathetic and parasympathetic pathways, or to transsynaptic degeneration of the pupillomotor fibers if the cortical lesion is prenatal.[218] On the basis of clinical evidence derived from patients with congenital homonymous hemianopia due to congenital occipital lesions, it appears that the pupillomotor fibers, which do not synapse at the lateral geniculate nucleus but at the pretectal area, may also be susceptible to transsynaptic degeneration.[218] Third, affected patients

may display intermittent, *unsustained* bursts of nystagmus. Characteristic wandering eye movements seen in severe CVI should not be mistaken for nystagmus. Finally, the eye examination may reveal coexistent optic atrophy due to associated anterior pathway disease or transsynaptic degeneration of the retinogeniculate pathway.

Causes of Cortical Visual Loss

Perinatal Hypoxia-Ischemia

The most common cause of CVI in children is hypoxic brain insult (asphyxia). Ischemic brain damage tends to involve different regions of the brain in premature infants as compared with full-term infants. This is so since the watershed areas (i.e., the areas that have the most tenuous vascular supply) are different in premature and term brains. In premature infants, meningeal anastomosis bridges the watershed zone between the major cerebral arteries; parasagittal infarctions are therefore rare. Instead, the periventricular region represents a transient watershed zone in premature brains between the ventriculopetal and ventriculofugal branches of deep penetrating arteries (so the optic radiations are more involved). This explains why periventricular leukomalacia is a common pathological finding in premature infants. In full-term infants, the watershed zones lie in the regions between the anterior and middle cerebral arteries and between the middle and posterior cerebral arteries. The resulting watershed area is termed the parasagittal region. Ischemic lesions most commonly involve either the frontal region or the parieto-occipital region at the posterior parasagittal area (so that the visual cortex is particulary susceptible to injury). Many watershed zones between two arteries exist in the brain, but the only triple watershed areas are the parieto-occipital areas and the area of the body of the caudate nucleus. It is in these watershed zones that tissues are most vulnerable to hypoxia and hypotension. It should be noted that damage to the radiations carries a worse prognosis than damage to the cortical areas.[140] Ischemic brain damage may occur perinatally or at any time after birth, as may occur following respiratory or cardiac arrest.

The precise nature of posthypoxic cerebral dysfunction is unknown. Perinatal hypoxia may interrupt protein synthesis in neural or glial cells, leading to cell death. Other effects may include delayed dendrite formation and synaptogenesis and abnormal myelination of the visual pathways. Some infants with perinatal hypoxic-ischemic encephalopathy and CVI may show improvement of visual function on follow-up. This has been demonstrated by longitudinal studies of such infants with utilization of forced preferential looking techniques.[80] Mechanisms accounting for such improvement include reactive synaptogenesis, rerouting of axons, or interruption of axon retraction.

Postnatal Hypoxia-Ischemia

There are a large number of causes of ischemic brain disorders in infants. Postnatal hemodynamic changes associated with generalized hypotension, cerebral angiography, cardiac surgery, cardiac arrest, and air embolism may result in CVI by diminishing the blood supply to the posterior visual pathway. Hypertensive crisis may result in occlusion of the posterior cerebral arteries, causing a similar problem. Transtentorial herniation may cause compression of the posterior cerebral arteries. Infarcts may also result from vascular malformations or from congenital central nervous system (CNS) tumors directly compressing cranial vessels. The most common cause of embolic phenomenon in the neonatal brain is congenital cyanotic heart disease. Thrombotic disorders may result from polycythemia, trauma, meningitis, and obliterative arteritis associated with neurofibromatosis and sickle cell disease. Anoxia might have been the etiology of cortical blindness in a patient with acute intermittent porphyria.[132]

Periventricular and Intraventricular Hemorrhages

Intracranial hemorrhages are especially common in premature infants, occurring most often within the first few days of life. They arise from poorly supported small vessels in the subependymal germinal matrix (the metabolically very active area within the ventricular wall in which the cells that compose the brain are produced), either spontaneously or as a result of hypoxia or hypertensive crisis. When ischemic brain tissue is reperfused, the weakened blood vessels frequently rupture, resulting in parenchymal hemorrhage. The hemorrhage extends into the ventricles and may eventually result in hydrocephalus and may dissect into the brain parenchyma, causing direct damage to neural structures, including the posterior visual pathways. During the last trimester, the germinal matrix diminishes in activity and begins to involute; germinal matrix hemorrhages are therefore unusual after 34 weeks of gestation. Choroid plexus hemorrhages are also common in premature infants, often accompanying hemorrhages of the germinal matrix. It should therefore be evident that the consequences of hypoxia-ischemia in premature infants result in damage located deep in the brain, represented largely by periventricular leukomalacia and hemorrhages.

Cerebral Malformations

A variety of cerebral malformations may be associated with CVI or congenital homonymous hemianopia. These include occipital or parietal encephaloceles, Chiari malformations, Dandy-Walker complex, hydranencephaly, porencephalic cysts (from either vascular compromise, infective processes, or hemorrhagic dissection),[206] or neuronal migrational abnormalities.[10]

During the 7th week of gestation, a neural layer known as the germinal matrix is formed by proliferation of neurons in the subependymal layer of the walls of the lateral ventricle. In the 8th gestational week, these neurons begin to migrate centrifugally from the germinal matrix to form the cerebral cortex. The route of neuronal migration is guided by radial glial fibers extending from the germinal matrix to the cortex. Events that interfere with this migration (e.g., infections, ischemia, metabolic derangements) can cause a migrational abnormality. A migrational anomaly shows normal neurons in an abnormal location, somewhere between the walls of the lateral ventricles and the cortex. The clinical manifestations of migrational abnormalities depend on the severity, nature (diffuse versus focal), and location of the abnormalities. Differences in the timing and severity of the migrational arrest result in different categories of abnormalities. The most severe of the migrational anomalies is lissencephaly, which includes agyria (absence of gyra on the surface of the brain) or pachygyria (a few broad, flat gyri) or both (Figure 1.5). In polymicrogyria, the neurons reach the cortex but distribute abnormally, forming multiple small gyri. Neuronal heterotopias are focal collections of neurons in abnormal locations. Schizencephaly denotes gray matter–lined clefts extending from the lateral ventricles to the surface of the brain. Unilateral megalencephaly consists of a hamartomatous overgrowth of all or part of one cerebral hemisphere, with migrational anomalies (pachygyria, polymicrogyria, and neuronal heterotopia) and gliosis of the affected hemisphere.

Strictly speaking, porencephaly refers to a focal cavity devoid of surrounding glial reaction resulting from localized brain destruction that occurs during the first 20 weeks of gestation (Figures 1.6 through 1.8). It differs from schizencephaly, a migrational anomaly resulting from destruction of a portion of the germinal matrix and consisting of a gray matter–lined cavity. Porencephaly also differs from encephalomalacia, which occurs later in pregnancy or anytime thereafter. These forms of cerebral dysgenesis are detailed in Chapter 11.

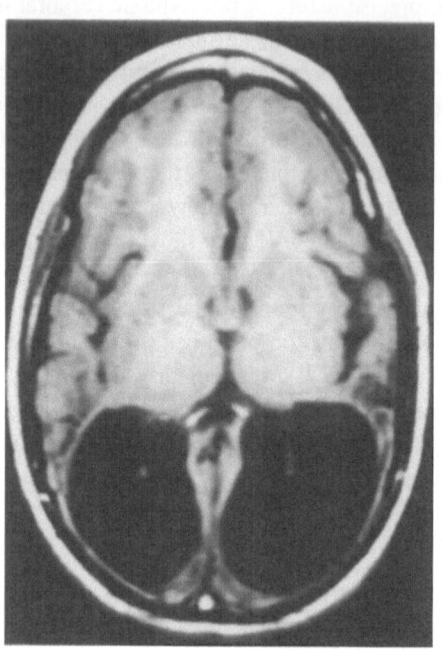

FIGURE 1.6. Axial MRI scan showing large, bilateral porencephalic cysts in a 6-year-old boy with cerebral palsy and cortical blindness.

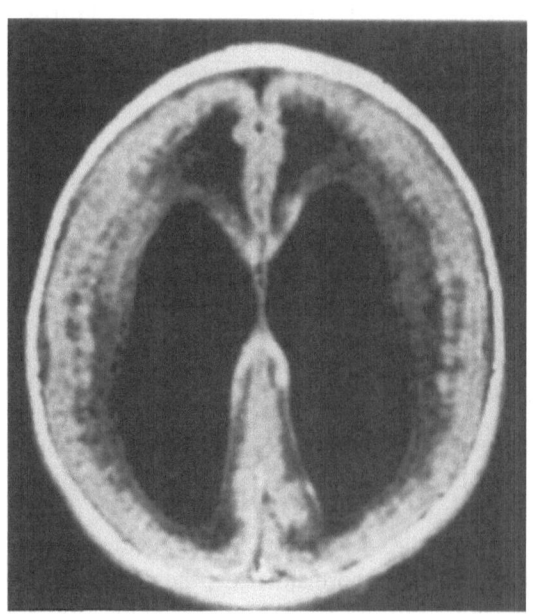

FIGURE 1.5. Proton density axial MRI scan from a child with cortical blindness and Walker–Warburg syndrome demonstrating lissencephaly (agyria) and hydrocephalus.

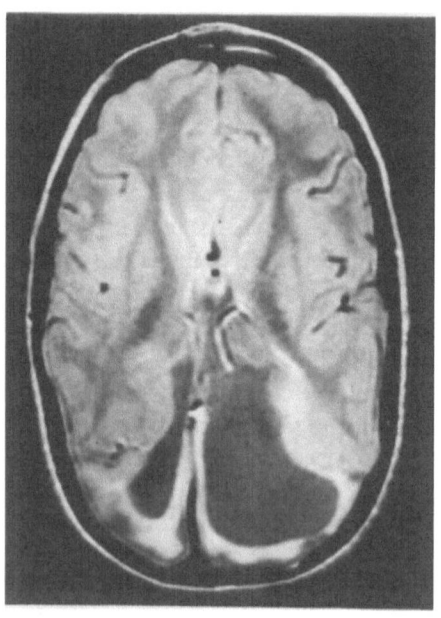

FIGURE 1.7. MRI scan of a 7-year-old boy with spastic diplegia, mental retardation, betaketothiolase deficiency, and severe CVI. Note the posterior, porencephalic-like dilatation of the occipital horns of the lateral ventricles. Only a thin margin of overlying cortex remains.

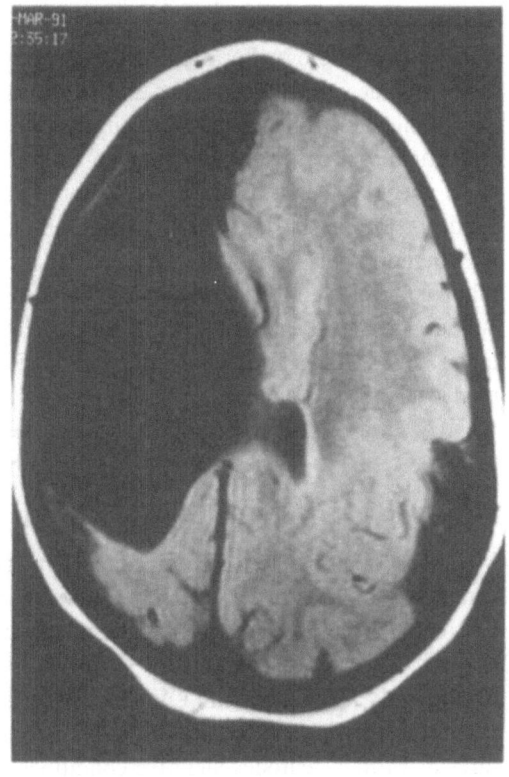
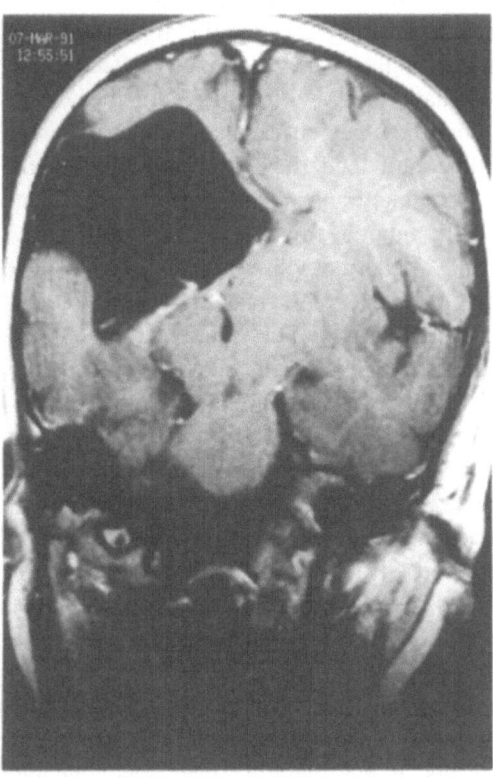

FIGURE 1.8. (A) Axial and (B) coronal MRI scans of a 3-year-old girl with left homonymous hemianopia and questionable history of a viral infection at approximately 8-weeks gestation. Note large, right cerebral porencephalic cyst, compensatory hemihypertrophy of the left cerebral hemisphere, and macrogyria with limited sulcal formation.

Head Trauma

The spectrum of traumatic head injury may range from mild concussion to a severe contusion, laceration, or diffuse axonal damage. The injury may also cause or be followed by epidural, subdural, subarachnoid, or intracerebral hemorrhage. Visual loss is typically noted immediately after the trauma or shortly thereafter (15 to 45 minutes), or it may be noted when a patient regains consciousness after recovering from coma. The CVI may be permanent, or it may resolve either partially or totally after a period ranging from a few minutes to several weeks. It is useful to separate cases occurring after minor or trivial trauma, which have a benign course, from those occurring after severe head trauma that often suffer permanent neurological and visual sequelae. Patients in the latter category usually show external or radiological signs of trauma (e.g., skull fracture, frank cerebral injury, intracranial hemorrhages, hemotympanum). For example, a 13-year-old boy was hit with a baseball bat on his occiput, losing consciousness for 4 minutes. On recovering consciousness, he was noted to be agitated, disoriented, and blind. Neuroimaging displayed comminuted skull fractures and contusion of both occipital lobes and right parietal lobe. Various neurological complications, including papilledema, developed. Vision recovered in 10 days, but visual field defects persisted. Follow-up CT showed atrophy of the previously injured lobes.[121] In patients with severe trauma, neuroimaging of the brain may demonstrate cerebral edema, massive brain swelling, hemorrhage, or resulting hydrocephalus.

Children with transient CVI after minor or apparently trivial trauma may have total or partial blindness, homonymous hemianopia, palinopsia, a patchy visual loss, or a "whiteout" of the visual fields, or they may describe fine flickering of vision resembling a snow storm.[51,86] Affected children usually have an otherwise normal examination, but they may occasionally show soft tissue swelling and tenderness corresponding to the area of cranial trauma. Neuroimaging studies are typically nonrevealing. In all reported cases, blindness occurred within several hours of head injury and lasted less than 24 hours. Patients characteristically do not experience loss of consciousness. They typically show visual recovery, which may occur from minutes to days after injury (on average, a few hours).[79,86] Such patients may have EEG findings that initially show either generalized or posterior, bioccipital, slowing that subsequently normalizes. The younger child may not report visual loss and may not recognize blindness but, rather, may display any combination of the following signs and symptoms: agitation, restlessness, uncooperativeness, confusion, irritability, disorientation, headaches, vomiting, drowsiness, or an unsteady gait. To avoid underdiagnosis, it has therefore been recommended that traumatic cortical blindness should be suspected in trauma patients who exhibit such findings.[231] Whether the associated agitation and restlessness are a psychological reaction to the blindness or a result of traumatic brain dysfunction is uncertain.

The nature of traumatic cerebral dysfunction may include a concussive cerebral injury, localized edema, ischemia, or epilepsy. Damage to the posterior visual pathway may occur via a coup or contracoup mechanism. Patients with transient blindness after minor trauma often have a family history of migraine, implicating a possible vascular role (a migraine equivalent), possibly local cerebral vasospasm.[51] The visual snow storms described in some patients are also described with migraine, and many of the above-mentioned associated symptoms and signs are common in migraines. The occasional patient who loses vision after voluntarily striking a soccer ball with his head[86] shows close clinical resemblance to the phenomenon of "footballers migraine."[148] One reported case of a child who might have had as many as four separate episodes of transient posttraumatic blindness suggests a possible predisposition to this syndrome in some patients.[231]

Some cases of transient posttraumatic blindness reported in the literature are inconsistent with a pure cortical etiology. For example, several cases have been described with either unilateral visual loss or bilaterally dilated and fixed pupils.[231]

Cortical visual impairment may be caused by child abuse as a sign of either the battered child syndrome or the shaken baby syndrome. Intracranial hemorrhages or concussive cerebral injury may be present in affected infants. In some cases, subdural hemorrhages may occur as a delayed event several days following injury. Associated physical signs of trauma or diffuse retinal hemorrhages warrant consideration of these diagnoses.

Metabolic and Neurodegenerative Conditions

Metabolic disturbances (e.g., profound hypoglycemia, carbon monoxide poisoning, nitrous oxide poisoning, cocaine, lead poisoning, uremia, hemodialysis, dialysis disequilibrium syndrome) are occasionally associated with CVI.[162,165] Cortical visual impairment may be one of the clinical features of various neurodegenerative conditions, including metabolic encephalopathy, lactic acidosis, and strokelike episodes (MELAS), Leigh's disease, and X-linked adrenoleukodystrophy. In metachromatic leukodystrophy, one-third of cases are associated with optic atrophy, but a component of CVI is not infrequent.

Byrd et al[28] described three children who experienced transient cortical blindness while receiving vincristine therapy for various malignancies. The cortical blindness in these patients, attributed to vincristine neurotoxicity, recovered completely after 1, 3, and 14 days.

Meningitis, Encephalitis, and Sepsis

Bacterial meningitis in infancy is an uncommon cause of CVI, accounting for only 5% of severe cases.[229] The most common organisms include hemophilus influenza, pneumococci, and streptococci. The CVI occurs within a week of onset of meningitis in about half the cases, and within 1 month of onset in almost all cases. Hemophilus influenza meningitis shows a predilection to damaging the occipital cortex,[42,146] with some cases showing CVI after recovery. A variety of neurologic or visual defects have been associated with meningitis, including mental retardation, seizures, hemiplegia, quadraplegia, homonymous hemianopia, double hemianopia with macular sparing, visual hallucinations, and CVI.[177] The postmeningitic CVI may be permanent or may show partial or complete recovery. The pathogenesis of postmeningitic CVI may be mediated by venous sinus thrombosis, thrombophlebitis, hydrocephalus, or hypoxic-ischemic insult in the watershed areas.[214]

Neonatal herpes simplex infection is frequently associated with severe CVI.[50] Eighty percent of these infections are caused by type 2 herpes simplex virus. The majority of affected children have severe brain damage, due to necrotizing encephalopathy and demyelination, with diffuse neurological disease including quadriplegia. Computed tomography findings in patients with neonatal herpetic encephalitis typically show extensive destruction of hemispherical white matter.[207] El Azazi et al[50] found 12 of 30 children with neonatal herpes simplex virus infection to have severe visual impairment, presumed due to cortical damage, although many of these also showed optic atrophy.

Granulomas, hydatid cyst infestation, syphilis, cerebral malaria, AIDS-related encephalopathy, or sepsis may result in cortical blindness (Figure 1.9).

Hydrocephalus, Ventricular Shunt Failure

Patients with hydrocephalus may show a spectrum of visual impairment with a variety of visual field defects, including homonymous hemianopia. Mixed anterior and posterior visual damage is frequently encountered in patients with hydrocephalus,[5] either primarily or following shunt malfunction. Damage to the anterior visual pathway may result from postpapilledema optic atrophy, chiasmal traction, a markedly dilated third ventricle that compresses the chiasm, compression of the optic tracts by the tentorial edge during herniation of the hippocampus, associated developmental anomalies, or from other vascular effects on the visual pathways. Damage to the posterior visual pathway due to hydrocephalus or shunt malfunction presumably results from compression of the posterior cerebral arteries against the tentorium.[5] This is thought to produce laminar necrosis of the visual cortex[33] but

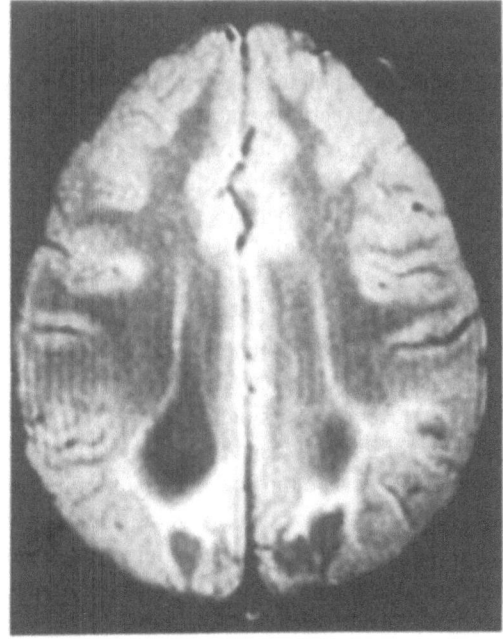
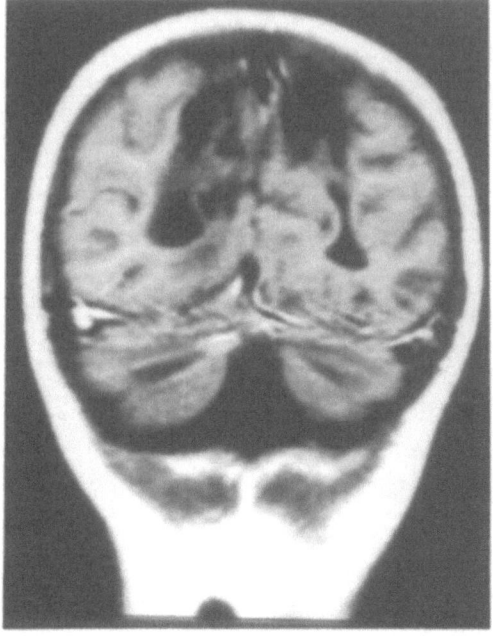

A   B

FIGURE 1.9. (A) Axial and (B) coronal MRI scan of a 3-year-old girl who suffered an episode of gram-negative sepsis at 1 year of age that resulted in complete blindness for 2 weeks. Subsequent gradual recovery of vision occurred to 20/20 in each eye, despite persistence of occipital lesions on MRI.

may also be related to coexisting congenital abnormalities or other structural alterations of the brain. In infants and young children, the visual impairment may resolve either partially or completely with time after shunt revision, usually over a period of several years (Figure 1.10). Rare instances with dramatic visual improvement occurring within a few hours to days of shunt revision have also been described.[32] The CVI due to hydrocephalus may be transient or episodic,[217] presumably due to a vascular dysfunction mediated by the intracranial hypertension.

Rabinowicz[179] examined visual perception in 100 hydrocephalic patients and found constructional apraxia, dyscalculia, and homonymous field defects in some of the patients, suggesting disorders of the posterior visual pathway and the parietal lobe.

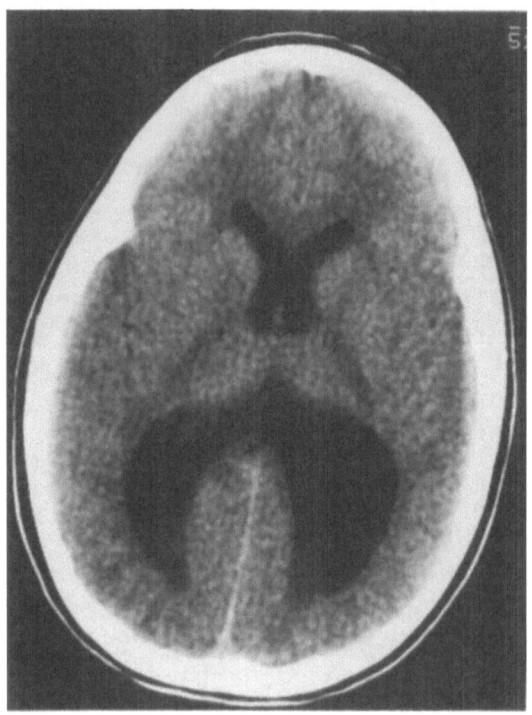

FIGURE 1.10. Axial CT scan of an 11-year-old boy, born 3 months prematurely, who had hydrocephalus and 20/30 vision bilaterally. Deterioration of vision to 20/200 bilaterally over several weeks was associated with shunt dysfunction and enlarging occipital horns of the lateral ventricles. Vision improved after shunt revision.

Hydrocephalus should not be confused with hydranencephaly. The latter denotes a severe process wherein there is nearly complete destruction and reabsorption of the cerebral hemispheres, with replacement by cerebrospinal fluid. Affected infants are uniformly blind.

Preictal, Ictal, or Postictal Phenomena

Neuro-ophthalmologic signs and symptoms of seizures include excessive eyelid blinking, fluttering, or spasms, nystagmus, contraversive gaze deviations or head deviations, spasms of the near reflex, unilateral pupillary dilatation, dyschromatopsia, altered stereopsis, unformed (elementary) hallucinations, hemianopsia and other transient or permanent visual field defects, and transient or permanent cortical blindness.[3,12,194]

A history of seizures is commonly found in children presenting with visual impairment, especially on the basis of cortical disease. The loss of vision may occur as an aura,[13] as the direct manifestation of the seizure itself,[111] or as a postictal phenomenon,[13] or it may be attributed to altered alertness due to the side effects of seizure medications.

Cases of blindness due to seizure activity directly may present a diagnostic quandary and are probably underrepresented in the literature, although some authors have speculated that unexplained cortical blindness may represent unrecognized seizure activity more often than may be inferred from reported cases.[12] Blindness due to seizure activity may be complete or may manifest as homonymous hemianopia.[12] Strauss[205] described an 11-year-old boy who had complete blindness associated with bilateral occipital spike-wave activity without affecting consciousness. This so-called status epilepticus amauroticus has been documented in a handful of cases.[12] Barry et al[12] described a 13-year-old girl who experienced episodic blindness, usually while walking to school, and was found to have light-stimulated bioccipital spike-wave activity. Jaffe and Roach[111] described three youths with intermittent blindness due to occipital seizures that improved with anticonvulsant medication. The symptoms included headaches and vomiting, rendering differentiation from basilar migraine difficult. Zung and Margalith[237] described a 7-year-old boy who experienced episodic blindness, accompanied by gastrointestinal symptoms and a sensation of fright, but with no alteration of consciousness. Computed tomography of the brain was normal; interictal electroencephalogram (EEG) showed bioccipital epilepsy. It is recommended that an EEG evaluation be included in the ancillary diagnostic testing of patients who present with cryptogenic acute blindness, even in the absence of obvious clinical symptoms of epilepsy. Infants with infantile spasms or constant seizures may seem blind because the seizure activity precludes visual attentiveness. The EEG in infants with infantile spasms shows hypsarrhythmia; affected infants sometimes show hundreds of small seizures daily. If visual pathway abnormalities are excluded with neuroimaging studies, the visual function may be expected to improve, sometimes dramatically, once the seizures are controlled.

Postictal blindness in infants was described as early as 1884 by Nettleship.[168] Kosnik et al[127] found an occipital focus in approximately 50% of children with seizures. They explained the predilection of occipital involvement in children with seizures by the presence of unstable electrical activity due to a putative relative immaturity of the occipital cortex in children. This high incidence of occipital lobe seizure activity in children explains why postictal blindness is more common in children. The precise pathophysiologic basis of postictal blindness is unknown, but a mechanism similar to Todd's paralysis has been suggested (Figure 1.11). Todd's paralysis denotes the postictal occurrence of focal neurologic deficits, which are mostly motor, but sensory deficits may also be associated. The mechanism of Todd's paralysis itself also remains speculative, with Jasper[119] suggesting, and Miller[159] supporting as the best available explanation, the occurrence of "neuronal exhaustion" due to hypoxia or high metabolic demands postictally. This notion is supported by the observation of one patient with postictal blindness who demonstrated marked hyperperfusion in both occipital regions on an ictal SPECT, carried out at the onset of the seizure.[13]

Occasionally, the seizure activity itself may be associated with drug toxicity. For example, a young patient with a blood cyclosporine level almost six times the therapeutic value suffered transient cortical blindness associated with continuous focal occipital EEG discharge.[187] Cortical blind-

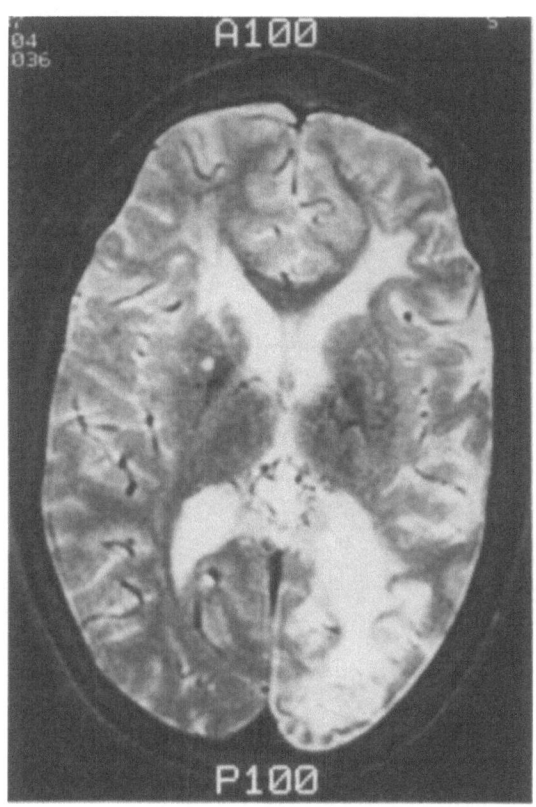

FIGURE 1.11. MR imaging in a 21-month-old girl with cerebral palsy and seizure disorder secondary to perinatal asphyxia who developed status epilepticus. The MRI scan obtained after control of status shows edema of nearly the entire cerebral hemisphere, especially posteriorly, presumably as a result of status epilepticus and sustained metabolic demands placed on the left hemisphere as a result.

ness and seizures have also been reported following cisplatin treatment.[94,224]

Visual disturbances are recognized as common side effects of anticonvulsant therapy.[182] Side effects of common antiseizure medications usually include sedation with a decreased level of alertness that may adversely affect visual performance during the examination. Other visual disturbances associated with anticonvulsant therapy include vertical or horizontal diplopia and oscillopsia, as well as pursuit and gazeholding disorders. These symptoms may be ascribed to ophthalmoplegia, vertical nystagmus, or abnormalities of the vestibulo-ocular reflex.[182]

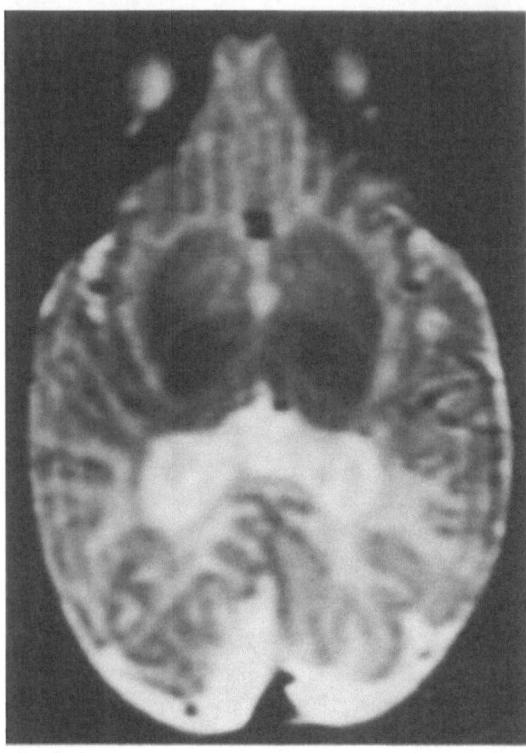

FIGURE 1.12. T2-weighted MRI of a 1-year-old girl with congenital profound CVI and developmental delay reveals marked atrophy of the occipital regions of uncertain etiology.

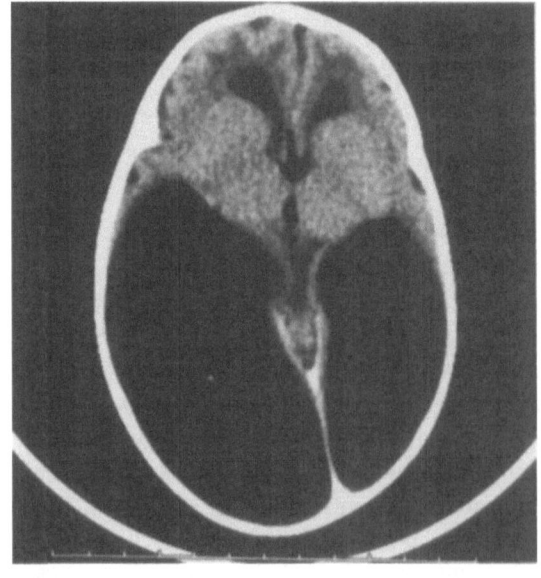

FIGURE 1.13. Axial CT scan from an infant with cerebral palsy, CVI, seizures, and deafness, demonstrating absence of occipital cortex. The etiology was unknown.

Despite best efforts to uncover the cause of cortical damage in patients with CVI, some cases elude classification into any of the etiologies previously detailed (Figures 11.12 and 11.13).

Associated Neurologic and Systemic Disorders

Cortical visual impairment may be rarely isolated, affecting children who are otherwise healthy. More commonly, CVI is found in association with other neurological or systemic diseases. Associated disorders may directly arise from the same event that caused the CVI (e.g., trauma, hypoxia) or may represent a constellation of findings characteristic of a syndrome that also exhibits CVI (e.g., MELAS, meningomyelocele with hydrocephalus, X-linked adrenoleukodystrophy). Associated disorders include cerebral palsy, mental retardation, learning disabilities, seizure disorders, microcephaly, hydrocephalus, and myelomeningocele. It should be noted, however, that some children with mental retardation or autism may be mistakenly diagnosed as having CVI because they display visual inattention, with lack of interest and detachment from their environment. An intact visual system can often be demonstrated in such patients with the use of forced preferential looking techniques,[76] but the limitations of such techniques should be borne in mind, as mentioned earlier.[130]

Characteristics of Visual Function

The degree of CVI in a given child can range from a defect that is barely detectable to complete blindness. The visual acuity may be spared in unilateral cortical lesions or bilateral lesions with sparing of cortical regions subserving the macula. In patients with profound visual impairment, appropriate methods of visual function assessment must be employed. Generally, it is very difficult to distinguish whether an infant is unable to see or simply unable to interpret visual input (visual agnosia). Snellen acuity measurements and similar methods have little to no utility in visual assessment of children with severe CVI. It is more relevant to obtain a measure of overall visual function than to simply attempt measurement of visual acuity. Can the child recognize various objects in the environment, navigate effectively, and interact visually with other people? Obtaining a visual history from the parents and spending some time playing with these children provides valuable information about the children's overall visual function.[114]

Children with CVI typically see better in a familiar environment. They often use touch to identify objects of interest.[114] They prefer to view objects at close range (independent of refractive errors) and appear to have a crowding phenomenon wherein individual objects are seen better than groups of objects. The preference of close viewing may be to produce linear magnification (by shortening the focal length) or to reduce crowding by viewing the object singly at close range.

Patients with CVI display on-again, off-again vision with wide fluctuations. Their visual function may be noted to vary widely from day to day and even from hour to hour.[114] This variability may correspond to changes in lighting conditions, attentiveness, tiredness, medications, illness, seizures, or environmental changes (noise, colors, etc.) but may also parallel the variable performance in other neurologic spheres that is characteristic of brain-damaged children. In some instances, variability of visual test results may arise from the presence of a "Swiss-cheese" visual field wherein an object may or may not be seen, depending upon whether or not it falls within a region of intact field. The extreme variability of visual function found in some patients with CVI may sometimes lead to the impression that the child is "faking." To be differentiated from true CVI is the visual disregard and intermittent visual inattention often seen in patients with developmental delay and other neurological disorders with intact posterior visual pathway. The phenomenon of decreased visual attention to novel stimuli in infants who later prove to be mentally retarded or autistic should also be borne in mind.[53]

Children may show a tendency to gaze at room lights, especially fluorescent lights, or other bright objects, including the sun (light gazing).[116] The precise explanation for this phenomenon is unknown, but it has been considered by some investigators to be a bad sign, indicating severe visual loss. Paradoxically, instead of light gazing, some degree of photophobia may be present in about one-third of children,[115] but this is usually much less than the severe photophobia so characteristic of retinal conditions, such as congenital achromatopsia. The cause of this photophobia is unknown, but damage to retinal, thalamic, or cortical structures may be responsible. It is possible that in some cases it may be of a retinal origin, arising from a hypoxia-damaged retina. Nickel and Hoyt[171] have shown that hypoxic insults can cause transient but notable electroretinographic changes in children. The photophobia may be a result of associated damage to the thalamus, a phenomenon called "thalamic dazzle."[34] The majority of cases exhibiting photophobia are thought to arise from damage to the striate cortex itself.[115] This may be analogous to the photophobia observed in Macaque monkeys when the occipital lobes are amputated.[40]

The visual performance of affected patients is better for moving objects than static objects. Parents may note that affected children see better when traveling in a car.[114] Some ambulatory children with CVI may show better visual function in terms of navigating successfully and avoiding obstacles than performing near-vision tasks. Jan et al[114,118] postulated that the most plausible explanation for this discrepancy is the presence of an extrageniculo-striate (collicular) visual system. However, the existence of an accessory system in man remains speculative (see "blindsight" below).

Patients are often able to identify the color of objects better than the form and shape of objects. This discrepancy has been attributed to several factors: (1) Color perception requires fewer neurons than form perception.[227] (2) Color perception, unlike form perception, is bilaterally represented in the cerebral hemispheres (but with dominance in one hemisphere), so it is more resilient to injuries that may affect form perception. (3) Color perception is diffusely represented in the striate cortex and the lingual and fusiform gyri. (4) Color perception may be preserved within the extrageniculostriate visual system.[204]

Some children with CVI turn their head a certain way or look away to either side, usually with a slight downward gaze, when reaching out for an object.[114] They display preference for peripheral vision over central vision, viewing objects eccentrically. This may result from bilateral central scotomas associated with sparing of the temporal crescent, which is represented by the most anterior portion of the striate cortex.

Accurate evaluation of the visual fields is notoriously difficult in children with CVI. Clinical clues may be obtained by moving colorful toys in their visual fields while observing the child's reaction. Even children with severe visual impairment often show asymmetric involvement with preferential relative sparing of either the right or the left visual fields.[114] Visual evoked potential recordings with separate hemispheric electrodes may help assess the presence of relative hemianopic defects in some children. When fields can be done, many children with CVI show severely constricted peripheral visual fields.[223]

Absence of Nystagmus

Patients with CVI usually show either no nystagmus or occasional, unsustained beats of nystagmus. The reason that patients with CVI typically show no nystagmus is not well known. Bilateral occipital lobectomy in monkeys results in latent, but not manifest, nystagmus.[233] Fielder and Evans[55] have speculated that an intact geniculostriate pathway may be a prerequisite for the development of congenital nystagmus. This is corroborated by the observation of Jan et al[112] of disappearance of nystagmus in a patient with anterior visual pathway dysfunction after onset of cerebral disease. It is also supported by the observation that horizontal nystagmus, due to various disorders of the eye or anterior visual pathway, appears to develop at an age when the geniculostriate system is emerging functionally (around 2 to 3 months of age). Fielder and Evans[55] argued that patients with CVI who, by definition, do not have a normally functioning geniculostriate pathway would not be expected to develop nystagmus. Tusa et al[216] suggested that "sensory" nystagmus results from interference with gaze-holding mechanisms, probably via visual deafferentation of the flocculus by the inferior olivary nucleus.

Patients with CVI and a few beats of nystagmus are likely to have coexisting anterior visual pathway dysfunction or to have developed the visual loss before the first year of life. Patients with "mixed mechanism" visual loss with both anterior as well as posterior visual pathway dysfunction are not uncommon. The degree and characteristics of nystagmus in these visually impaired children may theoretically be used as a rough assessment of the severity of the anterior visual pathway dysfunction. However, in light of evidence suggesting that the geniculostriate pathway is a prerequisite for the development of nystagmus,[55] a patient with mixed mechanism visual loss may not show significant nystagmus even in the presence of severe anterior visual pathway damage if significant posterior pathway damage coexists. Alternatively, finding sustained nystagmus in patients with anterior and posterior pathway disease indicates that the posterior component is not severe.

Associated Ocular Abnormalities

The ocular examination is commonly said to be otherwise normal in patients with CVI, but involvement of the retina, optic nerves, or chiasm is not unusual, arising from the same disease process that caused the cerebral damage. Some children with poor vision that may be readily attributable to other developmental ophthalmologic abnormalities may harbor at least a component of CVI as well. For example, approximately 20% of children with optic nerve hypoplasia also show hemispheric abnormalities[25,26] that may involve the posterior visual pathway. Four of 50 children diagnosed with permanent CVI had concurrent optic nerve hypoplasia.[229] The presence of optic atrophy in patients with CVI due to hypoxia-ischemia should not be surprising;[74] it may be argued that the reportedly low prevalence of concurrent optic atrophy may itself be surprising. Six of 30 children with hypoxic cortical visual impariment described by Lambert et al[40] showed mild optic atrophy. In a series of infants with significant hypoxic encephalopathy, Good et al[74] found less than 15% of infants with optic atrophy. The fact that many children with severe ischemic cortical damage do not show optic atrophy signifies that the anterior visual pathways are more resistant to the effects of hypoxia than the posterior visual pathways. However, it may be argued that concurrent anterior visual pathway involvement is underreported, in part due to mistakenly considering such defects to be the sole cause of the visual impairment.

Coexisting CVI should be suspected when the degree of visual deficit is not fully explained by the ocular defects.[229] Associated optic atrophy may be due to concomitant anterior pathway insult or retrograde transsynaptic degeneration of the retinogeniculate pathway. Patients with "mixed mechanism" visual loss with both anterior as well as posterior visual pathway dysfunction are not uncommon. This "mixed" category has been largely underemphasized in the literature but represents a diagnostic challenge in terms of determining the weighted contribution to the visual impairment of each insult. Alternatively, associated optic atrophy may reflect retrograde transsynaptic degeneration of the retinogeniculate pathway.[188]

Retrograde transsynaptic degeneration of the retinogeniculate pathway is known to occur in nonhuman primates following cerebral lesions even in adult life.[45] In contrast, retrograde transsynaptic degeneration in humans is said to occur only if the cortical lesion occurred *in utero*.[41,102,133] However, the presence of even severe prenatal cortical insults or malformations does not appear to be solely sufficient for the occurrence of transsynaptic degeneration. For instance, the literature contains well-described cases of severe occipital lesions, even tomographic absence of the occipital cortex[209] with normal fundus and optic disc appearance. In general, descriptions of normal optic discs in children with CVI may be explained by one of the following: (1) Cortical damage may involve the visual association areas without significant damage to the geniculostriate pathway.[6] (2) Subtle mild optic nerve pallor may be overlooked in infants and young children. (3) The nature, location, timing, or extent of the cerebral lesion is not sufficient to cause transsynaptic degeneration. (4) Other heretofore undetermined factors that are necessary for development of transsynaptic degeneration may be lacking.

Generally, optic disc pallor found in association with cortical damage may be due to the same process that caused the cortical damage, subsequent hydrocephalus, transsynaptic degeneration, or an entirely unrelated process. A primary insult to the retinogeniculate pathway with optic atrophy may be theoretically distinguishable from transsynaptic degeneration by the following means: (1) Documentation of healthy optic disc appearance shortly after the cortical insult with subsequent corresponding optic atrophy (typically, years afterward)

not explicable by other interceding disorders would argue for transsynaptic degeneration. (2) Since significant primary anterior visual pathway disease in early life may be accompanied or followed by nystagmus, one may be tempted to use this sign to distinguish between primary versus transsynaptic optic atrophy. However, it has been argued that an intact visual cortex is necessary for the development of such nystagmus[55] so that children with combined anterior and posterior pathway insults may not show nystagmus. Hence, we lose the opportunity to use nystagmus as a relatively reliable sign of profound anterior pathway disease in early life. (3) Scrutiny of optic discs in patients with unilateral or asymmetric postgeniculate pathway disease for signs of corresponding band atrophy would provide strong evidence of transsynaptic degeneration, assuming that the original damage did not involve the geniculate nucleus or optic tract on the same side. (4) Patients with pure cortical blindness usually show normal pupillary reactions. However, it appears that the pupillomotor fibers, which do not synapse at the lateral geniculate nucleus but at the pretectal area, may also be susceptible to transsynaptic degeneration.[218] On the basis of this evidence, the pupillary examination may not be sufficient in distinguishing anterior visual pathway disease from CVI in all instances.

Transsynaptic degeneration has been proposed to occur in humans after lesions during adult life in a variety of other locations in the nervous system. For instance, reduction in the number of lower motor units and electromyographic denervation activity have been found following upper motor neuron lesions caused by injury to the spinal cord or by cerebral hemorrhage; transsynaptic dysfunction has been presumed responsible.[18,27,126,151] Crossed cerebellar atrophy has been demonstrated on neuroimaging following cerebral hemorrhage or infarction; transsynaptic degeneration of the corticopontocerebellar tract and the cerebellorubrothalamic tract has been proposed as an explanation.[84] Oculopalatal myoclonus is thought to result from hypertrophy of the inferior olive because of transsynaptic degeneration.[142] Nerve fiber layer atrophy may also occur in conditions affecting outer retinal elements, presumably due to transsynaptic degeneration.[110,169] Iris heterochromia has been demonstrated in patients with acquired Horner's syndrome; transsynaptic degeneration of postganglionic sympathetic fibers has been suggested as an explanation.[43] Transsynaptic degeneration of postganglionic parasympathetic fibers has been suggested as an explanation for cholinergic supersensitivity of the iris sphincter noted after preganglionic oculomotor nerve lesions.[109] Transsynaptic degeneration of the visual pathways may also be antegrade. For example, the cells of the lateral geniculate nucleus showed transsynaptic degeneration following injury to the optic nerve in adult patients.[193,201]

Transsynaptic degeneration was postulated to affect the retinal ganglion cells of humans after postnatal cerebral damage as early as 1880. However, reported cases have had confounding findings, such as papilledema,[81,222] intraocular hypertension, or optic disc cupping,[52] raising doubt as to the contribution of transsynaptic degeneration. Beatty and associates[15] presented compelling histopathologic data that retrograde transsynaptic degeneration of the retinal ganglion cells with optic atrophy may occur after cerebral damage during adulthood. They presented a patient who died 40 years after surgical removal of one occipital hemisphere. The vascular supply of the lateral geniculate nucleus and ipsilateral optic tract were not damaged. Using specialized staining techniques of histopathologic specimens, they demonstrated striking asymmetry of the appearance of the retinogeniculate pathway: only the lateral geniculate nucleus and optic tract on the affected side showed atrophy and axonal degeneration. This is in contradistinction to what is found in cases of optic nerve damage, where both optic tracts demonstrate atrophic axons and both lateral geniculate nuclei show atrophy in the laminae corresponding to the damaged nerve.

Band atrophy of the optic disc is most often encountered in patients with compressive lesions of the anterior visual pathway (e.g., pituitary adenomas, craniopharyngiomas).[156,221] Concurrent damage to the optic tract or lateral geniculate body should be ruled out in patients who are suspected to show transsynaptic degeneration after *acquired* cerebral lesions. For example, observation of band atrophy of the contralateral optic disc in three patients with cerebral arteriovenous malformations might have been thought to represent transsynaptic degeneration across the optic tract. However, neuroimaging studies revealed abnormal deep venous drainage involving the optic tract, presumably causing direct axonal damage.[128]

Diagnostic and Prognostic Considerations

Improvement of vision occurs to varying degrees in most patients with CVI. In two large series of patients with CVI, over half of the children showed a significant improvement of vision on follow-up.[140,229] When the etiology of the CVI is taken into consideration, a more accurate prediction of visual prognosis may be made. For instance, ischemic and traumatic cases are more likely to show improvement than those due to neurometabolic disorders (e.g., X-linked adrenoleukodystrophy). The full scope of visual recovery may in some cases take several years to be realized.[80] However, improvement of vision that occurs after a year from initial injury may reflect better ability to accurately test older children and increased ability of these children to use their limited vision with time.[140] The sequence of visual recovery includes color vision, form vision, and then, finally, visual acuity.

Residual visual function despite apparently severe cortical damage may be due to a variety of possibilities, such as the following: (1) Children may still have residual cortex with some sparing of vision since central vision is widely represented in the occipital cortex. (2) Some visual recovery may be attributable to the plasticity of the brain in children, with other parts of the brain taking over via rewiring of neuronal connections, reactive synaptogenesis, rerouting of axons, or neurochemical adaptations.[60] This may be interpreted by clinicians, parents, and teachers as simply learning to better "interpret" poor images. (3) Residual vision may be due to the so-called "blindsight" phenomenon. The collicular system, the putative center for blindsight, may be the area in the CNS that subserves vision even in patients with little or no cortical tissue. (4) Finally, it is theoretically possible that residual vision may stem from heterotopic cortex.

Currently, the extent of cortical damage can best be studied with anatomical neuroimaging modalities, such as CT or MRI.[63] The neuroimaging abnormalities found in patients with CVI range from essentially normal to highly abnormal imaging studies, demonstrating virtual absence of the posterior visual pathway (Figure 1.13). Frequent findings on neuroimaging studies include diffuse cerebral atrophy, biooccipital lobe infarctions, periventricular leukomalacia, cerebral dysgenesis, and parieto-occipital and parasagittal "watershed" infarctions. In children with hypoxic cortical insults, Lambert et al demonstrated a significant positive correlation between a poor visual outcome, an early age of hypoxic damage, and the degree of damage to the optic radiation.[140] There was no statistically significant correlation between the visual outcome and the degree of damage to the striate and parastriate cortex. Difficulties in establishing clinical-neuroimaging correlation may reflect the fact that anatomy and function are not one and the same; areas that may appear relatively spared on anatomic neuroimaging may have considerable dysfunction, and areas that appear damaged may still have residual function. Also, Horton and Hoyt[95] have recently demonstrated that central macular vision is more widely represented in the occipital cortex than previously thought. This was demonstrated by correlating occipital lesions demonstrated with MRI with homonymous field defects. Therefore, even an extensive lesion of the occipital cortex is sometimes compatible with some degree of macular sparing.

Functional neuroimaging studies, such as positron emission tomography (PET)[20] and single photon emission tomography (SPECT),[172,196] have the added advantage of providing information regarding the functional, as opposed to anatomic, integrity of the brain based on the underlying biochemistry. These studies may help delineate the site of dysfunction in cases where anatomical neuroimaging shows little or no abnormality and vice versa. They also may enhance our understanding of the pathophysiology in cases where results of clinical, electrophysiologic, and imaging studies appear incongruent. For instance, the clinical utility of SPECT has been documented in patients with CVI in whom MRI was either normal or inconclusive.[196] The advent of functional brain imaging such as PET and SPECT scanning has shown that areas of the brain that are remote from the location of the primary insult may show concurrent impaired function, a phe-

nomenon called diaschisis.[4] This phenomenon infers that some patients with acute hemispheric injuries affecting the visual pathway may experience bilateral hemispheric symptoms through transhemispheric diaschisis. Functional neuroimaging may be particularly useful in cases with widespread nonocclusive cerebral ischemia and diffuse axonal injury from trauma in which the functional defect may be considerably greater than the anatomical lesion.[197]

Visual evoked potentials may be helpful in monitoring visual recovery, but they have some limitations, they are fraught with technical and interpretational pitfalls, and their value remains controversial. Early reports stressed the absence or marked attenuation of VEP responses in patients with acute cortical blindness, with recovery of VEP responses as vision improved over time.[185] However, significant VEP signals may be recorded in some infants who are cortically blind.[6] For example, Bodis-Wollner et al[19] found normal VEPs to flash, pattern, and sinusoidal gratings in a blind child who had CT evidence of loss of the visual association cortex. This emphasizes the point that VEPs may be valuable in testing that the primary visual pathways are intact, but they do not test perception.[65] Frank and Torres[69] recorded VEPs in 30 cortically blind children as well as 30 sighted children who had a similar CNS disease. They found some degree of abnormality in all recordings but no significant difference between the two groups. In patients with neurologic disorders, flash VEPs are often abnormal even when the patient is well-sighted.[211] Thus, they have little prognostic value when cortical blindness is present in children with neurological disease, with the possible exception of perinatal asphyxia.[152,153] Electroretinography is not of clinical value in CVI, except to exclude concomitant retinal disease.[70]

Taylor and McCulloch[212] have reported that flash VEPs may have a prognostic value in following young children with acute cortical blindness, who have no preexisting neurologic disorders, irrespective of etiology. They demonstrated that an intact flash VEP in a previously normal child with cortical visual loss carries a favorable prognostic significance for visual recovery. Conversely, absent VEP signals carry a poor prognosis.[212,213] Whiting et al[229] reported that VEP mapping might be more helpful than traditional VEP recordings in the investigation of cortical blindness. In their study of 50 children with permanent cortical visual impairment, the VEP map was always abnormal and showed good correlation with the CT scan results, whereas the conventional VEP recordings were abnormal in only 50% of cases. In addition to their utility as a tool to evaluate visual function, VEPs may have some value in predicting the neurodevelopmental outcome. Muttitt et al[166] performed serial VEPs in a series of term infants with birth asphyxia and found good correlation between the VEPs and the neurodevelopmental outcome.

Hemianopic Visual Field Defects in Children

Children may display pure hemianopic defects, with normal fields on the contralateral side, or asymmetric (albeit bilateral) visual field involvement. Children with pure hemianopic defects usually have normal visual acuity, and if the defect is congenital, it may go unnoticed for many years. The congenital variety is often discovered on a routine eye examination.[218] Patients may have a history of being involved in accidents with automobiles approaching from the affected side or of being tackled frequently by players approaching from the affected side when playing football, etc. Overall, patients with congenital hemianopia have minimal visual disability, whereas adults with acquired hemianopias are often severely disabled. This difference may hypothetically arise from the ability of the developing nervous system, but not the adult brain, to develop compensatory rewiring after prenatal damage, a phenomenon that has been well demonstrated in kittens[200,226] but not in man. It may also arise from differences in the adaptive strategies that hemianopic patients develop to fixate targets within the blind areas of the visual field (see below). Finally, an extrageniculostriate system may, theoretically, also play a role.[97]

The majority of cases of congenital homonymous hemianopia are due to unilateral or asymmetric cerebral lesions, but congenital optic tract syndromes may rarely occur.[145] Common structural causes are congenital lesions, such as porencephaly, arteriovenous malformations, and gan-

gliogliomas. Cases of congenital hemianopia may be isolated or associated with other neurological abnormalities. Associated lesions include a variety of hemispheric cortical lesions, including cerebral hemiatrophy, porencephaly of the posterior cerebral hemispheres, occipital lobe dysplasia,[218] vascular malformations (e.g., Sturge–Weber syndrome, occipital arteriovenous malformations), colpocephaly, polymicrogyria, as well as prenatal injury to the periventricular white matter.[101,181] Congenital homonymous hemianopia should be suspected in patients with congenital hemiplegia, both findings stemming from the same lesion. Sturge–Weber syndrome may cause homonymous hemianopia due to leptomeningeal malformations involving one occipital lobe with or without facial port-wine stains[101] (Figure 1.14). Congenital homonymous hemianopia with occipital porencephaly is now a recognized complication of neonatal isoimmune thrompocytopenia.[37a] Porencephalic cysts often show a distribution corresponding to a territory perfused by one of the major cerebral arteries, suggesting a vascular etiology (Figures 6 through 8). They may also arise in areas of the brain into which intracerebral hemorrhages have dissected. Most of these abnormalities can be elucidated with CT, but occasionally, this modality may be falsely negative. Tychsen and Hoyt,[218] described two patients with congenital hemianopia in whom the results of CT were normal. Magnetic resonance imaging disclosed focal occipital dysplasia involving the striate cortex and underlying white matter in each.

Highly characteristic optic disc and nerve fiber layer changes termed homonymous hemioptic atrophy may be seen in some patients as a result of transsynaptic degeneration.[100–102] These consist of band-shaped pallor or atrophy of the contralateral disc; the ipsilateral disc shows temporal pallor. Corresponding hemiretinal patterns of nerve fiber layer dropout are characteristically present. The contralateral eye shows intact arcuate nerve fibers above and below the disc but absent or sparse nerve fibers in the retinal sectors nasal and temporal to the disc. The ipsilateral eye shows sparse nerve fiber layers in retinal sectors above and below the disc. Current evidence supports the notion that the presence of these disc changes attests to the timing of the cortical lesion as being

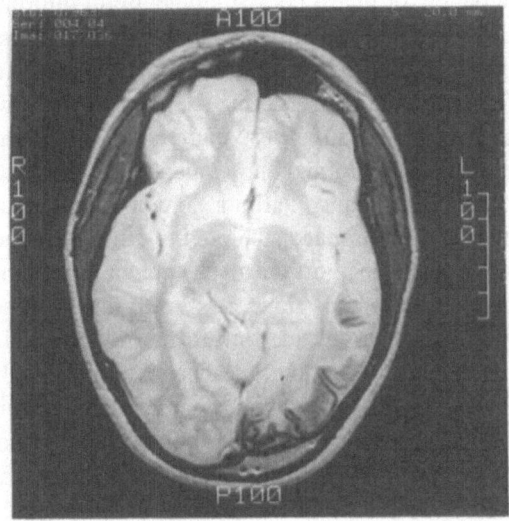
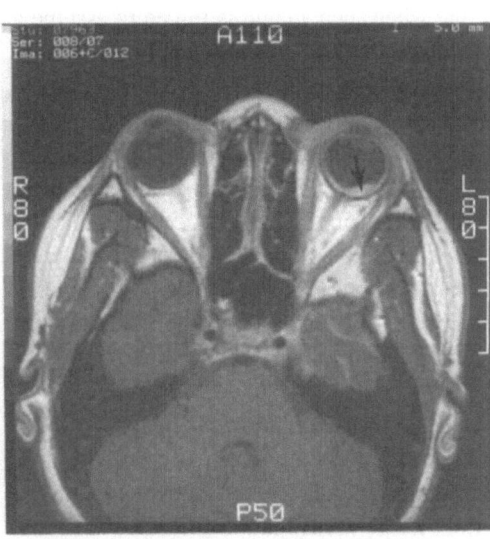

FIGURE 1.14. MRI scan of a 12-year-old girl with Sturge–Weber syndrome and right homonymous hemianopia. (A) Note severe atrophic foci over parietal and occipital areas with overlying venous malformation.

(B) The left globe shows thickened choroid (arrow) corresponding to the choroidal venous malformation seen on fundus examination.

prenatal[101,160] or perinatal rather than acquired later on in life. The clinical elucidation of transsynaptic degeneration of the retinogeniculate pathway has been used to ascribe a prenatal onset to associated cerebral lesions. For example, Fletcher et al[61] described a 24-year-old patient with recent onset of seizures who was found to have homonymous quadrantanopia with underlying occipital lobe ganglioglioma. Because the patient showed transsynaptic atrophy of retinal nerve fibers, the authors reasoned that these findings indicated that gangliogliomas may arise *in utero* and exist for many years before causing symptoms.

Patients with congenital homonymous hemianopia may show an afferent pupillary defect on the side contralateral to the cerebral lesion. These defects are rather small, measuring around 0.3 log units with a neutral density filter. This afferent pupillary defect has been attributed to transsynaptic degeneration of the pupillomotor fibers. It appears that the pupillomotor fibers, which do not synapse at the lateral geniculate nucleus but at the pretectal area, may also be susceptible to transsynaptic degeneration.[218] However, when an afferent defect is encountered in a patient with hemianopia, involvement of the contralateral lateral geniculate nucleus or optic tract should be considered.[17,170]

Generally, patients with congenital hemianopia appear to cope better with their deficit than those with lesions acquired in adult life. Patients with homonymous hemianopia may exhibit a variety of adaptive strategies to mitigate their visual handicap. Patients with either congenital or acquired lesions show diminished or absent head movements when fixating an eccentric target.[232] The saccadic strategy for fixating eccentric targets appears somewhat different between patients with congenital and acquired lesions. Congenital hemianopes often produce a single large saccadic movement into the blind field that overshoots the intended visual target and then "finds it" as the eyes drift back. This may be a more effective adaptation than that often seen in patients with acquired hemianopia wherein the patient makes multiple small saccades into the blind field until the target of interest is found.[154] Acquired hemianopes, though, may also learn the single large saccade strategy.

Patients with congenital, but not acquired, hemianopia frequently manifest a face turn.[96,97] We have examined a 12-year-old boy with a left homonymous hemianopia who turns his chin far over his left shoulder when batting right-handed during baseball games. Some authorities have noted that when such a child is forced to assume a normal head position, certain visual tasks, especially those related to mobility, become more difficult, which suggests that such head turns have a compensatory adaptive function. It is not clear, however, whether the head turn is an attempt to use peripheral vision rather than central vision in certain visually guided behaviors or whether it is an attempt to rotate the remaining field into a more midline position.[97] Since the fixation point of the eyes does not change with this maneuver, this adaptation may serve to centralize the remaining visual field with respect to the body.

It has been noted that some children with congenital hemianopic defects also show an exotropic deviation. Some investigators who theorized that the exotropic deviation represents a compensatory phenomenon to enable the patient to have panoramic vision in the presence of harmonious anomalous retinal correspondence cautioned that strabismus surgery may therefore be counterproductive.[92] The finding of the exotropia may also be coincidental, since neurologically damaged children are predisposed to strabismus.[97]

Patients with CVI from any cause may show asymmetric involvement of the cerebral hemispheres with corresponding asymmetry in their visual fields, with one hemianopic field allowing better visual function than the other. In infants and young children with lesions of the visual area of one cerebral hemisphere, a marked VEP asymmetry has been demonstrated for both flash and pattern testing.[137] Patients suspected of hemianopic defects on the basis of cerebral lesions should be tested for the presence of smooth pursuit asymmetry either with an optokinetic retinopathy of prematurity (OKN) target, spinning of the patient, or eye movement recording. Saccadic tracking to the side of the lesion is a helpful diagnostic sign in patients with large lesions involving the parietal lobe.[108]

Increasingly, younger patients are prone to acquire cortical blindness or hemianopic defects as either a presenting feature or an associated symptom of AIDS. The causative lesion is most commonly progressive multifocal leukoencephalopathy, but opportunistic infections and neoplastic lesions are not unusual.

Evaluation of the visual fields in infants and small children is more difficult than in adults, especially when neurological disorders, mental re-

tardation, or illness coexist. Some useful information about the visual fields can be gleaned utilizing a modification of confrontational methods referred to as evoked saccadic techniques. When we suspect that an infant or young child with hemiplegia or neuroimaging evidence of posterior hemispheric injury harbors homonymous hemianopia, we introduce a colored toy into the superior or inferior portion of the potentially hemianopic field and move it toward the vertical meridian. If a saccade toward the toy is consistently seen as the object reaches the midline, the diagnosis of homonymous hemianopia is confirmed. Kinetic perimetry has also been performed in infants.[80,163,223] Mayer et al[150] utilized a modified perimetric technique with LED stimuli and a forced-choice observation procedure to quantitatively record the visual fields of normal infants, ages 6 to 7 months. They also demonstrated the applicability of this technique to infants at risk of harboring field defects, such as those with hydrocephalus. However, such methods have not received widespread application and remain investigational at this point. As mentioned earlier, VEP measurements with hemispheric recordings can help delineate preferential or asymmetric hemispheric disorders associated with hemianopic field defects.[137]

Delayed Visual Maturation

Delayed visual maturation (DVM) is diagnosed when a child fails to show the expected visual function for his age, but does so spontaneously after a period of time. These infants may initially appear to have cortical blindness, with poor or no fixation, normal pupillary responses, and no nystagmus, but neuroimaging studies show no underlying cerebral insult. Some of these children may have a history of prematurity, delayed motor development, or small size for gestational age. Since improvement of vision is mandatory to make the diagnosis, the condition can only be suspected initially, with confirmation of the diagnosis made retrospectively following visual improvement. It should be evident then that there is no such entity as delayed visual maturation that does not show visual improvement. When an ophthalmologist "hedges" when giving a visual prognosis to the parents of an apparently blind infant, he is, at least partially, acknowledging the entity of delayed visual maturation.[83,85,105]

A brief summary of some developmental aspects of vision is relevant as background information for this topic.[21] The globe reaches adult size only after the first decade of life. The fovea is not mature at birth. The cone photoreceptors are immature, and the ganglion cells have not moved aside to form the foveal pit. The fovea reaches full maturity at 4 years of age.[89] Myelination of the optic nerves begins at the lateral geniculate nucleus, reaching the orbital part of the optic nerve at term, and continues over the following 2 years.[144] Myelination of the geniculostriate pathway begins in the 10th fetal month and is fully mature about 4 months postnatally.[230] The rate of myelination appears to be hastened by light exposure.[155] Thus, a preterm infant on reaching chronological term will have more-advanced myelination than a full-term newborn.[98] The parvocellular layers of the lateral geniculate nucleus (color vision and high-grade acuity) reach adult maturity at 6 months of age; the magnocellular layers (low-contrast sensitivity and motion detection) reach maturity at 2 years of age.[93] Postnatal growth and development of the brain is not associated with an increase in cell number, but rather reflects an increase in the size of individual cells, synaptic density, and interconnections. Synaptic density in the striate cortex increases over the first 8 months and then begins declining, reaching adult density at age 11 years.[104] Cortical ocular dominance columns become adult-like at 6 months.[7]

Functional, behavioral, and neurophysiological aspects of visual function emerge to some extent in a parallel manner with the aforementioned anatomical and physiological developmental aspects. Pupillary reaction to light becomes apparent in 30-week premature infants.[106] Accommodation and stereopsis begin to emerge at about 3 months of age.[7] Ocular pursuit movements in neonates are saccadic, becoming smooth at 2 to 3 months of age.[1] Rapid changes in the configuration of the VEPs occur in the first few months of life, so that abnormal-looking responses may be normal for age. Most newborn infants demonstrate fixation and following of a near object, such as the examiner's face. However, some neonates show significant delays in developing fixation and following.

It is these visual "late bloomers" that typify the entity of DVM.

The pathogenesis of DVM is controversial. Lambert et al[139] reported nine cases of "pure" DVM, excluding cases with ocular abnormalities, perinatal asphyxia, or structural cerebral abnormalities. With one exception, all infants showed normal VEPs to flash and to pattern stimulation (despite being behaviorally blind), and all these showed normalization of vision at the end of the follow-up period, usually within a few months. Despite the selection criteria, the children showed mild to moderate developmental delay on follow-up. The authors reported that intact pattern VEPs strongly indicate a good visual prognosis in such behaviorally blind infants. Skarf,[199] in a discussion of the paper by Lambert and colleagues,[139] advised that absence of a pattern or even a flash VEP in meeting the study's criteria should not, however, necessarily be interpreted as a dismal prognostic sign. Lambert et al[139] felt that the visual recovery could not be explained by foveal immaturity and delay in myelination and synaptogenesis of the posterior visual pathway.[139] Moreover, in view of the normal pattern visual evoked responses in all but the one patient who did not attain normal vision, delay in the maturation of the striate cortex was also considered to be an unlikely explanation of the poor vision. Lambert et al[139] suggested immaturity of the visual association areas as the possible explanation.

This suggestion may be supported by the observation that the phylogenetically older systems are myelinated first, with myelination proceeding roughly in a rostral direction; the cortical association fibers are myelinated last.[230] The overall myelination process appears to be delayed, on MRI studies, in developmentally delayed infants as compared with normal age-matched infants.[44] This is not to say that the delay in myelination is solely responsible for the developmental delay (or associated abnormalities including DVM), but that the delay in myelination may parallel other maturational processes occurring in the developing brain.

As a diagnostic label, DVM may be used in the narrow sense previously described or may be applied more broadly to include patients with various developmental abnormalities and ocular disorders. A trend for a broader application of the term emerged as experience has accumulated to justify this. Tresidder et al[215] reported 26 cases of DVM but had a different inclusion criteria, including all cases of blindness without an ophthalmological cause. They subdivided the cases into three groups: Group 1 included infants with isolated DVM. This group was further subdivided on the basis of the presence or absence of perinatal problems. Group 2 included infants with neurodevelopmental abnormalities. Group 3 included infants with nystagmus. Visual recovery was fastest in group 1 infants without perinatal problems of whom seven out of eight recovered normal vision between the third and fourth month of life. None in group 2 attained normal vision, while patients of group 3 did so but later than group 1. All groups developed nystagmus concurrent with visual recovery; the nystagmus disappeared in group 1 with complete visual recovery but persisted in group 3. The timing of visual recovery in this study (between the third and fourth month of life) has been noted to be synchronous with the emergence of geniculostriate-mediated visual functions, such as binocular vision, some orientation-specific responses, and smooth eye movements.

It has also been suggested that vision in infancy is subcortically mediated and that DVM may represent malfunction of the extrageniculostriate system (colliculus-pulvinar-parietal system), which subserves responses in neonates relating to detection, location, and orientation.[56] This is supported by the observation that visual function of premature infants with cortical lesions is similar to that of infants without such lesions.[48] This implies that a subcortical, possibly collicular, extrageniculostriate system is responsible for vision in the neonate, a postulate supported by the clinical observation that vision is indeed abnormal in infants with subcortical lesions.[49] According to this concept, visual recovery in DVM represents the emergence of a functioning geniculostriate system that takes place around 2 to 4 months of age.[39]

To reemphasize, if the notion is adopted that vision within the first two months of life is subcortical, two important clinical correlates emerge. First, a blind neonate with normal globes and optic nerves probably harbors some subcortical dysfunction. The cause may be demonstrable on neuroimaging (e.g., intracranial hemorrhage dissecting into the diencephalic structures) or it may

not be (e.g., pure DVM). Second, an isolated lesion of the geniculostriate pathway probably shows little effect on visual function of a neonate. Indeed, case reports supporting these concepts are available.

As the foregoing studies indicate, DVM is most widely thought of as representing an isolated anomaly with total eventual recovery of vision. However, as early as 1947, Beauvieux[16] pointed out that DVM may be further complicated by superimposed ocular or neurodevelopmental disorders that may render the eventual visual outcome variable. Fielder et al[56,57] modified the classification of DVM provided by Uemura and colleagues[219,220] and divided DVM into the following three types:

Type 1.   Isolated DVM is diagnosed when the child is otherwise healthy, with no associated ocular or systemic disease. Visual recovery usually occurs within a year of age.

Type 2.   This second type is diagnosed when the child has associated systemic disease, mental retardation, or other neurodevelopmental disorders. This type includes infants who may be small for gestational age or premature children[124] with associated delays in their general motor development.[31] Also included are children with organic brain damage, such as anoxia, hypoglycemia, Aicardi syndrome, tuberous sclerosis, etc. Infants in this group usually improve partially.

Type 3.   The third type is diagnosed when the child has associated ocular disease, such as bilateral cataracts, severe corneal opacities, colobomas, retinal dystrophy, optic nerve hypoplasia, or albinism. Affected children often have associated nystagmus. The visual impairment in such children may appear early on to be out of proportion to the ocular defect per se but improves proportionally with time. Not all patients with the aforementioned disorders show improved vision over time, and no clinical features help distinguish those who improve from those who do not.[58] The visual improvement has been postulated to result from posterior visual pathway maturation.[58]

As mentioned previously, many children with obvious ocular causes for their vision loss (e.g., coloboma, optic nerve hypoplasia, Leber's amaurosis) may have a superimposed component of DVM as attested to by the observation that the vision in many of such children improves somewhat within the first year of life. Of 11 such patients, Fielder et al[58] reported significant, albeit limited, visual improvement in eight. It is tempting in this context to speculate on the pathophysiologic basis of visual improvement reported in infants with unilateral ocular disease (e.g., optic nerve hypoplasia, congenital glaucoma) after patching therapy.[129,131] Could the visual improvement be due, at least in part, to a maturational phenomenon of the posterior visual pathway? Stated differently, is the partial recovery of vision observed in some patients with significant ocular disorders limited to those with bilateral disease, or can it also occur in unilateral ocular disorders? It is impossible to answer this question without an appropriately designed clinical trial.

Finally, DVM may in some cases represent a mild form of CVI. The underlying neuroanatomic abnormalities may be too subtle to be detected with current neuroimaging techniques. However, the much better visual prognosis than in patients with demonstrable cortical insults justifies a separate classification from the typical CVI.

The majority of patients with DVM show unremarkable optic disc appearance. However, it has been noted that some patients with DVM may show gray discoloration of the optic discs.[24] Such children are usually either immature or have ocular albinism, with the grayish tint presumably reflecting either deficient myelin of the optic nerve or "the effect of contrast" between a normally pigmented disc and an albinotic fundus, respectively. This discoloration should be distinguished from the grayish discoloration of the disc that may occur due to pigment on or within the disc substance that may be noted with melanocytoma or in several chromosomal abnormalities.

Follow-up studies of children with DVM reveal some tendency to show developmental problems, including global developmental delay as well as speech and language delay.[98] Some children who manifest DVM in infancy reportedly manifest autistic tendencies either concurrently or following visual improvement.[77] Kivlin et al[124] suggested that visual inattentiveness in a preterm infant is a harbinger of generalized neurological problems more so than in full-term infants.

Some children initially diagnosed with DVM may later prove to have congenital ocular motor apraxia. Infants with ocular motor apraxia may act blind before acquiring head and neck control, which is a prerequisite to manifest the characteristic head thrusts.[186] This is so since infants normally employ the saccadic system (which is defective in congenital ocular motor apraxia) to follow objects of regard (saccadic pursuit). Checking the vestibulo-ocular reflex by spinning such children around would produce only a slow phase of nystagmus; the fast phase would be expected to be defective. Only when the neck musculature and head control are sufficiently mature do the characteristic head thrusts emerge to strongly suggest the diagnosis. Children with ocular motor apraxia would be expected to have normal VEPs and ERGs.

Horizons

It should be apparent that our clinical understanding of CVI in children, although incomplete, has improved greatly over the last two decades. Unfortunately, therapy for the underlying disorders has lagged behind considerably, the role of the clinician is often limited to providing information, counseling, and support. Therapeutic interventions such as placement of a shunt for hydrocephalus or antibiotic treatment for meningitis are of obvious importance to limit the extent of neuronal damage. Unfortunately, many underlying conditions do not have such readily evident treatments.

Visual stimulation is a therapeutic modality that, generally speaking, is not popular with ophthalmologists. However, some authorities who work regularly with visually impaired children believe that certain techniques of visual stimulation may result in visual improvement but acknowledge that this reflects their clinical experience rather than results of scientific research (Jan JE, personal communication, 1994). Visual stimulation rests on the premise that vision is a learned skill, and like physical therapy, good visual stimulation helps the child use his residual sight more efficiently. This may occur as a result of recruiting neurons, increasing the synapses, or other means.[199a]

Refinement of preventive measures and early treatment of underlying causes to prevent neuronal damage can reduce the incidence of CVI. Rescuing sick axons to prevent their death is assuming an important role in areas of research concerned with brain injury.[14,90] Research to prevent transsynaptic degeneration after brain damage also holds promise,[195] although it is not clear whether or not such prevention would have a clinically desirable outcome.

Blindsight

There is considerable controversy regarding the existence in man of an extrageniculostriate visual system that subserves a cruder form of visual discrimination (blindsight).[29,147,175,235,236] The precise function of such a system is debatable, but it is thought to be integrated with the geniculostriate system and to mediate the unconscious awareness of motion in the peripheral field, spatial localization, and visuospatial orientation.[118] Neuroanatomically, it is estimated that 20% to 30% of the optic nerve fibers in humans terminate in structures other than the lateral geniculate body.[30] In primates, some such fibers go to the pretectal area and others to the superior colliculus, which in turn, project to the secondary, parastriate visual cortex (areas 18 and 19) and other areas of the brain via the pulvinar.[23] The function of the pretectal fibers is to mediate pupillary reaction to light, while collicular-pulvinar-parastriate fibers are presumed to subserve a subcortical form of vision that bypasses the geniculostriate pathway (blindsight).

The term *blindsight* refers to unconscious residual visual ability detected within a visual field defect corresponding to a lesion of the striate cortex. In humans, data supporting the existence of blindsight has been largely derived from studies demonstrating the ability of some patients with cortical blindenss or hemianopia to detect and localize stimuli that they do not report seeing within a perimetrically blind hemifield, as well as the ability to determine the orientation, motion, or color of such stimuli.[180] For example, when an image is flashed in the blind hemifield, affected patients are able to point to the location of the image or to guess correctly when it appeared. Despite insistence on seeing nothing, the

typical patient scores better than would be expected from chance alone. The results of such studies are open to question on the basis that some residual cortical function may still remain in the area subserving the blind fields due to incomplete destruction of the striate cortex[9,22,29,54] or that they may represent an artifact of poor fixation or light scattering.[29] Even in experimental studies after bilateral occipital lobectomy in primates, residual visual function may stem from subtotal resection of the anterior striate cortex.[40] The phenomenon of blindsight is unconscious. Conscious awareness of residual visual function in a patient with cortical blindness renders the possibility[109] of an underlying blindsight mechanism, which is subcortically mediated, quite unlikely.

Campion et al[29] summarized the existing evidence for and against the existence of extrageniculo-striate pathways in humans, and their study was followed by numerous peer commentaries. Most investigators seemed to believe the existence of an extrageniculostriate system that subconsciously mediates body orientation during traveling. This pathway is thought to involve the peripheral retina, the Y ganglion cells, the optic nerves, the superior colliculus, the pulvinar, and the occipitoparietal regions.

The notion of blindsight revolves around the idea that the extrageniculostriate system may act as a backup visual system if the geniculostriate system is defective. Human adults with acquired complete destruction of both areas 17 are usually totally blind,[23,30] "despite a preserved tectal system."[37] Whether a similar generalization applies to prenatal or neonatal lesions in humans is unknown. The age at the time of insult is important since many animal studies have suggested that the immature brain has a greater potential for recovery than the adult brain. Evidence derived from experiments with cats indicates that visual cortex damage in neonatal kittens, but not in adult cats, is followed by significant compensatory rewiring of the nervous system that reduces the otherwise expected visual handicap. A similar adaptability of the human embryonic CNS may underlie some cases that defy ready explanation on the basis of electrophysiologic and neuroimaging evidence. Summers and MacDonald[209] described a 14-month-old infant who showed intact central vision despite absent patterned VEPs and tomographic absence of the occipital cortex. The cerebral lesion might have resulted from a prenatal developmental defect. The authors speculated that the intact central vision may be explained on the basis of a heterotopic occipital cortex, a subcortical collicular system, or rewiring of the brain after the prenatal lesion.

Unlike humans, primates show preservation of visuospatial orientation and recognition of moving targets after bilateral destruction of both areas 17.[103] The interspecies difference may be theoretically explained from a phylogenetic viewpoint, that is, the greater the development of the newer cortical visual structures, the less the contribution of the older tectal and collicular structures to visual function. In lower vertebrates, the superior colliculus is the major visual processing center. It remains to be proven that the phylogenetically older collicular system maintains any function in man where the visual cortex is highly developed.

In summary, the phenomenon of blindsight remains controversial, especially in humans. However, the quest to settle the controversy has led to some intriguing questions about the nature of consciousness and the potential role of the extrageniculostriate system in visual performance.

It should be noted that while the phenomenon of blindsight (the ability to detect an object despite apparent lack of vision) has been rarely described in children, probably due to difficulty in testing for it, the converse (apparent inattentiveness or the inability to detect an object despite intact normal visual acuity and fields) is commonly seen in brain-damaged children. This resembles some of the findings in Balint syndrome,[87] which is caused by bilateral superior parieto-occipital lesions in the watershed areas resulting from anoxia, hypotension, or infarction. The features of Balint syndrome that may occur together or separately[225] include the following: (1) despite normal range of ocular movements, the patients seem unable to fixate an object voluntarily and, if fixated, gaze tends to involuntarily drift away ("psychic paralysis of gaze"); (2) inability to guide arm and hand movements by using visual feedback, with inaccurate reaching and grasping ("optic ataxia"); and (3) inability to attend to more than one visual stimulus, within the whole visual field, at a time

("piecemeal vision") and, often, unawareness of extramacular stimuli (bilateral visual neglect). The visual acuity is intact, and visual agnosia is absent (i.e., the patient recognizes what he sees), since the parietal and temporal association areas are intact. Balint syndrome has not been reported in children, possibly due to difficulty in testing of this age group.

The Effect of Total Blindness on Circadian Regulation

In the current cost-conscious climate of medical practice, the contribution of expensive and complicated surgical procedures to the overall quality of life is coming under increasing scrutiny. A case in point would be the patient with stage 5 retinopathy of prematurity (ROP) who undergoes extensive vitreoretinal surgery only to achieve "anatomical success," sometimes with no better than light perception vision. A question then arises whether the low functional vision attained with surgery contributes sufficiently to the patient's overall quality of life to justify the total cost. While questions like this are difficult to answer, there is increasing evidence to suggest that restoring any visual input may have significant impact on the overall well-being of the child in a manner unrelated to the meager improvement in visual function.[192] This evidence derives from recent studies demonstrating the importance of light input in the entrainment of circadian timing systems.[125] From the clinical standpoint, these adverse effects of blindness may manifest as sleep disturbances or depression following the visual loss, among other disorders.

Research on circadian timing systems in mammals have shown that three components of such a system exist: (1) a visual pathway connected to the circadian pacemaker, (2) a pacemaker (which in mammals, including possibly, humans, is the suprachiasmatic nucleus of the hypothalamus), and (3) efferent pathways coupling the pacemaker to effector systems that display circadian function.[164] Disruption in any of these components would result in circadian dysfunction. Total elimination of environmental light input may result in loss of circadian entrainment with subsequent free-running circadian rhythms. The endogenous, free-running, sleep-wake rhythms of humans is about 25 hours, a shift of 1 hour from the normal, entrained rhythm. This shift results in sleep disturbances, wherein affected patients are periodically awake at night and sleep during the day. The importance of retinohypothalamic connections in circadian rhythm regulation has been amply demonstrated in experimental animals. Retinohypothalamic fibers apparently project directly from the optic nerves to the suprachiasmatic nucleus of the hypothalamus, the putative circadian pacemaker. For example, bilateral transection of the optic nerves in rats resulted in loss of synchronized endogenous circadian rhythm, while bilateral transection of the optic tracts had no such effect. The recent demonstration of retinofugal projections to the suprachiasmatic nucleus of the hypothalamus in man suggests that much of what has been learned in experimental animals may be applicable to man. Blind people have a high incidence of sleep complaints, with some suffering intractable sleep disorders, suggesting that circadian disruption may be at fault.[157,158,174] Patients with congenital blindness have been shown to have abnormalities of other circadian rhythm regulation.[167,174] Many totally blind people have free-running temperature, cortisol, melatonin, and sleep-activity rhythms.[189,190] Melatonin, the so-called hormone of darkness,[221a] is a hormone actively secreted by the pineal gland and functions by providing a hormonal signal regarding the length of the night. The release of melatonin is controlled by an endogenous circadian system that is synchronized by the light–dark cycle, so that melatonin levels are high in darkness and low in light.

In mammals, retinohypothalamic projections to the pineal gland are the primary stimulus that serves to regulate melatonin secretion. Plasma melatonin levels rise at night and plummet during the day. Melatonin free running may explain why blind patients have chronic insomnia. Preliminary findings from Czeisler et al[35a] suggest that blind patients without chronic insomnia maintain normal melatonin levels while those with insomnia are found to have lost their ability to regulate these levels. Melatonin is now available in a synthetic form for investigational use. Recent studies have shown promising results for the possibility of treating certain sleep disorders by entraining the circadian pacemaker with external administration of melatonin.[111a,191]

Current evidence suggests that the perception of light is very important, if not essential, for the normal regulation of the human circadian pacemaker and that the quantity of light needed may be very small. Total elimination of light input into the hypothalamus may, accordingly, have far-reaching consequences on various circadian systems with potentially significant negative impact on the patient's health and well-being. Sadun et al[192] state, "In the future, ophthalmologists may consider the potential impact on the neuro-endocrine system when assessing the relative risks and benefits of therapy. Salvaging light perception vision may be of greater significance than previously thought."

References

1. Ablin RN, Salapatek P. Saccadic localization of peripheral targets by the very young human infant. Percept Psychophys 1975;17:293-302.
2. Aikawa J, Noro T, Tada K, et al. The heterogeneity of Leber's congenital amaurosis. J Inherit Metab Dis. 1989;12 (suppl 2):361-364.
3. Aldrich MS, Vanderzant CW, Alessi AG, et al. Ictal cortical blindness with permanent visual loss. Epilepsia 1989;30:116-120.
4. Andrews RJ. Transhemispheric diaschisis. A review and comment. Stroke. 1991;22:943-949.
5. Arroyo HA, Jan JE, McCormick AQ, et al. Permanent visual loss after shunt malfunction. Neurology 1985;35:25-29.
6. Atkin A, Raab E, Wolkstein M. Visual association cortex and vision in man: pattern-evoked occipital potentials in a blind boy. Science 1977;198:629-631.
7. Atkinson J. Human visual development over the first 6 months of life. A review and a hypothesis. Human Neurobiol 1984;3:61-74.
8. Babel J, Klein D, Roth A. Leber's congenital amaurosis associated with high hyperopia in four sisters. Ophthalmic Paediatr Genet. 1989;10:55-61.
9. Barinaga M. Unraveling the dark paradox of "blindsight." Science 1992;258:1438-1439.
10. Barkovich AJ, Maroldo TV. Magnetic resonance imaging of normal and abnormal brain development. Topics Magnet Resonance Imaging 1993; 5:96-122.
11. Barricks ME, Flynn JT, Kushner BJ. Paradoxical pupillary responses in congenital stationary night blindness. Arch Ophthalmol 1977;95:1800-1804.
12. Barry E, Sussman NM, Bosley TM, et al. Ictal blindness and status epilepticus amauroticus. Epilepsia 1985;26:577-584.
13. Bauer J, Schuler P, Feistel H, et al. Blindness as an ictal phenomenon: investigations with EEG and SPECT in two patients suffering from epilepsy. J Neurol 1991;238:44-46.

14. Baughler JM, Hall ED. Current application of "high dose" steroid therapy for CNS injury. J Neurosurg 1985;62:806-810.
15. Beatty RM, Sadun AA, Smith L, et al. Direct demonstration of transsynaptic degeneration in the human visual system: a comparison of retrograde and anterograde changes. J Neurol Neurosurg Psychiatry 1982;45:143-146.
16. Beauvieux M. La cecite apparente chez le nouveau-ne la pseudo-atrophie grise du nerf optique. Arch Ophthalmol 1947;7:241-249.
17. Bell RA, Thompson HS. Relative afferent pupillary defect in optic tract hemianopia. Am J Ophthalmol 1978;85:538-540.
18. Benecke R, Berthold A, Conrad B. Denervation activity in the EMG of patients with upper motor neuron lesions: time course, local distribution and pathogenetic aspects. J Neurol 1983;230:143-151.
19. Bodis-Wollner I, Atkin A, Raab E, et al. Visual association cortex and vision in man: pattern-evoked occipital potentials in a blind boy. Science 1977;198:629-630.
20. Bosley TM, et al. Ischemic lesions of the occipital cortex and optic radiations: positron emission tomography. Neurology 1985;35:470-484.
21. Brazelton TB, Scholl ML, Robey JS. Visual responses in the newborn. Pediatrics 1966;37:284-290.
22. Bridgeman B, Staggs B. Plasticity in human blind sight. Vis Res 1982;22:1199-1203.
23. Brindley GS, Gautier-Smith PC, Lewin W. Cortical blindness and the functions of the non-geniculate fibers of the optic tracts. J Neurol Neurosurg Psychiatry 1969;32:259-264.
24. Brodsky MC, Buckley EG, McConkie-Rosell A. The case of the gray optic disc! Surv Ophthalmol 1989;33:367-372.
25. Brodsky MC, Glasier CM, Pollock SC, et al. Optic nerve hypoplasia. Identification by magnetic resonance imaging. Arch Ophthalmol 1990;108:1562-1567.
26. Brodsky MC, Glasier CM. Optic nerve hypoplasia. Clinical significance of associated central nervous system abnormalities on magnetic resonance imaging. Arch Ophthalmol 1993;111:66-74.
27. Brown WF, Snow R. Denervation in hemiplegic muscles. Stroke 1990;21:1700-1704.
28. Byrd RL, Rohrbaugh TM, Raney RB Jr, et al. Transient cortical blindness secondary to vincristine therapy in childhood malignancies. Cancer 1981;47:37-40.
29. Campion J, Latto R, Smith YM. Is blind sight an effect of scattered light, spared cortex, and near-threshold vision? Behav Brain Sci 1983;6:423-486.
30. Celesia GG, Archer CR, Kuroiwa Y, et al. Visual function of the extrageniculo-calcarine system in man. Relationship to cortical blindness. Arch Neurol 1980;37:704-706.
31. Cole GF, Hungerford J, Jones RB. Delayed visual maturation. Arch Vis Child 1984;59:107-110.
32. Connolly MB, Jan JE, Cochrane DD. Rapid recovery from cortical visual impairment following correction of prolonged shunt malfunction in congenital hydrocephalus. Arch Neurol 1991;48:956-957.
33. Courville CB. Cerebral Anoxia. Los Angeles, CA: San Lucas Press; 1953:221-236.
34. Cummings JL, Gittinger JW Jr. Central dazzle: a thalamic syndrome? Arch Neurol 1981;38:372-374.
35. Curless RG, Flynn JT, Olsen KR, et al. Leber congenital amaurosis in siblings with diffuse dysmyelination. Pediatr Neurol 1991;7:223-225.
35a. Czeisler CA, Shanahan TL, Klerman EB, et al. Suppression of melatonin secretion in some blind patients by exposure to bright light. N Engl J Med 1995;332:6-11.
36. Dagi LR, Leys MJ, Hansen RM, et al. Hyperopia in complicated Leber's congenital amaurosis. Arch Ophthalmol 1990;108:709-712.
37. Daroff R. In discussion: Botez MI. Two visual systems in clinical neurology: the readaptive role of the primitive tectal system in visual agnosic patients. Trans Am Neurol Assoc 1972;97:63-65.
37a. Davidson JE, McWilliam DC, Evans TH, et al. Porencephaly and optic hypoplasia in neonatal thrombocytopenia. Arch Dis Child 1989;64:858-860
38. De Laey JJ. Leber's congenital amaurosis. Bull Soc Belge Ophtalmol 1991;241:41-50.
39. Delayed visual maturation. Lancet 1991;20;337 (8747):950-952. Editorial.
40. Denny-Brown D, Chambers RA. Physiological aspects of visual perception, I: functional aspects of visual cortex. Arch Neurol 1976;33:219-227.
41. de Sa LCF, Hoyt CS. Optic nerve and cortical blindness. In: Isenberg SJ, ed. The Eye in Infancy. St. Louis, MO: Mosby; 1994:413-425.
42. DeSousa AL, Kleiman MD, Mealey J. Quadraplegia and cortical blindness in Hemophilus influenzae meningitis. J Pediatr 1978;93:253-254.
43. Diesenhouse MC, Palay DA, Newman NJ, et al. Acquired heterochromia with Horner syndrome in two adults. Ophthalmology 1992;99(12):1815-1817.
44. Dietrich RB, Bradley WG, Zaragoza EJ, et al. MR evaluation of early myelination patterns in normal and developmentally delayed infants. AJNR 1988;9:69-76.
45. Dineen J, Hendrickson A, Keating EG. Alterations of retinal inputs following striate cortex removal in adult monkey. Exp Brain Res 1982;47:446-456.
46. Dobson V, Quinn GE, Biglan AW, et al. Acuity card assessment of visual function in the cryotherapy for retinopathy of prematurity trial. Invest Ophthalmol Vis Sci 1990;31:1702-1708.
47. Droste PJ, Archer SM, Helveston EM. Measurement of low vision in children and infants. Ophthalmology 1991;98:1513-1518.

48. Dubowitz LMS, Mushin J, De Vries L, et al. Visual function in the newborn infant: is it cortically mediated? Lancet 1986;(i):1139-1141.

49. Dubowitz LMS, Mushin J, Morani FA, et al. The maturation of visual acuity in neurologically normal and abnormal newborn infants. Behav Brain Res 1983;10:39-46.

50. el Azazi M, Malm G, Forsgren M. Late ophthalmologic manifestations of neonatal herpes simplex virus infection. Am J Ophthalmol 1990;109:1-7.

51. Eldridge PR, Punt JAG. Transient traumatic cortical blindness in children. Lancet 1988;1(8589): 815-816.

52. Euziere J, Viallefont H, Vidal J. Double atrophie optique et hemianopsie gauche consecutives a une blessure occipitale droite. Arch Soc Sci Med Biol Montpellier 1943;14:212-215.

53. Fagan JF III, Singer LT, Montie JE, et al. Selective screening device for the early detection of normal or delayed cognitive development in infants at risk for later mental retardation. Pediatrics 1986;78: 1021-1026.

54. Fendrich R, Wessinger CM, Gazzaniga MS. Residual vision in a scotoma: implications for blindsight. Science 1992;258:1489-1491.

55. Fielder AP, Evans NM. Is the geniculo-striate system a pre-requisite for nystagmus? Eye 1988;2: 380-382.

56. Fielder AR, Mayer DL. Delayed visual maturation. Semin Ophthalmol 1992;6:182-193.

57. Fielder AR, Russell-Eggitt IR, Dodd KL, et al. Delayed visual maturation. Trans Opthalmol Soc UK 1985;104:653-661.

58. Fielder AR, Fulton AB, Mayer DL. Visual development of infants with severe ocular disorders. Ophthalmology. 1991;98(8):1306-1309.

59. Fielder AR, Mayer DL, Fulton AB. Delayed visual maturation. Lancet. 1991;337(8753):1350. Letter.

60. Finger S, Almli CR. Brain damage and neuroplasticity: mechanisms of recovery or development? Brain Res Rev 1985;10:177-186.

61. Fletcher WA, Hoyt WF, Narahara MH. Congenital quadrantanopia with occipital lobe ganglioglioma. Neurology 1988;38:1892-1894.

62. Flett P, Saunders B. Ophthalmic assessment of physically disabled children attending a rehabilitation centre. J Paediatr Child Health 1993;29:132-135.

63. Flodmark O, Jan JE, Wong KHP. Computed tomography of the brains of children with cortical visual impairment. Dev Med Child Neurol 1990; 32:611-620.

64. Flynn JT, Kazarian E, Barricks M. Paradoxical pupil in congenital achromatopsia. Int Ophthalmol 1981;3:91-96.

65. Foley J. Central visual disturbances. Dev Med Child Neurol 1987;29:110-120.

66. Folz SJ, Trobe JD. The peroxisome and the eye. Surv Ophthalmol 1991;35:353-368.

67. Foxman SG, Wirtschafter JD, Letson RD. Leber's congenital amaurosis and high hyperopia: a discrete entity. In: Henkind P, ed. *ACTA. XXIV International Congress of Ophthalmology.* New York, NY: JB Lippincott;1983;1:55-58.

68. Frank JW, Kushner BJ, France TD. Paradoxic pupillary phenomena. A review of patients with pupillary constriction to darkness. Arch Ophthalmol 1988;106:1564-1566.

69. Frank Y, Torres F. Visual evoked potentials in the evaluation of "cortical blindness" in children. Ann Neurol 1979;6:126-129.

70. Fulton AB, Hansen RM. Electroretinography: application to clinical studies of infants. J Pediatr Ophthalmol Strabismus 1985;22:251-255.

71. Gelbart SS, Hoyt CS. Congenital nystagmus: a clinical perspective in infancy. Graefe's Arch Clin Exp Ophthalmol 1988;226:178-180.

72. Good PA, Searle AET, Campbell S, et al. Value of the ERG in congenital nystagmus. Br J Ophthalmol 1989;73:512-515.

73. Good WV, Crain LS, Quint RD, et al. Overlooking: a sign of bilateral central scotomata in children. Dev Med Child Neurol 1992;34:61-79.

74. Good WV, Hoyt CS, Lambert SR. Optic nerve atrophy in children with hypoxia. Invest Ophthalmol Vis Sci 1987;28(suppl):309. Abstract.

75. Good WV, Hoyt CS. Behavioral correlates of poor vision in children. Int Ophthalmol Clin 1989;29: 57-60.

76. Good WV, Jan JE, DeSa L, Barkovich AJ, et al. Cortical visual impairment in children. Surv Ophthalmol 1994; 38: 351-364.

77. Goodman R, Ashby L. Delayed visual maturation and autism. Dev Med Child Neurol 1990;32:814-819.

78. Gottlob I. Eye movement abnormalities in carriers of blue-cone monochromatism. Invest Ophthalmol Vis Sci 1994;35:3556-3560.

79. Griffith JF, Dodge PR. Transient blindness following head injury in children. N Engl J Med 1968; 278:648-651.

80. Groenendaal F, Duin v Hof-van. Partial visual recovery in two full-term infants after perinatal hypoxia. Neuropediatrics 1990;21:76-78.

81. Haddock JN. Transsynaptic degeneration in the visual system. Arch Neurol Psychiatr 1950;64:66-73.

82. Haginoya K, Aikawa J, Noro T, et al. Two siblings of Leber's congenital amaurosis with an increase in very long chain fatty acid in blood: relationship between peroxisomal disorders and Leber's congenital amaurosis [in Japanese]. No To Hattatsu. 1989;21(4):348-353.

83. Hall D. Delayed visual maturation. Dev Med Child Neurol 1991;33(2):181. Letter, comment.

84. Hanyu H, Arai H, Katsunuma H, et al. Crossed cerebellar atrophy following cerebrovascular lesions [in Japanese]. Nippon Ronen Igakkai Zasshi 1991;28:160-165.

85. Harel S, Holtzman M, Feinsod M. The late visual bloomer. In: Harel S, Anastasion N, eds. The At-Risk Infant: Psycho/Social/Medical Aspects. Baltimore, MD: Paul H. Brooks Publishing Co, Inc; 1985;359-362.

86. Harrison DW, Walls RM. Blindness following minor head trauma in children: a report of two cases with a review of the literature. J Emerg Med 1990;8:21-24.

87. Hecaen H, Ajuriaguerra J. Balint syndrome (psychic paralysis of visual fixation) and its minor forms. Brain 1954;77:373-400.

88. Heher KL, Traboulsi EI, Maumenee IH. The natural history of Leber's congenital amaurosis. Age-related findings in 35 patients. Ophthalmology 1992;99:241-245.

89. Hendrickson AE, Yuodelis C. The morphological development of the human fovea. Ophthalmology 1984;91:603-612.

90. Hernandez TD, Schallert T. Behavioural recovery following medial cortex damage is chronically impaired by transient GABA agonist infusion into adjacent sensorimotor cortex. Restorative Neurol Neurosci 1995. In press.

91. Hertz BG, Rosenberg J. Effect of mental retardation and motor disability on testing with visual acuity cards. Dev Med Child Neurol 1992;34:115-122.

92. Herzau V, Bleher I, Joos-Kratsch E. Infantile exotropia with homonymous hemianopia: a rare contraindication for strabismus surgery. Graefe's Arch Ophthalmol 1988;226:148-149.

93. Hickey TL. Postnatal development of the human lateral geniculate nucleus. Relationship to a critical period for the visual system. Science 1977; 198:836-838.

94. Highley M, Meller ST, Pinkerton CR. Seizures and cortical dysfunction following high-dose cisplatin administration in children. Med Pediatr Oncol 1992;20:143-148.

95. Horton JC, Hoyt WF. The representation of the visual field in human striate cortex: a revision of the classic Holmes map. Arch Ophthalmol 1991; 109:816-824.

96. Hoyt C. Neurovisual adaptations to subnormal vision in children. Aust New Z J Ophthalmol 1987; 15:57-63.

97. Hoyt CS, Good WV. Ocular motor adaptations to congenital hemianopia. Binocular Vision 1993; 8:125-126. Guest editorial.

98. Hoyt CS, Jastrzebski G, Marg E. Delayed visual maturation in infancy. Br J Ophthalmol 1983; 67:127-130.

99. Hoyt CS. Cryotherapy for retinopathy of prematurity: 3 1/2-year outcome for both structure and function. Arch Ophthalmol 1993;111:319-320.

100. Hoyt WF, Rios-Montenegro EN, Behrens MM, et al. Homonymous hemioptic hypoplasia. Funduscopic features in standard and red-free illumination in three patients with congenital hemiplegia. Br J Ophthalmol 1972;56:537-545.

101. Hoyt WF. Congenital occipital hemianopia. Neuro-Ophthalmol Jpn 1985;2:252-259.

102. Hoyt WF. Ophthalmoscopy of the retinal nerve fibre layer in neuro-ophthalmologic diagnosis. Aust J Ophthalmol 1976;4:14.

103. Humphrey NK, Weiskrantz L. Vision in monkeys after removal of the striate cortex. Nature 1967; 215:595-597.

104. Huttenlocher PR, deCourten C, Carey LJ, et al. Synaptogenesis in human visual cortex. Evidence for synapse elimination during normal development. Neurosci Letter 1982;33:247-252.

105. Illingworth RS. Delayed visual maturation. Arch Dis Child 1961;36:407-409.

106. Isenberg SJ, Molarte A, Vazquez M. The fixed and dilated pupils of premature neonates. Am J Ophthalmol 1990;110:168-171.

107. Ivarsson SA, Bjerre I, Brun A, et al. Joubert syndrome associated with Leber amaurosis and multicystic kidneys. Am J Med Genet. 1993;45:542-547.

108. Jacobs M, Shawkat F, Harris CM, et al. Eye movement and electrophysiological findings in an infant with hemispheric pathology. Dev Med Child Neurol 1993;35:431-448.

109. Jacobson DM. Pupillary responses to dilute pilocarpine in preganglionic 3rd nerve disorders. Neurology 1990;40:804-808.

110. Jacobson DM, Thompson HS, Bartley JA. X-linked progressive cone dystrophy. Clinical characteristics of affected males and female carriers. Ophthalmology. 1989;96:885-895.

111. Jaffe SJ, Roach ES. Transient cortical blindness with occipital lobe epilepsy. J Clin Neuroophthalmol. 1988;8:221-224.

111a. Jan JE, Espezel H, Appleton RE. The treatment of sleep disorders with melatonin. Dev Med Child Neurol 1994;36:97, 107.

112. Jan JE, Farrell K, Wong PK, et al. Eye and head movements of visually impaired children. Dev Med Child Neurol 1986;28:285-293.

113. Jan JE, Freeman RD, McCormick AQ, et al. Eye-pressing by visually impaired children. Dev Med Child Neurol 1983;25:755-762.

113a. Jan JE, Good WV, Freeman RD, et al. Eye-poking. Dev Med Child Neurol 1994;36:321-325.

114. Jan JE, Groenveld M, Sykanda AM, et al. Behavioral characteristics of children with permanent cortical visual impairment. Dev Med Child Neurol 1987;29:571-576.

115. Jan JE, Groenveld M, Anderson DP. Photophobia and cortical visual impairment. Dev Med Child Neurol 1993;35:473-477.

115a. Jan JE, Groenveld M, Connolly MB. Head shaking by visually impaired children: a voluntary neurovisual adaptation which can be confused with spasmus nutans. Dev Med Child Neurol 1990; 32:1061-1066.

116. Jan JE, Groenveld M, Sykanda AM. Light-gazing by visually impaired children. Dev Med Child Neurol 1990;32:755-759.

117. Jan JE, McCormick AQ, Hoyt CS. The unequal nystagmus test. Dev Med Child Neurol 1988; 30:441-443.

118. Jan JE, Wong PKH, Groenveld M, et al. Travel vision: "Collicular visual system?" Pediatr Neurol 1986;2:359-362.

119. Jasper H. Electrical activity in the depths of the cortex as compared to that on the surface. Trans Am Neurol Assoc 1955;80:21-22.

120. Joubert M, Eisenring J, Robb JP, et al. Familial agenesis of the cerebellar vermis. Neurology 1969; 19:813-825.

121. Kaye EM, Herskowitz J. Transient post-traumatic cortical blindness: brief v. prolonged syndromes in childhood. J Child Neurol 1986;1:206-210.

122. Kendall B, Kingsley D, Lambert SR, et al. Joubert syndrome: a clinico-radiological study. Neuroradiology 1990;31:502-506.

123. King MD, Dudgeon J, Stephenson JBP. Joubert's syndrome with retinal dysplasia: neonatal tachypnea as the clue to the genetic brain-eye malformation. Arch Dis Child 1984;59:709-718.

124. Kivlin JD, Bodnar A, Ralston CW, et al. The visually inattentive preterm infant. J Pediatr Ophthalmol Strabismus 1990;27:190-195.

125. Klein DC, Moore RY, Reppert SM, eds. Suprachiasmatic Nucleus. The Mind's Clock. New York, NY: Oxford University Press; 1991.

126. Kondo A, Nagara H, Tateishi J. A morphometric study of myelinated fibers in the fifth lumbar ventral roots in patients with cerebrovascular diseases. Clin Neuropathol 1987;6:250-256.

127. Kosnik E, Paulson GW, Laguna JF. Postictal blindness. Neurology 1976;26:248-250.

128. Kupersmith MJ, Vargas M, Hoyt WF, et al. Optic tract atrophy with cerebral arteriovenous malformations. Direct and transsynaptic degeneration. Neurology 1994;44:80-83.

129. Kushner BJ. Functional amblyopia associated with abnormalities of the optic nerve. Arch Ophthalmol. 1984;102:683-685.

130. Kushner BJ. Grating acuity tests should not be used for social service purposes in preliterate children. Arch Ophthalmol 1994;112:1030-1031.

131. Kushner BJ. Successful treatment of functional amblyopia associated with juvenile glaucoma. Graefe's Arch Clin Exp Ophthalmol. 1988;226: 150-153.

131a. Kusher BJ, Lucchese NJ, Morton GV. Grating visual acuity with Teller cards compared with Snellen visual acuity in literate patients. Arch Ophthalmol 1995;113:485-493.

132. Lai CW, Hung T, Lin WSJ. Blindness of cerebral origin in acute intermittent porphyria. Arch Neurol 1977;34:310-312.

133. Lambert SL, Hoyt C. Brain problems. In: Taylor D, ed. *Pediatric Ophthalmology*. Boston, MA: Blackwell Scientific Publications; 1990:507.

134. Lambert SR , Kriss A, Gresty M, et al. Joubert syndrome. Arch Ophthalmol 1989;107:709-713.

135. Lambert SR, Hoyt CS , Narahara MH. Optic nerve hypoplasia. Surv Ophthalmol 1987;32:1-9.

136. Lambert SR, Kriss A, Taylor D, et al. Follow-up and diagnostic reappraisal of 75 patients with Leber's congenital amaurosis. Am J Ophthalmol 1989;107:624-631.

137. Lambert SR, Kriss A, Taylor D. Detection of isolated occipital lobe anomalies during early childhood. Dev Med Child Neurol 1990;32:451-455.

138. Lambert SR, Taylor D, Kriss A. The infant with nystagmus, normal appearing fundi, but an abnormal ERG. Surv Ophthalmol 1989;34:173-186.

139. Lambert SR, Kriss A, Taylor D. Delayed visual maturation. A longitudinal clinical and electrophysiological assessment. Ophthalmology 1989;96:524-529.

140. Lambert SR, Hoyt CS, Jan JE, et al. Visual recovery from hypoxic cortical blindness during childhood. Computed tomographic and magnetic resonance imaging predictors. Arch Ophthalmol 1987; 105(10):1371-1377.

141. Lanska DJ, Lanska MJ. Visual "release" hallucinations in juvenile neuronal ceroid-lipofuscinosis. Pediatr Neurol. 1993;9:316-317.

142. Lapresle J. Palatal myoclonus. Adv Neurol. 1986; 43:265-273.

143. Lewis RA, Holcomb JD, Bromley WC, et al. Mapping X-linked ophthalmic diseases. III: provisional assignment of the locus for blue cone monochromacy to xq28. Arch Ophthalmol 1987;105:1055-1059.

144. Magoon EH, Robb RM. Development of myelin in human optic nerve and tract. A light and electron microscope study. Arch Ophthalmol 1981;99:655-659.

145. Margo C, Hamed LM, McCarty J. Congenital optic tract syndrome. Arch Ophthalmol 1991;109:1120-1122.

146. Margolis LH, Shaywutz BA. Cortical blindness associated with occipital atrophy: a complication of influenza meningitis. Dev Med Child Neurol 1978;20:490-493.

147. Marshall JC, Halligan PW. Blindsight and insight in visuo-spatial neglect. Nature. 1988; 336(6201):766-767.

148. Matthews WB. Footballer's migraine. Br Med J 1972;2:326-327.

149. Mayer DL, Fulton AB, Sossen PL. Preferential looking acuity of pediatric patients with developmental disabilities. Behav Brain Res 1983;10:189-198.

150. Mayer DL; Fulton AB; Cummings MF. Visual fields of infants assessed with a new perimetric technique. Invest Ophthalmol Vis Sci. 1988; 29:452-459.

151. McComas AJ. Invited review: motor unit estimation: methods, results, and present status. Muscle Nerve 1991;14: 585-597.

152. McCulloch DL, Taylor MJ, Whyte HE. Visual evoked potentials and visual prognosis following perinatal asphyxia. Arch Ophthalmol 1991;109: 229-233.

153. McCulloch DL; Taylor MJ. Cortical blindness in children: utility of flash VEPs. Pediatr Neurol 1992;8:156-157.

154. Meienberg O, Zangemeister WH, Rosenberg M, et al. Saccadic eye movement strategies in patients with homonymous hemianopia. Ann Neurol 1981; 9:537-544.

155. Mellor DH, Fielder AR. Dissociated visual development: electrodiagnostic studies in infants who are "slow to see." Dev Med Child Neurol 1980; 22:327-335.

156. Mikelberg FS; Yidegiligne HM. Axonal loss in band atrophy of the optic nerve in craniopharyngioma: a quantitative analysis. Can J Ophthalmol 1993;28:69-71.

157. Miles LEM, Raynal DM, Wilson MA. Blind man living in normal society has circadian rhythms of 24.9 hours. Science 1977;198:421-423.

158. Miles LEM, Wilson MA. High incidence of cyclic sleep/wake disorders in the blind. Sleep Res 1977; 6:192.

159. Miller NR, ed. *Walsh and Hoyt Clinical Neuro-Ophthalmology*. 4th ed. Baltimore, MD: Williams & Wilkins; 1982;1:142-149.

160. Miller NR, Newman SA. Transsynaptic degeneration. Arch Ophthalmol 1981;99:1654. Letter.

161. Miyake Y, Yagasaki K, Horiguchi M, et al. Congenital stationary night blindness with negative electroretinogram. A new classification. Arch Ophthalmol 1986;104:1013-1020.

162. Moel DI, Kwun YA. Cortical blindness as a complication of haemodialysis. J Pediatr 1978;93:890-891.

163. Mohn GJ, von-Hof-van D. Development of the binocular and monocular visual fields of human infants during the first year of life. Clin Vision Sci 1986;1:51-64.

164. Moore RY. Disorders of circadian function and human circadian timing system. In: Klein DC, Moore RY, Reppert SM, eds. *Suprachiasmatic Nucleus. The Mind's Clock*. New York, NY: Oxford University Press; 1991:429-441.

165. Mukamel M, Weitz R, Nissenkorn E, et al. Acute cortical blindness associated with hypoglycemia. J Pediatr 1981;98:583-584.

166. Muttitt SC, Taylor MJ, Kobayashi JS, et al. Serial visual evoked potentials and outcome in term birth asphyxia. Pediatr Neurol 1991;7:86-90.

167. Nakagawa H, Sack RL, Lewy AJ. Sleep propensity free-runs with the temperature, melatonin and cortisol rhythms in a totally blind person. Sleep. 1992; 15:330-336.

168. Nettleship E. On cases of recovery from amaurosis in young children. Trans Ophthalmol Soc UK 1883-1884:4:243-266.

169. Newman NM, Stevens RA, Heckenlively JR. Nerve fibre layer loss in diseases of the outer retinal layer. Br J Ophthalmol 1987;71:21-26.

170. Newman SA, Miller NR. Optic tract syndrome. Neuro-ophthalmologic considerations. Arch Ophthalmol 1983;101:1241-1250.

171. Nickel BL, Hoyt CS. The hypoxic retinopathy syndrome. Am J Ophthalmol 1982;93:589-593.

172. Nunn AD. Is nuclear medicine viable and can it measure viability? J Nucl Med 1993;34:924-926. Editorial.

173. O'Donnell FE Jr, Pappas HR. Autosomal dominant foveal hypoplasia and presenile cataracts. Arch Ophthalmol 1982;100:279-281.

174. Okawa M, Nanami T, Wada S, et al. Four congenitally blind children with circadian sleep-wake rhythm disorder. Sleep 1987;10:101-110.

175. Perenin MT, Ruel J, Hecaen H. Residual visual capabilities in a case of cortical blindness. Cortex 1980;16:605-612.

176. Poll-The BT, Saudubray JM, Ogier H, et al. Infantile Refsum's disease: biochemical findings suggesting multiple peroxisomal dysfunction. J Inherited Metab Dis 1986;9:169-174.

177. Pomeroy SL, Holmes SJ, Dodge PR, et al. Seizures and other neurologic sequelae of bacterial meningitis in children. N Engl J Med 1990; 323:1651-1657.

178. Price MJ, Thompson HS, Judisch GF, et al. Pupillary constriction to darkness. Br J Ophthalmol 1985;69:205-211.

179. Rabinowicz IM. Visual function in children with hydrocephalus. Trans Ophthalmol Soc UK 1974; 94:353-366.

180. Rafal R, Smith J, Krantz J, et al. Extrageniculate vision in hemianopic humans: saccade inhibition by signals in a blind field. Science 1990;250:118-121.

181. Ragge NK, Hoyt WF, Lambert SR. Big discs with optic nerve hypoplasia. J Clin Neuro Ophthalmol 1991;11:137. Letter.

182. Remler BF, Leigh RJ, Osorio I, et al. The characteristics and mechanisms of visual disturbances associated with anticonvulsant therapy. Neurology 1990;40:791-796.

183. Repka MX, Miller NR. Optic atrophy in children. Am J Ophthalmol 1988;106:191-193.

184. Rogers SJ; Newhart-Larson S. Characteristics of infantile autism in five children with Leber's congenital amaurosis. Dev Med Child Neurol. 1989; 31:598-608.

185. Ronen S, Nawratski I, Yanko L. Cortical blindness in infancy: a followup study. Ophthalmologica 1983;187:217-221.

186. Rosenberg ML, Wilson E. Congenital ocular motor apraxia without head thrusts. J Clin Neuro-Ophthalmol 1987;7:26-28.

187. Rubin AM. Transient cortical blindness and occipital seizures with cyclosporine toxicity. Transplantation 1989;47:572-573.

188. Sachdev MS, Kumar H, Jain AK, et al. Transsynaptic neuronal degeneration of optic nerves associated with bilateral occipital lesions. Indian J Ophthalmol 1990;38:151-152.

189. Sack RL, Lewy AJ. Human circadian rhythms: lessons from the blind. Ann Med. 1993;25:303-305. Editorial.

190. Sack RL, Lewy AJ, Blood ML, et al. Circadian rhythm abnormalities in totally blind people: incidence and clinical significance. J Clin Endocrinol Metab. 1992;75:127-134.

191. Sack RL, Lewy AJ, Blood ML, et al. Melatonin administration to blind people: phase advances and entrainment. J Biol Rhythms 1991;6:249-261.

192. Sadun AA, Johnson BM, Schaecter J. Neuroanatomy of the human visual system, Part III: three retinal projections to the hypothalamus. Neuro-Ophthalmol 1986;6:371-379.

193. Sadun AA, Smythe BA, Schaechter JD. Optic neuritis or ophthalmic artery aneurysm? Case presentation with histopathologic documentation utilizing a new staining method. J Clin Neuroophthalmol 1984;4:265-273.

194. Salanova V, Andermann F, Olivier A, et al. Occipital lobe epilepsy: electroclinical manifestations, electrocorticography, cortical stimulation and outcome in 42 patients treated between 1930 and 1991. Surgery of occipital lobe epilepsy. Brain 1992;115(pt 6):1655-1680.

195. Schallert T, Lindner MD. Rescuing neurons from transsynaptic degeneration after brain damage: helpful, harmful, or neutral in recovery of function? Can J Psychol 1990;44:276-292.

196. Silverman IE, Galetta SL, Alavi A, et al. SPECT in patients with cortical visual loss. J Nucl Med 1993;34:1447-1451.

197. Silverman IE, Galetta SL, Grossman M. SPECT and MRI in posterior cerebral artery infarction and related visual field defects. J Nucl Med 1993;34:1009-1012.

198. Skarf B, Hoyt CS. Optic nerve hypoplasia in children. Association with anomalies of the endocrine and CNS. Arch Opthalmol 1984;102:62-67.

199. Skarf B. In discussion: Lambert SR, Kriss A, Taylor D. Delayed visual maturation. A longitudinal clinical and electrophysiological assessment. Ophthalmology 1989;96:524-529.

199a. Sonksen PM, et al. Promotion of visual development in severely visually impaired babies. Evaluation of a developmentally based programme. Dev Med Child Neurol 1991;33:320-335.

200. Spear PD, Tong L, McCall MA. Functional influence of areas 17, 18, and 19 on lateral suprasylvian cortex in kittens and adult cats: implications for compensation following early visual cortex damage. Brain Res 1989;447:79-91.

201. Stefani FH, Asiyo MN, Mehraein P, et al. Histopathology of the retina, optic fascicle and lateral geniculate body in chronic, bilateral symmetric ischemic Schnabel's cavernous optic atrophy [in German]. Klin Monatsbl Augenheilkd 1990;197:162-165.

202. Steinberg A, Ronen S, Zlotogorski Z, et al. Central nervous system involvement in Leber congenital amaurosis. J Pediatr Ophthalmol Strabismus. 1992;29:224-227.

203. Steinlin M; Martin E; Schenker K; et al. Myelination of the optic radiation in Leber congenital amaurosis. Brain Dev. 1992;14:212-215.

204. Stoerig P, Cowey A. Increment-threshold spectral sensitivity in blindsight: Evidence for colour opponency. Brain 1991;114:1487-1512.

205. Strauss H. Paroxysmal blindness. Electroencephalogr Clin Neurophysiol 1963;15:921.

206. Strefling AM; Urich H. Prenatal porencephaly: the pattern of secondary lesions. Acta Neuropathol Berl 1986;71:171-175.

207. Sugimoto T, Woo M, Okazaki H, et al. Computed tomography in young children with herpes simplex virus encephalitis. Pediatr Radiol 1985;15:372-376.

208. Sullivan TJ, Lambert SR, Buncic JR, et al. The optic discs in Leber congenital amaurosis. J Pediatr Ophthalmol Strabismus 1992;29:246-249.

209. Summers CG, MacDonald JT. Vision despite tomographic absence of the occipital cortex. Surv Ophthalmol 1990;35:188-190.

210. Taylor D, Lake BD, Stephens R. Neurolipidoses. In: Taylor D, Wybareds K, eds. Pediatric Ophthalmology. New York, NY: Marcel Dekker; 1983:810-813.

211. Taylor MJ. Evoked potentials in pediatrics. In: Halliday AM, ed. Evoked Potentials in Clinical Testing. 2nd ed. London: Churchill Livingstone; 1992.

212. Taylor MJ, McCulloch DL. Prognostic value of VEPs in young children with acute onset of cortical blindness. Pediatr Neurol 1991;7:111-115.

213. Taylor MJ, McCulloch DL. Visual evoked potentials in infants and children. J Clin Neurophysiol 1992;9:357-372.

214. Thun-Hohenstein L, Schmitt B, Steinlin H, et al. Cortical visual impairment following bacterial meningitis: magnetic resonance imaging and visual evoked potentials findings in two cases. Eur J Pediatr 1992;151:779-782.

215. Tresidder J, Fielder AR, Nicholson J. Delayed visual maturation: ophthalmic and neurodevelopmental aspects. Dev Med Child Neurol 1990;32:872-881.

216. Tusa RJ, Repka MX, Smith CB, et al. Early visual deprivation results in persistent strabismus and nystagmus in monkeys. Invest Ophthalmol Vis Sci 1991;32:134-141.

217. Tychsen L, Hoyt WF. Hydrocephalus and transient cortical blindness. Am J Ophthalmol 1984;98:819-821.

218. Tychsen L, Hoyt WF. Occipital lobe dysplasia. Magnetic resonance findings in two cases of isolated congenital hemianopia. Arch Ophthalmol 1985;103:680-682.

219. Uemura Y. The assessment of visual ability in children. In: Francois J, Maione M, eds. *Pediatric Ophthalmology*. Chichester: John Wiley; 1979: 329-331.

220. Uemura Y, Oguchi Y, Katsumi O. Visual developmental delay. Ophthal Paediatr Genet 1981;1:49-58.

221. Unsold R, Hoyt WF. Band atrophy of the optic nerve. The histology of temporal hemianopsia. Arch Ophthalmol 1980;98:1637-1638.

221a. Utinger RD. Melatonin—the hormone of darkness. N Engl J Med 1992;327:1377-1379.

222. Van Buren JM. Transsynaptic retrograde degeneration in the visual system of primates. J Neurol Neurosurg Psychiatry 1963;26:402-409.

223. Van Hof-van Duin J, Mohn G. Visual defects in children after cerebral hypoxia. Behav Brain Res 1984;14:147-155.

224. van Gelder T, Geurs P, Kho GS, et al. Cortical blindness and seizures following cisplatin treatment: both of epileptic origin? Eur J Cancer. 1993; 29A(10):1497-1498. Letter.

225. Vighetto A, Perenin MT. Ataxie optique. Rev Neurol 1981;137:357-372.

226. Vito W, Spear PD, Tong L. How complete is physiological compensation in extrastriate cortex after visual cortex damage in kittens? Exp Brain Res 1992;91:455-466.

227. Weisel TN. The postnatal development of the visual cortex and the influence of environment. Biosci Rep 1982;2:351-377.

228. Weiss AH, Biersdorf WR. Visual sensory disorders in congenital nystagmus. Ophthalmology 1989; 96:517-523.

229. Whiting S, Jan JE, Wong PKH, et al. Permanent cortical visual impairment in children. Dev Med Child Neurol 1985;27:730-739.

230. Yakovlev PI, Lecours A. The myelogenetic cycles of regional maturation of the brain. In: Minkowski A, ed. *Regional Development of Brain in Early Life*. Oxford: Blackwell Scientific; 1967:3.

231. Yamamoto LG, Bart RD Jr. Transient blindness following mild head trauma. Criteria for a benign outcome. Clin Pediatr 1988;27:479-483.

232. Zangemeister WH, Mienberg O, Stark L, et al. Eye head coordination in homonymous hemianopia. J Neurol 1982;226:243-254.

233. Zee DS, Tusa RJ, Herdman SJ. Effects of occipital lobectomy upon eye movements in primates. J Neurophysiol 1987;58:883-907.

234. Zellweger H. The cerebro-hepato-renal (Zellweger) syndrome and other peroxisomal disorders. Dev Med Child Neurol 1987;29:821-829.

235. Zihl J, Von Cramon D. The contribution of the "second" visual system to directed visual attention in man. Brain 1979;102:835-856.

236. Zihl J. "Blindsight": improvement of visually guided eye movements by systematic practice in patients with cerebral blindness. Neuropsychologica 1980;18:71-77.

237. Zung A, Margalith D. Ictal cortical blindness: a case report and review of the literature. Dev Med Child Neurol. 1993;35:921-926.

2

Congenital Optic Disc Anomalies

Introduction

Ophthalmologists and neurologists are frequently called upon to evaluate infants and children with decreased vision resulting from congenital anomalies of the optic disc. A comprehensive evaluation necessitates an understanding of the ophthalmoscopic features, associated neuro-ophthalmologic findings, pathogenesis, and appropriate ancillary studies for each anomaly. Over the past decade, new ocular and systemic associations have emerged, and theories of pathogenesis for many optic disc anomalies have been revised. Our increasing ability to subclassify different forms of excavated optic disc anomalies that were previously lumped together as colobomatous defects has further refined our ability to predict the likelihood of associated central nervous system (CNS) anomalies based solely on the appearance of the optic disc. Added to this has been the widespread clinical application of magnetic resonance (MR) imaging, which has refined our ability to identify subtle associated CNS anomalies and to predict the likelihood of associated neurodevelopmental and endocrinological problems. Based largely upon information that has emerged over the past decade, this chapter will examine the optic disc anomalies, summarize our current understanding of their pathogenesis and treatment, and detail associated neuroimaging findings that predicate the general medical management of affected children.

We have found the following four general concepts particularly useful in evaluating and managing children with congenital optic disc anomalies:

1. Children with bilateral optic disc anomalies generally present in infancy with poor vision and nystagmus; those with unilateral optic disc anomalies generally present during their preschool years with sensory esotropia.

2. CNS malformations are common in patients with malformed optic discs. Small discs are associated with a variety of malformations involving the cerebral hemispheres, pituitary infundibulum, and midline intracranial structures (e.g., septum pellucidum, corpus callosum). Large optic discs of the morning glory configuration are associated with the transsphenoidal form of basal encephalocele, whereas large optic discs with a colobomatous configuration may be associated with systemic anomalies in a variety of coloboma syndromes.[74,148] Magnetic resonance imaging is advisable in all infants with small optic discs (unilateral or bilateral) and in infants with large optic discs (unilateral or bilateral) who have either neurodevelopmental deficits or midfacial anomalies suggestive of basal encephalocele.

3. Color vision is relatively preserved in an eye with a congenitally anomalous optic disc (i.e., limited only by the visual acuity) in contradistinction to the severe dyschromatopsia that characterizes most acquired optic neuropathies.

4. Any structural ocular abnormality that reduces visual acuity in infancy may lead to superimposed amblyopia. A trial of occlusion therapy is therefore warranted in most patients with unilateral optic disc anomalies and decreased

vision. The finding of an afferent pupillary defect should not discourage this effort.[115]

5. The finding of a discrete V- or tongue-shaped zone of infrapapillary retinochoroidal depigmentation in an eye with an anomalous optic disc should prompt a search for a transsphenoidal encephalocele.[27]

Optic Nerve Hypoplasia

Optic nerve hypoplasia is an anomaly that, until recently, escaped the scrutiny of even the most meticulous observers.[22] It was not until the late 1960s that its clinical description became commonplace. Optic nerve hypoplasia is now the most common optic disc anomaly encountered in ophthalmologic practice. The dramatic increase in prevalence of optic nerve hypoplasia primarily reflects its greater recognition by clinicians. Until recently, many cases of optic nerve hypoplasia undoubtedly went unrecognized or were misconstrued as congenital optic atrophy. However, some investigators have argued that drug and alcohol abuse, which have become more widespread in recent years, may also be contributing to the increasing prevalence of optic nerve hypoplasia.[22,116]

Ophthalmoscopically, the hypoplastic disc appears as an abnormally small optic nerve head. It may appear gray or pale in color and is often surrounded by a yellowish mottled peripapillary halo, bordered by a ring of increased or decreased pigmentation ("double-ring" sign, Figure 2.1).[94] The major retinal vessels are often tortuous. Histopathologically, optic nerve hypoplasia is characterized by a subnormal number of optic nerve axons with normal mesodermal elements and glial supporting tissue.[92,136] The double-ring sign has been found histopathologically to consist of a normal junction between the sclera and lamina cribrosa, which corresponds to the outer ring, and an abnormal extension of retina and pigment epithelium over the outer portion of the lamina cribrosa, which corresponds to the inner ring.[92,136] Visual acuity in optic nerve hypoplasia ranges from 20/20 to no light perception, and affected eyes show localized visual field defects, often combined with a generalized constriction of the visual fields.[67] Since visual acuity is determined primarily by the integrity of the papillo-

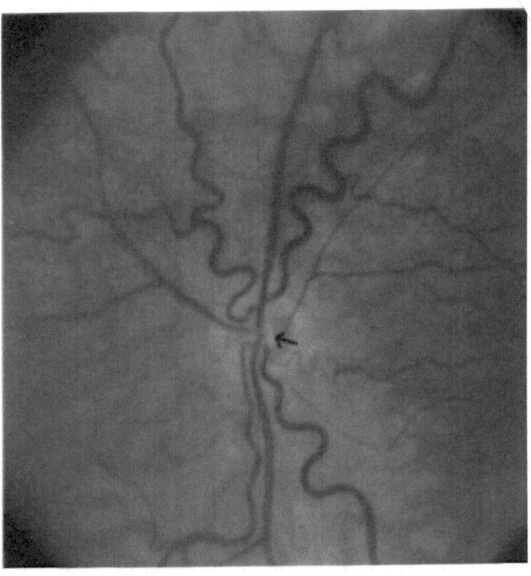

FIGURE 2.1. Optic nerve hypoplasia with double-ring sign. Arrow denotes true margin of the hypoplastic disc. Note associated retinal vascular tortuousity. (Photograph from Brodsky MC, Glasier CM, Pollock SC, et al: Optic nerve hypoplasia: identification by magnetic resonance imaging. Arch Ophthalmol 1990;108:562-567, with permission. Copyright 1990, American Medical Association.)

macular nerve fiber bundle, it does not necessarily correlate with the overall size of the disc. The strong association of astigmatism with optic nerve hypoplasia warrants careful attention to correction of refractive errors.[205]

While moderate or severe optic nerve hypoplasia can be recognized ophthalmoscopically, the diagnosis of mild hypoplasia continues to be problematic in infants and small children whose visual acuity cannot be accurately quantified. Several techniques have been devised to directly measure fundus photographs of the optic disc in an attempt to apply quantitative criteria to the diagnosis of optic nerve hypoplasia.[103] Jonas et al have defined "microdiscs" statistically as the mean disc area minus two standard deviations.[105] In their study of 88 patients, the mean optic disc area measured 2.89 mm^2 and the diagnosis of a microdisc corresponded to a disc area smaller than 1.4 mm^2. Romano has advocated the simple method of directly measuring the optic disc diameter using a hand ruler and a 30° transparency (both under magnification) and has concluded that a horizontal disc diameter of less than 3.4 mm constitutes optic nerve hypoplasia.[156] This quick and simple technique is limited to eyes with minimal spherical refractive error. Zeki et al[206] have found that a disc-to-macula/disc diameter ratio of 2.94 provides a one-tailed upper population limit of 95%, while individuals with optic nerve hypoplasia have a mean ratio of 3.57. Calculation of this ratio has the important advantage of eliminating the magnification effect of high refractive errors (myopic refractive errors can make a hypoplastic disc appear normal in size, whereas hyperopic refractive errors can make a normal disc appear abnormally small). While the Zeki technique is especially useful in patients with high refractive errors, the notion that one can establish an unequivocal dividing line between the normal and hypoplastic disc based strictly upon size is inherently flawed. As discussed later, large optic discs can be axonally deficient,[128,152] and small optic discs do not preclude normal visual function. In evaluating small optic discs, we have grown accustomed to drawing inferences about axon counts based upon size. While it is reasonable to infer that an extremely small disc must be associated with a diminution in axons, the application of this reasoning to mild or borderline cases is limited by additional variables, including the size of the central cup, the percentage of the nerve occupied by axons (as opposed to glial tissue and blood vessels), and the cross-sectional area and density of axons. Furthermore, segmental forms of optic nerve hypoplasia (described later) may affect a sector of the disc without producing a diffuse diminution in size. As such, it would seem prudent to reserve the diagnosis of optic nerve hypoplasia for patients with small optic discs who have reduced vision or visual field loss with corresponding nerve fiber bundle defects.

The use of the term "hypoplasia" to describe a congenitally small, axonally deficient optic nerve may erroneously imply that this abnormality results from a primary failure of optic axons to develop.[95,116,167] The timing of other CNS anomalies, which often coexist with optic nerve hypoplasia, would suggest that many, if not all, cases of optic nerve "hypoplasia" represent an intrauterine degenerative phenomenon rather than a primary failure of axons to develop. In human fetuses, Provis et al[150] found a peak of 3.7 million axons at 16 to 17 weeks of gestation, with a subsequent decline to 1.1 million axons by the 31st gestational week. This massive degeneration of supernumerary axons (termed "apostosis") occurs as part of the normal development of the visual pathways and may serve to establish the correct topography of the visual pathways.[116] Toxins or associated CNS malformations may, in some instances, augment or interfere with the usual processes by which superfluous axons are eliminated from the developing visual pathways.[116]

Optic nerve hypoplasia is often associated with a wide variety of CNS abnormalities. Septo-optic dysplasia (de Morsier syndrome) refers to the constellation of small anterior visual pathways, absence of the septum pellucidum, and thinning or agenesis of the corpus callosum.[50] The clinical association of septo-optic dysplasia and pituitary dwarfism was documented by Hoyt et al in 1970.[96]

MR imaging is currently the optimal noninvasive neuroimaging modality for delineating associated CNS malformations in patients with optic nerve hypoplasia.[21] MR imaging provides high contrast resolution and multiplanar imaging capability, allowing the anterior visual pathways to be visualized as distinct, well-defined structures.[21] In optic nerve hypoplasia, coronal and sagittal T1-weighted MR images consistently demonstrate thinning and attenuation of the corresponding prechiasmatic intracranial optic nerve (Figure 2.2). Coronal T1-weighted MR imaging in bilateral optic nerve hypoplasia shows diffuse thinning of the optic chiasm in bilateral optic nerve hypoplasia (Figure 2.2) and focal thinning or absence of the side of the chiasm corresponding to the hypoplastic nerve in unilateral optic nerve hypoplasia. When MR imaging shows a decrease in intracranial optic nerve size accompanied by other features of septo-optic dysplasia, the presumptive diagnosis of optic nerve hypoplasia can be made neuroradiologically.[21]

Over the past decade, the concept of septo-optic dysplasia as a distinct nosological entity has been called into question, as MR imaging has demonstrated associated structural abnormalities involving the cerebral hemispheres and the pituitary infundibulum.[22,23] Cerebral hemispheric abnor-

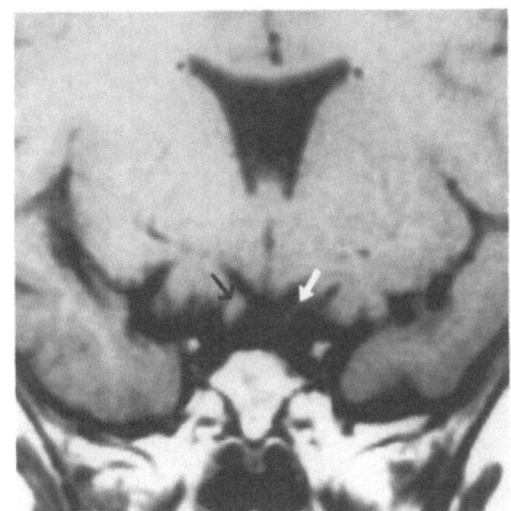
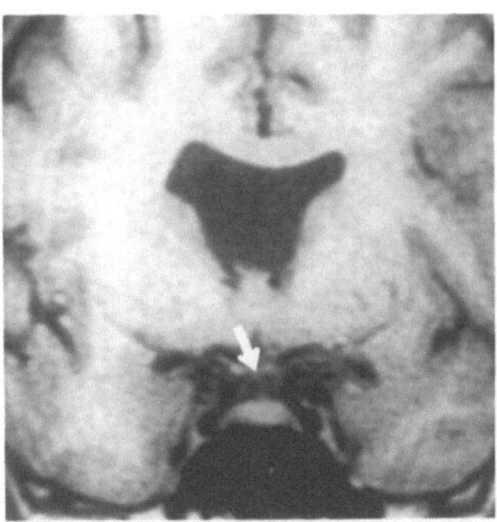

A
B

FIGURE 2.2. Magnetic resonance imaging in optic nerve hypoplasia. (A) T1-weighted coronal MR imaging in a patient with left optic nerve hypoplasia. Black arrow denotes the normal right optic nerve. White arrow denotes the thin, attenuated signal corresponding to the hypoplastic left optic nerve. (From Williams J, Brodsky MC, Griebel M, et al. Septo-optic dysplasia: the clinical insignificance of an absent septum pellucidum. Dev Med Child Neurol 1993;35:490-501, with permission.)

(B) T1-weighted coronal MR imaging demonstrating diffuse thinning of the optic chiasm (arrow) in a patient with absence of the septum pellucidum and bilateral optic nerve hypoplasia. (From Brodsky MC, Glasier CM, Pollock SC, et al. Optic nerve hypoplasia: identification by magnetic resonance imaging. Arch Ophthalmol 1990;108:562-567, with permission. Copyright 1990, American Medical Association.)

malities (Figure 2.3), which are evident on MR imaging in approximately 45% of patients with optic nerve hypoplasia, may consist of hemispheric migration anomalies (e.g., schizencephaly, cortical heterotopia) or intrauterine or perinatal hemispheric injury (e.g., periventricular leukomalacia, encephalomalacia).[23] Evidence of perinatal injury to the pituitary infundibulum (seen on MR imaging as posterior pituitary ectopia) is found in approximately 15% of patients with optic nerve hypoplasia.[23] Normally, the posterior pituitary gland appears bright on T1-weighted images, probably because of the chemical composition of the vesicles contained within it.[23] In posterior pituitary ectopia, MR imaging demonstrates absence of the normal posterior pituitary bright spot, absence of the pituitary infundibulum, and an ectopic posterior pituitary bright spot where the upper infundibulum is normally located (Figure 2.4).[22,23] Posterior pituitary ectopia is thought to result from a perinatal injury to the hypophyseal, portal system that results in necrosis of the infundibulum.[107] In the patient with optic nerve hypoplasia, posterior pituitary ectopia is virtually pathognomonic of

anterior pituitary hormone deficiency, whereas cerebral hemispheric abnormalities are highly predictive of neurodevelopmental deficits.[23] Absence of the septum pellucidum alone does not portend neurodevelopmental deficits or pituitary hormone deficiency.[198] Thinning or agenesis of the corpus callosum is predictive of neurodevelopmental problems only by virtue of its frequent association with cerebral hemispheric abnormalities. The finding of unilateral optic nerve hypoplasia does not preclude coexistent intracranial malformations.[23] Therefore, MR imaging can be used to provide specific prognostic information regarding the likelihood of neurodevelopmental deficits and pituitary hormone deficiency in the infant or young child with unilateral or bilateral optic nerve hypoplasia.[23]

Some forms of optic nerve hypoplasia are segmental. A pathognomonic superior segmental optic hypoplasia with an inferior visual field defect occurs rarely in children of insulin-dependent diabetic mothers (Figure 2.5).[108,138,146,147] Despite the multiple teratologic effects of maternal diabetes early in the first trimester,[89] superior segmental hy-

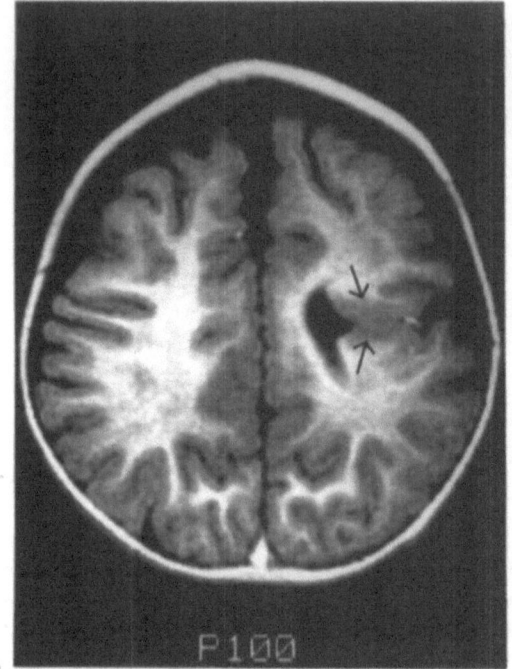

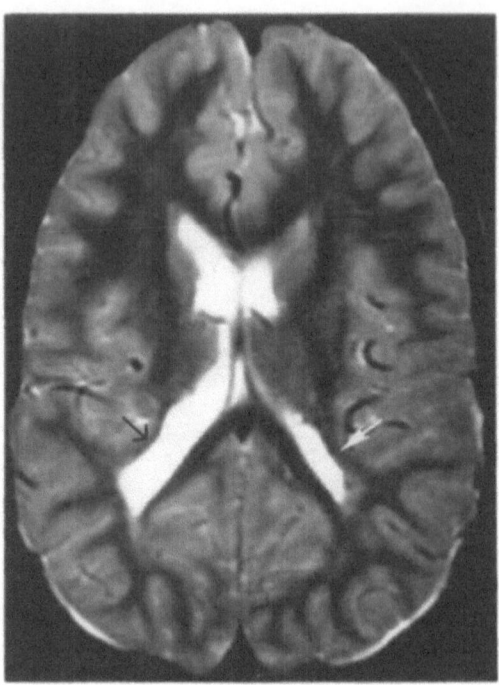

FIGURE 2.3. Cerebral hemispheric abnormalities associated with optic nerve hypoplasia. (A) Axial T1-weighted inversion recovery MR image demonstrating schizencephaly in a patient with optic nerve hypoplasia. The schizencephalic cleft (arrows) consists of an abnormal band of dysmorphic gray matter in the left cerebral hemisphere extending from the cortical surface to the lateral ventricle.(B) T2-weighted axial MR image demonstrating asymmetrical periventricular leukomalacia, worse in the right hemisphere (left side of picture), in a child with optic nerve hypoplasia. Note enlargement and irregular contour of the posterior aspect of the lateral ventricle. The black arrow denotes loss of posterior periventricular white matter with direct apposition of cortical gray matter to the trigone of the lateral ventricle. The white arrow indicates greater volume of posterior periventricular white matter in the left hemisphere. (From Brodsky MC, Glasier CM. Optic nerve hypoplasia: clinical significance of associated central nervous system abnormalities on magnetic resonance imaging. Arch Ophthalmol 1993;111:66-74, with permission. Copyright 1993, American Medical Association.)

poplasia is usually diagnosed in patients with no other systemic anomalies.[24] Kim et al have noted that the inferior visual field defects in superior segmental optic hypoplasia differ from typical nerve fiber bundle defects and questioned whether a regional impairment in retinal development could play a role in the pathogenesis.[108] The teratologic mechanism by which insulin-dependent diabetes mellitus selectively interferes with the early gestational development of superior retinal ganglion cells or their axons remains elusive.[24]

Congenital lesions involving the retina, optic nerve, chiasm, tract, or retrogeniculate pathways are associated with segmental hypoplasia of the corresponding portions of each optic nerve (Figure 2.6).[131,139] Hoyt et al coined the term "homo-nymous hemioptic hypoplasia" to describe the asymmetrical form of segmental optic nerve hypoplasia seen in patients with unilateral congenital hemispheric lesions involving the postchiasmal afferent visual pathways.[97] In this setting, the nasal and temporal aspects of the optic disc contralateral to the hemispheric lesion show segmental hypoplasia and loss of the corresponding nerve fiber layers (Figure 2.6 (B)). This may be accompanied by a central band of horizontal pallor across the disc. The ipsilateral optic disc may range from normal in size to frankly hypoplastic.[139] Homonymous hemioptic hypoplasia in retrogeniculate lesions results from transsynaptic degeneration of the optic tract that is usually seen in the setting of a congenital hemispheric lesion.[97,98,139]

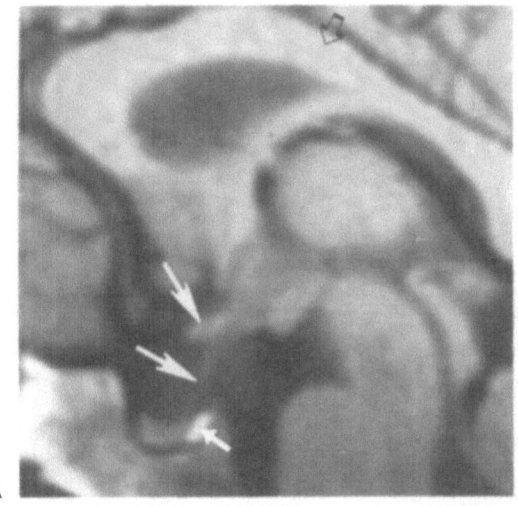 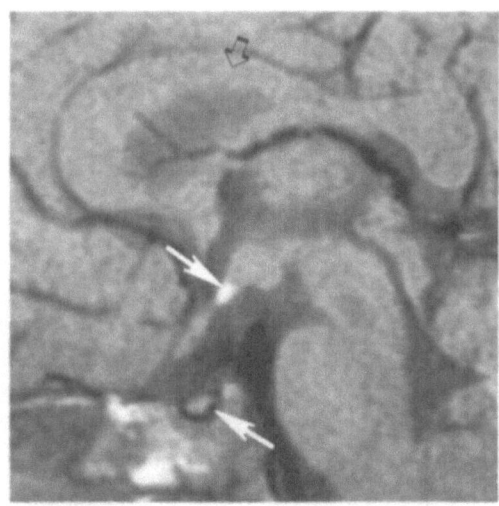

FIGURE 2.4. Posterior pituitary ectopia. (A) T1-weighted sagittal MR image demonstrating the normal hyperintense signal of posterior pituitary gland (lower black arrow), normal pituitary infundibulum (lower white arrow), optic chiasm (upper right arrow). Open arrow denotes the normal corpus callosum. (B) T1-weighted sagittal MR image demonstrating posterior pituitary ectopia (upper white arrow) which appears as an abnormal focal area of increased signal intensity at the tuber cinereum. Note absence of the pituitary infundibulum and absence of the normal posterior pituitary bright spot (lower arrow). Upper white arrow denotes optic chiasm. This child had a normal septum pellucidum and corpus callosum (open arrow). (From Brodsky MC, Glasier CM. Optic nerve hypoplasia: clinical significance of associated central nervous system abnormalities on magnetic resonance imaging. Arch Ophthalmol 1993;111:66-74, with permission. Copyright 1993, American Medical Association.)

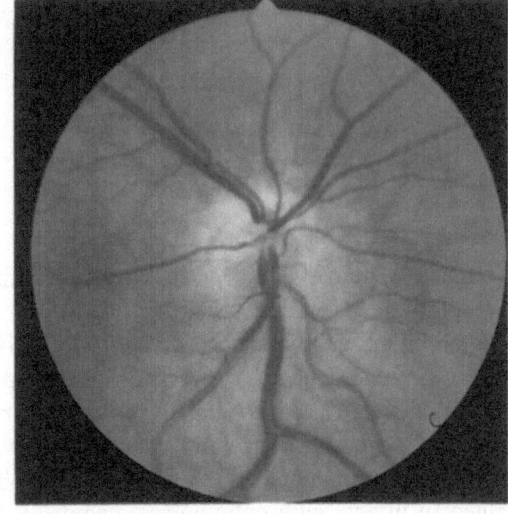 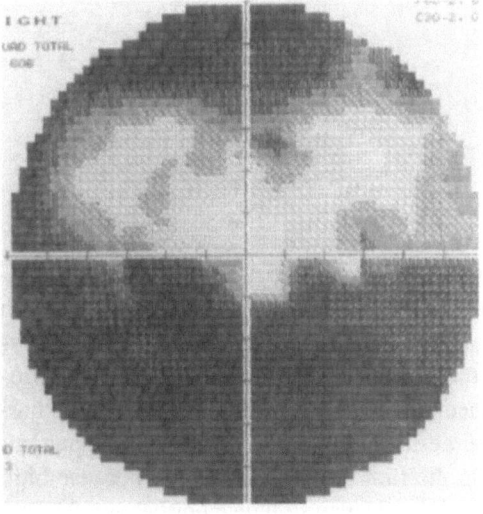

FIGURE 2.5. Superior segmental optic hypoplasia. (A) Right optic disc demonstrating an abnormal superior entrance of the central retinal artery, relative pallor of the superior disk, and a superior peripapillary halo. The superior nerve fiber layer is absent while the inferior nerve fiber layer is clearly seen. (B) Corresponding Humphrey 60-2 visual field demonstrating a nonaltitudinal inferior defect with mild superior constriction. (From Brodsky MC, Schroeder GT, Ford R. Superior segmental hypoplasia in identical twins. J Clin Neuro-ophthalmol 1993;13:152-154, with permission.)

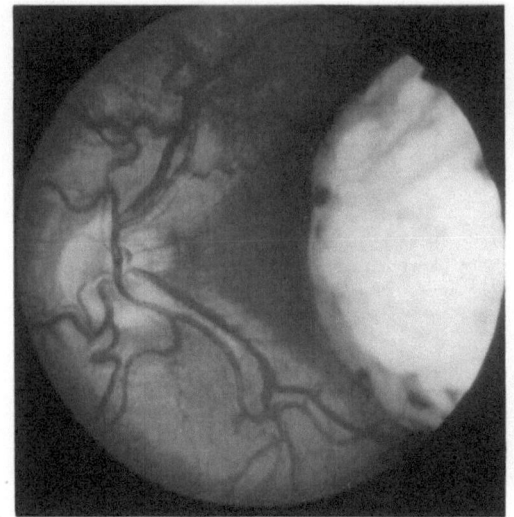
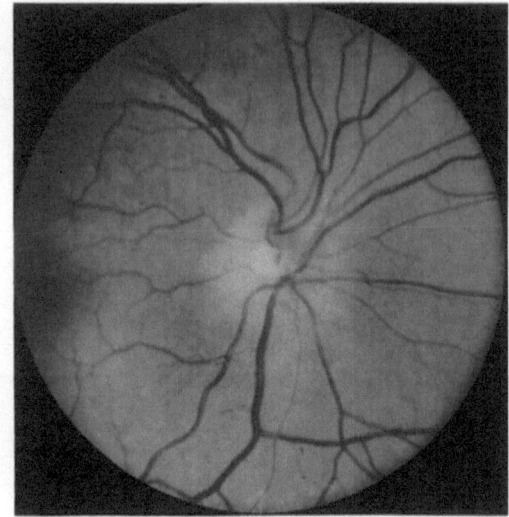

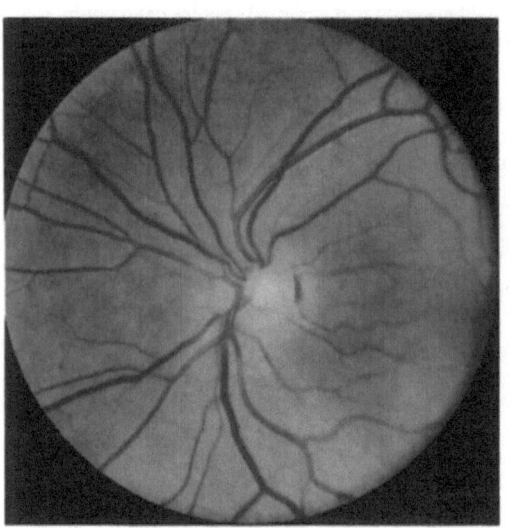

FIGURE 2.6. Segmental optic nerve hypoplasia. (A) Segmental hypoplasia of the temporal optic disc with focal absence of the temporal nerve fiber layer in a patient with a "macular coloboma." (B) and (C) Homonymous hemioptic hypoplasia in a patient with a right occipital porencephalic cyst. Both optic discs are hypoplastic. The left optic disc (C) shows a relative loss of disc substance and peripapillary nerve fiber layer nasally and temporally. (From Novakovic P, Taylor DSI, Hoyt WF. Localizing patterns of optic nerve hypoplasia-retina to occipital lobe. Br J Ophthalmol 1988;72:176-182, with permission. Published by BMJ Publishing Group. Photographs courtesy of William F. Hoyt, MD.)

Growth hormone deficiency is the most common endocrinologic abnormality associated with optic nerve hypoplasia. Hypothyroidism, panhypopituitarism, diabetes insipidus, and hyperprolactinemia may also occur.[6,94,101,130] Growth hormone deficiency may be clinically inapparent within the first 3 to 4 years of life because high prolactin levels may stimulate normal growth over this period.[46] Puberty may be precocious or delayed in children with hypopituitarism.[81] Sherlock and McNicol have noted that subclinical hypopituitarism can manifest as acute adrenal insufficiency following general anesthesia and suggested that it may be prudent to empirically treat children

who have optic nerve hypoplasia with perioperative intravenous corticosteroids.[164]

In an infant with optic nerve hypoplasia, a history of neonatal jaundice suggests congenital hypothyroidism, while neonatal hypoglycemia or seizures suggests congenital panhypopituitarism.[116] A serum thyroxine level can be easily obtained in infants with optic nerve hypoplasia to rule out neonatal hypothyroidism. Because of inherent difficulties in measuring normal physiologic growth hormone levels, which vary widely over a 24-hour period, most patients with optic nerve hypoplasia are followed clinically and only investigated biochemically if growth is subnormal. However, when MR imaging shows posterior pituitary ectopia, or when a clinical history of neonatal jaundice or neonatal hypoglycemia is obtained, anterior pituitary hormone deficiency is probable, and more extensive endocrinologic testing becomes mandatory.[22]

Early investigators understandably attributed optic nerve hypoplasia to a primary failure of retinal ganglion cell differentiation at the 13- to 15-mm stage of embryonic life (four to six weeks of gestation).[162] This hypothesis, however, fails to account for the frequent coexistence of multiple CNS abnormalities with optic nerve hypoplasia.[167] With the advent of high-resolution noninvasive neuroimaging, it is now recognized that gestational CNS injury can disrupt optic nerve development by both direct and indirect mechanisms.[22,23,139,167] For example, Taylor has documented optic nerve hypoplasia in patients with congenital suprasellar lesions, suggesting that the space-occupying effects of a prenatal suprasellar tumor can directly interfere with the normal migration of optic axons to their target sites.[184] Similarly, Skarf and Hoyt hypothesized that, in patients who fit the traditional diagnosis of septo-optic dysplasia, early gestational injuries to midline CNS structures (e.g, septum pellucidum, pituitary infundibulum) may either directly injure adjacent optic axons or secondarily disrupt their migration.[167] The frequent association of cerebral hemispheric anomalies with optic nerve hypoplasia is believed to result from disruption of normal neuronal guidance mechanisms involved in the migration of both hemispheric neurons and optic axons in utero, preventing them from forming appropriate connections at their target sites.[9,23,83,95] As previously mentioned, prenatal hemispheric injuries or malformations that directly involve the optic tracts or radiations can lead to direct or transsynaptic retrograde degeneration and segmental hypoplasia of both optic nerves.[23,97,139,153]

Systemic and teratogenic associations with optic nerve hypoplasia are summarized in Table 2.1.

Excavated Optic Disc Anomalies

Optic disc coloboma, the morning glory disc anomaly, and peripapillary staphyloma are examples of excavated anomalies involving the optic

TABLE 2.1. Systemic and teratogenic associations with optic nerve hypoplasia. (Modified from Zeki and Dutton.[207])

Systemic associations	Teratogenic agents
Albinism	Dilantin
Aniridia	Quinine
Duane syndrome	PCP
Median facial cleft syndrome	LSD
Klippel–Trenauney–Weber syndrome	Alcohol
Goldenhar syndrome	Maternal diabetes
Linear sebaceous nevus syndrome	
Meckel syndrome	
Hemifacial atrophy	
Blepharophimosis	
Osteogenesis imperfecta	
Chondrodysplasia punctata	
Aicardi syndrome	
Apert syndrome	
Trisomy 18	
Potter syndrome	
Chromosome 13q⁻	
Neonatal isoimmune thrombocytopenia	
Fetal alcohol syndrome	
Dandy–Walker syndrome	
Delleman syndrome	

disc. In the latter two conditions, an excavation of the posterior globe surrounds and incorporates the optic disc. In an elegant review article, Pollock has detailed the clinical features that distinguish the excavated optic disc anomalies.[149] He points out that the terms morning glory disc, optic disc coloboma, and peripapillary staphyloma are often transposed in the literature, which has propagated tremendous confusion regarding their diagnostic criteria, associated systemic findings, and pathogenesis. From his analysis, it is clear that optic disc colobomas, morning glory optic discs, and peripapillary staphylomas are distinct anomalies, each with its own specific embryological origin, and not simply clinical variants along a broad phenotypic spectrum.

Morning Glory Disc Anomaly

The morning glory disc anomaly is a congenital, funnel-shaped excavation of the posterior fundus that incorporates the optic disc.[149] It was so named by Kindler in 1970 because of its resemblance to the morning glory flower.[109] Ophthalmoscopically, the disc is markedly enlarged, it is orange or pink in color, and it may appear to be recessed or elevated centrally within the confines of a funnel-shaped peripapillary excavation (Figure 2.7).[105] A wide annulus of chorioretinal pigmentary disturbance surrounds the disc within the excavation.[149] A white tuft of glial tissue overlies the central portion of the disc. The blood vessels appear increased in number and often arise from the periphery of the disc.[149] They often curve abruptly as they emanate from the disc and then run an abnormally straight course over the peripapillary retina. It is often difficult to distinguish arterioles from venules. Close inspection occasionally reveals the presence of small peripapillary artenovenous communications.[26a] The macula may be incorporated into the excavation (macular capture, Figure 2.7).[14,149] Computed tomography (CT) scanning shows a funnel-shaped enlargement of the distal optic nerve at its junction with the globe (Figure 2.8).[125,188]

The morning glory disc anomaly usually occurs as a unilateral condition, but several bilateral cases have been reported.[14,149] Visual acuity usually ranges from 20/200 to finger counting in the morning glory disc anomaly, but cases with 20/20 vision as well as no light perception have been reported. As in all congenital optic disc anomalies, functional amblyopia may contribute to visual loss in unilateral cases, and a trial of occlusion therapy is warranted in infants and small children.[115] Unlike optic disc colobomas that have no racial or gender predilection, morning glory discs are conspicuously more common in females and rare in blacks.[78,149,175] With rare exceptions,[140] the morning glory disc anomaly does not present as part of a multisystem genetic disorder.[149]

The association of morning glory disc anomaly with the transsphenoidal form of basal encephalocele is well established.[14,35,74,91,110,148,188] Transsphenoidal encephalocele is a rare midline congenital malformation in which a meningeal pouch, often containing the chiasm and adjacent hypothalamus, protrudes inferiorly through a large, round defect in the sphenoid bone (Figure 2.9). Children with this occult basal meningocele have a wide head, a flat nose, mild hypertelorism, a midline notch in the upper lip, and sometimes a midline cleft in the soft palate (Figure 2.10). The meningocele protrudes into the nasopharynx, where it may obstruct the airway. Symptoms of transsphenoidal encephalocele in infancy may include rhin-

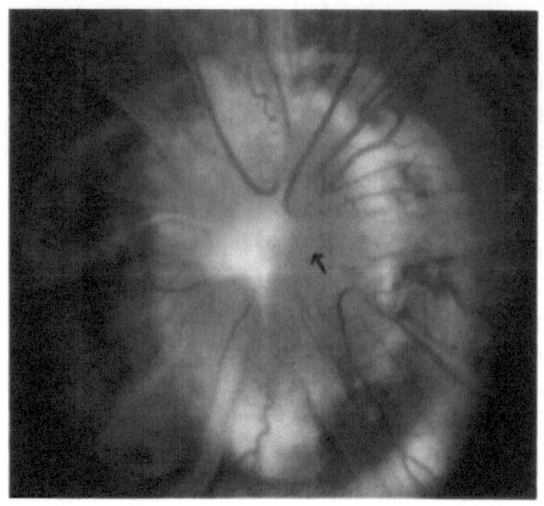

FIGURE 2.7. Morning glory optic disc. A large optic disc is surrounded by an annular zone of pigmentary disturbance. The retinal vessels appear increased in number as they emerge from the disc and have an abnormally straight, radial configuration. There is radial folding of the peripapillary retina. Arrow denotes focal yellowish discoloration that corresponds to macula lutea pigment (macular capture). (From Goldhammer Y, Smith JL. Optic nerve anomalies in basal encephalocoele. Arch Ophthalmol 1975;93:115-118, with permission. Copyright 1975, American Medical Association. Photograph courtesy of Stephen C. Pollock, MD.)

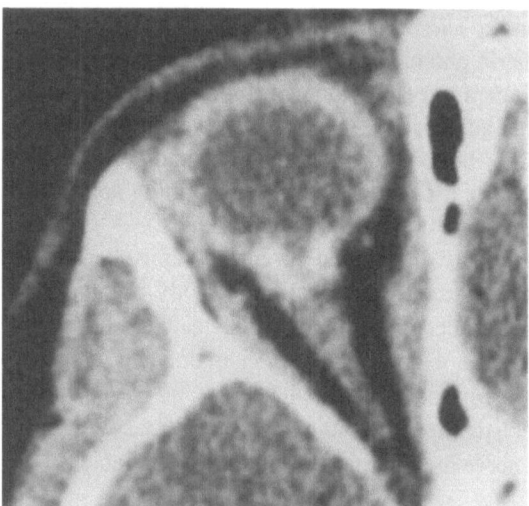

FIGURE 2.8. CT scan of morning glory disc anomaly. Note calcified, funnel-shaped enlargement of the distal optic nerve at its junction with the globe. (From Brodsky MC. Congenital optic disk anomalies. Surv Ophthalmol 1994;39:89–112, with permission.)

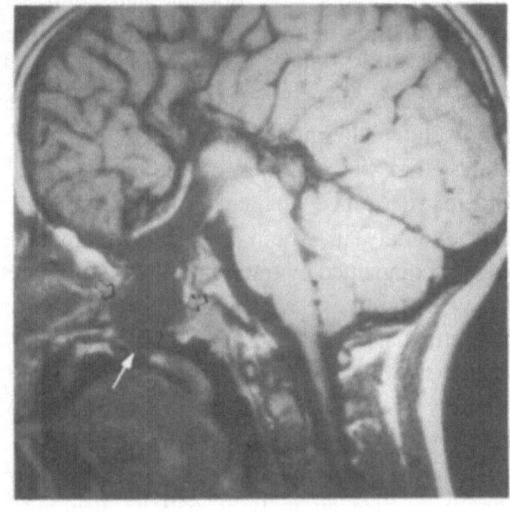 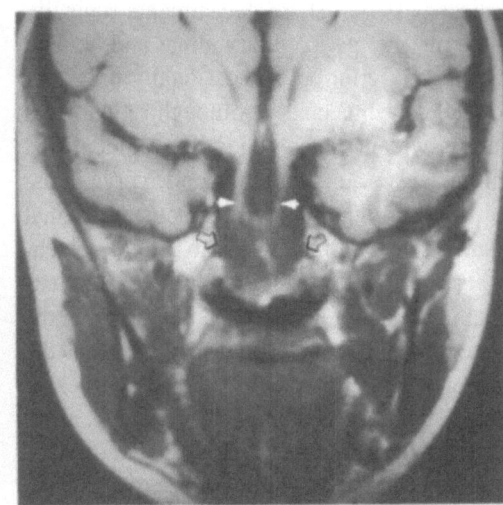

A   B

FIGURE 2.9. Transsphenoidal encephalocele. (A) T1-weighted sagittal MR image shows an encephalocele (delimited by open arrows) extending down through the sphenoid bone into the nasopharynx with impression on the hard palate (white arrow). (B) T1-weighted coronal MR image shows the third ventricle and hypothalamus (white arrowheads) extending inferiorly into the encephalocoele (delimited inferiorly by open arrows). (From Barkovich AJ. *Pediatric Neuroimaging*. New York, NY: Raven Press; 1990;1:89 with permission. Photographs courtesy of A. James Barkovich, MD.)

orrhea, nasal obstruction, mouth breathing, or snoring.[52,148,203] These symptoms may be overlooked unless the associated morning glory disc anomaly or the characteristic facial configuration is recognized. A transsphenoidal encephalocele may appear clinically as a pulsatile posterior nasal mass or as a "nasal polyp" high in the nose; surgical biopsy or excision can have lethal consequences.[148] Associated brain malformation include agenesis of the corpus callosum and posterior dilatation of the lateral ventricles. Absence of the chiasm is seen in approximately one-third of patients at surgery or autopsy. Most of the affected children have no overt intellectual or neurological deficits, but panhypopituitarism is common.[52,148] Surgery for transsphenoidal encephalocele is considered by many authorities to be contraindicated, since herniated brain tissue may include vital structures, such as the hypothalamic-pituitary system, optic nerves and chiasm, and anterior cerebral arteries, and because of the high postoperative mortality reported, particularly in infants.

Patients with morning glory disc anomaly are also at increased risk for acquired visual loss. Serous retinal detachments have been estimated to occur in 26% to 38% of eyes with morning glory

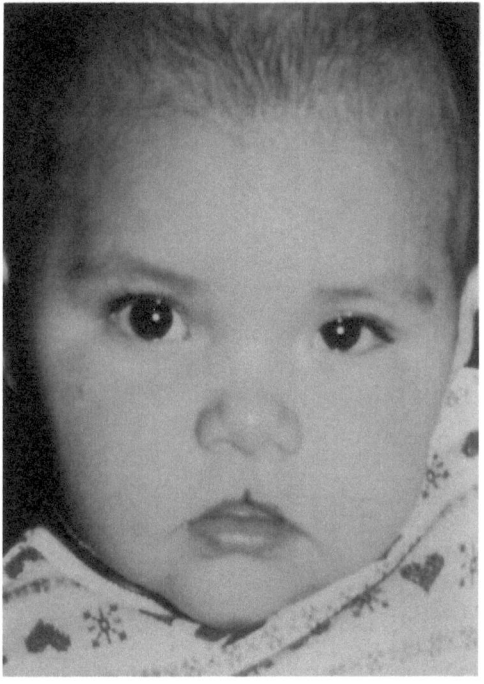

FIGURE 2.10. Infant with transsphenoidal encephalocele. Note hypertelorism, depressed nasal bridge, and mid–upper–lip defect. (Photograph courtesy of Thomas P. Naidich, MD.)

optic discs.[78,175,183] These detachments typically originate in the peripapillary area and extend through the posterior pole, occasionally progressing to total detachments.[192] Although retinal tears are rarely evident, three reports have identified small retinal tears adjacent to the optic nerve in patients with morning glory disc–associated retinal detachments.[3,82,192] In addition to retinal detachments, careful fundus examination reveals nonattachment and radial folding of the retina within the excavated zone in a substantial percentage of the remaining cases (Figure 2.7).[149] The sources of subretinal fluid may be multiple.[100] Irvine et al reported a patient with a morning glory disc–associated retinal detachment who was treated with optic nerve fenestration followed by gas injection into the vitreous cavity.[100] Following the procedure, gas was seen to bubble out through the dural window, demonstrating an interconnection between the vitreous cavity and the subarachnoid space through the anomalous disc. Chang et al also reported resolution of a morning glory–associated serous retinal detachment following optic nerve sheath fenestration.[39] Spontaneous resolution of morning glory–associated retinal detachments have also been reported.[78]

Several authors have documented contractile movements in a morning glory optic disc (Figure 2.11).[149,181,193] Pollock attributed the contractile movements in his case to fluctuations in subretinal fluid volume altering the degree of retinal separation within the confines of the excavation.[149] Graether described a patient with a morning glory disc anomaly in whom episodes of amaurosis were accompanied by transient dilation of the retinal veins in an eye with a morning glory disc.[76] Subretinal neovascularization may occasionally develop within the circumferential zone of pigmentary disturbance adjacent to a morning glory disc.[48,172]

The embryological defect leading to the morning glory disc anomaly is widely disputed.[188] Histopathological reports have unfortunately lacked clinical confirmation,[43,129,145,151] although Cogan detailed a case in which the gross morphological appearance was highly suggestive of this anomaly.[43] Some authors have hypothesized that the morning glory disc anomaly results from defective closure of the embryonic fissure and is but one phenotypic form of a colobomatous (i.e., embryonic fissure-related) defect.[69,125] Others have interpreted the clinical findings of a central glial

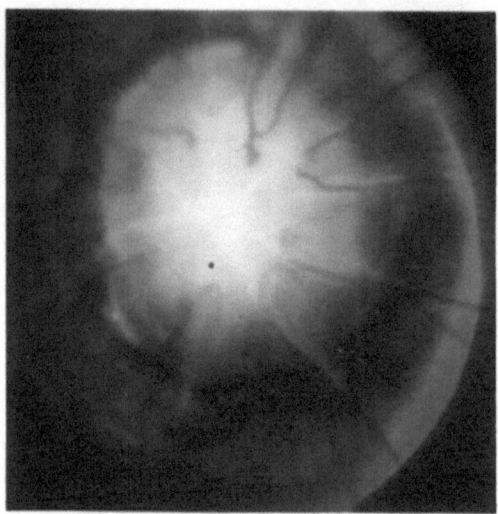 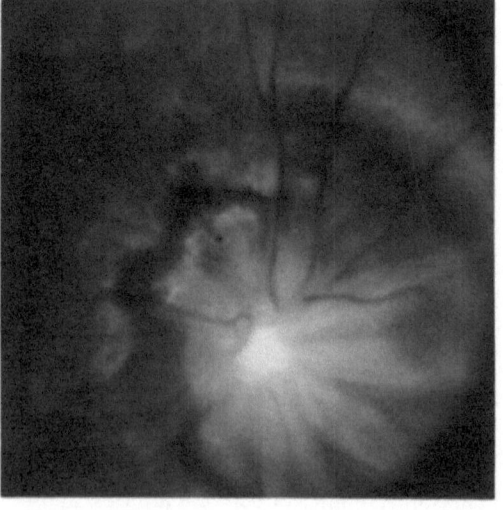

A   B

FIGURE 2.11. Contractile morning glory optic disc. (A) Morning glory disc prior to contraction. Note minor retinal elevation with radial folding of the peripapillary retina. (B) Same morning glory disc during contraction. There is now greater elevation of the retina and encroachment of the peripapillary retinal folds upon the central glial tuft. (From Pollock S. The morning glory disc anomaly: contractile movement, classification, and embryogenesis. Doc Ophthalmol 1987;65:439-460. Reprinted by permission of Kluwer Academic Publishers. Photograph courtesy of Stephen C. Pollock, MD.)

tuft, vascular anomalies, and a scleral defect, together with the histological findings of adipose tissue and smooth muscle within the peripapillary sclera in presumed cases of the morning glory disc, to signify a primary mesenchymal abnormality and have suggested that the associated midfacial anomalies in some patients further support the concept of a primary mesenchymal defect, since most of the cranial structures are derived from mesenchyme.[188] Dempster has attempted to reconcile these two views by proposing that the basic defect is mesodermal but that some clinical features of the defect may result from a dynamic disturbance between the relative growth of mesoderm and ectoderm.[51,188]

Pollock has argued that the fundamental symmetry of the fundus excavation with respect to the disc implicates an anomalous funnel-shaped enlargement of the distal optic stalk at its junction with the primitive optic vesicle, as the primary embryological defect.[149] In this setting, invagination of the optic vesicle proceeds normally, leading to formation of an embryonic fissure, which extends from the newly formed optic cup into the expanded distal optic stalk. Complete closure of the embryonic fissure follows, but because of the increased dimensions of the distal optic stalk, the process of normal closure fails to obliterate the space within the dysgenetic distal stalk, resulting in a persistent excavated defect at the site of entry of the optic nerve into the eye. According to this hypothesis, the glial and vascular abnormalities that characterize the morning glory disc anomaly would be explainable as the secondary effects of a primary neuroectodermal dysgenesis on the formation of mesodermal elements that arise later in embryogenesis.[149]

Optic Disc Coloboma

The term coloboma, of Greek derivation, means curtailed or mutilated.[127,143] It is used only with reference to the eye. Colobomas of the optic disc result from incomplete or abnormal coaptation of the proximal end of the embryonic fissure. In optic disc coloboma, a sharply delimited, glistening white, bowl-shaped excavation occupies an enlarged optic disc (Figure 2.12). The excavation is decentered inferiorly, reflecting the position of the embryonic fissure relative to the primitive epithe

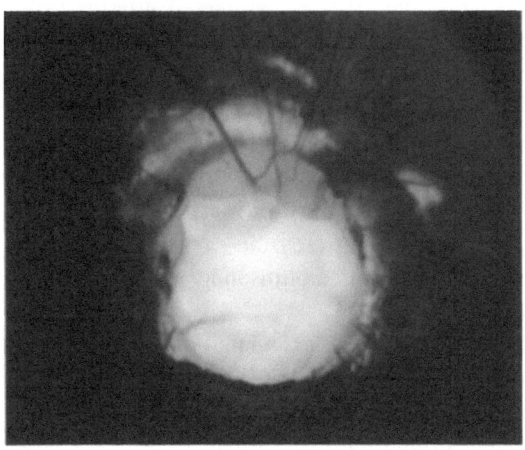

FIGURE 2.12. Optic disc coloboma. The disc is enlarged. A deep white excavation occupies most of the disc but spares its superior aspect. Note chronic serous retinal elevation (seen best at 11 o'clock) that has caused subretinal fibrosis. Otherwise, there is minimal peripapillary pigment disturbance (in contrast to the morning glory disc anomaly). (From Brodsky MC, Congenital optic disk anomalies. Surv Ophthalmol 1994; 39:89–112, with permission.)

lial papilla.[149] The inferior neuroretinal rim is thin or absent while the superior neuroretinal rim is relatively spared. Rarely, the entire disc may appear excavated; however, the colobomatous nature of the defect can still be appreciated ophthalmoscopically since the excavation is deeper inferiorly.[149] The defect may extend further inferiorly to involve the adjacent choroid and retina, in which case microphthalmia is frequently present.[64] Iris and ciliary colobomas often coexist. Axial CT scanning shows a craterlike excavation of the posterior globe at its junction with the optic nerve.[69,125]

Visual acuity, which depends primarily upon the integrity of the papillomacular bundle, may be mildly to severely decreased and is difficult to predict from the appearance of the disc. Unlike the morning glory disc anomaly, which is usually unilateral, optic disc colobomas occur unilaterally or bilaterally with approximately equal frequency.[149] As with uveal colobomas, optic disc colobomas may arise sporadically or be inherited in an autosomal dominant fashion. Ocular colobomas may also be accompanied by multiple systemic abnormalities in myriad conditions including the CHARGE association,[40,144,155,159] Walker–Warburg syndrome,[143] Goltz focal dermal hypoplasia,[143,185] Aicardi syndrome,[36,93] Goldenhar sequence,[119,195] and linear sebaceous nevus syndrome.[143,185] Rarely, large orbital cysts can occur in conjunction with atypical excavations of the disc, which are probably colobomatous in nature.[34,169,197] A communication between the excavation and the cyst was documented ultrasonographically in one case.[169]

Histopathological examination in optic disc coloboma has demonstrated the presence of intrascleral smooth muscle strands oriented concentrically around the distal optic nerve.[61,200] Presumably, this pathological finding accounts for the contractility of the optic disc seen in rare cases of optic disc coloboma.[62]

Eyes with isolated optic disc colobomas are prone to develop serous macular detachments (Figure 2.12) (in contrast to the rhegmatogenous retinal detachments that complicate retinochoroidal colobomas).[120,161] In a clinicopathologic study of an optic disc coloboma and associated macular detachment in a rhesus monkey, Lin et al noted disruption of the intermediary tissue of Kuhnt with diffusion of retrobulbar fluid from the orbit into the subretinal space.[120] A variety of treatment modalities have been applied to the associated sensory retinal detachments including patches, bedrest, corticosteroids, vitrectomy, scleral buckling procedures, gas-fluid exchange, and photocoagulation.[17,161] Schatz and McDonald have advocated waiting 3 months before treating coloboma-associated macular detachments since spontaneous reattachment may occur.[17,161]

Unfortunately, many uncategorizable dysplastic optic discs are indiscriminantly labeled as optic disc colobomas. This practice continues to complicate the nosology of coloboma-associated genetic disorders. It is therefore crucial that the diagnosis of optic disc coloboma be reserved for discs

that show an inferiorly decentered, white-colored excavation with minimal peripapillary pigmentary changes. For example, the purported association between optic disc coloboma and basal encephalocele[118,148,178] is deeply entrenched in the literature; however, a critical review reveals only two photographically documented cases.[45,178] In striking contrast to the numerous well-documented reports of morning glory optic discs occurring in conjunction with basal encephaloceles, cases of optic disc coloboma with basal encephalocele are conspicuous by their absence.

In the early 1900s, von Szily, in his monumental study of colobomas, stated "with certainty" that "all the true morphological malformations of the optic disc, including true colobomas . . . are only different manifestations of the same developmental anomaly, namely, a different form and degree of malformation of the primitive or epithelial optic papilla."[74,194] Despite the multiple ophthalmoscopic findings that distinguish optic disc coloboma from the morning glory disc anomaly (Table 2.2), many authors still consider these two anomalies as merely different phenotypic expressions of the same embryological defect, namely, failure of closure of the superior aspect of the embryonic fissure.[29,74,125,154,157,160] Savell and Cook's widely quoted report of a family with optic disc colobomas, some of whom had tan or glial tissue within the excavation, is frequently invoked to support the position that the morning glory optic disc anomaly may actually be a colobomatous defect.[160] Although the phenotypic profiles of optic disc coloboma and the morning glory disc anomaly may occasionally overlap, the ophthalmoscopic features of optic disc coloboma (Table 2.2) are most consistent with a primary structural dysgenesis involving the proximal embryonic fissure, as opposed to an anomalous dilatation confined to the distal optic stalk in the morning glory disc anomaly.[149] The profound differences in as-

TABLE 2.2. Ophthalmoscopic findings that distinguish the morning glory disc anomaly from optic disc coloboma.[149]

Morning glory disc anomaly	Optic disc coloboma
Optic disc lies within the excavation	Excavation lies within the optic disc
Symmetrical defect (disc lies *centrally* within the excavation)	Asymmetrical defect (excavation lies *inferiorly* within the disc)
Central glial tuft	No central glial tuft
Severe peripapillary pigmentary disturbance	Minimal peripapillary pigmentary disturbance
Anomalous retinal vasculature	Normal retinal vasculature

TABLE 2.3. Associated ocular and systemic findings that distinguish isolated optic disc coloboma from the morning glory disc anomaly.[149]

Morning glory disc anomaly	Optic disc coloboma
More common in females, rare in blacks	No sex or racial predilection
Rarely familial	Often familial
Rarely bilateral	Often bilateral
No iris, ciliary, or retinal colobomas	Iris, ciliary, and retinal colobomas common
Rarely associated with multisystem genetic disorders	Often associated with multisystem genetic disorders
Basal encephalocele common	Basal encephalocele rare

sociated ocular and systemic findings between the two anomalies (Table 2.3) lend further credence to this hypothesis.[26] As previously mentioned, anomalous optic discs with overlapping features of the morning glory disc anomaly and optic disc coloboma are occasionally seen.[157,160] These "hybrid" anomalies could easily represent instances of early embryonic injury involving both the proximal embryonic fissure and the distal optic stalk. Their existence should not obscure the fact that colobomatous and morning glory optic discs appear as clinically distinct anomalies in the great majority of cases. The concept of "an optic disc coloboma with a morning glory configuration" should be abandoned.

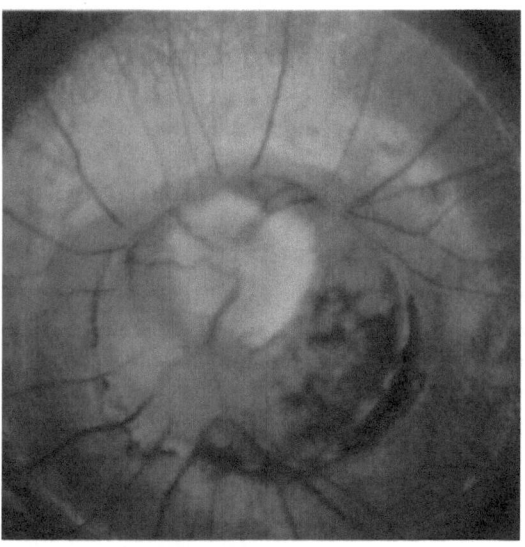

FIGURE 2.13. Peripapillary staphyloma. A relatively normal disc is seen within the recess of a deep peripapillary excavation. The normal optic disc appearance, absence of vascular anomalies, absence of a central glial tuft, and depth of the lesion distinguish this condition from the morning glory optic disc. (From Apple DJ, Raab MF, Walsh PJ. Congenital anomalies of the optic disc. Surv Ophthalmol 1982;27:3-41, with permission.)

Peripapillary Staphyloma

Peripapillary staphyloma is an extremely rare, usually unilateral anomaly, in which a deep fundus excavation surrounds the optic disc.[29,166] In this condition, the disc is seen at the bottom of the excavated defect and may appear normal or shows temporal pallor (Figure 2.13).[149,201] The walls and margin of the defect may show atrophic pigmentary changes in the retinal pigment epithelium (RPE) and choroid.[201] Unlike the morning glory disc anomaly, there is no central glial tuft overlying the disc, and the retinal vascular pattern remains normal, apart from reflecting the essential contour of the lesion.[149] The staphylomatous excavation in peripapillary staphyloma is also notably deeper than that seen in the morning glory disc anomaly. Several cases of contractile peripapillary staphyloma have been documented.[37,111,112,201] Seybold and Rosen described a patient who had transient visual obscurations in an eye with an atypical peripapillary staphyloma.[163]

Visual acuity is usually markedly reduced, but cases with nearly normal acuity have also been reported.[33] Affected eyes are usually emmetropic or slightly myopic.[29] Eyes with decreased vision frequently have centrocecal scotomas.[29] Although peripapillary staphyloma is clinically and embryologically distinct from morning glory optic disc, these conditions are frequently transposed in the literature.[53,76,181] Table 2.4 contrasts the ophthalmoscopic features that distinguish these two anomalies.

The relatively normal appearance of the optic disc and retinal vessels in peripapillary staphyloma suggest that the development of these structures is

TABLE 2.4. Ophthalmoscopic findings that distinguish peripapillary staphyloma from morning glory disc anomaly.[149]

Peripapillary staphyloma	Morning glory disc anomaly
Deep, cup-shaped excavation	Less depth, funnel-shaped excavation
Relatively normal, well-defined optic disc	Grossly anomalous, poorly defined optic disc
Absence of glial and vascular anomalies	Central glial bouquet, anomalous vascular pattern

complete prior to the onset of the staphylomatous process.[149] Pollock has argued that the clinical features of peripapillary staphyloma are most consistent with diminished peripapillary structural support, perhaps resulting from incomplete differentiation of sclera from posterior neural crest cells in the fifth month of gestation. Staphyloma formation presumably occurs when establishment of normal intraocular pressure leads to herniation of unsupported ocular tissues through the defect.[149] Thus, peripapillary staphyloma and the morning glory disc anomaly appear to be pathogenetically distinct both in the timing of the insult (five months gestation versus four weeks gestation) as well as the embryological site of structural dysgenesis (posterior sclera versus distal optic stalk) (Figure 2.13).

Miscellaneous Anomalies

Megalopapilla

Franceschetti and Bock originally assigned the term megalopapilla to a patient who had enlarged optic discs with no other morphological abnormalities.[63] Since that time, megalopapilla has become a generic term that connotes an abnormally large optic disc that lacks the inferior excavation of optic disc coloboma or the numerous anomalous features of the morning glory disc anomaly. In its current usage, megalopapilla comprises two phenotypic variants. The first is a relatively common variant in which an abnormally large optic disc (greater than 2.1 mm in diameter) retains an otherwise normal configuration.[29,63] This form of megalopapilla is usually bilateral and often associated with a large cup-to-disc ratio, which almost invariably raises the diagnostic consideration of normal-tension glaucoma (Figure 2.14 (A)).[134] However, the optic cup is usually round or horizontally oval with no vertical notching or encroachment, so that the quotient of horizontal to vertical cup-to-disc ratio remains normal, in contradistinction to the decreased quotient that characterizes glaucomatous optic atro-

phy.[104] Because the axons are spread over a larger surface area, the neuroretinal rim may also appear pale, mimicking optic atrophy.[32] Less commonly, a unilateral form of megalopapilla is seen in which the normal optic cup is replaced by a grossly anomalous noninferior excavation that obliterates the adjacent neuroretinal rim (Figure 2.14 (B)). The inclusion of this rare variant under the rubric of megalopapilla serves the nosologically useful function of distinguishing it from a colobomatous defect with its attendant systemic implications. Cilioretinal arteries are more common in megalopapilla.[104] A high prevalence of megalopapilla has been observed in natives of the Marshall Islands.[126]

Two recent reports have documented large optic discs in patients with optic nerve hypoplasia associated with a congenital homonymous hemianopia.[128,152] This rare combination of findings suggests that a prenatal loss of optic nerve axons leading to optic nerve hypoplasia may not always alter the genetically predetermined size of the scleral canals.[153]

Visual acuity in megalopapilla is usually normal but may be mildly decreased in some cases. Visual fields are usually normal, except for an enlarged blind spot, allowing the examiner to effectively rule out normal tension glaucoma or compressive optic atrophy. Colobomatous discs are distinguished from megalopapilla by their predominant excavation of the inferior optic disc. Aside from glaucoma and optic disc coloboma, the differential diagnosis of megalopapilla includes orbital optic glioma, which in children can cause progressive enlargement of a previously normal-sized optic disc.[77]

Pathogenetically, most cases of megalopapilla may simply represent a statistical variant of normal. However, it is likely that megalopapilla can occasionally result from altered optic axonal migration early in embryogenesis, as evidenced by a report of megalopapilla in a child with basal encephalocoele.[74] The rarity of this association, however, would suggest that neuroimaging is unwarranted in megalopapilla, unless midfacial

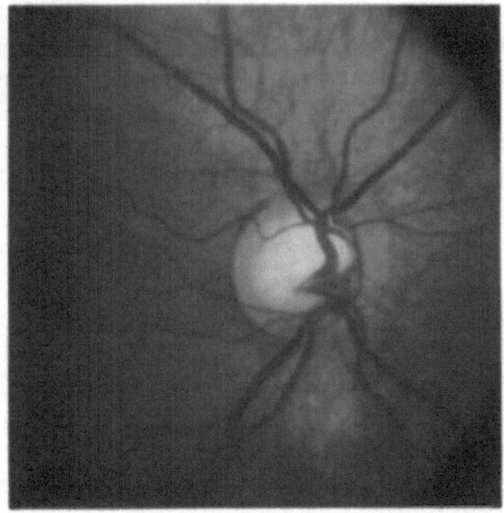

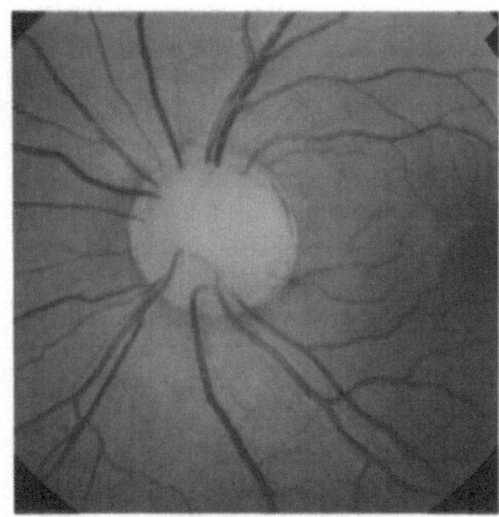

FIGURE 2.14. Megalopapilla. **(A)** A common variant of megalopapilla in which an abnormally large optic disc contains a large central cup. Unlike glaucomatous optic atrophy, the cup is horizontally oval with an intact neuroretinal rim, and there is no nasalization of vessels at their point of origin. **(B)** An uncommon variant of megalopapilla in which an anomalous superior excavation obliterates much of the temporal neuroretinal rim. (From Brodsky MC. Congenital optic disk anomalies. Surv Ophthalmol 1994;39:89–112, with permission. Photograph courtesy of William F. Hoyt, MD.)

anomalies (e.g., hypertelorism, cleft palate, cleft lip, depressed nasal bridge) coexist.

Optic Pit

An optic pit is a round or oval, gray, white, or yellowish depression in the optic disc (Figure 2.15). Optic pits commonly involve the temporal optic disc but may be situated in any sector.[30] Temporally located pits are often accompanied by adjacent peripapillary pigment epithelial changes. One or two cilioretinal arteries are seen to emerge from the bottom or the margin of the pit in greater than 50% of cases.[29,187] Although optic pits are typically unilateral, bilateral pits are seen in 15% of cases.[29] In unilateral cases, the involved disc is slightly larger than the normal disc. Visual acuity is typically normal in the absence of subretinal fluid. Although visual field defects are variable and often correlate poorly with the location of the pit, the most common defect appears to be a paracentral arcuate scotoma connected to an enlarged blind spot.[30,113] Optic pits do not portend additional CNS malformations, although rare exceptions exist.[191] Acquired depressions in the optic disc that are indistinguishable from optic pits have been documented in normal-tension glaucoma.[102]

Serous macular elevations have been estimated to develop in 25 to 75% of eyes with optic pits.[18,30,113,180] Optic pit–associated maculopathy generally becomes symptomatic in the third and fourth decade of life. Numerous investigators have suggested that vitreous traction on the margins of the pit and tractional changes in the roof of the pit may be the inciting events that ultimately lead to late-onset macular detachment.[18,60,187]

Until recently, all optic pit–associated macular elevations were thought to represent serous detachments. Recent observations by Lincoff et al have led to a better understanding of optic pit–associated maculopathy.[121] These investigators have proposed that careful stereoscopic examination of the macula in conjunction with kinetic perimetry demonstrates the following progression of events:

1. A schisis-like inner-layer retinal separation initially forms in direct communication with the optic pit, which produces a mild, relative, centrocecal scotoma.
2. An outer-layer macular hole develops beneath the boundaries of the inner-layer separation and produces a dense central scotoma.
3. An outer-layer retinal detachment develops around the macular hole (presumably from

influx of fluid from the inner-layer separation). This outer-layer detachment ophthalmoscopically resembles an RPE detachment but fails to hyperfluoresce on fluorescein angiography.

4. The outer-layer detachment may eventually enlarge and obliterate the inner-layer separation. At this stage, it is no longer ophthalmoscopically or histopathologically distinguishable from a primary serous macular detachment.

Figure 2.15 depicts the retinal findings that can be observed in the evolution of an optic pit–associated macular detachment. The finding of a sensory macular detachment in histopathologically studied eyes with optic pits presumably represents the endstage of this sequence of events. Whether this sequence of events leads to all optic pit–associated macular detachments is unclear.

The risk of optic pit–associated macular detachment is greater in eyes with large optic pits and in eyes with temporally located pits.[30] Spontaneous reattachment is seen in approximately 25% of cases.[30,173] Sugar's early report of spontaneous resolution of most optic pit–associated macular de-

tachments with good visual recovery[180] differs from the experience of subsequent investigators who have noted permanent visual loss in untreated patients, even when spontaneous reattachment occurs.[70,173] Bedrest and bilateral patching have led to retinal reattachment in some patients, presumably by decreasing vitreous traction.[47,161] Laser photocoagulation to block the flow of fluid from the pit to the macula has been largely unsuccessful, perhaps due to the inability of laser photocoagulation to seal a retinoschisis cavity.[18,47,70,117,121,133,161,171] Vitrectomy with internal gas tamponade laser photocoagulation has recently been shown to produce long-term improvement in acuity in several independent studies.[4,47,121,133,161] The initial intent of this treatment was to compress the retina at the edge of the disc to enhance the effect of laser treatment.[122] However, Lincoff et al have postulated that internal gas tamponade functions to mechanically displace subretinal fluid away from the macula, allowing a shallow, inner-layer separation to persist, which is associated with a mild scotoma and relatively good visual acuity.[122] Based upon clinical and perimetric observations following treatment, Lincoff et al have concluded that laser photo-

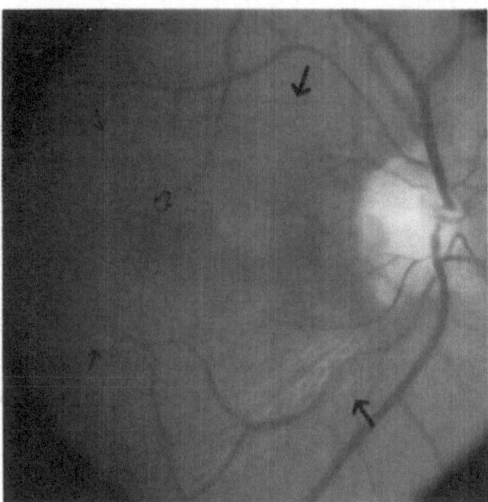
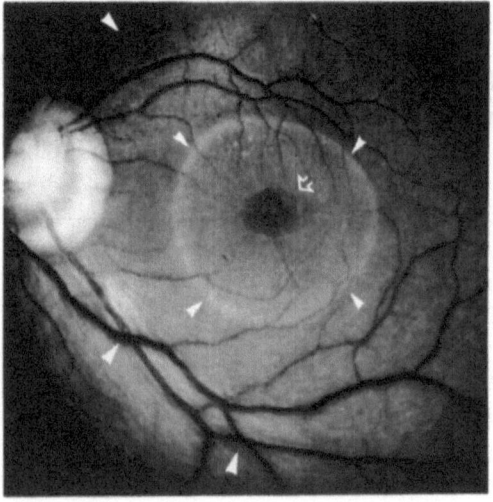

FIGURE 2.15. Optic pit showing each stage in the evolution of a serous macular detachment. (A) The abnormal radial striations between the disc and macula (delimited by large arrows) correspond to the schisis-like inner-layer retinal separation. There is also an outer-layer hole (open arrow) surrounded by an outer-layer macular detachment (delimited by small arrows). (B) Black and white photograph demonstrating an inner-layer separa-

tion (delimited by large arrowheads), macular hole (open arrowhead), and an outer-layer sensory detachment (delimited by small arrowheads). (From Lincoff H, Lopez R, Kreissig I, et al. Retinoschisis associated with optic pits. Arch Ophthalmol 1988;106:61-67, with permission. Copyright 1988, American Medical Association. Photograph courtesy of Harvey Lincoff, MD.)

coagulation probably does not contribute to the success of this procedure.[122]

The source of intraretinal fluid in eyes with optic pits is controversial. Possible sources include (1) vitreous cavity via the pit, (2) the subarachnoid space, (3) blood vessels at the base of the pit, and (4) the orbital space surrounding the dura.[5,18,29,120] Although fluorescein angiography shows early hypofluorescence of the pit followed in many cases by late hyperfluorescent staining,[18,30,38,133] optic pits do not generally leak fluorescein, and there is no extension of fluorescein into the subretinal space toward the macula.[5,158] The finding of late hyperfluorescent staining has been shown to correlate strongly with the presence of cilioretinal arteries emerging from the pit.[187] Careful slit-lamp biomicroscopy often reveals a thin membrane overlying the pit[30] or a persistent Cloquet's canal terminating at the margin of the pit.[2] In collie dogs, active flow of fluid from the vitreous cavity through the pit to the subretinal space has been demonstrated.[28] This mechanism has never been conclusively demonstrated in humans.

Histologically, optic pits consist of herniations of dysplastic retina into a collagen-lined pocket extending posteriorly, often into the subarachnoid space, through a defect in the lamina cribrosa.[29,60,100,133] Friberg and McLellan demonstrated a pulsatile communication of fluid between the vitreous cavity and a retrobulbar cyst through an optic pit.[66] Rarely, macular holes can develop in eyes with optic pits or optic disc colobomas and lead to rhegmatogenous retinal detachment.[15,186]

Although the pathogenesis of optic pits is unclear, the great majority of authors view optic pits as the mildest variant in the spectrum of optic disc colobomas.[5,30,70,100,113,120,125,154,158,161,179,180] It should be noted, however, that this widely accepted hypothesis is inconsistent with the preponderance of clinical evidence:

1. Optic pits are usually unilateral, sporadic, and unassociated with systemic anomalies. Colobomas are bilateral as often as unilateral, commonly autosomal dominant, and may be associated with a variety of multisystem disorders.
2. It is rare for optic pits to coexist with iris or retinochoroidal colobomas.
3. Optic pits usually occur in locations unrelated to the embryonic fissure.

Following a review of 75 eyes with optic pits, Brown et al concluded that "the sparsity of inferonasal pits (none among our cases) casts doubt as to whether the pits are truly colobomas resulting from incomplete closure of the embryonic fissure. Certain authors have thought that pits are colobomas and the finding of pits in three of our patients in association with true optic nerve colobomas, along with similar reports by others, indicates more than an incidental relationship. However, if pits are colobomatous defects they are certainly atypical."[30] While it is true that colobomas may contain focal craterlike deformations that resemble optic pits[5,73] and that the distinction between an inferiorly located pit and a small optic disc coloboma is difficult at times, there appears to be sufficient evidence to conclude that most optic pits are fundamentally distinct from colobomas in their pathogenesis. The observation that one or more cilioretinal arteries emerge from the majority of optic pits suggests that this finding must somehow be pathogenetically related.[30,85]

Congenital Tilted Disc Syndrome

The tilted disc syndrome is a nonhereditary, bilateral condition in which the superotemporal optic disc is elevated and the inferonasal disc is posteriorly displaced, resulting in an oval-appearing optic disc, with its long axis obliquely oriented (Figure 2.16). This configuration is accompanied by situs inversus of the retinal vessels, congenital inferonasal conus, thinning of the inferonasal RPE and choroid, and bitemporal hemianopia.[204] The anomalous optic disc appearance is secondary to a posterior ectasia of the inferonasal fundus and optic disc. Because of the regional fundus ectasia, affected patients have myopic astigmatism, with the plus axis oriented parallel to the ectasia. The cause of the condition is unknown, but the inferonasal or inferior location of the excavation is at least vaguely suggestive of a pathogenetic relationship to retinochoroidal coloboma.[5]

Familiarity with the tilted disc syndrome is crucial for the ophthalmologist, since affected patients may present with bitemporal hemianopia or optic disc elevation.[5,134] The bitemporal hemianopia in affected patients, which is typically incomplete and confined primarily to the superior quadrants, represents a refractive scotoma, secondary to regional myopia localized to the inferonasal retina (Figure

2.16). Unlike the visual field loss from chiasmal lesions, the field defects seen in the tilted disc syndrome fail to respect the vertical meridian on careful kinetic perimetry. Furthermore, the superotemporal depression is selectively confined to the midsize isopter while the large and small isopters remain fairly normal, due to the marked ectasia of the midperipheral fundus (Figure 2.16). Repeat perimetry after addition of a −4.00 lens often eliminates the visual field abnormality, confirming the refractive nature of the defect. In some cases, retinal sensitivity may be decreased in the area of the ectasia, and the defect persists to some degree despite appropriate refractive correction.[204]

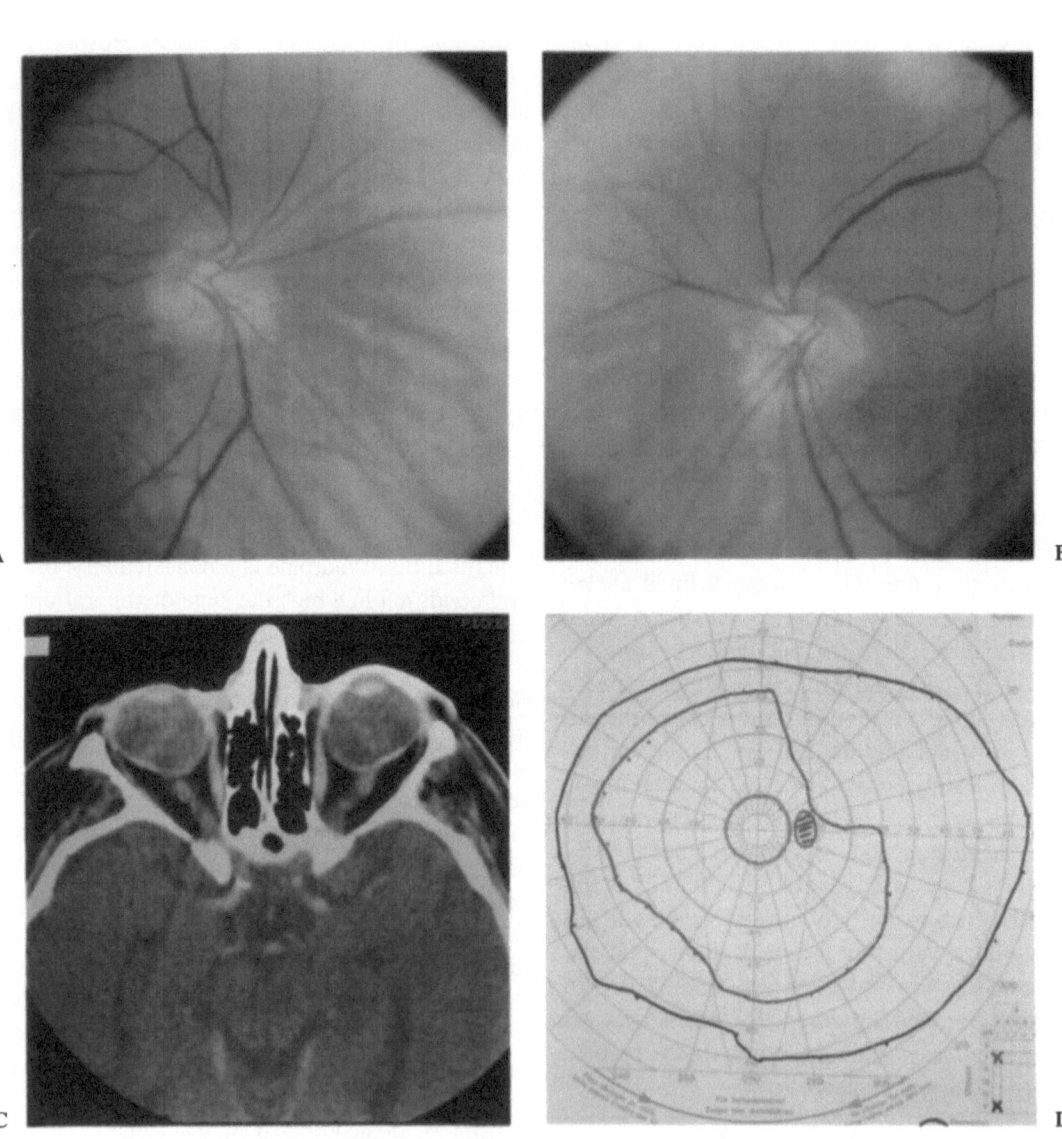

FIGURE 2.16. Congenital tilted disc syndrome. (A) and (B) The optic discs appear obliquely oval. There is elevation of the superonasal discs and posterior displacement of the inferonasal disc. Note subtle inferonasal peripapillary crescent, albinotic appearance of the inferonasal retina, and situs inversus of the vessels as they emerge from the disc. (C) Axial CT scan through lower aspect of globes. The nasal aspects of both globes protrude posteriorly. (D) Goldmann visual field of the right eye demonstrates a superotemporal visual field defect confined to the midperipheral isopter that does not respect the horizontal meridian. (Photographs A–C courtesy of William F. Hoyt, MD.) (From Brodsky MC. Congenital optic disk anomalies. Surv Ophthalmol 1994;39:89–112, with permission.)

It should be emphasized that the tilted disc syndrome has been associated with true bitemporal hemianopia in several patients who were found to harbor a congenital suprasellar tumor. As with optic nerve hypoplasia, these two seemingly disparate findings may reflect the disruptive effect of the suprasellar tumor on optic axonal migration during embryogenesis.[106,142,184] This sinister association makes neuroimaging mandatory in any patient with a tilted disc syndrome whose bitemporal hemianopia either respects the vertical meridian or fails to preferentially involve the midperipheral isopter on kinetic perimetry.[80,83] The tilted disc syndrome has also been reported in patients with X-linked congenital stationary night blindness.[84,86]

Optic Disc Dysplasia

The term "optic disc dysplasia" should be viewed not as a diagnosis but as a descriptive term that connotes a markedly deformed optic disc that fails to conform to any recognizable diagnostic category (Figure 2.17). The distinction between an uncategorizable "anomalous" disc and a "dysplastic" disc is somewhat arbitrary and based primarily

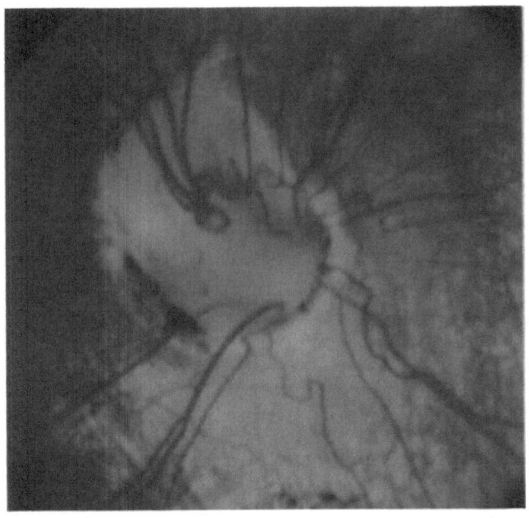

FIGURE 2.17. Optic disc dysplasia. This optic disc is vertically elongated and grossly anomalous. The retinal vessels emerge from the disc in an anomalous pattern. (Photograph courtesy of Stephen C. Pollock, MD.) (From Brodsky MC. Congenital optic disk anomalies. Surv Ophthalmol 1994;39:89–112, with permission.)

upon the severity of the lesion. In the past, the term optic disc dysplasia has been applied to cases that are now recognizable as the morning glory disc anomaly.[74,80] Conversely, many dysplastic optic discs have been indiscriminately labeled as optic disc colobomas. It is likely that additional variants of optic disc dysplasia will be recognized and identified as distinct anomalies. Dysplastic optic discs can occur in association with transsphenoidal encephalocoele.[27,31,59,134,190]

Congenital Optic Disc Pigmentation

Congenital optic disc pigmentation is a condition in which melanin deposition anterior to or within the lamina cribrosa imparts a gray appearance to the optic disc (Figure 2.18). True congenital optic disc pigmentation is extremely rare, but it has been described in a child with an interstitial deletion of chromosome 17 and in Aicardi syndrome.[20,185] Congenital optic disc pigmentation is compatible with good visual acuity but may be associated with coexistent optic disc anomalies that decrease vision.[20] Silver and Sapiro have demonstrated that, in developing mice and rats, a transient zone of melanin in the distal developing optic stalk influences migration of the earliest optic nerve axons.[165] The effects of abnormal pigment deposition on optic nerve embryogenesis could explain the frequent coexistence of congenital optic disc pigmentation with other anomalies, particularly optic nerve hypoplasia.

The great majority of patients with gray optic discs do not have congenital optic disc pigmentation. For reasons that are poorly understood, optic discs of infants with delayed visual maturation and albinism may have a diffuse gray tint when viewed ophthalmoscopically (Figure 2.19). In these conditions, the gray tint often disappears within the first year of life without visible pigment migration. Beauvieux observed gray optic discs in premature infants and in albinotic infants who were apparently blind but who later developed good vision as the gray color disappeared.[11,12] He attributed the gray appearance of these neonatal discs to delayed optic nerve myelination with preservation of the "embryonic tint." It should be noted, however, that gray optic discs may also be seen in normal neonates and are therefore a nonspecific finding of little diagnostic

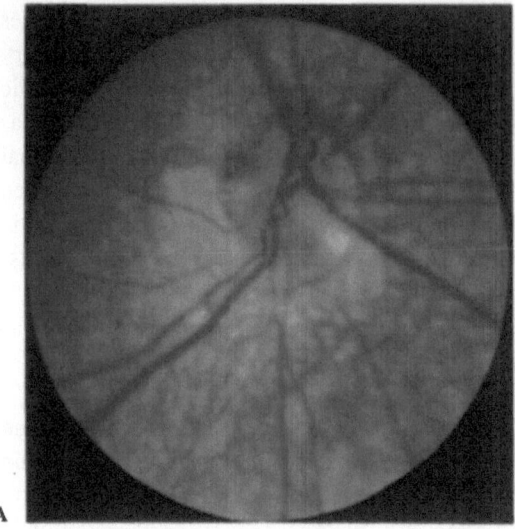

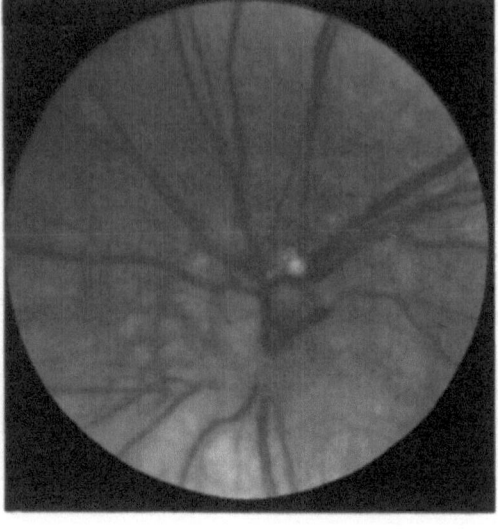

A

B

FIGURE 2.18. Congenital optic disc pigmentation. **(A)** Right optic disc. A circular area of patchy pigmentation surrounds a severely hypoplastic, elevated, central tuft of optic nerve substance, producing the appearance of a gray optic disc. The arteries and veins overlying the disc are anomalous. **(B)** Left optic disc. The disc is elevated and uniformly gray in appearance. Note anomalous superior vasculature and anomalous venous trunk along the 2 o'clock meridian of the disc. (From Brodsky MC, Buckley EG, Rosell-McConkie A. The case of the gray optic disc! Surv Ophthalmol 1989;33:367-372, with permission.)

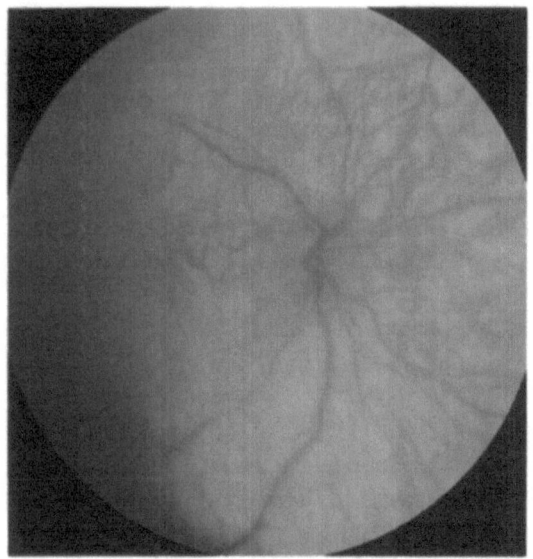

FIGURE 2.19. Optic disc from an infant with albinism and delayed visual maturation demonstrating a diffuse gray cast unrelated to pigmentation. (From Brodsky MC. Congenital optic disk anomalies. Surv Ophthalmol 1994;39:89–112, with permission.)

value, except when accompanied by other clinical signs of delayed visual maturation or albinism.

Despite their fundamental differences, "optically gray optic discs" and congenital optic disc pigmentation have unfortunately been lumped together in many reference books. These two conditions can usually be distinguished ophthalmoscopically, since melanin deposition in true congenital optic disc pigmentation is often discrete, irregular, and granular in appearance.[20]

Aicardi Syndrome

Aicardi syndrome is a cerebroretinal disorder of unknown etiology. Its salient clinical features are infantile spasms, agenesis of the corpus callosum, a characteristic electroencephalographic pattern termed hypsarrhythmia, and a pathognomonic optic disc appearance consisting of multiple depigmented "chorioretinal lacunae" clustered around the disc (Figure 2.20).[36,54,93] Histologically, chorioretinal lacunae consist of well-circumscribed, full-thickness defects limited to

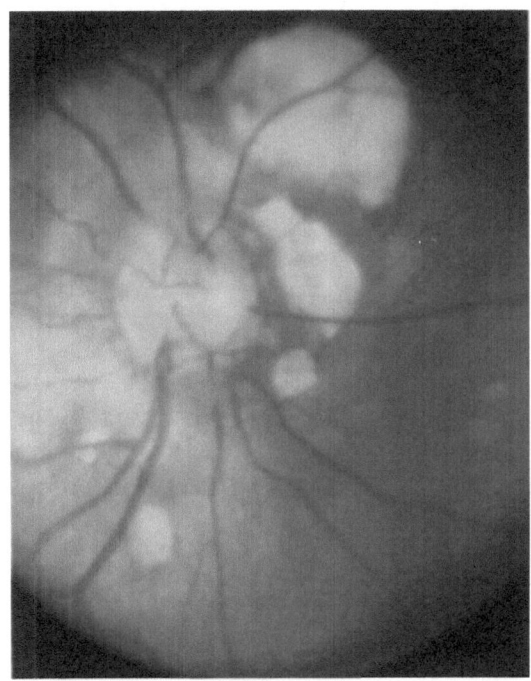

FIGURE 2.20. Aicardi syndrome. A cluster of peripapillary lacunae surround an enlarged, anomalous right optic disc. (From Brodsky MC. Congenital optic disk anomalies. Surv Ophthalmol 1994;39:89–112, with permission.)

the RPE and choroid. The overlying retina remains intact but is often histologically abnormal.[36]

Congenital optic disc anomalies, including optic disc coloboma, optic nerve hypoplasia, and congenital optic disc pigmentation, may accompany chorioretinal lacunae.[36,41] Other ocular abnormalities include microphthalmos, retrobulbar cyst, pseudoglioma, retinal detachment, macular scars, cataract, pupillary membranes, iris synechiae, and iris colobomas.[41,93] The most common systemic findings associated with Aicardi syndrome are vertebral malformations (e.g., fused vertebrae, scoliosis, spina bifida) and costal malformations (e.g., absent ribs, fused or bifurcated ribs).[41,93] Other systemic associations include muscular hypotonia, microcephaly, dysmorphic facies, and auricular anomalies. Severe mental retardation is almost invariable.[36,41] The intriguing association between choroid plexus papilloma and Aicardi syndrome has been documented in five patients.[182]

Central nervous system anomalies in Aicardi syndrome include agenesis of the corpus callosum, cortical migration anomalies (e.g., pachygyria, polymicrogyria, cortical heterotopias), and multiple structural CNS malformations (e.g., cerebral hemispheric asymmetry, Dandy–Walker variant, colpocephaly, midline arachnoid cysts) (Figure 2.21).[8,72,79,99] An overlap between Aicardi syndrome and septo-optic dysplasia has been recognized in several patients.[36]

Aicardi syndrome is thought to result from an X-linked mutational event that is lethal in males.[41,137] Parents should therefore be asked about a previous history of miscarriages. In 1986, Chevrie and Aicardi suggested that all cases of Aicardi syndrome represent fresh gene mutations since no cases of affected siblings had been reported.[41] A recent report of Aicardi syndrome in two sisters challenges the notion that Aicardi syndrome always results from a de novo mutation in the affected infant and indicates that parental gonadal mosaicism for the mutation may be an additional mechanism of inheritance.[135] Although early infectious CNS insults can lead to severe CNS anomalies, tests for infective agents have been consistently negative. No teratogenic drug or other toxin has yet been associated with Aicardi syndrome. Based on the pattern of cerebroretinal malformations in Aicardi syndrome, it is speculated that an insult to the CNS must take place between the fourth and eighth week of gestation.[41]

Doubling of the Optic Disc

Doubling of the optic disc is a rare anomaly in which two discs appear to be in close proximity to one another.[55] This ophthalmoscopic finding is presumed to result from a duplication or separation of the distal optic nerve into two fasciculi.[55] Most reports describe a "main" disc and a "satellite" disc, each with its own vascular system (Figure 2.22). Doubling of the optic disc is usually unilateral and associated with decreased vision in the involved eye.[55]

The majority of clinical reports antedate the era of high resolution neuroimaging and have relied upon the roentgenographic demonstration of two optic nerves in the same orbit, results of fluorescein angiography, synchronous pulsations of each major

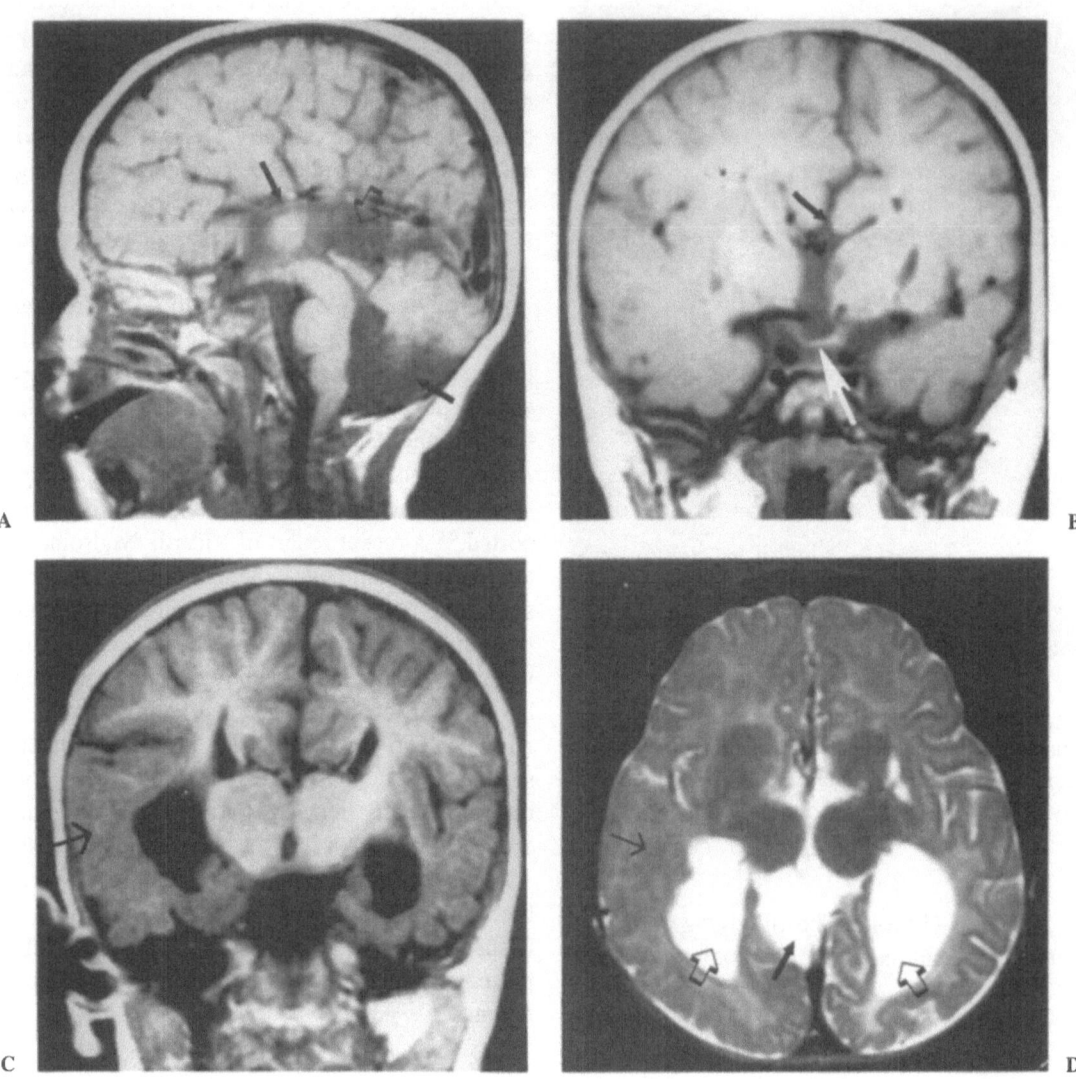

FIGURE 2.21. MR imaging in Aicardi syndrome. (A) Sagittal T1-weighted MR image demonstrating agenesis of the corpus callosum (upper solid arrow denotes normal position of the corpus callosum), an arachnoid cyst in the region of the quadrigeminal cistern (open arrow), and hypoplasia of the cerebellar vermis with cystic dilatation of the fourth ventricle (Dandy–Walker variant) (white arrow). (B) Coronal T1-weighted image demonstrating absent corpus callosum (black arrow denotes the normal position of the corpus callosum) and chiasmal hypoplasia (white arrow). (C) Coronal inversion recovery image (arrow) demonstrating pachygyria (thickened dysmorphic cortex with decreased cortical gyri and sulci). (D) Axial T1-weight MR image demonstrating gray matter heterotopias in the right temporal lobe (upper arrow), small areas of probable polymicrogyria just medial to the occipital poles (greater in the left hemisphere), dilatation of the posterior horns of the lateral ventricles (also known as colpocephaly) (open arrows), and an arachnoid cyst in the region of the quadrigeminal cistern (lower arrow). (From Carney SH, Brodsky MC, Good WV, et al. Aicardi Syndrome: more than meets the eye. Surv Ophthalmol 1993;37:419-424, with permission.)

disc artery, dual blind spots, and angioscotomas to provide indirect evidence of optic nerve diastasis.[55] In some cases, an apparent doubling of the optic disc results from a focal, juxtapapillary retinochoroidal coloboma that displays an abnormal vascular anastomosis with the optic disc.[55]

Separation of the optic nerve into two or more strands (Figure 2.22) is rare in humans but common in lower vertebrates.[55] However, separation of various portions of an intracranial or orbital optic nerve has been documented in a handful of autopsy cases.[44,68,141,168,170] Magnetic resonance imaging should allow in vivo confirmation of optic nerve diastasis in some individuals with doubling of the optic disc.

Optic Nerve Aplasia

Optic nerve aplasia is a rare nonhereditary malformation, which is usually seen in a unilaterally malformed eye of an otherwise healthy person.[196] In its current usage, the term optic nerve aplasia comprises complete absence of the optic nerve (including the optic disc), retinal ganglion and nerve fiber layers, and optic nerve vessels.[132] Histopathological examination usually demonstrates a vestigial dural sheath entering the sclera in its normal position, as well as retinal dysplasia with rosette formation[196] (Figure 2.23). Some early reports of optic nerve aplasia actually described patients with severe hypoplasia at a time when the latter entity was not clearly recognized.[123,132]

Ophthalmoscopically, optic nerve aplasia may take on any of the following appearances:[16]

absence of a normally defined optic nerve head or papilla in the ocular fundus, without central blood vessels and with an absence of macular differentiation;

a whitish area corresponding to the optic disc, without central vessels or macular differentiation; or

a deep avascular cavity in the site corresponding to the optic disc, surrounded by a whitish annulus.

Optic nerve aplasia seems to fall within a malformation complex that is fundamentally distinct from that seen with optic nerve hypoplasia, as evidenced by its tendency to occur unilaterally, and its frequent association with malformations that are otherwise confined to the involved eye (microphthalmia, malformations in the anterior chamber angle, hypoplasia or segmental aplasia of the iris, cataracts, persistent hyperplastic primary vitreous, colobomas, and retinal dysplasia), as opposed to the brain.[16,71] The pathogenesis of optic nerve aplasia is unknown. When it occurs bilaterally, optic nerve aplasia is usually associated with other CNS malformations.[10,132,176,202]

In patients with unilateral optic nerve aplasia, the intracranial course of the "intact" optic nerve may vary. Hoff et al[90] reported a patient with

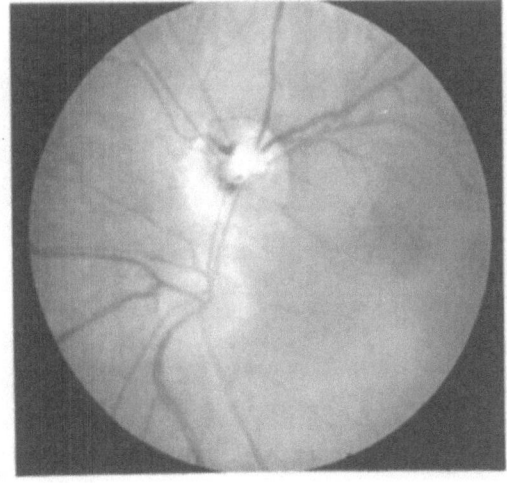

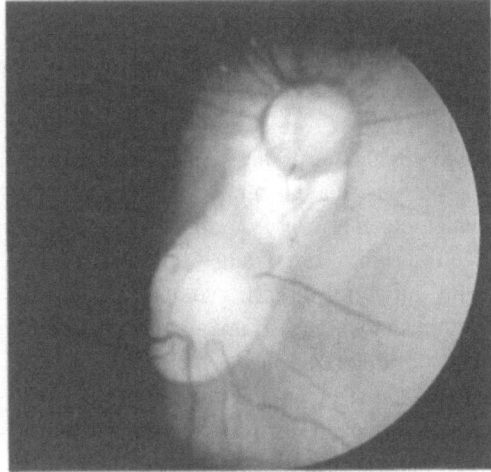

FIGURE 2.22. Doubling of the optic disc (A) Note superior retinal vasculature arising from the upper disc, and inferior retinal vasculature arising from the lower disc, with interconnecting vessels between the two discs. (B) Major optic disc and superotemporal "accessory optic disc" (right eye). Note "bridging tissue" between the discs. (From Donoso LA, Magargal LE, Eiferman RA, Meyer D. Ocular anomalies simulating double optic discs. Can J Ophthalmol 1981;16:84-87. Photographs courtesy of Larry Donoso, MD, with permission.)

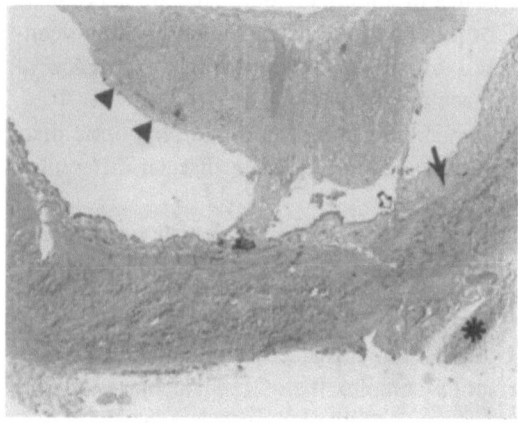

FIGURE 2.23. Histopathologic section of an eye with optic nerve aplasia. Note the mass of gliotic retina (arrowheads) filling the vitreous cavity. The RPE ends abruptly (open arrow) in the area where the optic nerve should be. The choroid (solid arrow) is replaced with gliotic tissue. A residual tag of dura (asterisk) is attached to the outer sclera. (Courtesy of Curtis Margo, MD.)

unilateral anophthalmos and optic nerve aplasia associated with a congenital giant suprasellar aneurysm. The remaining optic nerve was identified at craniotomy as passing posteriorly as a single cord to form an optic tract with no adjoining chiasm. It was speculated that the absent optic nerve and chiasm may have formed initially and then degenerated in a retrograde fashion. Hotchkiss and Green[92] provided necropsy findings from a patient with a Hallerman-Streiff–like syndrome and left optic nerve hypoplasia in whom the geniculate bodies and optic tracts appeared grossly normal bilaterally, but only a single nerve emerged anteriorly from the chiasm that deviated to the right. Margo et al[132] described a patient with unilateral optic nerve aplasia and microphthalmos in whom MR imaging demonstrated unilateral optic nerve aplasia, hemichiasmal hypoplasia on the affected side, and bilateral optic tracts. Visual evoked cortical responses demonstrated increased signals over the occipital lobe contralateral to the intact optic nerve, suggesting chiasmal misdirection of axons from the temporal retina of the normal eye, as seen in albinos. The authors speculated that this abnormal decussation may represent an atavistic form of neuronal reorganization.[132]

Myelinated (Medullated) Nerve Fibers

Myelination of the afferent visual pathways begins at the lateral geniculate body at 5 months of age and terminates at the lamina cribrosa at term or shortly thereafter.[134] Oligodendrocytes, which are responsible for myelination of the CNS, are not normally present in the human retina. Histological studies have confirmed the presence of presumed oligodendrocytes and myelin in areas of myelinated nerve fibers and their absence in other areas.[177] Myelinated retinal nerve fibers have been found in approximately 1% of eyes examined at autopsy[189] and in 0.3% to 0.6% of routine ophthalmic patients.[57]

Ophthalmoscopically, myelinated nerve fibers usually appear as white striated patches at the upper and lower poles of the disc (Figure 2.24). In this location, they may simulate papilledema, both by elevating the involved portions of the disc and by obscuring the disc margin and the underlying retinal vessels.[134,199] Distally, they have an irregular fan-shaped appearance that facilitates their recognition. Small slits or patches of normal-appearing fundus color are occasionally visible within an area of myelination.[134] Myelinated nerve fibers are bilateral in 17% to 20% of cases, and clinically, they are discontinuous with the op-

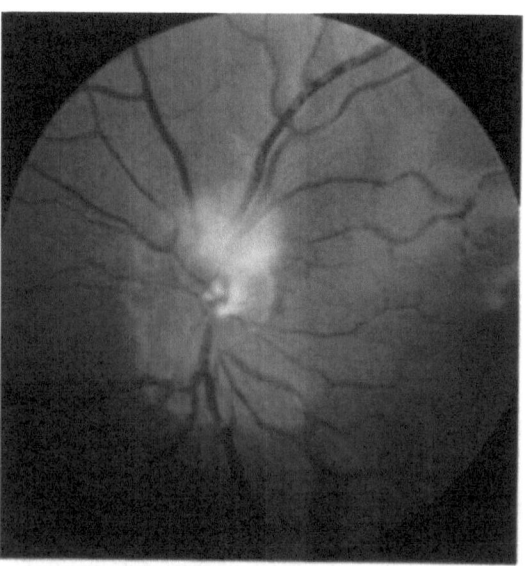

FIGURE 2.24. Myelinated nerve fibers.

tic nerve head in 19%. Isolated patches of myelinated nerve fibers in the peripheral retina are rarely found nasal to the optic nerve head.[199]

The pathogenesis of myelinated nerve fibers remains largely speculative, but several recent hypotheses advanced by Williams[199] provide a useful conceptual framework and seem particularly plausible in light of recent reports. It is known that animals with little or no evidence of lamina cribrosa tend to have deep physiological cups and extensive myelination of retinal nerve fibers, while animals with a well-developed lamina cribrosa tend to show fairly flat nerve heads and no myelination of retinal nerve fibers. Williams[199] has used this animal model to question whether the following factors could play a critical role in the pathogenesis of myelinated nerve fibers:

1. A defect in the lamina cribrosa may allow oligodendrocytes to gain access to the retina and produce myelin there.
2. There may be fewer axons relative to the size of the scleral canal, producing enough room for myelination to proceed into the eye. In eyes with remote, isolated peripheral patches of myelinated nerve fibers, an anomaly in the formation or timing of formation of the lamina cribrosa permits access of oligodendrocytes to the retina. These cells then migrate through the nerve fiber layer until they find a region of relatively low nerve fiber layer density, where they proceed to myelinate some axons.[199]
3. Late development of the lamina cribrosa may allow oligodendrocytes to migrate into the eye. The sclera begins to consolidate in the limbal region, then proceeds posteriorly toward the lamina cribrosa. As stated by Williams, "In a sense, it is possible to imagine a race going on, with the oligodendrocytes myelinating their way toward the retina and the mesodermal tissue consolidating its way to make the lamina cribrosa. If scleral consolidation is retarded, then some retinal myelination may occur."[199]

Extensive unilateral (or rarely bilateral) myelination of nerve fibers can be associated with high myopia and severe amblyopia (Figure 2.25). Unlike other forms of unilateral high myopia that characteristically respond well to occlusion therapy, many children with myelinated nerve fibers are notoriously refractory to rehabilitation.[58] In

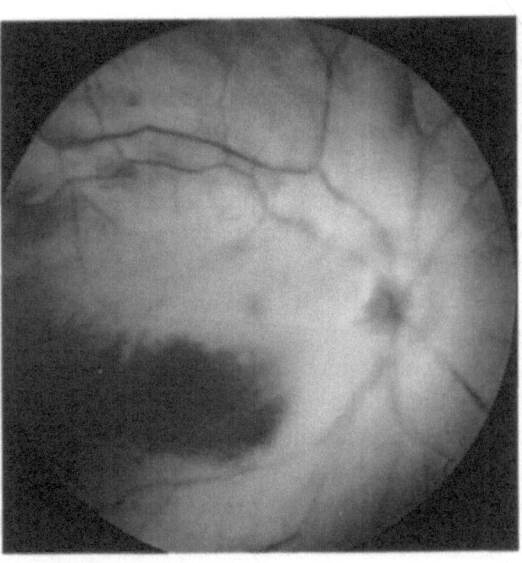

FIGURE 2.25. Diffuse myelination of nerve fibers in an eye with high myopia and refractory amblyopia.

such patients, myelin envelops most or all of the circumference of the disc. Additionally, the macular region (although unmyelinated) usually appears abnormal, showing a dulled reflex or pigment dispersion.[88] Hittner and Antoszyk[88] found the appearance of the macula to be the best direct correlate of response to occlusion therapy.

Myelinated nerve fibers occur in association with the Gorlin (multiple basal cell nevi) syndrome.[49] This autosomal dominant disorder can often be recognized by the finding of numerous tiny pits in the hands and feet that produce a "sandpaper" irregularity. Multiple cutaneous tumors develop in the second to third decade, but they may occasionally develop in the first few years of life. When present in childhood, these lesions remain quiescent until puberty, then increase in number and demonstrate a more rapid and invasive growth pattern.[114] Additional features include jaw cysts (which are found in approximately 70% of patients and often appear in the first decade of life), and mild mental retardation.[114] Rib anomalies (bifid ribs, splaying, synostoses, and partial agenesis) are found in approximately 50% of patients. Facial characteristics include hypertelorism, prominent supraorbital ridges, frontoparietal bossing, a broad nasal root, and mild mandibular prognathism.[114] Ectopic calcification, especially of the falx cerebri, is an almost constant finding.[49] Medulloblastomas have developed in several children with this condition. This disorder should be considered in children with myelinated nerve fibers since small lesions can be treated with curettage, electrophotocoagulation, cryosurgery, and topical chemotherapy to forestall the development of aggressive and invasive lesions.[114]

Traboulsi et al[189] recently described an autosomal dominant vitreoretinopathy characterized by congenitally poor vision, bilateral extensive myelination of the retinal nerve fiber layer, severe vitreal degeneration, high myopia, a retinal dystrophy with night blindness, reduction of the electroretinographic responses, and limb deformities.

Myelinated nerve fibers may also be familial, in which case the trait is usually inherited in an autosomal dominant fashion.[65] Isolated cases of myelinated nerve fibers have also been described in association with abnormal length of the optic nerve (oxycephaly),[13] effects in the lamina cribrosa (tilted disc),[42] anterior segment dysgenesis,[87,199] and NF-2.[75] Although myelinated nerve fibers are purported to be associated with neurofibromatosis, many authorities feel that this association is questionable at best.[134]

Rarely, areas of myelinated nerve fibers may be acquired after infancy and even in adulthood.[1,7] Trauma to the eye (a blow to the eye in one patient and an optic nerve sheath fenestration in the other) seems to be a common denominator in these cases. Williams has suggested that "perhaps there was sufficient damage to the lamina cribrosa in these patients to permit oligodendrocytes to enter the retina, whereupon they moved to the nearest area of relatively loose nerve fibers and myelinated them." Myelinated nerve fibers have also been known to disappear as a result of tabetic optic atrophy, pituitary tumor, glaucoma, central retinal artery occlusion, and optic neuritis.[134]

The Albinotic Optic Disc

The optic discs of albinos have a number of distinct ophthalmoscopic appearance that has gone largely unrecognized. Albino optic discs often have a diffuse gray tint when viewed ophthalmo-

scopically within the first few years of life. This discoloration must somehow be related to optical effects resulting from surrounding chorioretinal depigmentation since it is no longer evident in older children and adults.

Schatz and Pollock[161a] have identified the following five ophthalmoscopic findings that characterize the majority of albino optic discs: (1) small disc diameter; (2) absence of the physiological cup; (3) oval shape with long axis oriented obliquely; (4) origin of the retinal vessels from the temporal aspect of the disc; and (5) abnormal course of retinal vessels consisting of initial nasal deflection followed by abrupt divergence and reversal of direction to form the temporal vascular arcades (Figure 2.26). We routinely scrutinize the optic disc for these characteristic ophthalmoscopic features of albinism when evaluating an infant with nystagmus whose cutaneous and ocular findings are equivocal.

The purported association between optic nerve hypoplasia and albinism is controversial. Although histopathological verification is lacking in humans, some circumstantial evidence supports this association. Clinically, it has been observed that the optic discs appear small in some

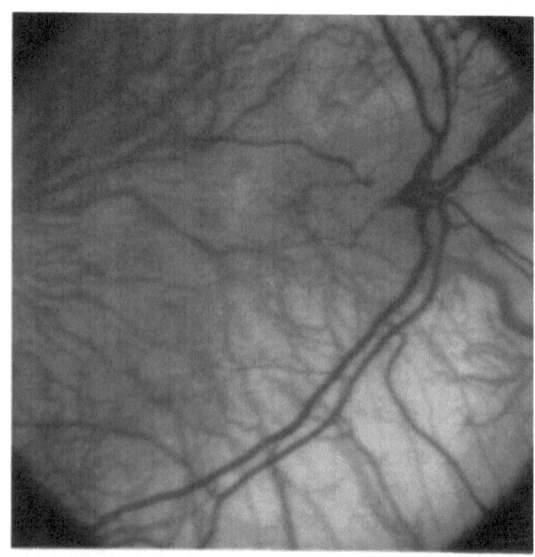

FIGURE 2.26. Albinotic optic disc. Note small size, situs inversus of vessels and abnormal course of retinal vessels.

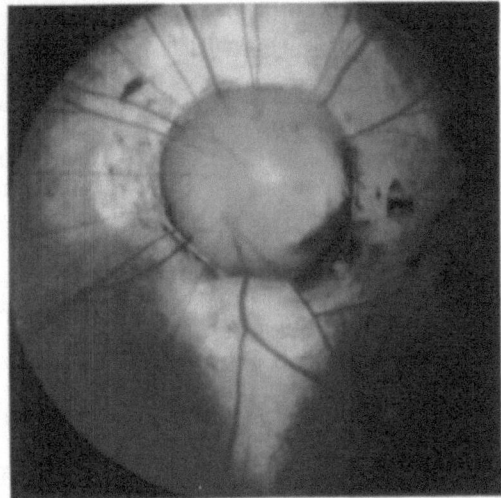
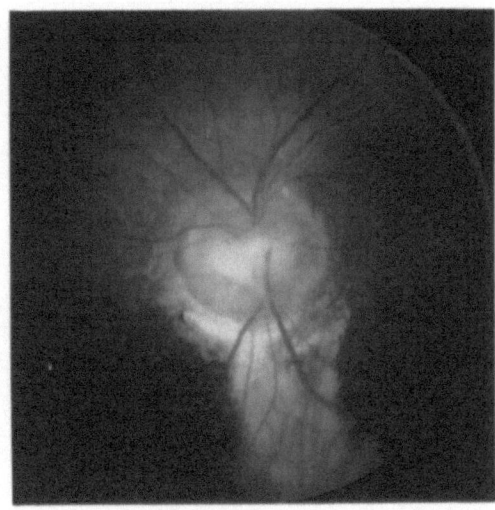

A

B

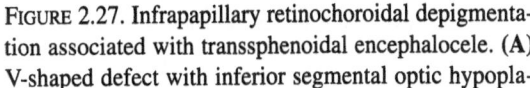

FIGURE 2.27. Infrapapillary retinochoroidal depigmentation associated with transsphenoidal encephalocele. (A) V-shaped defect with inferior segmental optic hypoplasia. (B) Tongue-shaped infrapapillary depigmentation with dysplastic optic disc.

human albinos.[174] Since the macula is poorly developed in albinos, it is plausible that a decreased number of macular ganglion cells would reduce the total number of optic nerve axons from the papillomacular nerve fiber bundle. Optic nerve hypoplasia would then be inevitable, unless other nerve fiber bundles contained a proportionately larger number of axons. Several histological studies have estimated that animals with albinism have approximately 7% fewer optic nerve fibers than their normally pigmented counterparts.[19,56] These findings raise the possibility that optic nerve hypoplasia is a component of albinism. However, high resolution MR imaging of the intracranial optic nerves in human albinos shows no diminution in size.[25] Clinically, the diagnosis of mild optic nerve hypoplasia is usually predicated on finding either subnormal visual acuity or visual field abnormalities, which are usually present in albinos by virtue of the associated macular hypoplasia and nystagmus. Since neither ophthalmoscopy or MR imaging alone can definitively distinguish mild forms of optic nerve hypoplasia from variants of normal, resolution of this controversy awaits neuropathological examination of human albino optic nerves.[25]

V- or Tongue-Shaped Infrapapillary Depigmentation

A discrete infrapapillary zone of V- or tongue-shaped retinochoroidal depigmentation has been described in five patients with anomalous optic discs and transsphenoidal encephalocele[27] (Figure 2.27). These juxtapapillary defects differ from typical retinochoroidal colobomas, which widen inferiorly and are not associated with basal encephalocele. Unlike the typical retinochoroidal coloboma, this distinct juxtapapillary defect is associated with minimal scleral excavation and no visible disruption in the integrity of the overlying retina. In patients with anomalous optic discs, the finding of this V- or tongue-shaped infrapapillary retinochoroidal anomaly should prompt neuroimaging to look for transsphenoidal encephalocele.[27]

References

1. Aaby AA, Kushner BJ. Acquired and progressive myelinated nerve fibers. Arch Ophthalmol 1985; 103:542-544.
2. Akiba J, Kakehashi A, Hikichi T, Trempe CL. Vitreous findings of optic nerve pits and serous macular detachment. Am J Ophthalmol 1993;116:38-41.

3. Akiyama K, Azuma N, Hida T, Uemura Y. Retinal detachment in morning glory syndrome. Ophthal Surg 1984;15:841-843.

4. Alexander TA, Billson FA. Vitrectomy and photo-coagulation in the management of serous detachment associated with optic nerve pits. Aust J Ophthalmol 1984;12:139-142.

5. Apple DJ, Rabb MF, Walsh PM. Congenital anomalies of the optic disc. Surv Ophthalmol 1982;27:3-41.

6. Arslanian SA, Rothfus WE, Foley TP, Becker DJ. Hormonal, metabolic, and neuroradiologic abnormalities associated with septo-optic dysplasia. Acta Endocrinol 1984;139:249-254.

7. Baarsma GS. Acquired medullated nerve fibers. Br J Ophthalmol 1980;64:651.

8. Baieri P, Markl A, Thelen M, et al. MR imaging in Aicardi syndrome. AJNR 1988;9:805-806.

9. Barkovich AJ, Lyon G, Evrard PL. Formation, maturation, and disorders of white matter. AJNR 1992;13:447-461.

10. Barry DR. Aplasia of the optic nerves. Int Ophthalmol 1985;7:235-242.

11. Beauvieux J. La pseudo-atrophie optique dés nouveau-nes (dysgénésie myélinique des voies optiques). Ann Ocul (Paris) 1926;163:881-921.

12. Beauvieux J. La cécité apparente chez le nouveau-né: la pseudoatrophie grise du nerf optique. Arch Ophthalmol (Paris) 1947;7:241-249.

13. Bertelsen TI. T: The Premature Synostosis of the Cranial Sutures. Acta Ophthalmol 1958;51 (suppl): 65.

14. Beyer WB, Quencer RM, Osher RH. Morning glory syndrome: a functional analysis including fluorescein angiography, ultrasonography, and computerized tomography. Ophthalmology 1982; 89:1362-1364.

15. Biedner B, Klemperer I, Dagan M, Yassur Y. Optic disc coloboma associated with macular hole and retinal detachment. Ann Ophthalmol 1993;25:350-352.

16. Blanco R, Salvador F, Galan A, Gil-Gibernau JJ. Optic nerve aplasia: report of three cases. J Pediatr Ophthalmol Strabis 1992;29:228-231.

17. Bochow TW, Olk RJ, Knupp JA, Smith ME. Spontaneous reattachment of a total retinal detachment in an infant with microphthalmos and an optic nerve coloboma. Am J Ophthalmol 1991;112:347-349.

18. Bonnet M. Serous macular detachment associated with optic nerve pits. Arch Clin Exp Ophthalmol 1991;229:526-532.

19. Breusch SR, Arey LB. The number of myelinated and unmyelinated fibers in the optic nerves of vertebrates. J Comput Neurol 1942;77:631-665.

20. Brodsky MC, Buckley EG, Rosell-McConkie A. The case of the gray optic disc! Surv Ophthalmol 1989;33:367-372.

21. Brodsky MC, Glasier CM, Pollock SC, et al. Optic nerve hypoplasia: identification by magnetic resonance imaging. Arch Ophthalmol 1990;108:562-567.

22. Brodsky MC. Septo-optic dysplasia: a reappraisal. Semin Ophthalmol 1991;6:227-232.

23. Brodsky MC, Glasier CM. Optic nerve hypoplasia: clinical significance of associated central nervous system abnormalities on magnetic resonance imaging. Arch Ophthalmol 1993;111:66-74.

24. Brodsky MC, Schroeder GT, Ford R. Superior segmental optic hypoplasia in identical twins. J Clin Neuro-Ophthalmol 1993;13:152-154.

25. Brodsky MC, Glasier CM, Creel DJ. Magnetic resonance imaging of the visual pathways in human albinos. J Pediatr Ophthalmol Strabis 1993;30: 382-385.

26. Brodsky MC. Morning glory disc anomaly or optic disc coloboma. Arch Ophthalmol 1994;112:153. Letter.

26a. Brodsky MC, Wilson RS. Retinal arteriovenous communications in the morning glory disk anomaly. Arch Ophthalmol 1995;115:410-411.

27. Brodsky MC, Hoyt WF, Hoyt CS, et al. Atypical retinochoroidal coloboma in patients with dysplastic optic discs and transsphenoidal encephalocele. Arch Ophthalmol 1995;113:624-628.

27a. Brodsky MC. Congenital optic disc anomalies. Surv Opthamol 1994;39:89-112.

28. Brown BC, Shields JA, Patty BE, Goldberg RE. Congenital pits of the optic nerve head. I: experimental studies in collie dogs. Arch Ophthalmol 1979;97:1341-1344.

29. Brown G, Tasman W. Congenital Anomalies of the Optic Disc. New York, NY: Grune & Stratton; 1983:31-215.

30. Brown GC, Shields JA, Goldberg RE. Congenital pits of the optic nerve head. II. clinical studies in humans. Ophthalmology 1980;87:51-65.

31. Bullard DE, Crockard HA, McDonald WI. Spontaneous cerebrospinal fluid rhinorrhea associated with dysplastic optic discs and a basal encephalocoele. J Neurosurg 1981;54:807-810.

32. Bynke H, Holmdahl G. Megalopapilla: a differential diagnosis in suspected optic atrophy. Neuro-ophthalmology 1981;2:53-57.

33. Caldwell JBH, Sears ML, Gilman M. Bilateral peripapillary staphyloma with normal vision. Am J Ophthalmol 1971;71:423-425.

34. Calhoun FP. Bilateral coloboma of the optic nerve associated with holes in the disc and a cyst of the optic nerve sheath. Arch Ophthalmol 1930;3:71-79.

35. Caprioli J, Lesser RL. Basal encephalocoele and morning glory syndrome. Br J Ophthalmol 1983; 67:349-351.

36. Carney SH, Brodsky MC, Good WV, et al. Aicardi syndrome: more than meets the eye. Surv Ophthalmol 1993;37:419-424.

37. Cennamo G, Sammartino A, Fioretti F. Morning glory syndrome with contractile peripapillary staphyloma. Br J Ophthalmol 1983;67:346-348.
38. Chang M. Pits and crater-like holes of the optic disc. Ophthal Semin 1976;1:21-61.
39. Chang S, Haik BG, Ellsworth RM, et al. Treatment of total retinal detachment in morning glory syndrome. Am J Ophthalmol 1984;97:596-600.
40. Chestler RJ, France TD. Ocular findings in the CHARGE syndrome. Ophthalmology 1988;95:1613-1619.
41. Chevrie JJ, Aicardi J. The Aicardi syndrome. In: Pedley TA, Meldrum BS, eds. Recent Advances in Epilepsy. New York, NY: Churchill Livingston; 1986:189-210.
42. Cockburn DM. Tilted disc and medullated nerve fibers. Am J Optom Physiol Opt 1982;59:760-761.
43. Cogan DG. Coloboma of optic nerve with overlay of peripapillary retina. Br J Ophthalmol 1978;62:347-350.
44. Collier M. Communications sur le sujet du rapport les doubles papilles optiques. Bull Soc Optalmol Fr 1958;328-252.
45. Corbett JJ, Savino PJ, Schatz NJ, Orr LS. Cavitary developmental defects of the optic disc: visual loss associated with optic pits and colobomas. Arch Neurol 1980;37:210-213.
46. Costin G, Murphree AL. Hypothalamic pituitary dysfunction in children with optic nerve hypoplasia. AJDC 1985;143:249-254.
47. Cox MS, Witherspoon D, Morris RE, Flynn HW. Evolving techniques in treatment of macular detachment caused by optic nerve pits. Ophthalmology 1988;95:889-896.
48. Dailey JR, Cantore WA, Gardner TW. Peripapillary choroidal neovascular membrane associated with an optic disc coloboma. Arch Ophthalmol 1993; 111:441-442.
49. De Jong PTVM, Bistervels B, Cosgrove J, et al. Medullated nerve fibers: a sign of multiple basal cell nevi (Gorlin's) syndrome. Arch Ophthalmol 1985;103:1833-1836.
50. de Morsier G. Etudes sur les dysraphies crânio-encéphaliques. III. agénésis du septum lucidum avec malformation du tractus optique. La dysplasie septo-optique. Schweiz Arch Neurol Psychiatr 1956;77:267-292.
51. Dempster AG, Lee WR, Forrester JV, McCreath GT. The "morning glory syndrome." A mesodermal defect? Ophthalmologica 1983;187:222-230.
52. Diebler C, Dulac O. Cephalocoeles. clinical and neuroradiological appearance. Neuroradiology 1983;25:199-216.
53. Donaldson DD, Bennett N, Anderson DR, Eckelhoff R. Peripapillary staphyloma. Arch Ophthalmol 1969;82:704-705.
54. Donnenfeld AE, Packer RJ, Zackai EH, et al. Clinical, cytogenetic and pedigree findings in 18 cases of Aicardi syndrome. Am J Med Genet 1989;32:461-467.
55. Donoso LA, Magargal LE, Eiferman RA, Meyer D. Ocular anomalies simulating double optic discs. Can J Ophthalmol 1981;16:84-87.
56. Dreher B, Sefton AJ, Ni SYK, et al. The morphology, number, distribution, and central projections of class I retinal ganglion cells in albinos and hooded rats. Brain Behav Evol 1985;26:10-48.
57. Duke-Elder S. Congenital deformities. In: System of Ophthalmology. St. Louis, MO: C.V. Mosby Co; 1963;3:661.
58. Ellis GS, Frey T, Gouterman RZ. Myelinated nerve fibers, axial myopia, and refractory amblyopia: an organic disease. J Pediatr Ophthalmol Strabis 1987;24:111-119.
59. Eustis HS, Sanders MR, Zimmerman T. Morning glory syndrome in children. Arch Ophthalmol 1994;112:204-207.
60. Ferry AP. Macular detachment associated with congenital pit of the optic nerve head. Arch Ophthalmol 1963;70:346-357.
61. Font RL, Zimmerman LE. Intrascleral smooth muscle in coloboma of the optic disc. Am J Ophthalmol 1971;72:452-457.
62. Foster JA, Lam S. Contractile optic disc coloboma. Arch Ophthalmol 1991;109:472-473.
63. Franceschetti A, Bock RH. Megalopapilla: a new congenital anomaly. Am J Ophthalmol 1950;33:227-235.
64. Francois J. Colobomatous malformations of the ocular globe. Int Ophthalmol Clin 1968;8:797-816.
65. Francois J. Myelinated Nerve Fibers. Heredity in Ophthalmology. St. Louis, MO: Mosby-Year Book; 1961:494-496.
66. Friberg TR, McClellan TG. Vitreous pulsations, relative hypotony, and retrobulbar cyst associated with a congenital optic pit. Am J Ophthalmol 1992;114:767-768.
67. Frisen L, Holmegaard L. Spectrum of optic nerve hypoplasia. Br J Ophthalmol 1975;62:7-15.
68. Fuchs E. über den anatomischen Befund einiger angeborener Anomalien der Netzhaut und des Sehnerven. Albrecht Von Graefes Arch Opthalmol 1917;93:1.
69. Gardner TW, Zaparackas ZG, Naidich TP. Congenital optic nerve colobomas: CT demonstration. J Comput Assisted Tomogr 1984;8:95-102.
70. Gass JDM. Serous detachment of the macula: secondary to congenital pit of the optic nervehead. Am J Ophthalmol 1969;67:821-841.
71. Ginsberg J, Bove KE, Cuesta MG. Aplasia of the optic nerve with aniridia. Ann Ophthalmol 1980;12:433-439.
72. Gloor P, Pulido JS, Judisch GF. Magnetic resonance imaging and fundus findings in a patient with Aicardi's syndrome. Arch Ophthalmol 1989;107:922-923.

73. Goldberg RE. Optic nerve pit and associated coloboma with serous detachment. Arch Ophthalmol 1974;91:160-161.

74. Goldhammer Y, Smith JL. Optic nerve anomalies in basal encephalocele. Arch Ophthalmol 1975; 93:115-118.

75. Goldsmith J. Neurofibromatosis associated with tumors of the optic papilla. Arch Ophthalmol 1949;41:718-729.

76. Graether JM. Transient amaurosis in one eye with simultaneous dilatation of retinal veins. Arch Ophthalmol 1963;70:342-345.

77. Grimson BS, Perry DD. Enlargement of the optic disk in childhood optic nerve tumors. Am J Ophthalmol 1984;97:627-631.

78. Haik BG, Greenstein SH, Smith ME, et al. Retinal detachment in the morning glory syndrome. Ophthalmology 1984;91:1638-1647.

79. Hall-Craggs MA, Harbord MG, Finn JP, et al. Aicardi syndrome: MR assessment of brain structure myelination. AJNR 1990;11:532-536.

80. Handmann M. Erbliche, vermutlich angeborene zentrale gliose entartung des sehnerven mit besonderer beteilgung der zentralgefasse. Klin Monatsbl Augenheilkd 1929;83:145.

81. Hanna CE, Mandel SH, LaFranchi SH. Puberty in the syndrome of septo-optic dysplasia. ADJC 1989;143:186-189.

82. Harris MJ, De Bustros S, Michels RG, Joondeph HC. Treatment of combined traction-rhegmatogenous retinal detachment in the morning glory syndrome. Retina 1984;4:249-252.

83. Hatten ME, Mason CA. Mechanisms of glial guided neuronal migration in vitro and in vivo. Experientia 1990;46:907-916.

84. Heckenlively JR, Martin DA, Rosenbaum AL. Loss of electroretinographic oscillatory potentials, optic atrophy, and dysplasia in congenital stationary night blindness. Am J Ophthalmol 1983;96: 526-534.

85. Henkind PL. Craterlike holes of the optic nerve. Am J Ophthalmol 1963;55:613-615.

86. Hittner HM, Borda RP, Justice J. X-linked recessive congenital stationary night blindness, myopia, and tilted discs. J Pediatr Ophthalmol Strabismus 1981;18:15-20.

87. Hittner HM, Kretzer FL, Antoszyk JH, et al. Variable expressivity of autosomal dominant anterior segment mesenchymal dysgenesis in six generations. Am J Ophthalmol 1982;93:57-70.

88. Hittner HM, Antoszyk JH. Unilateral peripapillary myelinated nerve fibers with myopia and/or amblyopia. Arch Ophthalmol 1987;105:943-948.

89. Hod M, Diamant YZ. The offspring of a diabetic mother: short and long-range implications. Isr J Med Sci 1992;28:81-86.

90. Hoff J, Winestock D, Hoyt WF. Giant suprasellar aneurysm associated with optic stalk agenesis and unilateral anophthalmos. J Neurosurg 1975;43: 495-498.

91. Hope-Ross M, Johnston SS. The morning glory syndrome associated with sphenoethmoidal encephalocele. Ophthal Pediatr Genet 1990; 2:147-153. 1990.

92. Hotchkiss ML, Green WR. Optic nerve aplasia and hypoplasia. J Pediatr Ophthalmol Strabismus 1979;16:225-240.

93. Hoyt CS, Billson F, Ouvrier R, et al. Ocular features of Aicardi's syndrome. Arch Ophthalmol 1978;96:291-295.

94. Hoyt CS, Billson FA. Optic nerve hypoplasia: changing perspectives. Aust New Zealand J Ophthalmol 1986;14:325-331.

95. Hoyt CS, Good WV. Do we really understand the difference between optic nerve hypoplasia and atrophy? Eye 1992;6:201-204.

96. Hoyt WF, Kaplan SL, Grumback MM, Glaser JS. Septo-optic dysplasia and pituitary dwarfism. Lancet 1970;2:893-894.

97. Hoyt WF, Rios-Montenegro EN, Behrens MM, Eckelhoff RJ. Homonymous hemioptic hypoplasia: funduscopic features in standard and red-free illumination in three patients with congenital hemiplegia. Br J Ophthalmol 1972;56:537-545.

98. Hoyt WF. Congenital occipital hemianopia. Neuroophthalmol Jpn 1985;2:252-259.

99. Igidbashian V, Mahboubi S, Zimmerman RA. Clinical Images: CT and MR findings in Aicardi syndrome. J Comput Assisted Tomogr 1987;11:357-358.

100. Irvine AR, Crawford JB, Sullivan JH. The pathogenesis of retinal detachment with morning glory disc and optic pit. Retina 1986;6:146-150.

101. Izenberg N, Rosenblum M, Parks JS. The endocrine spectrum of septo-optic dysplasia. Clin Pediatr 1984;23:632-636.

102. Javitt JC, Spaeth GL, Katz LJ, et al. Acquired pits of the optic nerve. Ophthalmology 1990;97:1038-1044.

103. Jonas JB, Gusek GC, Guggenmoss-Holzmann I, Naumann GO. Variability of the real dimensions of normal human optic discs. Graefes Arch Clin Exp Ophthalmol 1988;226:332-336.

104. Jonas JB, Zach FM, Gusek GC, Naumann GOH. Pseudoglaucomatous physiologic optic cups. Am J Ophthalmol 1989;107:137-144.

105. Jonas JB, Koniszewski G, Naumann GO. "Morning glory syndrome" and "Handmann's anomaly in congenital macropapilla." Extreme variants of confluent optic pits. Klin Monatsbl Augenheilkd 1989; 195:371-374.

106. Keane JR. Suprasellar tumors and incidental optic disc anomalies: diagnostic problems in two patients with hemianopic temporal scotomas. Arch Ophthalmol 1977;95:2180-2183.

107. Kelly WM, Kucharczyk W, Kucharczyk J, et al. Posterior pituitary ectopia: an MR feature of pituitary dwarfism. Am J Neuroradiol 1988;9:453-460.

108. Kim RY, Hoyt WF, Lessell S, Narahara MH. Superior segmental optic hypoplasia: a sign of maternal diabetes. Arch Ophthalmol 1989;107:1312-1315.

109. Kindler P. Morning glory syndrome: unusual congenital optic disk anomaly. Am J Ophthalmol 1970;69:376-384.

110. Koenig SP, Naidich TP, Lissner G. The morning glory syndrome associated with sphenoidal encephalocele. Ophthalmology 1982;89:1368-1372.

111. Konstas P, Katikos G, Vatakas LC. Contractile peripapillary staphyloma. Ophthalmologica 1971;172:379-381.

112. Kral K, Svarc D. Contractile peripapillary staphyloma. Am J Ophthalmol 1971;71:1090-1092.

113. Kranenburg EW. Crater-like holes in the optic disc and central serous retinopathy. Arch Ophthalmol 1960;64:912-924.

114. Kronish JW, Tse DT. Basal cell nevus syndrome. In: Gold DH, Weingeist, TA, eds. The Eye in Systemic Disease. Philadelphia, PA: J.B. Lippincott; 1990;583-585.

115. Kushner BJ. Functional amblyopia associated with abnormalities of the optic nerve. Arch Ophthalmol 1985;102:683-685.

116. Lambert SR, Hoyt CS, Narahara MH. Optic nerve hypoplasia. Surv Ophthalmol 1987;32:1-9.

117. Lee KJ, Peyman GA. Surgical management of retinal detachment associated with optic nerve pit. Int Ophthalmol 1993;17:105-107.

118. Lewin ML, Schuster MM. Transpalatal correction of basilar meningocele with cleft palate. Arch Surg 1965;90:687-693.

119. Limaye SR. Coloboma of the iris and choroid and retinal detachment in oculo-auricular dysplasia (Goldenhar's syndrome). Eye, Ear, Nose Throat Monthly 1972;51:28-31.

120. Lin CCL, Tso MOM, Vygantas CM. Coloboma of the optic nerve associated with serous maculopathy: a clinicopathologic correlative study. Arch Ophthalmol 1984;102:1651-1654.

121. Lincoff H, Lopez R, Kreissig I, et al. Retinoschisis associated with optic nerve pits. Arch Ophthalmol 1988;106:61-67.

122. Lincoff H, Yannuzzi L, Singerman L, et al. Improvement in visual function after displacement of the retinal elevation emanating from optic pits. Arch Ophthalmol 1993;111:1071-1079.

123. Little LE, Whitmore PV, Wells TW Jr. Aplasia of the optic nerve. J Pediatr Ophthalmol 1976;13:84-88.

124. Longfellow DW, Davis SD, Walsh FB. Unilateral intermittent blindness with dilation of retinal veins. Arch Ophthalmol 1962;67:554.

125. Mafee MF, Jampol LM, Langer BG, Tso MOM. Computed tomography of optic nerve colobomas, morning glory anomaly, and colobomatous cyst. Radiol Clin of North Am 1987;25:693-699.

126. Maisel JM, Pearlstein CS, Adams WH, Heotis DM. Large optic discs in the Marshallese population. Am J Ophthalmol 1989;107:145-150.

127. Mann I. Developmental Abnormalities of the Eye. Philadelphia, PA: JB Lippincott; 1957:74-91.

128. Manor RS, Kesler A. Optic nerve hypoplasia, big discs, large cupping, and vascular malformation embolized: 22 years of follow-up. Arch Ophthalmol 1993;111:901-902.

129. Manschot WA. Morning glory syndrome: a histopathological study. Br J Ophthalmol 1990;74: 56-58.

130. Margalith D, Tze WJ, Jan JE. Congenital optic nerve hypoplasia with hypothalamic-pituitary dysplasia. AJDC 1985;139:361-366.

131. Margo CE, Hamed LM, McCarty J. Congenital optic tract syndrome. Arch Ophthalmol 1991;109: 1120-1122.

132. Margo CE, Hamed LM, Fang E, and Dawson WW. Optic nerve aplasia. Arch Ophthalmol 1992;110: 1610-1613.

133. McDonald HR, Schatz H, Johnson RN. Treatment of retinal detachment associated with optic nerve pits. Int Ophthalmol Clin 1992;32:35-42.

134. Miller NR. Walsh and Hoyt's Clinical Neuro-ophthalmology. 4th ed. Baltimore, MD: Williams & Wilkins Co; 1982;I: 343-369.

135. Molina JA, Mateos F, Merino M, et al. Aicardi syndrome in two sisters. J Pediatr 1989;115:282-283.

136. Mosier MA, Lieberman MF, Green WR, Knox DL. Hypoplasia of the optic nerve. Arch Ophthalmol 1978;96:1437-1442.

137. Neidich JA, Nussbaum RL, Packer RJ, et al. Heterogeneity of clinical severity and molecular lesions in Aicardi syndrome. J Pediatr 1990;116: 911-917.

138. Nelson M, Lessell S, Sadun AA. Optic nerve hypoplasia and maternal diabetes mellitus. Arch Neurol 1986;43:20-25.

139. Novakovic P, Taylor DSI, Hoyt WF. Localizing patterns of optic nerve hypoplasia-retina to occipital lobe. Br J Ophthalmol 1988;72:176-182.

140. Nucci P, Mets MB, Gabianelli EB. Trisomy 4q with morning glory anomaly. Ophthalmic Pediatr Genet 1990;2:143-145.

141. Orcutt JC, Bunt AH. Anomalous optic discs in a patient with a Dandy-Walker cyst. J Clin Neuro-ophthalmol 1982;2:43-47.

142. Osher RH, Schatz NJ. A sinister association of the congenital tilted disc syndrome with chiasmal compression. In: Smith JL, ed. Neuro-ophthalmology Focus 1980. New York, NY: Masson;1979: 117-123.

143. Pagon RA. Ocular coloboma. Surv Ophthalmol 1981;25:223-236.

144. Pagon RA, Graham JM, Zonana J, Yong Sui-Li. Coloboma, congenital heart disease, and choanal atresia with multiple anomalies: CHARGE association. J Pediatr 1981;99:233-227.

145. Pedler C. Unusual coloboma of the optic nerve entrance. Br J Ophthalmol 1961;45:803-807.

146. Petersen RA, Walton DS. Optic nerve hypoplasia with good visual acuity and visual field defects: a

study of children of diabetic mothers. Arch Ophthalmol 1977;95:254-258.

147. Petersen RA, Holmes LB. Optic nerve hypoplasia
in infants of diabetic mothers. Arch Ophthalmol
1986;104:1587.

148. Pollock JA, Newton TH, Hoyt WF. Transsphenoidal and transethmoidal encephaloceles: a review of clinical and roentgen features in 8 cases.
Radiology 1968;90:442-453.

149. Pollock S. The morning glory disc anomaly: contractile movement, classification, and embryogenesis. Doc Ophthalmol 1987;65:439-460.

150. Provis JM, Van Driel D, Billson FA, Russell P. Human fetal optic nerve: overproduction and elimination of retinal axons during development. J Comput Neurol 1985;238:92-100.

151. Rack JH, Wright GF. Coloboma of the optic nerve
entrance. Br J Ophthalmol 1966;50:705-709.

152. Ragge N, Hoyt WF, Lambert SR. Big discs with
optic nerve hypoplasia. J Clin Neuro-ophthalmol
1991;11:137.

153. Ragge NK, Barkovich AJ, Hoyt WF, et al. Isolated
congenital hemianopia caused by prenatal injury to
the optic radiation. Arch Neurol 1991;48:1088-
1091.

154. Ribeiro-da-Silva J, Castanheira-Dinis A, Agoas V,
Dodinho-de-Matos J. Congenital optic disc defor-
mities. A clinical approach. Ophthalmic Pediatr
Genet 1985;5:67-70.

155. Risse JF, Guillaume JB, Boissonnot M, Bonneau
D. Un syndrome polymalformatif inhabituel: 1 <
association charge > à un < morning glory syndrome > Unilateral Ophtalmol 1989;3:196-198.

156. Romano PE. Simple photogrammetric diagnosis of
optic nerve hypoplasia. Arch Ophthalmol 1989;
107:824-826.

157. Rosenberg LF, Burde RM. Progressive visual loss
caused by an arachnoidal brain cyst in a patient
with an optic nerve coloboma. Am J Ophthalmol
1988;106:322-325.

158. Rubenstein K, Ali M. Complications of optic disc
pits. Trans Ophthalmol Soc UK 1978;98:195-200.

159. Russell-Eggitt IM, Blake KD, Taylor DSI, Wyse
RKH. The eye in the CHARGE association. Br J
Ophthalmol 1990;74:421-426.

160. Savell J, Cook JR. Optic nerve colobomas of autosomal dominant heredity. Arch Ophthalmol 1979;
94:395-400.

161. Schatz H, McDonald HR. Treatment of sensory
retinal detachment associated with optic nerve pit
or coloboma. Ophthalmology 1988, 95:178-186.

161a. Schatz MP, Pollock SC. Optic disc morphology in
albinism. Presented as a poster at the North American Neuro-ophthamology Society, Durango, CO,
February 27–March 3, 1994.

162. Scheie HG, Adler FH. Aplasia of the optic nerve.
Arch Ophthalmol 1941;26:61-70.

163. Seybold ME, Rosen PN. Peripapillary staphyloma
and amaurosis fugax. Ann Ophthalmol 1977;9:
139-141.

164. Sherlock DA, McNicol LR. Anesthesia and septo-
optic dysplasia. Anesthesia 1987;143:186-189.

165. Silver J, Sapiro J. Axonal guidance during development of the optic nerve: the role of pigmented
epithelia and other factors. J Comput Neurol 1981;
202:521-538.

166. Singh D, Verma A. Bilateral peripapillary staphyloma (ectasia). Ind J Ophthalmol 1978;25:50-51.

167. Skarf B, Hoyt CS. Optic nerve hypoplasia in children. Arch Ophthalmol 1984;102:255-258.

168. Slade HW, Weekley RD. Diastasis of the optic
nerve. J Neurosurg 1957;14:571-574.

169. Slamovits TL, Kimball GP, Friberg TR, Curtin
HD. Bilateral optic disc colobomas with orbital
cysts and hypoplastic optic nerves and chiasm. J
Clin Neuro-ophthalmol 1989;9:172-177.

170. Snead CM. Congenital division of the optic nerve
at the base of the skull. Arch Ophthalmol 1915;
44:418-120.

171. Snead MP, James N, Jacobs PM. Vitrectomy, argon
laser, and gas tamponade for serous retinal detachment associated with an optic disc pit: a case report. Br J Ophthalmol 1991;75:381-382.

172. Sobol WM, Bratton AR, Rivers MB, Weingeist
TA. Morning glory disk syndrome associated with
subretinal neovascularization. Am J Ophthalmol
1990; 110:93-94.

173. Sobol WM, Blodi CF, Folk JC, Weingeist TA.
Long-term visual outcome in patients with optic
nerve pit and serous retinal detachment of the macula. Ophthalmology 1990;97:1539-1542.

174. Spedick MJ, Beauchamp GR. Retinal vascular and
optic nerve abnormalities in albinism. J Pediatr
Ophthalmol Strabis 1986;23:58-62.

175. Steinkuller PG. The morning glory disc anomaly.
Case report and literature review. J Pediatr Ophthalmol Strabismus 1980;17:81-87.

176. Storm RL, PeBenito R. Bilateral optic nerve aplasia associated with hydroencephaly. Ann Ophthalmol 1984;16:988-992.

177. Straatsma BR, Foos FY, Heckenlively JR, Taylor
GN. Myelinated retinal nerve fibers. Am J Ophthalmol 1981;91:25-38.

178. Streletz LJ, Schatz NJ. Trassphenoidal encephalo-
cele associated with colobomas of the optic disc
and hypopituitary dwarfism. In: Smith JL, Glaser
JS, ed. *Neuro-Ophthalmology Symposium of the
University of Miami and the Bascom Palmer Eye
Institute.* St Louis, MO: CV Mosby;1973;7:78-86.

179. Sugar HS. Congenital pits of the optic disc with
acquired macular pathology. Am J Ophthalmol
1962;53:307-311.

180. Sugar HS. Congenital pits of the optic disc and
their equivalents (congenital colobomas and
colobomalike excavations) associated with submacular fluid. Am J Ophthalmol 1967;63:298-307.

181. Sugar HS, Beckman H. Peripapillary staphyloma with respiratory pulsations. Am J Ophthalmol 1969;68:895-897.
182. Tagawa T, Mimaki T, Ono J, et al. Aicardi syndrome associated with an embryonal carcinoma. Pediatr Neurol 1989;5:45-47.
183. Takida A, Hida T, Kimura C, et al. A case of bilateral morning glory syndrome with total retinal detachment. Folia Ophthalmol Japonica 1981;32:1177-1182.
184. Taylor D. Congenital tumors of the anterior visual pathways. Br J Ophthalmol 1982;66:455-463.
185. Taylor D. *Optic Nerve, Pediatric Ophthalmology.* Cambridge, MA: Blackwell Scientific Publications; 1990:441-466.
186. Theodossiadis G. Evolution of congenital pit of the optic disc and macular detachment in photocoagulated and non-photocoagulated eyes. Am J Ophthalmol 1977;84:620-631.
187. Theodossiadis GP, Kollia AK, Theodossiadis PG. Cilioretinal arteries in conjunction with a pit of the optic disc. Ophthalmologica 1992;204:115-121.
188. Traboulsi EI, O'Neill JF. The spectrum in the morphology of the so-called "morning glory disc anomaly." J Pediatr Ophthalmol Strabismus 1988;25:93-98.
189. Traboulsi EI, Lim JI, Pyeritz R, et al. A new syndrome of myelinated nerve fibers vitreoretinopathy and skeletal malformations. Arch Ophthalmol 1993;111:1543-1545.
190. Tuft SJ, Clemmet RS. Dysplastic optic disc in association with transphenoidal encephalocoele and hypopituitary dwarfism: a case report. Aust J Ophthalmol 1983;11:309-313.
191. Van Nouhuys JM, Bruyn GW. Nasopharyngeal transsphenoidal encephalocoele, craterlike hole in the optic disc and agenesis of the corpus callosum pneumoencephalographic visualisation in a case. Psychiat Neurol Neurochir 1964;67:243-258.
192. von Fricken MA, Dhungel R. Retinal detachment in the morning glory syndrome: pathogenesis and management. Retina 1984;4:97-99.
193. Vuori M-L. Morning glory disc anomaly with pulsating peripapillary staphyloma. A case history. Acta Ophthalmol 1987;65:602-606.
194. Von Szily A. Die Obntogenese der idiopathiachen (erbbildlichen Spaltbildungen des Auges des Mikrophthalmus und der Orbitalcysten), Z Anat Entwicklungsgesch 1924;74:1-230.
195. Warburg M. Update of sporadic microphthalmos and coloboma. Ophthalmic Pediatr Genet 1992;13:111-122.
196. Weiter JJ, McLean IW, Zimmerman LE. Aplasia of the optic nerve and disk. Am J Ophthalmol 1977;83:569-576.
197. Wiggins RE, von Noorden GK, Boniuk M. Optic nerve coloboma with cyst. A case report and review. J Pediatr Ophthalmol Strabismus 1991;28:274-277.
198. Williams J, Brodsky MC, Griebel M, et al. Septo-optic dysplasia: clinical significance of an absent septum pellucidum. Dev Med Child Neurol 1993;35:490-501.
199. Williams TD. Medullated retinal nerve fibers: speculations on their cause and presentation of cases. Am J Optometry Physiolog Optics 1986;63:142-151.
200. Willis R, Zimmerman LE, O'Grady R, et al. Heterotopic adipose tissue and smooth muscle in the optic disc, association with isolated colobomas. Arch Ophthalmol 1972;88:139-146.
201. Wise JB, Maclean AL, Gass JDM. Contractile peripapillary staphyloma. Arch Ophthalmol 1966;75:626-630.
202. Yanoff M, Rorke LB, Allman MI. Bilateral optic system aplasia with relatively normal eyes. Arch Ophthalmol 1978;96:97-101.
203. Yokota A, Matsukado Y, Fuwa I, et al. Anterior basal encephalocele of the neonatal and infantile period. Neurosurgery 1986;19:468-478.
204. Young SE, Walsh FB, Knox DL. The tilted disc syndrome. Am J Ophthalmol 1976;82:16-23.
205. Zeki SM. Optic nerve hypoplasia and astigmatism: a new association. Br J Ophthalmol 1990;74:297-299.
206. Zeki SM, Dudgeon J, Dutton GN. Reappraisal of the ratio of disc to macula/disc diameter in optic nerve hypoplasia. Br J Ophthalmol 1991;75:538-541.
207. Zeki SM, Dutton GV. Optic nerve hypoplasia in children. Brit J Ophthalmol 1990;74:300-304.

3

The Swollen Optic Disc in Childhood

Introduction

"Optic disc elevation" is a reason for neuro-ophthalmologic referral common in children. The nature of the underlying disorder can often be predicted from the wording of the referring physician's telephone call. Bilateral optic disc elevation without visual loss in a child with headaches, nausea, and vomiting of several months duration creates a high index of suspicion for papilledema (i.e., swelling of the optic discs secondary to elevated intracranial pressure). Blurring of the nasal disc margins which is noted as an incidental finding in an otherwise healthy child is usually found to be pseudopapilledema (i.e., real or apparent elevation of the optic discs due to local structural factors, which simulates swelling of the discs). Optic disc swelling in the setting of acute visual loss usually signifies optic neuritis.

When the child arrives for consultation, we first examine the optic discs with a direct ophthalmoscope through undilated pupils. Often, the diagnosis of pseudopapilledema is readily apparent. In this setting, parents and siblings should also be examined since anomalously elevated discs are frequently inherited as a dominant disorder. One can then reassure the concerned parents that their child is well. In the child with additional systemic anomalies, consideration must be given to the possibility that the pseudopapilledema may be related to an underlying genetic disorder.

In the child who has swollen optic discs and other symptoms of increased intracranial pressure, we uniformly obtain magnetic resonance (MR) imaging to look for an intracranial mass lesion. If no lesion is found, we perform a lumbar puncture to determine the opening pressure, to rule out meningitis, and to examine protein and cell count. Optic disc elevation in children may be associated with a wide variety of systemic disorders. Some conditions, such as neurosarcoidosis or leukemia, can produce optic nerve infiltration with visual loss in some cases and papilledema with little or no visual loss in others. Disorders such as mucopolysaccharidoses can be associated with either papilledema or pseudopapilledema.

This chapter will focus primarily upon the differential diagnosis of optic disc elevation in children. Its primary purpose will be to delineate the broad spectrum of neurological and systemic conditions that may manifest with optic disc swelling or pseudopapilledema in childhood.

Optic Disc Swelling

Swelling of the optic disc is due to interruption of axonal transport in the optic nerve head. Experimentally, interruption of axoplasmic transport can be associated with pressure changes at the level of the disc resulting from increased cerebrospinal fluid (CSF) pressure around the retrolaminar optic nerve. Anoxia, ischemia, cyanide toxicity, decreased temperature, methanol toxicity, and antimitotics also can cause optic disc swelling.[114]

Clinically, the terms *optic disc swelling* and *optic disc edema* are used interchangably. We prefer the term swelling to edema since, histopathologically, the degree of axonal distension usually exceeds the degree of edema (exceptions to this rule are seen in diabetic papillopathy and Leber idiopathic stellate neuroretinitis, in which severe edema may be present). Swelling of the optic disc may result from increased intracranial pressure, local inflammation or ischemia, local metabolic effects, compression of the retrobulbar optic nerve, hypotony, intraocular inflammation, or infiltration or inflammation. Narrowing of the scleral canal with crowding of axons is associated with diabetic papillopathy (a form of disc swelling) as well as pseudopapilledema. While the acute ischemic infarction characteristic of ischemic optic neuropathy does not occur in children,[41] a recurrent form of anterior ischemic optic neuropathy has been described in young adults with small cupless discs.[110]

It would appear that interruption of axonal transport with prelaminar accumulation of cytoskeletal elements is not a primary cause of visual loss, as evidenced by the fact that severe papilledema is compatible with normal vision. It is the underlying pathogenetic mechanism (inflammatory, vascular, infiltrative) that determines the nature and severity of visual loss, with interruption of axonal transport and swelling of the disc occurring as epiphenomena.

Swelling of the optic disc may or may not lead to optic atrophy and visual loss. Visual loss as a chronic effect of optic disc edema seems to depend, at least in part, upon the severity and duration of the disc edema. Conceptually, the effects of papilledema can be likened to those of elevated intraocular pressure. An intraocular pressure of 30 mm Hg may be tolerated for years with no adverse effect. An intraocular pressure of 60 mm Hg will inevitably produce axonal loss. Either ocular hypertension or chronic papilledema can exist for years without optic nerve injury, however, a threshold is assumed to exist for each condition above which axonal loss occurs. There likely exists a *duration* threshold for each level of severity of disc swelling as well as a *severity* threshold for any given duration. As with elevated intraocular pressure, severity and duration probably act as independent parameters.

Papilledema

By convention, the term *papilledema* has been assigned to optic disc swelling caused by elevated intracranial pressure. Ophthalmoscopic signs of papilledema include optic disc elevation, venous distension, obscuration of the major retinal vessels (particularly at the disc margin), hyperemia of the disc, opacification of the peripapillary nerve fiber layer, and absent venous pulsations. Later signs include flame-shaped hemorrhages, peripapillary subretinal hemorrhages, and cotton wool spots (Figure 3.1). From the ophthalmoscopic appearance of the disc alone, one cannot reliably distinguish papilledema from other forms of optic disc edema. Ophthalmoscopic signs of chronic papilledema and chronic atrophic papilledema have been detailed elsewhere.[179]

Elevated intracranial pressure produces a rise in CSF pressure surrounding the optic nerves, which increases tissue pressure within the nerves, leading to interruption of axonal transport at the lamina cribrosa and swelling of axons.[114] Vascular changes in papilledema are secondary to axonal distension, which compresses the retinal veins, leading to venous engorgement as well as capillary leakage and extracellular fluid accumulation. [114,268] Fluorescein angiography in papilledema shows dilated capillaries, microaneurysms, and flame-shaped hemorrhages in the arteriovenous phase, followed by diffuse prelaminar capillary

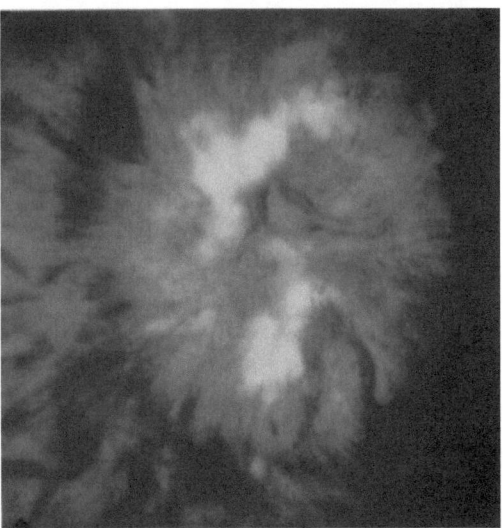

FIGURE 3.1. Papilledema. Note optic disc elevation, papillary and peripapillary hemorrhage, venous congestion, and cotton wool spots.

leakage and late staining of the nerve head and adjacent tissues (Figure 3.2). Interestingly, intraocular protrusion of the optic discs in papilledema does not produce a visible signal differential with the vitreous gel when viewed with routine MR imaging.[38] Occasionally, the swollen disc can be visualized within the globe on MR imaging following gadolinium enhancement (Figure 3.3).[38]

Unilateral papilledema is rare in children but not uncommon in adults. [160,241]

Headaches and transient visual obscurations are the major neuro-ophthalmologic symptoms resulting from elevated intracranial pressure. Nausea, vomiting, persistent visual loss, and diplopia are reported less commonly. A historical clue to the nature of these headaches is that they are fre-

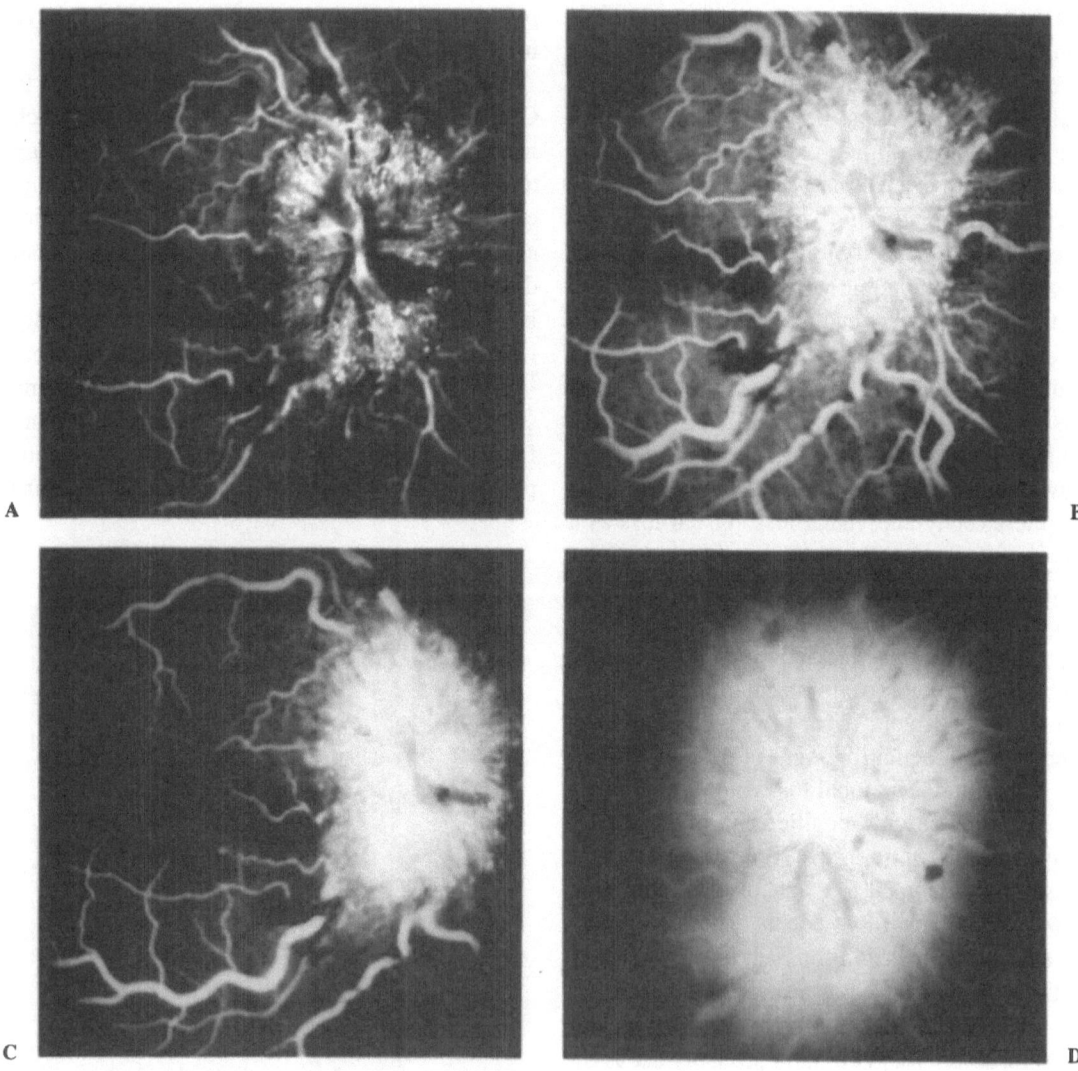

FIGURE 3.2. Fluorescein angiogram in papilledema. (A) Venous laminar phase demonstrating dilated capillaries, flame hemorrhages, and microaneurysms on the surface of the optic disc of an adjacent retina. (B) Arteriovenous phase demonstrating fluorescein leakage from dilated surface capillaries on disc, which masks deeper fluorescence. (C) Venous phase demonstrating increased leakage of fluorescein, which now obscures surface details on the optic disc. (D) Late phase demonstrating intense, kidney-shaped staining that extends into the peripapillary region. Fluorescein dye no longer fills the arteries and veins.

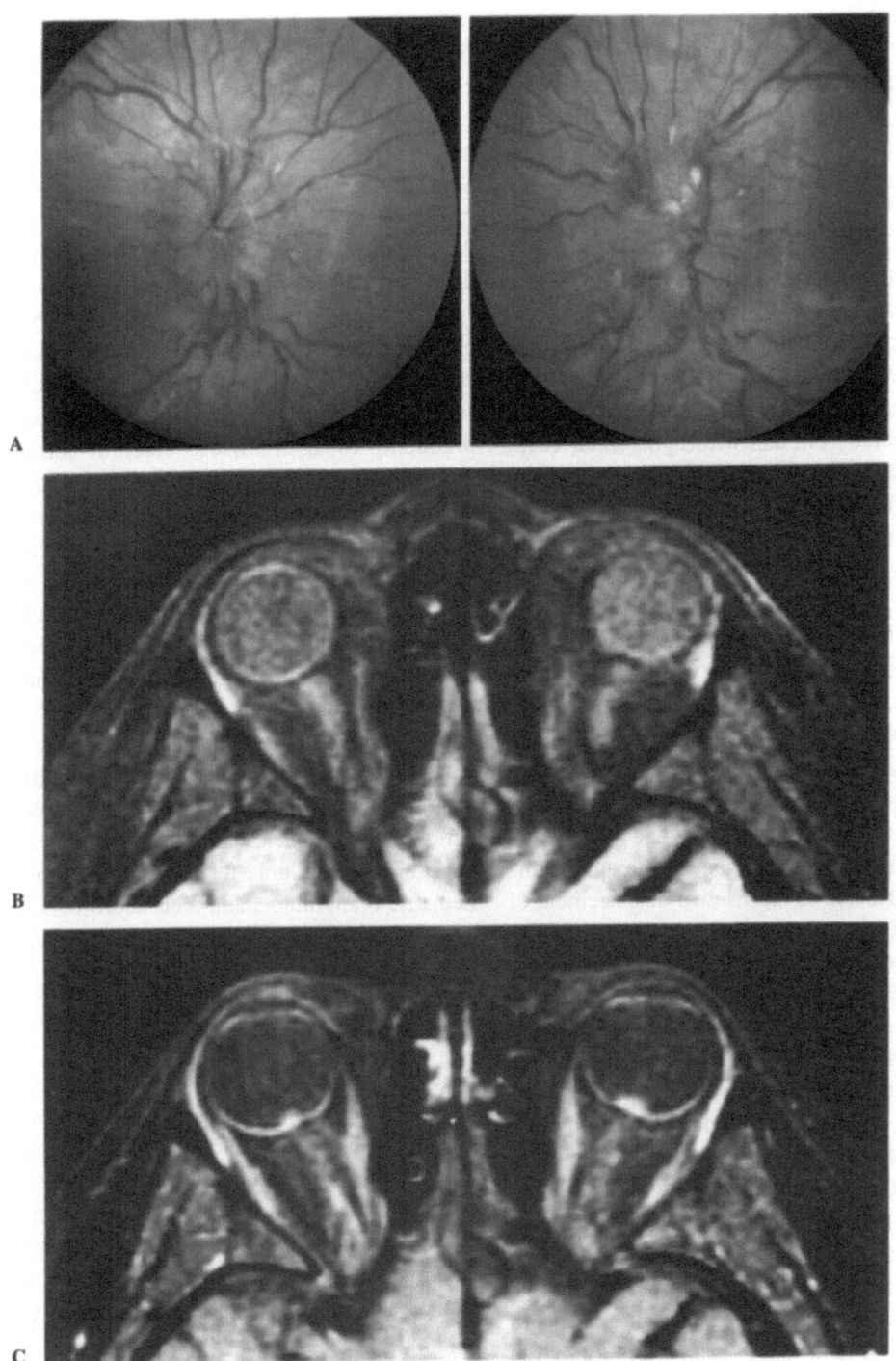

FIGURE 3.3. MR imaging in a child with pseudotumor cerebri. (A) Bilateral papilledema. (B) Intraocular signal abnormalities corresponding to the swollen discs are absent unenhanced MR images. (C) Following Gadolinium administration, the hyperintense signal corresponding to the swollen optic discs is visible within the vitreous cavities. (From Brodsky MC, Glasier CM. Magnetic resonance visualization of the swollen optic disk in papilledema. J Clin Neuro-ophthalmol 1994 in press, with permission.)

quently present upon awakening. Transient visual obscurations consist of "gray-outs" or "fuzz-outs" of vision, each lasting a few seconds. They occur from one or two to several hundred times per day and often occur upon bending over or standing up or with Valsalva pressure. Although they are thought to result from momentary ischemia, an electrochemical perturbation would seem equally plausible. Diplopia, when present, is usually horizontal and incomitant, reflecting the presence of unilateral or bilateral sixth nerve palsy. Sixth nerve palsies caused by elevated intracranial pressure are typically incomplete. Third and fourth nerve palsies have also rarely been attributed to increased intracranial pressure as have skew deviation and acute comitant esotropia. Such cases should be viewed as due directly to an intracranial mass lesion until proven otherwise.

Visual acuity is usually normal in the patient with papilledema, except in cases where signs of chronic disc swelling or atrophy are present. However, visual field defects are common even in early papilledema. When tested with Goldmann perimetry, concentric enlargement of the blind spot is the most common, and frequently the only, visual field defect in patients with papilledema. Automated static perimetry is more sensitive and frequently demonstrates inferonasal field loss and constriction of isopters. Blind spot enlargement in papilledema has been attributed to mechanical displacement of the peripapillary retina by the swollen disc. Recently, Corbett et al showed that the size of the enlarged blind spot could be reduced by addition of plus lenses, demonstrating that blind spot enlargement in papilledema is primarily refractive in nature.[52] Accurate visual field testing can be problematic in younger children, although close attention and frequent rest periods often enable one to surmount these difficulties. Progressive visual field loss usually evolves over months in patients with chronic and/or atrophic papilledema. Once central visual loss begins, it can progress rapidly, and blindness can ensue over a period of weeks to months. Visual field loss is usually severe by the time acuity begins to drop. The patient with papilledema whose visual acuity has decreased to 20/30 is therefore at grave risk for future visual loss, and surgical treatment is usually required.

It is important to document color vision whenever possible in children with papilledema. Sec-ondary macular pathology (e.g., choroidal folds, macular star figures, macular edema, macular pigmentary changes) can compromise vision in patients with papilledema[95,131,186] but tends to spare color vision. By contrast, an evolving optic neuropathy in the setting of chronic papilledema is virtually always associated with dyschromatopsia. Since decreasing visual acuity is an ominous sign in papilledema, the degree of dyschromatopsia assists the clinician in identifying those rare cases in which decreased acuity is due to macular pathology.

Intracranial mass lesions are the primary diagnostic consideration in the child or adult with papilledema. Brain tumors elevate intracranial pressure by acting as space occupying lesions, by producing focal or diffuse cerebral edema, by blocking the flow of cerebrospinal fluid, or by compressing a venous sinus.[179] Rarely, brain tumors, such as choroid plexus papilloma, can elevate intracranial pressure by producing excess CSF. Papilledema is more likely to develop in children with infratentorial than supratentorial tumors. Papilledema from infratentorial tumors usually results from compression of the aqueduct but may also be caused by pressure on the vein of Galen or occlusion of the posterior sagittal sinus.[179] The most common tumors associated with childhood papilledema are midbrain and cerebellar glioma, medulloblastoma, and ependymoma.[76] Pediatric brain tumors and their neuro-ophthalmologic sequelae will be detailed in chapter 10.

Pseudotumor Cerebri in Children

Pseudotumor cerebri is a condition characterized by symptoms and signs of increased intracranial pressure without evidence of a mass lesion or hydrocephalus.[55] It differs from other causes of increased intracranial pressure in that the level of consciousness is not altered. The diagnosis of *primary* pseudotumor cerebri is usually established when the following modified Dandy criteria are met:

1. Signs and symptoms of increased intracranial pressure.
2. Absence of localizing findings on neurological examination.
3. Absence of deformity, displacement, or obstruction of the ventricular system and other-

wise normal neurodiagnostic studies, except for increased CSF pressure.

4. Alert and oriented patient.
5. No other cause of increased intracranial pressure present.

In an elegant discussion of the numerous disorders of cerebrospinal fluid circulation causing intracranial hypertension without ventriculomegaly, Johnston et al[136] have proposed a classification of pseudotumor cerebri that reflects the concept of pseudotumor cerebri as a disorder of CSF outflow. We have modified this model (Table 3.1) to apply it to the different forms of pseudotumor cerebri of childhood. By expanding the diagnosis of pseudotumor cerebri to include intracranial hypertension without ventriculomegaly from a defect of CSF absorption (of any cause), one can begin to synthesize the numerous and disparate causes into a single conceptual framework in which the finding of clinical or neuroimaging abnormalities would not preclude the diagnosis of pseudotumor cerebri as long as the mechanism of decreased CSF absorption is present.

The accumulated evidence best supports a blockage of CSF absorption that presumably occurs at the level of the Pacchionian granulations. This hypothesis is consistent with the absence of tight junctions in the ependymal cells surrounding the lateral ventricles, which allows high-pressure fluid to move transependymally into the extracellular space. The absence of tight junctions in pial cells that cover the cerebral convexities allows high-pressure fluid to communicate from the lateral ventricles to the subarachnoid space and vice versa. This flow may lead to the establishment of an equilibrium between raised CSF outflow resistance and increased brain stiffness (occurring as a consequence of increased cerebral blood volume and/or mild interstitial cerebral edema), which would explain the absence of ventriculomegaly in pseudotumor cerebri. The development of such a steady state of CSF fluid migration would also help explain the inability of some studies to demonstrate increased periventricular brain water content on MR imaging.[50,250] Two other studies[188,257] found increased periventricular signal intensity (presumably signifying low-grade edema) in patients with

---

TABLE 3.1. Classification of pseudotumor cerebri in children. (Modified from Johnston et al.[136])

1. Primary pseudotumor cerebri
    A. No recognized cause (idiopathic pseudotumor cerebri or benign intracranial hypertension)
2. Secondary pseudotumor cerebri
    A. Pseudotumor cerebri associated with neurological disease
        Dural venous sinus thrombosis (associated with otitis media, mastoiditis, or head trauma)
        Altered CSF composition (meningitis)
        Arteriovenous malformation draining into a venous sinus
        Gliomatosis cerebri
    B. Pseudotumor cerebri secondary to systemic disease
        Malnutrition
        Systemic lupus erythematosis
        Polyangiitis overlap syndrome
        Addison disease
        Severe anemia (aplastic or iron deficiency)
    C. Pseudotumor cerebri secondary to ingestation or withdrawal of exogenous agents
        Corticosteroid withdrawal
        Malnutrition or renutrition
        Tetracycline or minocycline therapy (used in teenagers to suppress acne)
        Vitamin A intoxication—often in adolescents who take vitamin A or the synthetic vitamin A derivative isoretinoin for acne
        Nalidixic acid (used in the treatment of urinary tract infection and bacillary dysentery)
        Thyroxine replacement in hypothyroidism
        Danazol, danocrine (used for endometriosis or autoimmune hemolytic anemia)
3. Atypical pseudotumor cerebri
    A. Occult pseudotumor cerebri (no papilledema)
    B. Normal pressure pseudotumor cerebri
    C. Infantile pseudotumor cerebri

pseudotumor cerebri. In one of these studies,[188] however, the increased white matter signal intensity was demonstrable only by statistical analysis of periventricular signal intensities.[188]

Corbett[54] has proposed that elevated levels of free vitamin A in obese patients may be the underlying factor that damages arachnoidal granulations and leads to decreased CSF absorption in primary pseudotumor cerebri. The evidence of an adverse effect of high vitamin A intake on intracranial pressure is well recognized. Infants given large oral doses of vitamin A develop acute swelling of the anterior fontanelle with vomiting, agitation, and insomnia. These changes occur after only a few hours delay and usually subside 24 to 48 hours later.[173] While 98% of vitamin A is said to be stored in the liver, there is evidence that this fat-soluble vitamin may be stored in fat to a greater degree than generally appreciated. Unbound vitamin A (retinyl esters) is a toxic agent that triggers cell death by activating lysosomal enzymes. It is therefore attached to different carrier proteins throughout the body. In the blood, it is bound to retinol binding protein. In the CSF, it is attached to prealbumin (transthyretin), a carrier protein synthesized at the choroid plexus. Any condition leading to elevated levels of unbound vitamin A within the CSF, such as endogenous obesity, excess ingestion, or renal failure (which results in decreased excretion of retinol-binding protein and secondarily high levels of total vitamin A), could exceed the capacity of transthyretin to bind it. Free vitamin A within the CSF would then percolate out into the Pacchionian granulations where it produces damage to the endothelial cells, which eventuates in decreased CSF absorption. Since CSF transthyretin also binds thyroxine, the occurence of pseudotumor cerebri during thyroxine replacement in hypothyroidism (which would deplete CSF transthyretin and increase the level of unbound vitamin A in the CSF) is consistent with this hypothetical mechanism, as is the association of pseudotumor cerebri with obesity, and its occurrence in women (who have more body fat). The changing hormonal status at menarche may have a contributory effect upon vitamin A storage and binding. Drugs and toxins associated with pseudotumor cerebri may have an effect upon absorption, binding, storage, or transmission of vitamin A.

MR Imaging in Pseudotumor Cerebri

MR imaging shows an empty sella in 71% of adults with pseudotumor cerebri.[177] The incidence of empty sella in children with pseudotumor cerebri is unknown. Empty sella is thought to result from a pressure-induced, downward herniation of the suprasellar subarachnoid space into the sella, with secondary compression and flattening of the pituitary gland.[177] MR imaging in pseudotumor cerebri may also show tortuosity of the intraorbital optic nerves, with a widened perineural CSF signal. Intraocular protrusion of the swollen optic discs can occasionally be visualized following gadolinium enhancement (Figure 3.3). [38]

Primary Pseudotumor Cerebri in Children

Although pseudotumor cerebri is generally considered to be a disease of obese women of childbearing age, its occurrence in children has been documented in numerous studies.[13,15,162] Recent studies have noted that the clinical profile of pediatric pseudotumor cerebri differs in many respects from the adult variety (Table 3.2), which suggests that the precipitating factors may be different in children.

Unlike adults, in whom there is a strong female predominance, the male-female ratio for pseudotumor cerebri in prepubescent children is approximately equal.[13,15,162] Starting at puberty, however, there is a distinct female predominance. A self-limited form of pseudotumor cerebri may develop in girls following the onset of menstruation.[104] Obesity is less common in children than adults with pseudotumor cerebri. Spontaneous remission appears to be more common in children and may even follow a diagnostic lumbar puncture.[274]

Infants and young children may present with irritability, listlessness, and somnolence.[14,108,162] Dizziness or ataxia may also be evident.[108,162] Irritability, nervousness, or apathy may be observed in older children.[108] Generalized seizures have also been reported.[108] Infants with open fontanelles who have elevated intracranial pressure may still develop manifest papilledema.[162] Complaints of earache or roaring tinnitus are relatively common in children as well as adults.[101] These associated symptoms should raise the diagnostic consideration of lateral venous sinus thrombosis.[101] The incidence of certain neurological

TABLE 3.2. Clinical and epidemiological differences between pediatric and adult pseudotumor cerebri (intracranial hypertension).

	Pediatric	Adult
Potential for permanent visual loss	Yes	Yes
Sex ratio	50:50 before puberty; female predominance thereafter	10:1 female predominance
Obesity	Not a factor under age 10	Rare in non-obese females
Spontaneous remission	Common	Rare, often associated with residual intracranial pressure elevation even when papilledema resolves
Response to oral corticosteroids	Possibly better in children	Fair
Corticosteroid withdrawal	Possibly more causative in children	Rarely causative in adults
Indications for surgical intervention	Progressive visual loss regardless of whether a causative factor is defined	Same

deficits appear to be more common among children than adults. These include a higher incidence of lateral rectus paresis and atypical neurological manifestations, such as skew deviation, facial paresis, as well as neck, shoulder, and back pain.[162] It has been suggested that facial nerve paresis in pseudotumor cerebri results from traction on the extra-axial facial nerves associated with small brainstem shifts caused by elevated intracranial pressure.[245]

Until recently, the consensus from clinical studies was that young patients with pseudotumor cerebri tolerate chronic papilledema well and that visual loss from pseudotumor cerebri is extremely rare in the pediatric age group.[101–103,108,224,274] In summarizing 23 cases of childhood pseudotumor cerebri, Rose and Matson[224] concluded that "benign intracranial hypertension (in children) thus emerges as a clinical syndrome of varied etiology, generally with a short course, good prognosis, little tendency to recurrence, and only rarely requiring surgical intervention." It is now well established that permanent visual loss may occur in both the adult and pediatric variants of pseudotumor cerebri[13,14,55,162] and that children share similar risks as adults.[14,15,161] Recognition of this visual morbidity has led to discarding the term *benign intracranial hypertension* in favor of the term *idiopathic intracranial hypertension*.

Optic atrophy as a consequence of chronic papilledema is the cause of visual loss in pseudotumor cerebri. In severe cases, loss of vision may evolve over a period of weeks; the finding of decreased vision therefore demands aggressive and urgent intervention. In addition to chronic atrophic

papilledema, rarer causes of visual loss, such as central retinal artery occlusion, peripapillary subretinal neovascularization, anterior ischemic optic neuropathy, and macular edema, should also be sought.[14] The assessment of progressive visual loss is more difficult in children who are unable to cooperate for visual field testing.

Secondary Pseudotumor Cerebri

Once the diagnosis of pseudotumor cerebri has been established, one must exclude the presence of associated neurological disorders, systemic disease, or ingestion of vitamins or other medications that are known to precipitate pseudotumor cerebri (Table 3.2). The latter two categories merge together in patients for whom an exogenous agent is used to treat a systemic disease (e.g., thyroid replacement for hypothyroidism or danazol therapy for anemia).[111,162] The three most commonly recognized causes of childhood pseudotumor cerebri are dural venous thrombosis, steroid withdrawal, and malnutrition associated with refeeding.

Pseudotumor Cerebri Secondary
to Neurological Disease

The importance of otitis media, mastoiditis, and lateral sinus thrombosis in childhood pseudotumor cerebri has long been recognized.[102,264] Such cases of otitic hydrocephalus have decreased in recent decades as the incidence of mastoiditis has diminished with the advent of effective antibiotics.[55,162] The differential diagnosis of otitis media (with or without mastoiditis) associated with elevated intracranial pressure includes dural venous sinus thrombosis, venous sinus compression by a regional abscess, and contiguous meningitis.[102,264] It is the prevailing belief of most authorities that increased intracranial pressure may also follow an acute and uncomplicated otitis media.[55,101,264]

Several earlier studies identified otitis media with mastoiditis as a major cause.[101,102] At mastoidectomy in 11 such children, Greer consistently found compression of the junction between the lateral and sigmoid sinus by overlying necrotic material or abscess.[102] The primary channel for intracranial venous drainage is the sagittal sinus, which normally drains into the right lateral sinus. This explains the preponderance of right-sided infections in children with otitis-associated pseudotumor cerebri.[102] Lateral sinus thrombosis, although less frequent today, remains an important consideration in childhood pseudotumor cerebri since children with dural sinus thrombosis may be at increased risk for visual loss compared to those with primary pseudotumor cerebri.[14] Lateral sinus thrombosis, mastoiditis, and cerebral abscess can usually be identified on MR imaging (Figure 3.4). Obstruction of the transverse, sagittal, or straight sinus may follow seemingly insignificant head trauma in children and cause intracranial hypertension.[224,265]

Early investigators noted that pseudotumor cerebri in children may develop after a symptom-free period of weeks following bacterial or viral infections. They speculated that pseudotumor cerebri in such patients might be related to venous thrombosis within the pterygoid plexus, with propagation of the thrombus into the jugular vein (Figure 3.4).[224,265] It may also result from blockage of the arachnoid granulation by inflammatory material in predisposed individuals.

Papilledema may be seen in children with arteriovenous malformations who have no signs of hydrocephalus or recent subarachnoid hemorrhage. In this setting, papilledema probably results from decreased CSF absorption related to high pressure in the venous sinuses caused by arterial blood shunted directly into the cerebral veins, resulting in increased cerebral venous pressure.[155,275] Impairment of cranial venous outflow can theoreti-

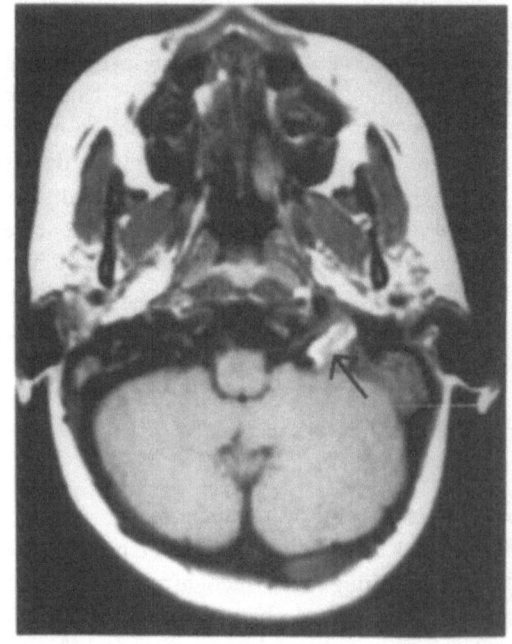
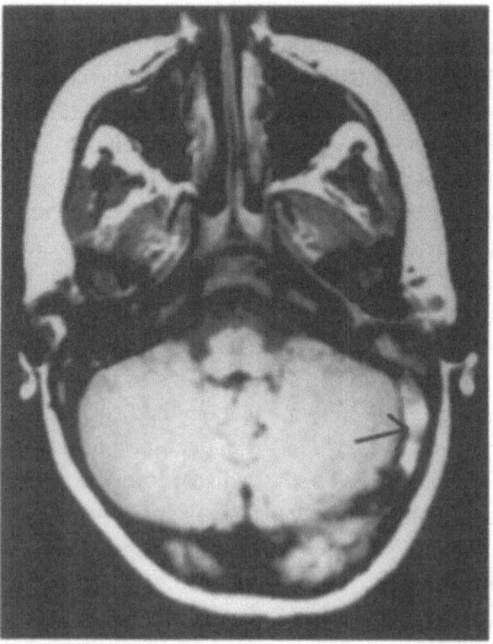

FIGURE 3.4. Pseudotumor cerebri following mastoiditis "otitic hydrocephalus." (A) Focal high-signal intensity area on T2-weighted MR imaging corresponds to thrombosis of the left jugular vein (arrow). (B) Hyperintense signal (arrow) in same patient corresponds to left transverse sinus thrombosis.

cally elevate intracranial pressure in the following three ways: (1) an increase in venous intracranial pressure may distend the capacitance component of the intracranial vasculature, leading to an increase in cerebral blood volume; (2) there may be brain edema with or without venous infarction; and (3) there may be impairment of CSF absorption due to reduction or reversal of the normal pressure gradient between the subarachnoid space and the superior sagittal sinus, which drives the bulk flow of CSF across the absorptive channels in the arachnoid villi.[136] Postoperative intracranial pressure elevation associated with cerebral edema and/or hemorrhage may also complicate embolization or surgical obliteration of large arteriovenous malformations (AVMs).[7,280]

Papilledema may also develop in children with meningitis or meningoencephalitis.[179] In most cases, elevated intracranial pressure is presumed to result from a secondary pseudotumor cerebri mechanism in which abnormal CSF composition impedes the absorption of CSF by cellular or macromolecular obstruction of channels in the arachnoid villi or by involvement of the narrow supracortical subarachnoid space over the cerebral convexities.[136] Meningitis can also be associated with an inflammatory optic neuritis, which should be suspected in the child with swollen discs and decreased acuity. It is impossible, however, to distinguish inflammatory disc swelling from papilledema on the basis of clinical findings alone.[179] Only when a lumbar puncture is performed and a normal opening pressure with increased protein and cellular contents is found can the diagnosis of inflammatory optic neuritis be established.[179]

Pseudotumor Cerebri Secondary to Systemic Disease

Systemic Lupus Erythematosis. Systemic lupus erythematosis is sometimes complicated by pseudotumor cerebri in children prior to commencement of corticosteroid therapy.[162] Pseudotumor cerebri has also been described in a child as a feature of polyangiitis overlap syndrome.[87] It is important to remember that pseudotumor cerebri can occasionally be the presenting sign of systemic vasculitis, and to be attuned to associated signs of systemic vasculitis in children with pseu-

dotumor cerebri so that early intervention can be initiated.

Severe Anemia. Papilledema is a rare but well-recognized complication of severe anemia in children as well as adults. Guiseffi et al[106] and Ireland et al[134] found similar frequencies of iron deficiency anemia between adults with pseudotumor cerebri and controls, suggesting that the purported association of iron deficiency (a common condition) with pseudotumor cerebri may be spurious. Nevertheless, some cases of childhood pseudotumor cerebri associated with severe iron deficiency anemia have been reported to resolve following iron supplementation.[105,133]

While few patients with iron deficiency anemia develop papilledema, this finding may be more common (albeit often overlooked) in patients with aplastic anemia.[164] In a review of 120 patients with aplastic anemia, Wang et al[272] found unequivocal disc swelling in 10 patients and blurred disc margins in an additional 34 patients. Papilledema in patients with immune hemolytic anemia may also be due to treatment with Danazol, an attenuated androgen derived from ethisterone.[70,111] Although it has been suggested that optic disc swelling in such patients could also result from local hypoxia associated with anemia (i.e., an "energy-deficient" optic neuropathy),[168] the cause of elevated intracranial pressure in the context of severe anemia is unknown.

Addison Disease

Although many purported cases of pseudotumor cerebri in Addison disease have been incompletely documented, Alexandrakis et al[6] recently provided convincing documentation of this association in a 12-year-old boy whose papilledema resolved following corticosteroid replacement. The findings of weakness, weight loss, hypotension, cutaneous or mucous membrane pigmentation, and abdominal symptoms should suggest this diagnosis.

Gliomatosis Cerebri

The development of gliomatosis cerebri in a 16-year-old child who presented with signs and symptoms of pseudotumor cerebri has recently been described.[283] Gliomatosis cerebri is an uncommon central nervous system (CNS) primary neoplasm that is characterized by proliferation of neoplastic glial cells, usually astrocytes with varying degrees of malignant potential. These cells infiltrate the cerebral cortex but do not destroy its cytoarchitecture.[283] Since the clinical presentation is usually neurologically nonfocal, the diagnosis is often delayed. Diffuse infiltration produces increased intracranial pressure with headache, nausea, vomiting, and papilledema. In the absence of a localized intracranial mass, these signs may lead to the diagnosis of pseudotumor cerebri.[283] The diagnosis of gliomatosis cerebri should be considered in a child with pseudotumor cerebri who develops progressive, neurological dysfunction or MR evidence of subtle signal abnormalities. The prognosis of gliomatosis cerebri is dismal, with survival ranging from a few weeks to several years after diagnosis. Responsiveness to radiation therapy presumably depends on the grade of the neoplasm. New chemotherapeutic regimens are currently under investigation.[283]

Childhood Pseudotumor Cerebri Associated with Administration or Withdrawal of Exogenous Agents

The phenomenon of childhood pseudotumor cerebri during or following corticosteroid withdrawal in children is well recognized.[103,169] Multiple reports of pseudotumor cerebri developing in children receiving thyroid replacement therapy leave little doubt that this association is valid. Nalidixic acid, a urinary tract antiseptic, has been reported to cause pseudotumor cerebri.[162] There are numerous reports implicating tetracycline and minocycline, which are bacteriostatic antibiotics.[162] Ciprofloxacin, a ubiquitous quinolone antibiotic whose parent compound is naladixic acid, has precipitated pseudotumor cerebri in a 14-year-old child with cystic fibrosis who was also receiving vitamin supplementation.[281] Vitamin A intoxication is well-established in the pathogenesis of some cases of pseudotumor cerebri (discussed earlier). This association should be considered in adolescents who take vitamin A for acne. Isotretoin, a synthetic retinoid used for the treatment of acne, has been implicated in the pathogenesis of pseudotumor cerebri in adolescents. Because of these associations, it is crucial to obtain a history regarding medical treatment for acne in the adolescent with pseudotumor cerebri.

Pseudotumor cerebri has also been recognized in malnourished children and immediately upon renourishment. Couch et al[55] found this to be the underlying cause in 26% of children with pseudotumor cerebri. They noted that nutritionally deprived children often display accelerated growth of the head when they are renourished. Animal models have shown malnutrition to severely impede bone growth. Refeeding presumably permits more rapid growth of the brain than the skull vault, which would explain the development of raised intracranial pressure.[55] Couch et al described a transient type of "nutritional pseudotumor cerebri" that occurs within days of starting treatment for cystic fibrosis. The rapid early onset and rapid resolution in this group suggests that some mechanism other than differential brain growth is occuring.[55]

Atypical Pseudotumor Cerebri in Children

A syndrome of *transient intracranial hypertension of infancy* exists in which the affected infant presents with a febrile illness associated with a bulging anterior fontanelle and irritability. Some infants present with an abnormal rate of head growth and a head circumference above the 90th percentile.[136] These infants are without neurological or developmental abnormalities and have normal imaging studies except for mild ventricular dilatation and distension of the subarachnoid space in some cases.[136] Papilledema is infrequently present. Symptoms may abate following a single lumbar puncture, and intracranial pressure typically normalizes over days. This condition has been attributed to a nonspecific infectious illness that interferes with absorption of cerebrospinal fluid by the arachnoid villi. When an infant with the diagnosis of transient intracranial hypertension fails to improve, the possibility of early meningitis that has failed to cause an initial pleocytosis must be considered, and a repeat lumbar puncture should be performed.[171]

Treatment of Pseudotumor Cerebri in Children

Spontaneous resolution of pseudotumor cerebri appears to be more common in children than adults. In some children, pseudotumor cerebri resolves following a single lumbar puncture. Because of the potential for permanent visual loss,[14,15] however, children with pseudotumor cerebri should not be followed with less vigilance than adults. Some investigators believe that oral steroids are more efficacious in children than in adults with pseudotumor cerebri and advocate their use.[274] Some have found the combination of furosemide and high-dose acetazolamide to be an effective nonsurgical intervention in children.[239]

Current surgical treatment of pseudotumor cerebri is limited to optic nerve sheath fenestration and lumboperitoneal shunt. Lumboperitoneal shunting is an effective means of reducing intracranial pressure, but shunt failures are frequent (particularly in obese individuals).[13] Shunt infection may be life-threatening, and acquired Chiari type I tonsillar herniation commonly occurs. Although successful lumboperitoneal shunting relieves headaches from elevated intracranial pressure, this form of headache may be traded for another due to hindbrain herniation.[13] Over the last 6 years, numerous studies have suggested that optic nerve sheath fenestration is the lowest-risk, most effective way to restore or preserve vision in pseudotumor cerebri,[13] and it has become the surgical treatment of choice. Optic nerve sheath fenestration is also efficacious in cases where lumboperitoneal shunting is unsuccessful. Optic nerve sheath fenestration relieves headaches in approximately two-thirds of patients.[53]

The finding of a potentially reversible cause of pseudotumor cerebri in a child (e.g. dural sinus thrombosis) should not lead to a false sense of security that the child is not at risk for blindness. Our indications for surgical intervention include the following:

1. Evidence of progressive optic neuropathy (i.e., loss of visual acuity or visual field despite maximal medical therapy, or worsening papilledema in a child who cannot cooperate with examination).
2. Severe optic neuropathy (i.e., chronic atrophic papilledema) that would seriously jeopardize the patient's ability to function normally if further visual loss occured.[15]

If these criteria are met, we believe that optic nerve sheath fenestration should be performed despite the fact that the underlying condition is expected to eventually resolve.

Optic Disc Swelling Secondary to Neurological Disease

Hydrocephalus

Papilledema is absent in the majority of infants with congenital hydrocephalus. Ghose[93] reviewed optic nerve changes in 200 consecutive cases of congenital hydrocephalus examined before shunt surgery and found papilledema in 12%. The absence of papilledema in the remaining cases has been attributed to the fact that open sutures permit the head to enlarge in response to increased intracranial pressure. However, the low prevalence of papilledema in infantile hydrocephalus is still perplexing since numerous studies have confirmed that infants with intracranial mass lesions still develop papilledema.[179] Despite the ability of the infant skull to enlarge and act as a "release valve" for elevated intracranial pressure, large or rapid elevations in intracranial pressure may exceed this response. In making the diagnosis of papilledema in an infant who appears to have hydrocephalus, it is important to consider the association of megalencephaly (a large heavy brain with normal to slightly dilated ventricles and normal intracranial pressure) and optic disc drusen in the differential diagnosis.[126]

Once a patient with hydrocephalus is shunted, the situation changes. Shunting allows the intracranial sutures to fuse, and subependymal gliosis may develop that can greatly reduce ventricular compliance. Subsequent shunt failure can produce marked papilledema, along with signs and symptoms of dorsal midbrain syndrome but no ventricular dilation.[51] Visual loss associated with postpapilledema optic atrophy remains a major morbidity in shunted congenital hydrocephalus. The neuro-ophthalmologic signs of shunt failure are discussed in Chapter 11.

Neurofibromatosis

Neurofibromatosis may produce optic disc swelling by several mechanisms. Most commonly, optic disc swelling in a child with neurofibromatosis signals the presence of an optic nerve glioma. Large chiasmal gliomas may also extend superiorly to compress the third ventricle and foramen of Monro and produce obstructive hydrocephalus.[179] Children with neurofibromatosis are also at higher risk for aqueductal stenosis. Spinal cord tumors, which can elevate intracranial pressure and produce papilledema, occur with increased frequency in patients with neurofibromatosis (see below).[176]

Spinal Cord Tumors

Spinal cord tumors are a well-recognized but easily missed cause of papilledema. Ependymomas constitute 40% of spinal cord tumors producing papilledema. Most spinal cord tumors associated with papilledema are located in the lumbar or thoracic region.[176] Symptoms of backache or gait disturbance should lead the clinician to check carefully for evidence of sensory or motor deficits. If present, further diagnostic evaluation (CT scanning, myelography) should be directed toward the possibility of an underlying spinal cord tumor.[176] The papilledema usually resolves following surgical excision of the lesion.[148]

Theories that have been put forth to explain the association of papilledema with spinal cord tumors are summarized in Table 3.3.

Subacute Sclerosing Panencephalitis

Subacute sclerosing panencephalitis (SSPE) is a fatal neurologic disease caused by the measles virus. It is more common in males and is usually associated with infection before 4 years of age.[231] Neurovisual symptoms first become apparent in late childhood or early adolescence. The diagnosis is suggested by the clinical picture of mental deterioration, myoclonus and seizures, often with a

TABLE 3.3. Potential causes of papilledema with spinal cord tumors.[148,176]

Protein molecules released into the CSF by the tumor may mechanically block the arachnoidal pores and prevent CSF absorption.

An aseptic arachnoiditis may develop secondary to protein leakage.

CSF hyperviscosity may follow release of products of protein disintegration, which slows CSF circulation from the cranial circulation to the spinal spaces.

Spinal cord tumors may hemorrhage into the subarachnoid space.

The spinal cord normally acts as an "elastic reservoir" for cerebrospinal fluid. Spinal cord tumors may reduce the capacitance of this reservoir by mechanical blockage and thereby cause papilledema.

---

characteristic maculopathy (see chapter 10).[231] Cortical visual loss, hemianopia, impaired visual spatial abilities, and visual hallucinations develop. The diagnosis is confirmed by elevated CSF and serum titers, measles titers, and immunoglobulin elevation. The classic electroencephalogram (EEG) changes are sharp wave complexes every 5 to 15 seconds in a "burst-suppression pattern."

Optic disc swelling has been reported frequently in SSPE and is generally ascribed to elevated intracranial pressure, although Hiatt et al[122] found optic neuritis in 6% of patients. A ground-glass whitening of the macula with mottling of the underlying pigment epithelium is commonly found. Over time, a gliotic retinal scar with contracture of the inner limiting membrane may develop. The SSPE is uniformly fatal.

Optic Disc Swelling Secondary to Systemic Disease

Diabetic Papillopathy

In 1971, Lubow and Makley reported three young patients with juvenile-onset diabetes and bilateral optic disc edema, with an intricate capillary network on the surface of the disc.[167] Visual disturbances were minimal (in two patients, the disc swelling was discovered on routine examination), and the disc edema resolved spontaneously in approximately 6 months. Twelve cases reported by Barr et al[17] exhibited a similar picture: bilateral superior disc swelling that may be segmental, minimal reduction in visual acuity, mild visual field abnormalities (e.g., inferior arcuate scotomas, blind spot enlargement, inferior depression with involvement of fixation), excellent recovery, predominant occurrence in the second or third decades of life, no clear correlation with background diabetic retinopathy, and variable presence of dilated superficial radial capillaries on the surface of the disc (Figure 3.5).[17,204]

Patients with diabetic papillopathy tend to have small cupless discs, as seen in most adults with ischemic optic neuropathy. Some authors have hypothesized that optic disc edema in young patients with juvenile-onset diabetes represents a form of ischemic optic neuropathy.[41,137,255] Slavin has suggested that younger patients may have sufficient collateral circulation to spare the axons from irreversible injury that would impair vision.[255]

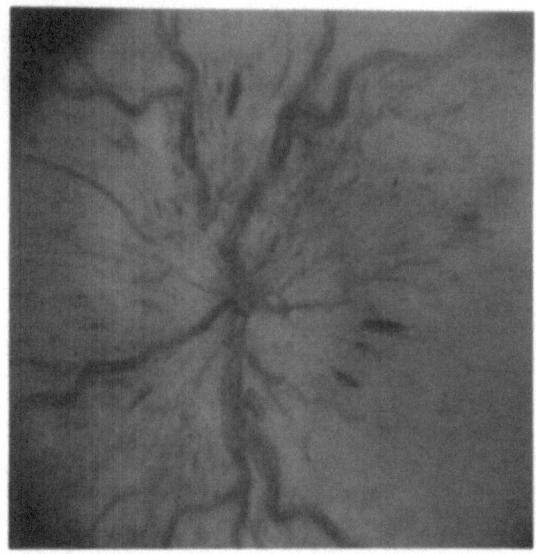

FIGURE 3.5. Diabetic papillopathy. Note bilateral optic disc edema and surface capillary dilation. (Courtesy of William F. Hoyt, MD.)

According to this hypothesis, the dilation of the superficial peripapillary capillary network would represent a compensatory mechanism to ameliorate the ischemic process.[41] Hayreh's finding of asymptomatic optic disc swelling in the contralateral eye of adults with typical nonarteritic ischemic optic neuropathy lends support to the hypothesis that this self-limited form of disc edema is secondary to axonal stasis from low-grade ischemia, which is insufficient to produce visual dysfunction.[115,140,255] Alternatively, disc swelling in young diabetics could result from a primary microangiopathy affecting the vascular bed subserving the distal optic nerve head, which would be influenced by local anatomic factors, such as axonal crowding due to the size of the surrounding scleral canal.[140,204]

Malignant Hypertension

Malignant hypertension in children is seen in several settings, including severe glomerulonephritis, vasculitis (lupus, polyarteritis), and renal artery stenosis, and in transplant patients with severe rejection. In the most widely used classification of hypertensive fundus changes, the presence of optic disc edema separates grades III and IV, with grade IV hypertension associated with a grave systemic prognosis. Disc swelling in malignant hypertension has been attributed to elevated CSF pressure due to cerebral edema, particularly in patients with hypertensive encephalopathy. Accordingly, optic disc swelling in this setting has been equated with papilledema.[116] However, Hayreh et al[118] have demonstrated that the optic disc swelling in hypertensive retinopathy is caused by local ischemia rather than by elevated intracranial pressure. The swollen optic disc characteristically shows either hyperemia or pallor. It is believed that leakage of high levels of angiotensin II from the choriocapillaris produces vasoconstriction in the choroid and choroidal occlusion. Additionally, diffusion of angiotensin through the border tissue of Elschnig and into the optic nerve head causes ischemia in the axons that reduces axoplasmic transport proximal to the ischemic site. This process causes disc swelling and, secondarily, more ischemia and occlusion with resultant swelling of the disc. In addition to the well-recognized signs of hypertensive retinopathy and choroidopathy, a pathognomonic finding—focal intraretinal periarteriolar transudates (FIPTs)—has been identified by Hayreh et al.[117] Blindness due to optic disc ischemia (AION) may occur if there is a precipitous reduction in blood pressure in patients with malignant hypertension.[118]

Sarcoidosis

Neurological complications of sarcoidosis are said to occur in 5% of patients, and autopsy studies have identified unrecognized CNS disease in 15%.[26,153] The CNS involvment in childhood sarcoidosis is less common than in adults. Neurosarcoidosis has a predilection for the base of the brain.[248] Granulomatous meningitis at the skull base with infiltration or compression of adjacent nerves is the most common intracranial manifestation.[141,288] Neurological manifestations include cranial nerve palsies, meningitis, hypothalamic and pituitary lesions, granulomatous basal meningitis, space-occupying masses (mimicking gliomas and meningiomas), peripheral neuropathy, spinal cord involvement, and progressive multifocal leukoencephalopathy.[240,248,291] Facial nerve palsy is the most common neurological manifestation of sarcoidosis, followed by involvement of the optic nerves and chiasm and, in descending order of frequency, the glossopharyngeal, vagus, and auditory nerves.[248] Localized granulomatous lesions have been found in practically every part of the CNS, including the meninges, the floor of the third ventricle, the lateral ventricle, the occipital, frontal, and temporal lobes, the optic chiasm, the optic nerves, the basal ganglia, the cerebellum, and the spinal cord.[240]

The evaluation of optic disc swelling in a child with sarcoidosis requires a detailed ocular and systemic evaluation. Optic disc edema in sarcoidosis may be due to infiltration of the disc (i.e., granulomatous optic neuritis), a local reaction to contiguous intraocular inflammation, or an indirect effect of neurosarcoidosis (hydrocephalus or mass effect) (Table 3.4). The characteristic irregular, cauliflower appearance of the infiltrated optic disc is a clue to the diagnosis of neurosarcoidosis (Figure 3.6).[19]

Magnetic resonance imaging and lumbar puncture combined with evaluation of the anterior and posterior chambers of the eye are useful in determining which mechanisms are primarily responsible for the optic disc edema.[68] Gadolinium increases the sensitivity of MR imaging if steroids have not been given, permitting detection of meningeal, parenchymal, optic nerve, and ependymal sarcoid lesions not visible on unenhanced scans.[62,246,291] Lumbar puncture serves to rule out elevated intracranial pressure and other infectious

TABLE 3.4. Causes of optic disc swelling in sarcoidosis.

Granulomatous infiltration of the optic nerve head.
Postlaminar granulomatous involvement of the optic nerve or surrounding meninges (retrobulbar neuritis).
Papilledema secondary to intracerebral masses, hydrocephalus, or granulomatous meningitis.
Ischemic optic nerve infarction associated with perivascular inflammation.
Pseudotumor cerebri associated with steroid withdrawal.
Disc swelling secondary to ocular hypotony.
Disc swelling secondary to contiguous intraocular inflammation.

and granulomatous disorders (tuberculosis, coccidioidomycosis, parasites, and lymphoma). Diagnostic tests with the highest yield and common clinical usage include chest X-ray, ACE level, serum lysozyme levels, limited gallium scan, and tissue biopsy.[26] Radiological evidence of bilateral hilar adenopathy, with or without parenchymal involvement, is a hallmark of the disease. Serum angiotensin converting enzyme is elevated in approximately 80% of children aged 8 to 15 with sarcoidosis, but this figure may be lower for children under 5 years of age.[125] Biopsy confirmation may be obtained from nodular areas of skin, conjunctiva, and lacrimal gland. Conjunctival biopsies yield positive results in only 10% to 28% of eyes without visible granulomas.[125]

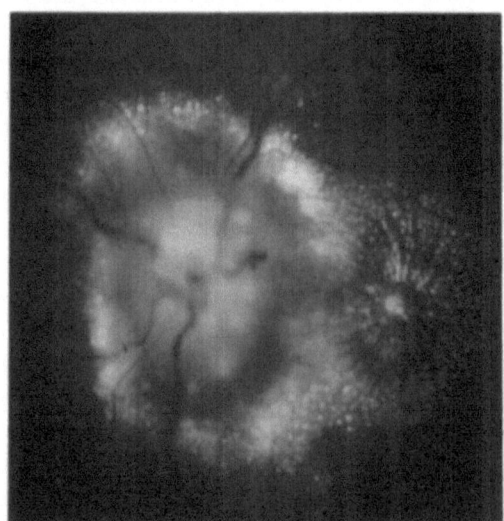 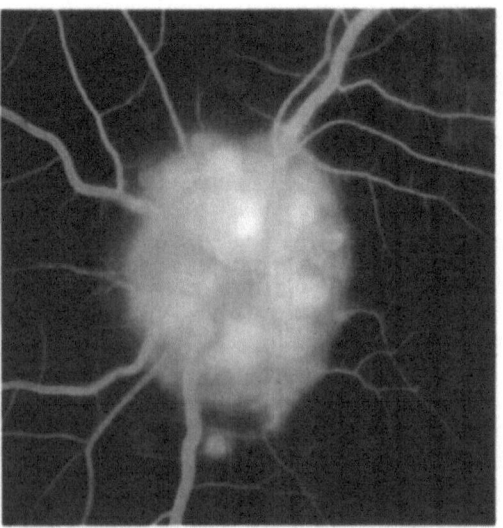

FIGURE 3.6. (A) Optic disc elevation secondary to granulomatous infiltration of the disc in sarcoidosis. (B) Fluorescein angiogram demonstrating nodular hyperfluorescence of the disc. (Courtesy of William F. Hoyt M.D.)

Sarcoid optic neuropathy is a very nasty and unforgiving problem. Chronic steroids or treatment with steroid-sparing agents may be required to prevent blindness. Methotrexate and cyclosporine have been used in some resistant cases with good results. The acute form of meningitis responds favorably to corticosteroids, whereas chronic meningitis may go through a cycle of remissions and exacerbations that require long-term steroid therapy.[248] Surgical therapy is indicated in cases of hydrocephalus, expanding mass lesions, or mass lesions causing increased intracranial pressure.[248] Seizure activity with neurosarcoidosis is a bad prognostic sign.[153]

Leukemia

The diverse spectrum of ocular involvement in childhood leukemia can be divided into three groups: neuro-ophthalmologic features associated with CNS involvement, vascular abnormalities reflecting changes in hematological status, and direct infiltration of ocular tissues.[215] The acute forms of leukemia are responsible for most of these ocular and CNS complications.[8,57,237] Since modern chemotherapy has prolonged survival and provided a possibility of cure in leukemic children, it has also increased the incidence of leukemic cell infiltration, especially of the CNS.[200] While optic nerve infiltration is usually related to CNS involvement, anterior segment infiltration frequently occurs in the absence of CNS disease.[198,215] Optic nerve infiltration occurs mainly in children with acute leukemia, with a proclivity for acute myelocytic leukemia.[226]

Several mechanisms have been defined by which leukemia can produce swelling of the optic nerve head (Table 3.5).[66] The differentiation between leukemic infiltration of the optic nerve and disc swelling due to increased CSF pressure remains the fundamental clinical distinction to be made as early cases of leukemic infiltration can be reversed with local irradiation.[57,66,127,216] Optic nerve infiltration may be predominantly prelaminar or retrolaminar.[226] Prelaminar leukemic infiltration of the optic nerve head appears as an elevated, fluffy, whitish swelling of the disc that progressively obscures the retinal vessels and is associated with edema and varying degrees of hemorrhage (Figure 3.7).[226] Larger infiltrates may

TABLE 3.5. Causes of optic disc swelling with leukemia.

Leukemic infiltration of the optic nerve head.

Papilledema secondary to leukemic CNS infiltrate, intracranial hemorrhage, steroid withdrawal following prolonged treatment, or opportunistic CNS infection.

Papilledema related to leukemic infiltrates in the CNS.

Ischemic optic neuropathy secondary to local vascular compromise from tumor infiltration of the optic nerve or orbit, to sludging of blood flow secondary to hyperviscosity, or to small vessel thrombosis in the microcirculation of the optic nerve in patients with thrombocytosis.

Optic neuropathy secondary to opportunistic infections of the CNS that are more common in leukemic patients.

extend into the peripapillary retina and produce sheathing of the contiguous retinal vessels. The leukemic cells are characteristically most numerous in the perioptic meninges and peripheral portions of the nerve, and then they extend along the optic septa to accumulate about the blood vessels within the optic nerve.[8,57] Direct leukemic invasion of the optic nerve head usually causes slowly progressive visual loss that occurs late in the course of the infiltration, although it can occasionally proceed rapidly.[57] When leukemic infiltration is primarily posterior to the lamina cribrosa, a profound decrease in vision is usually accompanied by swelling of the disc without visible infiltrate.[226] Leukemic infiltration of the optic nerve is

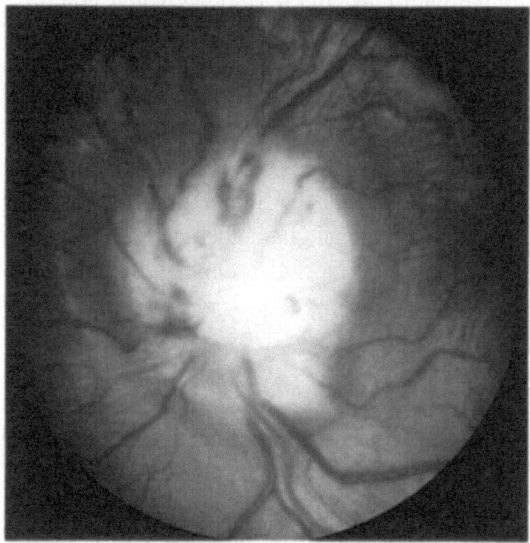

FIGURE 3.7. Leukemic infiltration of the optic disc. (Courtesy of William F. Hoyt, MD.)

a visual emergency requiring immediate local irradiation (approximately 2000 rads over a 1- to 2-week period), usually combined with intrathecal injection of cytotoxic drugs.[196] Optic atrophy is a frequent sequela of irradiation therapy, whether or not it is used in conjunction with chemotherapy. Leukemic patients may also develop optic disc edema following bone marrow transplantation,[11] believed to be a manifestation of cyclosporine toxicity. This swelling usually resolves without consequence following a decrease or discontinuation of cyclosporine. Lumbar puncture is essential, since irradiation therapy would not improve papilledema due to increased CSF pressure, while orbital irradiation is the treatment of choice for direct optic nerve infiltration.[226] Monoclonal typing of CSF lymphocytes may aid in the difficult clinical task of differentiating insidious optic nerve infiltration from infectious optic nerve damage.[57] The MR imaging shows promise in delineating leukemic optic nerve infiltration. Perineural enhancement within the subarachnoid space and leptomeninges has been accomplished with gadolinium and orbital fat suppression in a patient with leukemic invasion of the optic nerve.[127] The major forms of leukemic optic disc swelling are summarized in Table 3.5.

The prognostic implications of ophthalmic involvement in childhood leukemia are mostly negative.[200] In a 15-year study period, 28 of 131 children with leukemia developed ocular complications. Twenty seven of these patients died within 28 months from the onset of the ophthalmic involvement. All patients with ophthalmic manifestations had either bone marrow relapse or CNS involvement. Ocular involvement would appear, then, to be the harbinger of a relapse.[215] Newer investigational chemotherapeutic regimens may improve the morbid prognosis in this subgroup.

Cyanotic Congenital Heart Disease

A retinopathy consisting of dilated, tortuous retinal veins, and optic disc elevation has been described in patients with congenital heart disease. Petersen and Rosenthal[205] found optic disc elevation in 12 of 52 patients with cyanotic congenital heart disease. The severity of the fundus changes was closely related to the patient's arterial oxygen

saturation and hematocrit, but not to arterial PCO_2, pH, central venous pressure, type of cardiac malformation, or the patient's age. The retinopathy of cyanotic congenital heart disease resembles that seen in patients with polycythemia. Local hypoxemia, which causes retinal vasodilation, may also play a major role.[205] The role of elevated intracranial pressure, if any, has not been determined.

Craniosynostosis syndromes

Craniosynostosis syndromes primarily involve the cranium and upper face.[266] Each condition involves premature closure of one or more sutures that limits skull growth in the direction perpendicular to the suture and results in compensatory growth in the unrestricted direction to minimize the compressive effect of the growing brain.[267] When brain growth exceeds growth of the skull, elevated intracranial pressure develops.

Craniosynostosis syndromes are commonly associated with papilledema or optic nerve atrophy.[85,96] In a series of 244 patients with craniosynostosis, Dufier et al[63] found disc edema in 31% with Crouzon's disease, 23% with oxycephaly, and 9.5% with Apert's disease. Optic discs were considered either pale or atrophic in 50% with Crouzon's disease, 34% with oxycephaly, and 24% with Apert's disease. Fishman et al have stressed that hydrocephalus appears to be independently associated with premature synostosis rather than occuring as a direct consequence of it.[75] Papilledema in these conditions can therefore result from elevated intracranial pressure related directly to premature synostosis, or from hydrocephalus. Bertelsen[29] noted that papilledema had not been observed in any of his children who developed optic atrophy.

Child Abuse (Shaken Baby Syndrome)

The shaken baby syndrome is a unique but common form of child abuse in which intracranial injury and intraocular hemorrhage may exist in the absence of external signs of direct head trauma.[156,278] Shaken baby syndrome occurs when a screaming child with elevated jugular venous pressure is squeezed and forcefully shaken. This action produces a sudden instantaneous rise in intracranial pressure. This pressure is transmitted down the optic nerve sheath which abruptly elevates retinal venous pressure, producing retinal hemorrhages.[278] The infant brain is particularly prone to whiplash injuries because of the proportionately larger and unsupported head, the pliability of sutures and fontanelles that allows stretching of the calvarium, the greater deformability of the unmyelinated brain, and the greater percentage of cerebrospinal fluid.[44,142] The common finding of subdural hemorrhage in infants with shaken baby syndrome is thought to result from tearing of the bridging cerebral vessels.[94] Contusion, laceration, and edema of the brain may also occur. The retinal hemorrhages may precede the subdural hemorrhage by days; repeat neuroimaging is therefore warranted if clinical deterioration is observed.[94] Wilkinson et al[278] found the severity of the intraocular hemorrhages correlated with the severity of the acute neurological injury. Mental retardation and other permanent neurological dysfunction are common.[44] Caffey emphasized the deleterious effects of even mild whiplash and swinging activities in young children and conjectured that many cases of mental retardation, cerebral palsy, and congenital hydrocephalus represent undiagnosed "shaken baby" injuries to the CNS.[44]

The importance of the presence or absence of papilledema as a distinguishing clinical sign in the evaluation of a child with retinal hemorrhages cannot be overstated. The presence of papilledema in the infant with retinal hemorrhages usually signifies coexistent intracranial hemorrhage or cerebral edema, which may or may not be traumatic in nature. Although the presence or absence of papilledema are both consistent with shaken baby syndrome, the *absence* of papilledema in a healthy infant with retinal hemorrhages suggests that any elevation in intracranial pressure must have been brief and warrants systemic evaluation for other physical signs of shaken baby syndrome (such as midsternal ecchymosis).[156] It is important to remember that papilledema takes 1 to 5 days to develop after intracranial pressure rises.[114] White, ring-shaped retinal folds that encircle the macula outside the vascular arcades are also highly suggestive of the shaken baby syndrome.[92] The autopsy finding of hemorrhage within the optic nerve sheath seems to be a relatively specific retrospective marker for this mechanism of injury.[40] Because CNS injury often coexists, the diagnosis

of shaken baby syndrome imparts a poor neurological prognosis. Cortical visual loss and macular pucker are common residua that often limit the ultimate visual prognosis.

As there are many causes of retinal hemorrhages in infancy, it is the cumulative clinical evidence along with social factors that enable one to make the diagnosis of shaken baby syndrome.[142] The ophthalmologist should resist the temptation to draw judgmental conclusions prematurely when examining infants with retinal hemorrhages.

Cysticercosis

Cysticercosis is a common worldwide parasite that affects the CNS.[141a] Humans serve as intermediate hosts in the life cycle of the pork tapeworm Taenia solium, when eggs are ingested with contaminated food.[263] The disease is endemic in Mexico, Central and South America, India, and China.[58] In Mexico, the prevalence of neurocysticercosis may be as high as 2% to 3% based on patients autopsied at general hospitals.[58] Neurocysticercosis can develop in children and adults, but symptoms occur most often in young adults. Before modern neuroimaging, neurocysticercosis was included in the differential diagnosis of pseudotumor cerebri.[209]

Many patients remain asymptomatic until degenerating parenchymal cysts produce contiguous inflammation, at which time seizures, increased intracranial pressure, altered mental status, and focal neurological signs develop.[58,141a,145] Degenerating parenchymal cysts may produce chronic meningitis. Papilledema and pretectal signs (associated with hydrocephalus) are the usual neuro-ophthalmologic manifestations of neurocysticercosis, although other brainstem and cerebellar signs, such as trochlear nerve palsy, facial myokymia, upbeat nystagmus, periodic alternating nystagmus, and oculopalatal myoclonus, have been reported.[145] Blindness from postpapilledema optic atrophy occurs in some cases.

The MR imaging and CT scanning are now considered to be complementary in the diagnosis of neurocysticercosis (Figure 3.8). Suh et al[263] found MR to be more sensitive than CT scanning for visualization of the scolex within the cystic lesions but less sensitive for detection of small calcifications. Since it has been estimated that dead

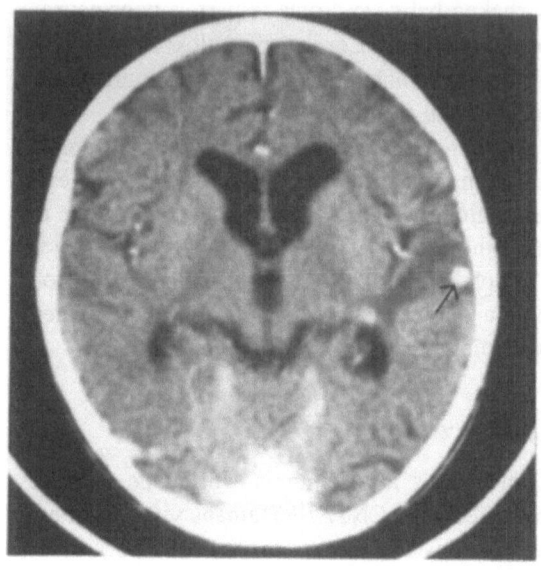

FIGURE 3.8. Neurocysticercosis. CT scan demonstrates multiple intracranial cysts.

cysticercal larvae take 4 to 7 years to calcify (and become visible on CT scanning), MR imaging appears to be preferable in children.[43] The location of cysticerci can be intraventricular, cisternal, parenchymal, or meningeal.[43] In the neurologically symptomatic patient, the diagnosis of neurocysticercosis is almost always made presumptively from neuroimaging studies.

Ten years ago, an enzyme-linked immunosorbent assay (ELISA) test became available that, when applied to the CSF of people with active disease, has a sensitivity of over 80% and a specificity of over 90%. More recently, the Centers for Disease Control have developed an immunoblot test that detects both IgM and IgG antibodies to cysticercosis antigens and has a specificity close to 100% and a sensitivity of approximately 98% in both serum and CSF.[58]

Treatment of active neurocysticercosis consists of praziquantel, which kills cysticerci by a mechanism that is poorly understood.[58] Patients with inactive disease and dead cysts do not respond to praziquantal. Surgical removal is occasionally indicated for intraventricular cysts, which may have become dislodged and produce obstructive hydrocephalus. Patients with multiple cystic lesions may develop increased CNS symptoms shortly after praziquantel is started, which appears to result from intense reactive inflammation in the surrounding brain following death of the cysticerci. During treatment, patients must therefore be observed closely for worsening of papilledema, which may necessitate acetazolamide and/or optic nerve sheath fenestration.

Mucopolysaccharidosis

Optic disc swelling is a common ocular finding in patients with systemic mucopolysaccharidosis. In a study of 108 patients with optic disc edema, Collins et al[49] found a greater than 40% incidence of optic disc edema in patients with Hurler, Hurler–Scheie, Maroteux–Lamy, and Sly syndrome, 19.7% in Hunter syndrome, and 4.6% in Sanfilippo syndrome. No patient with Scheie or Morquio syndrome had optic disc edema. Optic disc swelling in mucopolysaccharidosis can result from any one or a combination of several mechanisms.[49] (Table 3.6)

Beck and Cole provided ocular histopathology[22] from a patient with Hunter syndrome who had optic disc swelling without raised intracranial pressure.[21] They confirmed deposition of abnormal mucopolysaccharides within the sclera and lamina cribrosa that produced gross thickening of these structures and compression of the optic nerve.

Infantile Malignant Osteopetrosis

Osteopetrosis describes a group of hereditary metabolic bone diseases in which osteoclast dysfunction results in abnormal bone resorption, thickened cortical bone, structural skeletal defects, and frequent bone fractures.[228] Reduced bone marrow space and replacement of its normal contents by chondro-osseous tissue in the sclerotic bones results in anemia, hepatosplenomegaly,

TABLE 3.6. Causes of optic disc elevation with mucopolysaccharidosis.[98]

Narrowing of the scleral canal by thickened, infiltrated peripapillary sclera.
Increased intracranial pressure associated with hydrocephalus.
Accumulation of acid mucopolysaccharides in retinal ganglion cells.
Compression of the optic nerve by thickened infiltrated meninges.

thrombocytopenia, leukopenia, and increased susceptibility to infection.[228,285] Infantile malignant osteopetrosis is an autosomal recessive subtype of the juvenile-onset variety that develops in utero or within the first months of life.[228] Clinical signs in malignant infantile osteopetrosis include reduced vision in the first months of life, an enlarged skull with parietal and frontal bossing, hepatosplenomegaly, recurrent infections, failure to thrive, and bruising.[4] Neurologic abnormalities, including extreme irritability, cranial nerve palsies, developmental delay, hydrocephalus, mental retardation, and cerebral atrophy, are often the first manifestation of the disease.[228] Hydrocephalus in osteopetrosis may result from obstruction of cerebral venous outflow secondary to narrowed venous foramina.[150]

Neuro-ophthalmologic findings are common in malignant infantile osteopetrosis. They include optic atrophy, papilledema, nystagmus, strabismus, nasolacrimal duct obstruction, limited extraocular movements, and proptosis.[4,285] Papilledema in osteopetrosis has been attributed to hydrocephalus, although a pseudotumor cerebri mechanism related to venous outflow obstruction also seems plausible. Optic atrophy with severe visual loss is seen in approximately 80% of cases. Optic atrophy may be caused by either the compressive effects of narrowed optic canals or by long-standing papilledema.[228] Visual loss in osteopetrosis may also result from a primary retinal degeneration associated with diminished electroretinographic amplitudes. Some affected infants develop multiple lacunar areas of macular depigmentation.[228] The recent association of infantile malignant osteopetrosis with neuronal storage disease suggests that degenerative retinal changes in osteopetrosis may be secondary to neuronal storage disease. Lysosome dysfunction has been identified in both infantile malignant osteopetrosis and neuronal storage diseases.

Infantile malignant osteopetrosis is lethal if untreated within the first decade of life.[228] Bone marrow transplantation is the only definitive therapy, with a success rate approaching 50%.[285] In one child, the electroretinogram reportedly normalized following bone marrow transplantation while the visual evoked response remained undetectable.[4] Optic canal decompression may result in improved visual function when visual loss is associated with

CT evidence of narrowing of the optic canals, a normal electroretinogram, and subjective or objective evidence of decreased optic nerve function (such as progressive abnormality on serial visual evoked potential (VEP) examinations).[60,285]

Optic Disc Swelling in Primary Ocular Disease

Intraocular inflammation and hypotony are well-recognized causes of optic disc swelling. These two conditions often coexist in children with uveitis (juvenile rheumatoid arthritis, sarcoidosis, pars planitis) (Figure 3.9). Postoperative hypotony, particularly following glaucoma surgery, is also a common cause of transient optic disc swelling in children. Visual acuity is thought to be unaffected by disc swelling alone in inflamed or hypotonous eyes.[179] The finding of optic disc swelling and decreased acuity in an eye with uveitis should suggest the possibility of an associated anterior optic neuritis, whereas decreased acuity in a hypotonous eye is usually attributable to coexistent macular edema.[179] Beardsley et al[19] and Minckler and Bunt[183] have demonstrated compromised axoplasmic transport anterior to the lamina cribrosa in ocular hypotony just as in increased intracranial pressure. Interestingly, elevated intraocular pressure is also rarely associated

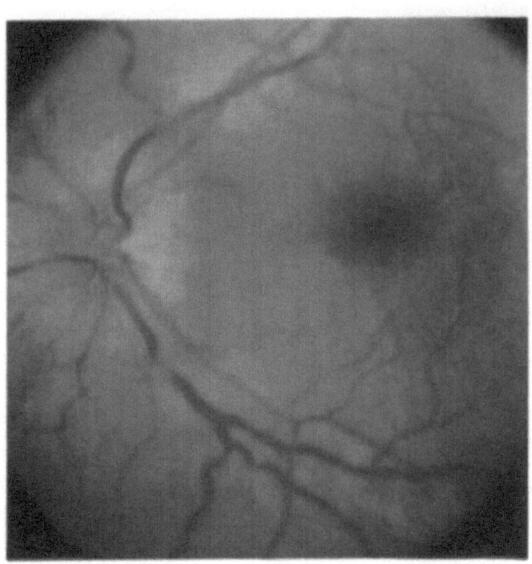

FIGURE 3.9. Disc swelling and macular edema in a 12-year-old girl with pars planitis and 20/25 vision.

with optic disc swelling.[182] The biochemical mechanisms by which any of these conditions eventuate in optic disc swelling are speculative.[114]

Posttraumatic Optic Disc Swelling

Traumatic optic neuropathy typically involves the intracanalicular segment of the optic nerve and is not associated with optic disc swelling. We have examined three young patients (two children and one young adult) in whom blunt ocular trauma caused an unusual form of optic neuropathy, characterized by prolonged optic disc swelling, negative orbital imaging studies, and slow visual recovery over weeks to months (Figure 3.10).[39] The associated findings of choroidal ruptures and peripapillary subretinal hemorrhages suggest contrecoup mechanism of injury to the optic nerve at its junction with the globe. The pathogenesis of this rare form of posttraumatic optic disc swelling is speculative. Possible inciting factors include chronic, low-grade ischemia secondary to traumatic posterior ciliary artery occlusion, axonal crowding secondary to edema of the peripapillary sclera, and posttraumatic posterior vitreous detachment in a young patient with strong vitreopapillary adhesions to the disc. The delayed visual recovery

may relate to the ability of young patients to withstand chronic, low-grade optic disc ischemia.

CT scanning should be obtained to rule out an intrasheath hemorrhage in any child with decreased vision and optic disc edema following blunt ocular trauma, as vision can be restored by optic nerve sheath fenestration in this setting.[107,132] Optic disc swelling secondary to intraocular inflammation or to hypotony (due to a cyclodialysis cleft or ciliary body hyposecretion) should also be considered in the context of posttraumatic optic disc swelling.

Intrinsic Optic Disc Tumors

Optic Disc Hemangioma

Capillary hemangiomas may occur within the substance of the disc as an isolated tumor (von Hippel's disease) or in association with cerebellar and visceral tumors (von Hippel–Lindau disease). "Endophytic" hemangiomas appear as reddish, spherical, slightly elevated "knobs" that lie anterior to the disc vasculature (Figure 3.11). The "endophytic" type of capillary hemangioma does not appear as a distinct mass but is typically seen as blurring and elevation of the disc margin, often associated with a serous detachment of the peripapillary retina.[179] Hemangiomas of the optic disc may leak lipoprotein exudates into the retina and may be mistaken for either neuroretinitis or juxtapapillary choroidal neovascularization (Figure 3.11).[90,179] Fluorescein angiography shows early and diffuse filling confined to the area of the tumor with late staining (Figure 3.11). Histopathologically, the disc hemangioma consists of multiple thin-walled interconnecting aneurysms of variable size.[90]

Tuberous Sclerosis

Astrocytic hamartomas of the optic disc or peripapillary retina may produce optic disc elevation in tuberous sclerosis.[199,279] These lesions typically protrude or overlie the optic disc and evolve from a gray or grayish-pink translucent appearance in infancy to a glistening, yellow, mulberry appearance later in childhood. Small calcified astrocytic hamartomas of the optic disc may be impossible to distinguish from disc drusen.[90] Blood vessels within the tumor are usually permeable to fluores-

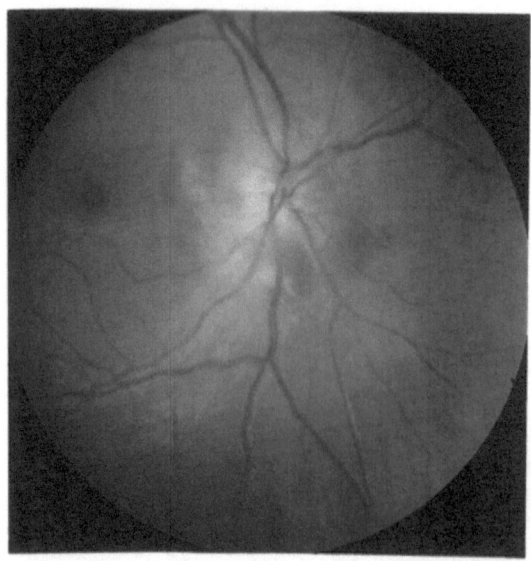

FIGURE 3.10. Posttraumatic optic disc swelling. Note peripapillary hemorrhages, choroidal striae, and segmental pallor of the inferior disc.

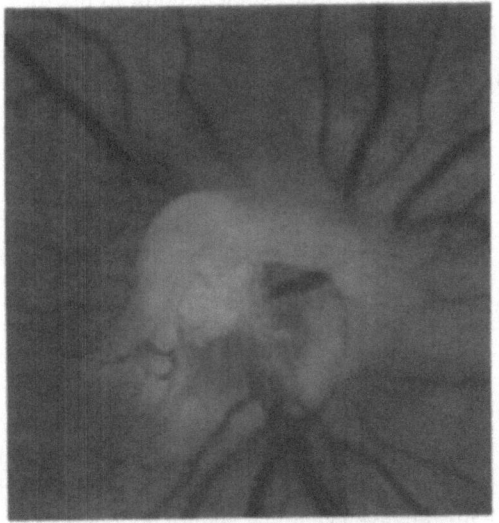

A

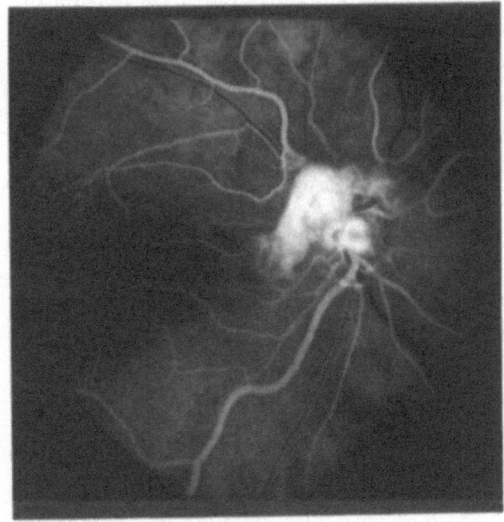

B

FIGURE 3.11. **(A)** Exophytic optic disc hemangioma in a patient with von Hippel–Lindau disease. An area of fibrovascular proliferation overlies the superior disc margin. **(B)** Early phase fluorescein angiogram showing discrete filling of the lesion. (Courtesy of Stephen C. Pollock, MD.) **(C)** Endophytic optic disc hemangioma with retinal exudate simulating neuroretinitis. (Courtesy of Stephen P. Christiansen, MD.)

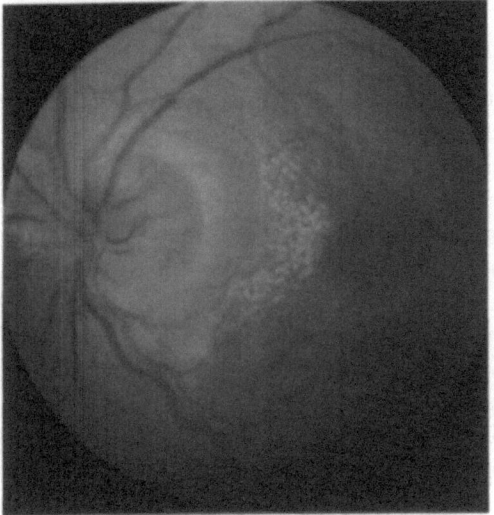

C

cein.[90] Depending upon their stage of evolution, these tumors are composed of either spindle-shaped astrocytes, or acellular, laminated calcific concretions.[90,179]

Intracranial lesions in children with tuberous sclerosis may cause obstructive hydrocephalus, papilledema, and eventually, optic atrophy.[198,267] The associated CNS and systemic signs of tuberous sclerosis are discussed in Chapter 11.

Optic Disc Glioma

Optic disc glioma is an extremely rare tumor that appears as a mass of whitish, gray, or yellow tissue protruding from the disc surface.[179] Visual acuity is variably affected. Dossetor et al[61] recently reviewed all previously reported cases and established the strong association of optic disc glioma with NF-2.

Combined Hamartoma of the Retina and RPE (CHRPE)

Combined hamartomas of the retina and retinal pigment epithelium (RPE) are irregular, elevated, variably pigmented lesions characterized by a proliferation of the RPE, retina, and overlying vitreous. They have a predilection for the juxtapapillary area and are often accompanied by significant wrinkling and distortion of the retina.

Combined hamartomas may elevate a portion of the optic disc and leak fluorescein. Conversely, chronic papilledema can rarely produce a constellation of juxtapapillary pigmentary, vascular, and glial changes, which is indistinguishable from a combined hamartoma.[131] Gass[90] described an older adult in whom a small depigmented juxtapapillary CHRPE produced elevation of the disc with segmental leakage on fluorescein angiography, simulating ischemic optic neuropathy. Landau et al[157] recently established the association of CHRPE with NF-2 that has been confirmed in subsequent studies.[100,143,254]

Retrobulbar Tumors

The finding of optic disc swelling in a proptotic eye (usually with decreased acuity) is highly suggestive of a retrobulbar tumor. Intrinsic optic nerve tumors may compress and/or infiltrate the optic nerve and interrupt axonal transport, leading to swelling of the optic disc. Optic nerve glioma is the most common retrobulbar tumor associated with optic disc swelling in children. While it has been found experimentally that extrinsic optic nerve compression must occur in close proximity to the globe to produce optic disc edema, many clinical exceptions to this rule have been documented.[179] Orbital venous stasis may be a predominant mechanism whereby mass lesions in the posterior orbit lead to optic disc edema.

Optic nerve sheath meningioma is rare in children. When present, it produces gradual visual loss, optic disc swelling, and proptosis. This tumor can usually be differentiated from orbital optic glioma based upon its neuroimaging characteristics (see Chapter 4). Optic nerve sheath meningioma is classically held to exhibit a more aggressive course in children than in adults, especially with regard to early intracranial extension.[9,287] There is no evidence, however, that this has any significant effect on prognosis for life or vision in the contralateral eye.[65] Children with optic nerve sheath meningioma should be evaluated by chromosome analysis for the possibility of occult NF-2 (see Chapter 11).

Optic Neuritis in Children

Pediatric optic neuritis is commonly held to be fundamentally different than adult optic neuritis.

Many reviews of this subject point to the following fundamental differences:

1. Pediatric optic neuritis is commonly bilateral; adult optic neuritis is usually unilateral.[147,178] (It is likely, however, that some unilateral cases of childhood optic neuritis are not brought to medical attention because young children either fail to note a problem or ignore the symptoms.)
2. Pediatric optic neuritis is usually associated with optic disc swelling;[147,178] adult optic neuritis is more often retrobulbar.[201]
3. Pediatric optic neuritis is usually a postinfectious condition that does not presage multiple sclerosis;[178] adult optic neuritis is usually a demyelinative event that augurs the onset of multiple sclerosis.[221]

History and Physical Examination

It is often difficult or impossible to obtain an accurate history of the onset of visual symptoms in children. Young children may not notice unilateral visual loss and may blithely accept bilateral visual loss until it is so severe as to become incapacitating.[147] In older children, a sense of panic may lead to denial of symptoms.[147] The vagaries of subjective symptoms in children detract from the overall reliability of the history. Headache appears to be more common in childhood optic neuritis.[147,152] As in adults, a history of pain with eye movements supports the diagnosis.

Postinfectious Optic Neuritis

A febrile or flulike illness commonly precedes pediatric optic neuritis by days or weeks. Diseases that have been specifically associated with optic neuritis in children include measles, mumps, chickenpox, rubella, brucella, pertussis, infectious mononucleosis, cat scratch disease, toxoplasmosis,[222] and Q fever.[35,67,71,144,206,207,212,244,247,252,261,262] DPT vaccines or other immunizations may also precipitate optic neuritis in children. The delayed onset of pediatric optic neuritis after recent infection or immunization, and the bilateral involvement in most cases of postinfectious optic neuritis suggest a generalized mechanism of injury (i.e., a systemic autoimmune demyelination) rather than random, viral invasion of each optic nerve.[244] Hierons and Lyle noted that encephalomyelitis typically occurs in the wake of viral infections and suggested that optic neuritis in children be viewed as localized form of encephalitis.[123]

Acute Disseminated Encephalomyelitis

When childhood optic neuritis is accompanied by multiple neurological signs, the primary diagnostic considerations are acute disseminated encephalomyelitis (ADE), multiple sclerosis (MS), and Devic disease (Table 3.7). The terms *postinfectious encephalomyelitis* and *acute disseminated encephalomyelitis* are used interchangably to describe an uncommon, inflammatory, demyelinating disease of the CNS that usually follows a viral illness or vaccination by days to weeks.[18,135] Children 6 to 10 years of age are most commonly affected, presenting with the acute onset of motor signs and symptoms, seizure activity, and sometimes, altered consciousness, headache, fever, and ataxia.[18] Cerebrospinal fluid analysis may show pleocytosis.[71,220,251] The histopathological hallmark of ADE is a zone of demyelination (with relative sparing of axons) around veins in association with infiltration of vessel walls and perivascular spaces by lymphocytes, plasma cells, and monocytes.[18] Acute disseminated encephalomyelitis is believed to result from an autoimmune reaction to myelin triggered by a virus or vaccine, since no virus has consistently been isolated.[18] Also, the temporal framework and pathological features of postinfectious encephalitis closely resemble those of experimental allergic encephalitis, a prototypical autoimmune demyelinating disease.[244]

The MR imaging in ADE shows moderate to large areas of increased signal intensity on T2-

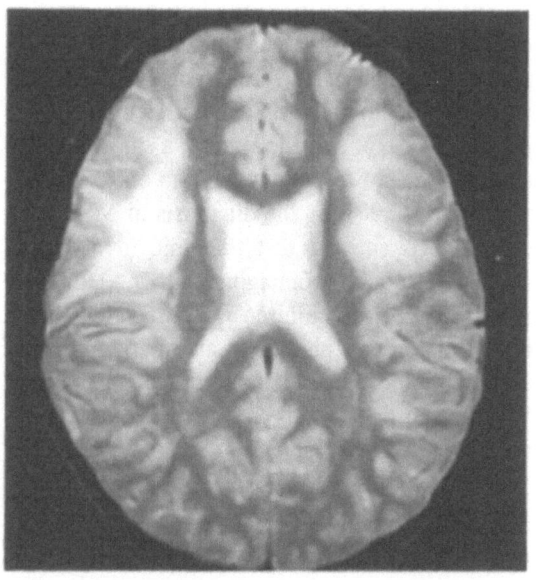

FIGURE 3.12. Acute disseminated encephalomyelitis. MR image shows patchy areas of prolonged T2 relaxation involving subcortical white matter and cortex. (Courtesy of A. James Barkovich, MD.)

weighted images corresponding to the inflammation and edema associated with demyelination (Figure 3.12).[10,18] These lesions involve subcortical white matter in a patchy distribution, but cortical and deep gray matter are also involved to a lesser extent. The lesions are bilateral but usually asymmetrical. Brain stem and cerebellar lesions are common.[10]

Despite the large size and subcortical location of the lesions, MR findings in ADE show significant overlap with those of MS.[18] Conclusive dif-

TABLE 3.7. Differential diagnosis of optic disc swelling with visual loss in children.

Isolated visual loss	Visual loss with additional neurological signs
Postinfectious optic neuritis	Accute disseminated encephalomyelitis
Early neuroretinitis	Multiple sclerosis
Leber hereditary neuroretinopathy	Devic disease
Nutritional deficiency	Meningitis
Pseudopapilledema with cortical visual loss	Neurosarcoidosis
Pseudopapilledema with psychogenic visual loss	Leukemia
Systemic vasculitis (e.g., lupus)	Optic glioma
AMPEE, MEWDS, and related disorders	Craniopharyngioma
	Shunt failure with hydrocephalus
	Adrenoleukodystrophy
	Drug toxicity

ferentiation of ADE from the initial presentation of childhood MS is not possible, even by a combination of clinical features, CSF analysis, and MR imaging.[18] Although ADE is classically considered to be a monophasic illness, a small but significant fraction of patients will go on to develop relapses, establishing the diagnosis of MS.[18] Recent reports suggest that thalamic involvement may be a useful neuroimaging sign of ADE, since it is rarely seen in children with MS.[18,112] Acute disseminated encephalitis is an emergent condition, with mortality estimated at 10% to 20%. Systemic corticosteroids are the mainstay of treatment.

Multiple Sclerosis and Pediatric Optic Neuritis

Recent evidence suggests that the distinction between postinfectious childhood optic neuritis and MS may not be absolute. Riikonen believes that a combination of abnormal immunological responses, possibly precipitated by infectious agents in a genetically susceptible individual, may lead either to MS or to optic neuritis.[217] Riikonen et al studied 18 children with optic neuritis, 10 of whom eventually developed MS.[220] More than half of the children had suffered a bacterial or viral infection within 2 weeks prior to the first symptoms of optic neuritis. Vaccinations with live or attenuated viruses (e.g., polio, vaccinia, rubella, influenza) preceded the first episode of optic neuritis in six patients. Subsequent vaccinations caused exacerbations of optic neuritis in several cases. Five of the recently vaccinated children eventually developed MS. Killed virus components such as those used for influenza vaccines do not produce this effect. Riikonen has recommended avoiding immunizations with live or attenuated viruses in children with MS. Bye et al[42] described five similar children with chronic, recurrent optic neuritis, three of whom had encephalomyelitis with optic neuritis as their initial episode. These findings corroborate those from the Riikonen study and confirm that postinfectious optic neuritis, with or without encephalomyelitis, may be a harbinger of MS in some children.[42] It is currently unclear whether concurrent encephalomyelitis effects the liklihood that MS will develop in the child with optic neuritis or whether the severity of the encephalomyelitis influences this prognosis.[202]

Devic Disease (Neuromyelitis Optica)

The diagnosis of early Devic disease should be considered in any child or adult who presents with acute bilateral optic neuritis. Such patients should be cautioned to return immediately if they develop a gait disturbance or bladder dysfunction. Unlike MS, Devic disease is usually an acute and often self-limiting disorder (a "once and for all" demyelination). Subsequent attacks of demyelination are rare. When relapses involve other neurological signs, the patient must be considered to have MS. The relative incidence of Devic disease to MS is much higher in Asia, particularly in Japan.[154] It is most common in young adults but may appear at any age from 5 to 60 years.[178] Most cases start with bilateral visual symptoms. Visual loss occurs acutely and becomes severe within a few days.[154] The optic discs may be normal or swollen.[178] Although many adults remain permanently blind after an attack of Devic disease, Jeffery and Buncic have found that children with Devic disease have an excellent prognosis for visual and neurological recovery with no recurrences or long-term sequelae.[134a] Occasionally, visual system and spinal cord involvement may be separated by months or years.[170]

Neurological involvement consists of a progressive and often ascending sensorimotor myelitis, affecting either the lower limbs or all four limbs and sometimes causing a complete transverse lesion of the cord.[178] Urinary retention or incontinence are common. The cerebrospinal fluid typically shows a pleocytosis and increased total protein. Patients with Devic disease have a high CSF albumin level with low serum/CSF albumin ratios, suggesting a permeability defect in the blood brain barrier. Most affected individuals are found to have absent oligoclonal bands, in contrast to the increased daily CSF IgG synthesis and oligoclonal bands that typify MS.[170] Devic disease is fatal in approximately 20% of cases.[154] Immunosuppressive therapies generally fail to benefit patients.[170]

The initial diagnosis of Devic disease rests on the recognition of concurrent acute optic neuritis and spinal cord dysfunction, with absence of brain white matter signal abnormalties on MR imaging. MR imaging in Devic disease typically demonstrates a normal-appearing brain with enlargement and cavitation of the spinal cord.[170] Unlike in MS, the cerebral hemispheres, brain stem, and cerebellum are generally unaffected in Devic disease.[170] The absence of white matter MR signal abnormalities within the brain hemispheres in Devic disease helps to distinguish it from multiple sclerosis.[170]

A necrotizing (rather than demyelinating) myelopathy is the histopathological hallmark of Devic disease.[170] Autopsy examination of the optic nerves and chiasm shows demyelination, with gliosis and cavitation in some cases.[170] The remainder of the brain is normal. Autopsy examination of the spinal cord shows a severe necrotizing myelopathy with involvement of both gray and white matter, thickening of blood vessels walls, and no lymphocytic infiltrate.[170] These findings constrast sharply with those of MS, in which multiple demarcated plaques are scattered throughout white matter in the brain and spinal cord.

Course of Visual Loss and Visual Recovery

Initial visual loss in pediatric optic neuritis is often profound; acuities of light perception and no light perception are not unusual. Despite the severity of visual loss, the prognosis for visual recovery is generally regarded as excellent (Table 3.8).[147, 152,178,244] Kennedy and Carroll[147] noted that "in most instances, improvement begins before the end of the third week after onset and reaches a maximum by six months. In a few cases, a year may pass before improvement is detectable.[11]

Kriss et al found the pattern-evoked VEP latency to be normal in 55% of children with recovered optic neuritis, as compared to a previously established figure of 10% in adults, and suggested that the greater potential for remyelination in the young than the old may account for these findings.[152] In most children, vision spontaneously recovers to 20/20, but some degree of optic disc pallor usually persists.[152,178,244]

Meadows stated that "the slower and more insidious the loss of function, the less the likelihood of visual improvement, and if this does occur it tends to be equally slow. In contrast, a more abrupt and catastrophic onset is sometimes followed by surprising recovery."[178] In offering an optimistic prognosis to the parents and child, it should be kept in mind that most series include descriptions of a few children whose vision either failed to improve or improved minimally.[120] Some children in the older series may have had a mutation for Leber hereditary neuroretinopathy. It is not known whether children who sustain permanent visual loss have a distinct form of optic neuritis or whether their failure to improve represents the low end in a broad spectrum of recovery.

Systemic Prognosis

It is classically held that optic neuritis is less likely to lead to MS in children than adults[152] (Table 3.8). In adults, Rizzo and Lessell reported that 58% of optic neuritis patients (69% of women and 33% of men) were diagnosed as having MS during an average follow-up of 14.9 years.[221] The incidence of MS following childhood optic neuritis has ranged from 5.2% to 55.5% in different studies.[146,152,220] There seems to be a greater predisposition for children with unilateral rather than bilateral optic neuritis to develop MS.[109,152,220] (Table 3.8) Conversely, optic neuritis is commonly reported in studies of children with MS; in a recent report by Bye et al, all five children with MS had this early sign.[42] Since the incidence of MS continues to increase with long-term follow-up in adults with optic neuritis, and since the length of follow-up is less than 15 years in most pediatric studies, one cannot conclude on the basis of present data that the incidence of demyelinating disease is less in children with optic neuritis than in adults.

Kriss et al found that MS developed in 3 of 29 children with bilateral optic neuritis and 3 of 10 children with unilateral optic neuritis, suggesting that, while bilateral cases have a lower incidence of MS than unilateral cases, the risk in bilateral cases is not negligible[152] (Table 3.9). In the 8 of

TABLE 3.8. Natural history of optic neuritis in children.

Study	Bilateral	Disc swelling	Visual recovery	Incidence of MS	Mean follow-up
Hierons and Lyle[123]	100%	—	92% "excellent"	7.6%	4 years
Kennedy and Carroll[147]	60%	87%	77% to 20/20	26%	8 years
Kriss et al[152]	74%	74%	78% to 20/20	15%	4.6 years
Riikonen et al[217]	65%	76%	80% to 20/30 or better	56%	7 years

TABLE 3.9. Incidence of MS in unilateral versus bilateral childhood optic neuritis.

Study	MS in bilateral cases	MS in unilateral cases	Mean follow-up
Kennedy and Carroll[147]	4/18 (22.2%)	4/12 (33.3%)	8 years
Haller and Patzold[109]	4/10 (40%)	3/9 (33%)	6 months to 30 years (no mean)
Kriss et al[152]	3/29 (10.3%)	3/10 (30%)	4.6 years
Riikonen et al[217]	2/13 (15.4%)	7/8 (87.5%)	7 years

30 patients from the Kennedy and Carroll series that developed MS, four had simultaneous bilateral disc swelling.[147] In the Riikonen study, MS developed in seven of eight patients with unilateral optic neuritis and in only 2 of 13 patients with bilateral optic neuritis.[217] Riikonen noted that all patients who later developed MS had a second attack of optic neuritis within 1 year of the first attack.

Systemic Evaluation of Pediatric Optic Neuritis

The diagnosis of bilateral optic neuritis is established by the finding of bilaterally decreased vision, decreased color vision, an afferent pupillary defect (if the visual loss is asymmetrical), swollen or normal discs, and the absence of space-occupying intracranial lesions, such as optic nerve glioma, craniopharyngioma, or hydrocephalus, on MR imaging. Using kinetic perimetry, cecocentral scotomas and large central scotomas are the most common visual field defects.

Once the diagnosis of optic neuritis is established, a diagnostic evaluation is undertaken to determine an underlying cause (Table 3.10). The MR imaging is exquisitely sensitive to the periventricular ovoid lesions that characterize MS in adults.[37] In the Optic Neuritis Treatment Trial, unenhanced MR imaging of the brain was performed as part of baseline diagnostic testing with a standardized protocol in 440 adults. The MR images in 418 of these patients were deemed acceptable for evaluation of signal intensity abnormalities.[24] At 2-year follow-up, the initial MR imaging findings were compared with the neurologic course in each patient to determine whether any association could be established. Results of this study showed initial MR findings to be a powerful predictor of MS.[24] Thirty-six percent of placebo-treated patients whose initial MR images revealed two or more signal-intensity abnormalities developed clinical signs and symptoms of MS within 2 years, compared with only 3% of patients whose MR images were normal.[25] Results of the study by Morrissey et al[187] support this finding and indicate that, with long-term follow-up, the risk of developing MS may approach 100% in adults with abnormal MR images, whereas the risk in patients with normal MR images is likely to remain low. Preliminary evidence from the Riikonen study suggests that MR imaging may be as useful in children as it is in adults for predicting which patients will subsequently develop MS.[218]

In children, a lumbar puncture is usually performed to rule out elevated intracranial pressure, meningitis, or a coexistent encephalitis. Riikonen and von Willebrandt found normal peripheral blood lymphocyte counts and function in most children with optic neuritis and MS.[219] A thorough history of recent infection or systemic disease, illness, recent immunizations, bee stings,[28] tick bites,[284] or neurological symptoms suggestive

TABLE 3.10. Infectious and noninfectious causes of childhood optic neuritis.

Infectious or postinfectious	Noninfectious
Rubeola (measles)	Multiple sclerosis
Paramyxovirus (mumps)	Devic disease
Varicella zoster (chicken pox)	Sarcoidosis
Pertussis (whooping cough)	Bee venom
Boriella burgdorferi (Lyme disease)	Vasculitis (e.g. lupus)
Epstein-Barr virus (infectious mononucleosis)	
Rochalimaea (cat scratch disease)	
Treponema pallidum (syphilis)	
Toxocara canis	
Toxoplasmosis	
Tuberculosis	
Rickettsia	
Coxiella burnetti	
Brucella	
Vaccinations	

of MS should be obtained. Symptoms of headache, malaise, lethargy, seizures, or fever should suggest the possibility of a coexistent encephalomyelitis. The findings of lymphadenopathy, hepatomegaly, or splenomegaly should suggest the possibility of infectious mononucleosis or cat scratch disease.[71] A chest X-ray (to rule out sarcoidosis and tuberculosis) and a tuberculin skin test can be predicated upon the index of suspicion. Systemic signs of vasculitis should be sought since systemic lupus erythematosis can occasionally cause a bilateral simultaneous optic neuritis in children that is usually associated with a poor visual outcome.[3] In children with a discrete white inflammatory mass on the disc, or prominent vitreous inflammation, serological testing for toxoplasmosis and toxocariasis should be obtained.[56,78] Table 3.10 summarizes the recognized infectious and noninfectious causes of childhood optic neuritis.

Treatment of Pediatric Optic Neuritis

There has been no controlled study to determine the efficacy of oral or intravenous steroids in the treatment of childhood optic neuritis.[120] Recommendations in the literature are largely anecdotal.[71] In typical demyelinating optic neuritis in adults, the Optic Neuritis Treatment Trial has found that neither oral nor intravenous steroids change the final visual outcome as measured at 1 year after onset of symptoms. However, adults who received intravenous steroids in high doses had more rapid recovery of vision. Adult patients who received oral corticosteroids alone for acute optic neuritis had twice the number of recurrent attacks of optic neuritis over the following 2 years.[25] In contrast, patients who were treated with intravenous corticosteroids had only half the number of systemic demyelinative episodes as the placebo or oral corticosteroid treated groups over the same 2-year period.[25] The protective effect of intravenous steroids was seen only in the subgroups with abnormal MR scans.[37] Based upon these results, some adults with optic neuritis and/or MS are now treated at 2-year intervals with intravenous high-dose steroids. These results may also be applicable to children with optic neuritis and signal abnormalities on MR imaging suggestive of MS or to children with MS. MR imaging is

also crucial to define the multiple bilateral large signal abnormalities of ADE, which is corticosteroid responsive.[112]

Leber Idiopathic Stellate Neuroretinitis

In 1916, Theodor Leber described the clinical syndrome of unilateral visual loss, optic disc swelling, macular star, and spontaneous resolution in otherwise healthy patients.[89,159] He referred to this condition as an idiopathic stellate neuroretinopathy, emphasizing the star figure that surrounded the fovea (Figure 3.13).

The onset of visual loss usually follows a viral prodrome by 2 to 4 weeks.[203] Visual loss may be accompanied by symptoms of floaters and ocular pain. Ophthalmoscopic examination at onset shows a swollen optic disc with peripapillary retinal striae extending from the disc toward the macula or extending radially from the fovea, frequent serous detachment of the peripapillary retina, and cells in the anterior vitreous. An associated iridocyclitis is seen in some cases. Within weeks, the disc swelling and peripapillary edema begin to subside, and a yellowish star-shaped pattern of macular exudate appears and becomes more prominent[89,229] (Figure 3.13).

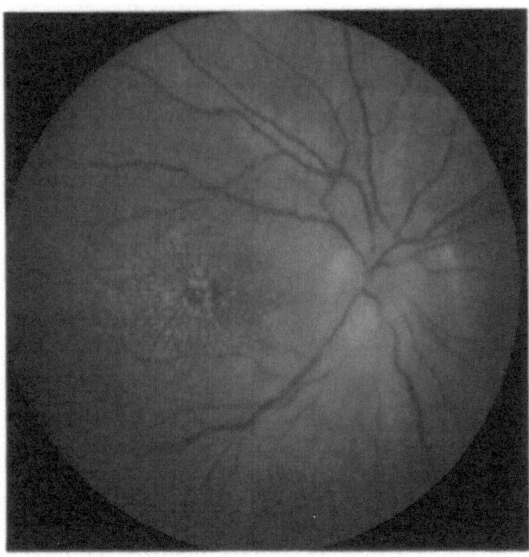

FIGURE 3.13. Leber stellate neuroretinitis. Note swelling of the optic disc and macular star-shaped exudates.

In most cases, visual acuity ranges from 20/50 to 20/200, and an afferent pupillary defect is present.[89] Visual field testing shows a central or centrocecal scotoma.[62] Fluorescein angiography shows evidence of abnormal capillary permeability, particularly from the capillaries deep within the optic disc.[89]

The disc swelling clears over 2 to 3 months, but the macular exudate may persist and be associated with retinopathic deficits for a longer period of time. A minority of patients with Leber stellate neuroretinitis have either focal neurological symptoms or elevated intracranial pressure at presentation; fulminant encephalitis or meningitis is not seen.[203,276] The ultimate level of visual recovery seems to be the same in Leber idiopathic stellate neuroretinitis as in optic neuritis, but the course of visual recovery is prolonged in neuroretinitis. During the period of months between the resolution of disc edema and the resolution of macular exudates, a dissociation between color vision and visual acuity may be apparent, with the former normalizing before the latter. Following resolution, patients are left with varying degrees of optic atrophy and mild macular pigmentary changes. As in optic neuritis, most patients recover near-normal vision, but occasional patients fail to recover or recover only minimally.[276]

The distinction between Leber stellate neuroretinitis and anterior optic neuritis bears tremendous prognostic significance, since the diagnosis of Leber stellate neuroretinitis essentially rules out the possibility of MS.[203] This fundamental difference can be predicted from the known pathophysiology of the disease. Gass originally suggested that Leber stellate neuroretinitis is due to a prelaminar disc vasculitis that results in a leakage of lipid and protein-rich exudate from the disc capillaries into the outer plexiform layer.[62,88,203] As the serous component is resorbed over days to weeks, lipid precipitates within Henle's fiber layer, forming a star figure.[62] Leber stellate neuroretinitis is thought to be fundamentally different from optic neuritis in that Leber stellate neuroretinitis presumably represents an autoimmune vasculitis confined to the nonmyelinated prelaminar optic disc.[276] In anterior optic neuritis, the target tissue is primarily retrolaminar myelin.[62] Although anterior optic neuritis can indirectly produce disc swelling, it does not cause the profuse leakage from the prelaminar disc capillaries necessary to produce a macular star.

The finding of angiomatous skin lesions (bacillary angiomatosis) resembling Kaposi sarcoma in the child with neuroretinitis or hepatosplenomegaly should also suggest the possibility of infection with the rickettsial organism Rochalimaea henselae, which has recently been implicated in the pathogenesis of cat scratch disease.[99,214,277] Infection with Rochalimaea henselae produces the triad of septicemia, bacillary angiomatosis, and hepatic and splenic peliosis (numerous small blood-filled cystic lesions).[277] Weiss and Beck[276] noted that the swollen optic disc usually had a yellowish-white nodular region located at the temporal aspect of the swollen disc.[276] Fish et al documented *peripapillary angiomatosis* on the surface of a swollen disc of a child with cat scratch disease.[73] Papillary angiomatosis may turn out to be a unique ocular manifestation of cat scratch disease that is analogous to the skin lesions of bacillary angiomatosis. In the past, a cat scratch skin test and/or a lymph node biopsy were the methods most commonly employed to establish the diagnosis. Previously reported cases of cat scratch–associated neuroretinitis must be considered at least somewhat presumptive, since a positive skin test only demonstrates acquired immunity to the infection, which could have occured months to years previously.[16] In patients with lymphadenopathy from cat scratch disease, a lymph node biopsy typically shows noncaseating necrosis and gram-negative coccobacilli with Warthin-Starry silver stain.[47,73] The cat scratch skin test was never approved by the FDA and has now been replaced by serological testing of acute and chronic IgG and IgM. Rochalimaea can also be cultured from blood or skin lesions.[99] Oral ciprofloxacin, or doxycycline, can be used to treat ocular and systemic cat scratch disease.[99] Oral steroid therapy is often empirically added in patients with optic neuritis or neuroretinitis.[270] Systemic corticosteroids, with and without systemic antibiotics, have been reported to be effective in the treatment of cat scratch disease.[73]

Lyme disease is another recognized cause of Leber stellate neuroretinitis.[163] Lyme disease is caused by the spirochete *Borrelia burgdorferi*, which is transmitted by the *Ixodidae* ticks.[1] Serological testing is therefore particularly important in children who have recently been camping or have a history of a tick bite. Clinical signs of erythema migrans, carditis, arthritis, or facial palsy should raise suspicion for this diagnosis.[1] Unfortunately, currently available serology for Lyme disease has problems with both false-positive and false-negative results, causing overdiagnosis and underdiagnosis, respectively.[259,282] Patients with syphilis can have positive Lyme serology.[282] Patients with Lyme disease who have early skin, joint, or cardiac involvement are often treated with oral antibiotic therapy, while those with neuroborreliosis (encephalitis, neuroretinitis, facial palsy) or chronic arthritis require longer-term intravenous third generation cephalosporins.

Other infectious and parainfectious causes of Leber stellate neuroretinitis in childhood include mumps,[79] leptospirosis,[62] infectious mononucleosis,[31,81] exudative tuberculous retinitis,[64] a toxocaral granuloma within the nerve head,[30,56] toxoplasmic neuroretinitis,[74] syphilis,[72,77] and influenza.[175] It also is important to remember that macular stars may rarely accompany disc swelling due to elevated intracranial pressure.[95] Tables 3.11 and 3.12 summarize the recognized infectious causes of Leber stellate neuroretinitis, along with suggested medical evaluations.

Gass described acute visual loss with optic disc swelling, peripapillary exudate, and a macular star in two children with progressive facial hemiatrophy (Parry–Romberg syndrome).[89] One of these children had angiographic evidence of increased peripheral retinal vascular permeability. Both patients developed optic atrophy as the peripapillary and macular exudation cleared, but neither demonstrated progressive loss of visual field. The pathogenesis of this acute neuroretinopathy is not known.[89]

TABLE 3.11. Infectious causes of Leber idiopathic stellate neuroretinitis in childhood.

Rochalimaea (cat scratch disease)
Mumps
Boriella burgdorferi (Lyme disease)
Toxocara optic neuritis
Toxoplasma optic neuropathy
Tuberculosis
Syphilis
Leptospirosis

TABLE 3.12. Suggested medical evaluation for neuroretinitis in childhood.

1. Cat scratch skin test
2. Tuberculin skin test
3. FTA-ABS
4. Serology for the following:
   Rochalimaea
   Lyme disease
   Toxoplasmosis
   Toxocara canis
   Epstein-Barr virus
   Leptospirosis

Other forms of childhood neuroretinitis include posterior scleritis and diffuse unilateral subacute neuroretinitis (DUSN). Posterior scleritis is an autoimmune disorder that is often associated with ocular pain, conjunctival injection, and ocular motility disturbances. Ophthalmoscopic abnormalities include optic disc edema, retinal and choroidal striae, exudative retinal detachment, annular choroidal detachment, and cystoid macular edema.[27] The disc swelling in posterior scleritis may be caused by narrowing of the scleral canal due to contiguous scleral inflammation and edema. The diagnosis can be confirmed by ultrasonography, which demonstrates a fluid-filled space within Tenon's tissue behind the globe, or by CT scanning, which demonstrates enhancement and thickening of the posterior sclera. Diffuse unilateral subacute neuroretinitis occurs in healthy patients and, in its acute stage, is characterized by mild to moderate swelling of the optic disc, vitreous cells, and transient crops of focal, gray-white or yellow-white lesions that involve the deep or external layers of the retina and RPE.[89,91] Rarely is DUSN associated with a macular star.[89] Over a period of weeks to months, depigmentation of the overlying RPE occurs, along with severe optic atrophy and marked retinal arteriolar attenuation.[89] DUSN is now considered to be a multietiologic syndrome caused by different species of nematodes.[97] It is believed that larval excretory-secretory products, including various enzymes and metabolic wastes produced by nematode larvae, cause localized toxic effects and/or stimulate an inflammatory response, especially one mediated by eosinophils.[97] Direct photocoagulation has proven successful in eradicating the nematode and halting the progression of visual loss.[91] Oral treatment with the antihelminthic agent thiabendazole has met with success in some patients and has been recommended for use in cases in which the worm cannot be located.[91]

Pseudopapilledema

Anomalous elevation of the optic disc is a primary diagnostic consideration in the child referred for papilledema.[129] Buried drusen within the optic disc is the most common form of pseudopapilledema in childhood and must be distinguished from other causes of pseudopapilledema, such as hyperopia, myelinated nerve fibers, epipapillary glial tissue, and hyaloid traction on the disc.[236]

Optic Disc Drusen

The word *drusen*, of Germanic derivation, originally meant tumor, swelling, or tumescence.[165] According to Lorentzen,[165] the word was used in the mining industry approximately 500 years ago to indicate a crystal-filled space in a rock. Other terms such as *hyaline* bodies and *colloid* bodies are occasionally used to describe drusen of the optic disc.[82]

The fact that drusen may closely simulate early or chronic papilledema, that they are associated with visual field defects, and that they may occasionally show solitary hemorrhages often serve to complicate the diagnostic picture and impart a sense of urgency to the diagnosis.[232] If buried drusen go unrecognized, the elevated optic discs may precipitate inappropriate diagnostic studies.[225]

The conceptual problem that persists in understanding the evolution of disc drusen comes from viewing drusen as the cause rather than the effect of an underlying configurational anomaly of the disc. This tendency carries over into our analysis of associated complications (e.g., the lack of correspondence between visual field abnormalities with the position of visible drusen on the disc has puzzled many). It is helpful to recognize at the outset that the time course of evolution of optic disc drusen and the histopathological findings suggest that disc drusen actually result from axonal degeneration, rather than encroaching upon adjacent axons to cause their degeneration. Disc

drusen signify a *chronic, low-grade optic neuropathy measured over decades.*

Epidemiology

Lorentzen examined 3200 routine cases from an ophthalmological practice in Denmark and found that 11 had drusen of the optic disc (for a prevalence of 0.34%). This prevalence increased by a factor of 10 in family members of patients with disc drusen.[165] Friedman et al examined 737 cadavers and found disc drusen in 15. The drusen were often minute and situated deep within the optic nerve tissue.[83] Francois, and later Lorentzen, concluded that familial drusen are transmitted as an autosomal dominant trait.[80,166] Subsequent studies have confirmed the familial nature of this anomaly.[128,166,253] Disc drusen are rare in blacks.[128,225] The early notion that disc drusen are associated with hyperopia has not been substantiated.[128,193,225] In one large study, visible disc drusen were bilateral in approximately two-thirds of cases, whereas pseudopapilledema associated with buried drusen were bilateral in 86% of cases.[225] Although Erkkila found a high prevalence of clumsiness, learning disabilities, and neurological problems in her Finnish population of children with drusen,[69] subsequent studies have failed to substantiate these findings.

Ophthalmoscopic Appearance in Children

In our experience, most childhood cases present initially with pseudopapilledema secondary to buried drusen (Figure 3.14). In this setting, the disc appears elevated, and its margins are blurred or obscured.[82] The elevated disc may have a gray or a yellow-white discoloration. Disc drusen tend to become more ophthalmoscopically conspicuous with age.[180] In older children, there is often a scalloped contour to the disc margins, due to the presence of partially buried drusen protruding from the edge of the disc into the peripapillary retina.[82]

Buried drusen are most visible at the margin of the disc, where they impart an irregular lumpy-bumpy contour to the line of demarcation between the elevated disc and the retina (Figure 3.15). Exposed drusen are more frequently found on the nasal side of the optic disc. Surface drusen appear as yellowish, globular, hemitranslucent formations

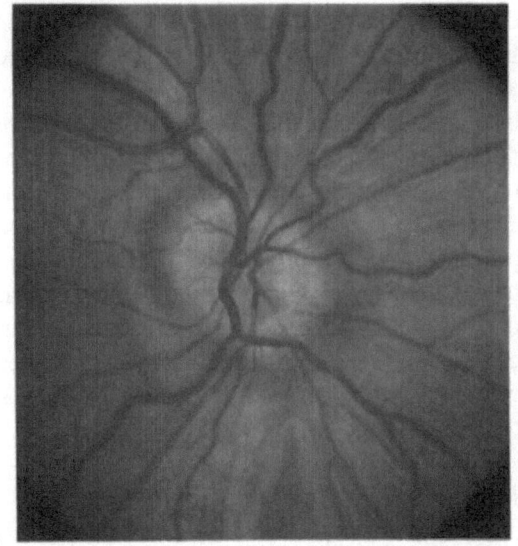
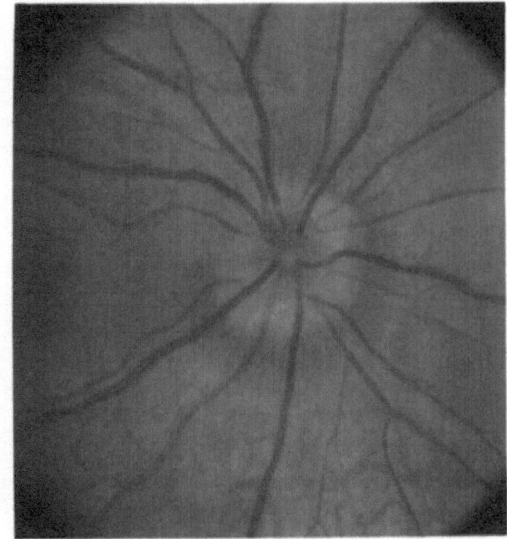

A

B

FIGURE 3.14. (**A, B**) Two examples of pseudopapilledema with buried drusen. Note cupless discs, anomalous vasculature, and crescentic circumpapillary light reflexes. A few surface drusen are visible in (**B**).

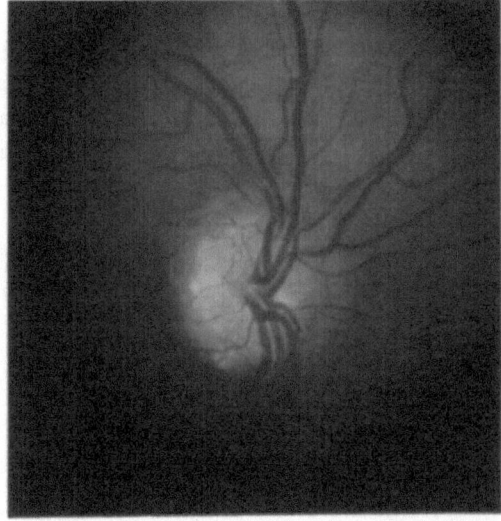
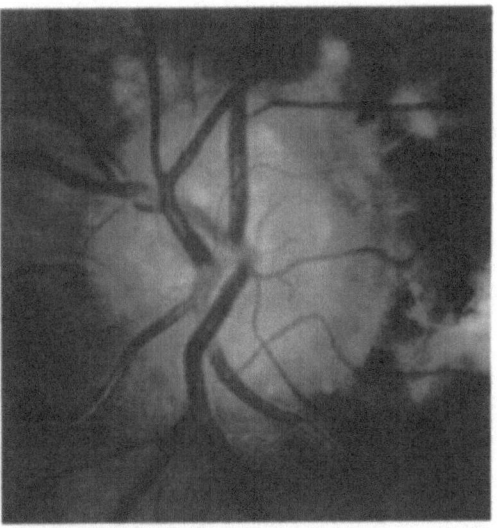

A

B

FIGURE 3.15. (**A, B**) Two examples of pseudopapilledema with surface drusen. Note peripapillary pigment atrophy in (**B**).

on the optic disc, often accumulated in larger or smaller conglomerations[165] (Figure 3.16). They may occur singularly, in grapelike clusters, or as fused conglomerations, varying in size from small dots to several vein widths in diameter.[82] By direct illumination, the central portion of each druse shines uniformly, while the border may appear as a glistening ring. With indirect illumination of the druse from light focused on the peripapillary retina, the druse shines uniformly, except for a brighter, semicircular marginal zone on the side opposite from the spot of light (known as inverse shading). In addition to the small size of the optic disc and the absence of a central physiological cup, the disc vasculature is anomalous (Figure 3.15). The major retinal vessels are increased in number and often tortuous (Figure 3.15). They tend to branch early and may trifurcate or quadrificate. The prevalence of cilioretinal arteries is also increased, with estimates ranging from 24.1%[193] to 43%.[69] Mustonen found peripapillary atrophy or pigment epithelial derangement in 29.7% of eyes (Figure 3.16).[193] Retinal venous loops or anomalous retinociliary shunt vessels are occasionally seen.

Distinguishing Buried Disc Drusen from Papilledema

The distinction between pseudopapilledema associated with buried drusen from papilledema (or other forms of optic disc edema) can at times be difficult, but there are several clinical signs that serve to distinguish these two conditions (Table 3.13).[129] In papilledema, the swelling extends into the peripapillary retina and obscures the peripapillary retinal vasculature. In pseudopapilledema, there is a discrete, sometimes grayish or straw-colored elevation of the disc without obscuration of vessels or opacification of peripapillary retina. Hoyt and Knight[130] have called attention to the graying or muddying of the peripapillary nerve fiber layer that occurs with swelling of the optic

disc from papilledema or other causes. In pseudopapilledema associated with buried drusen, light reflexes of the peripapillary nerve fiber layer appear sharp, and the elevated disc is often haloed by a crescentic peripapillary ring of light that reflects from the concave internal limiting membrane surrounding the elevation (Figure 3.14). This crescentic light reflex is absent in papilledema, due to diffraction of light from distended peripapillary axons.[69,124,130] Single splinter or subretinal optic disc hemorrhages are occasionally seen with disc drusen, but exudates, cotton wool spots, hyperemia, and venous congestion are conspicuously absent.[124,165]

Fluorescein Angiographic Appearance

Discs with ophthalmoscopically prominent drusen may exhibit autofluorescence in the preinjection phase.[82] This is followed by a true nodular hyperfluourescence corresponding to the location of the drusen. Hyperfluorescence, which typically is mild, begins in the arteriovenous phase and continues into the late phases. The superficial disc capillary network may show prominence in areas overlying buried drusen (Figure 3.16).[82] The late phases may be characterized by some minimal

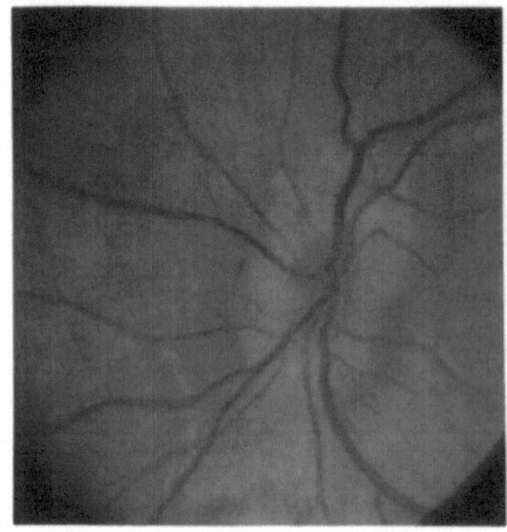
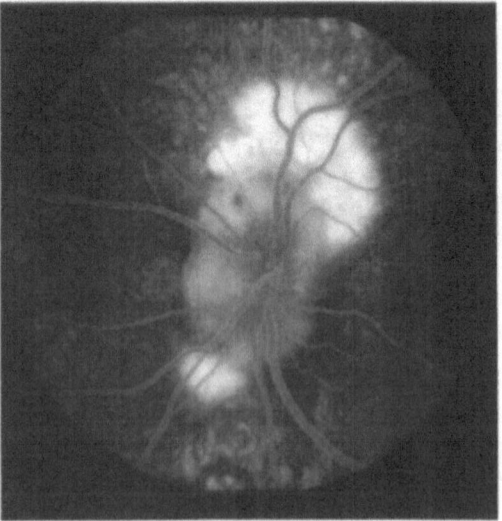

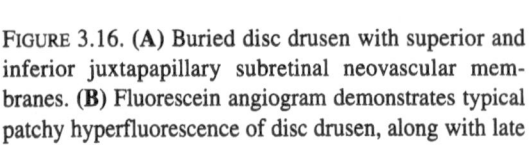

FIGURE 3.16. (A) Buried disc drusen with superior and inferior juxtapapillary subretinal neovascular membranes. (B) Fluorescein angiogram demonstrates typical patchy hyperfluorescence of disc drusen, along with late peripapillary staining corresponding to juxtapapillary subretinal neovascular membranes. (Courtesy of Stephen C. Pollock, MD.)

TABLE 3.13. Ophthalmoscopic features useful in differentiating optic disc swelling from pseudopapilledema associated with buried drusen in children.

Optic disc swelling	Pseudopapilledema with buried drusen
Disc vasculature obscured at disc margins	Disc vasculature remains visible at disc margins
Elevation extends into peripapillary retina	Elevation confined to optic disc
Graying and muddying of peripapillary nerve fiber layer	Sharp peripapillary nerve fiber reflexes
Venous congestion	No venous congestion
+/- exudates	No exudates
Loss of optic cup only in moderate to severe disc edema	Small cupless disc
Normal configuration of disc vasculature despite venous congestion	Increased major retinal vessels with early branching and anomalous trifurcations and quadrifurcations
No circumpapillary light reflex	Crescentic circumpapillary light reflex
Absence of spontaneous venous pulsations	Spontaneous venous pulsations may be present or absent

blurring of the drusen that may either fade or maintain fluorescence (staining). Unlike papilledema, however, there is no visible leakage along the major vessels.[232,253] Venous anomalies (venous stasis, venous convolutions, and retinociliary venous communications) and staining of the peripapillary vein walls are occasionally seen.[138]

Histopathology

Optic disc drusen are situated anterior to the lamina cribrosa; they occur nowhere else in the brain. They consist of homogenous, globular concretions, often collected in larger, multilobulated agglomerations. Individual druse usually exhibit a concentrically laminated structure, which is not encapsulated and contains no cells or cellular debris.[165] Drusen are often most concentrated within the nasal portion of the disc. The optic disc axons are atrophic adjacent to large accumulations of drusen.[33,84,165] Drusen take up calcium salts and must be decalcified before being cut into sections for histological study.[165]

Pathogenesis

The primary developmental expression of the genetic trait for drusen may be a smaller-than-normal scleral canal.[172,190] The peripapillary sclera forms after the optic stalk is complete.[190] Mesenchymal elements from the sclera then invade the glial framework of the primitive lamina, reinforcing it with collagen.[190] An abnormal encroachment of sclera, Bruch's membrane, or both upon the developing optic stalk would narrow the exit space of optic axons from the eye. The absence of a central

cup in affected eyes is consistent with the existence of axonal crowding. Drusen are often first detected clinically and histopathologically at the margins of the optic disc, which raises the possibility that the rigid edge of the scleral canal may be an aggravating factor in producing a relative mechanical interruption of axonal transport.[190]

In 1962, Seitz and Kersting first suggested that disc drusen may be the product of chronic degenerative changes in ganglion cell axons.[242] In 1968, Seitz concluded from a series of histochemical studies that drusen originate from axonal derivatives of disintegrating nerve fibers resulting from a slow degenerative process.[243] Sacks et al advanced an alternative hypothesis that formation of drusen is secondary to the associated abnormal disc vascular pattern, which is conducive to leakage of nonformed elements such as plasma proteins from the blood, and that these elements serve as a nidus for the deposition of other materials within the perivascular space, which then gradually increase in size and coalesce.[230] In his A.O.S thesis, Spencer hypothesized that axonal crowding may provide the anatomical substrate for impaired axoplasmic transport anterior to the lamina cribrosa that, over years, leads to intracellular mitochondrial calcification, axonal rupture, extrusion of mitochondria into the extracellular space, and the appearance of drusen on the surface of the disc.[258] Tso favored a similar mechanism but believed that abnormal axonal metabolism, rather than axonal transport, was responsible for the accumulation of disc drusen.[185,269] The lower prevalence of optic disc drusen in blacks, who have a larger disc area with less potential for axonal crowding, is consistent with the notion of axonal crowding as a fundamental anatomical substrate for formation of disc drusen.[172] Figure 3.17 summarizes our current understanding of the pathogenesis of optic disc drusen and their attendent complications.

Ocular Complications

Optic disc drusen should not be viewed as an innocuous condition. While the finding of disc drusen is generally compatible with preservation

Pathogenesis of Optic Disc Drusen

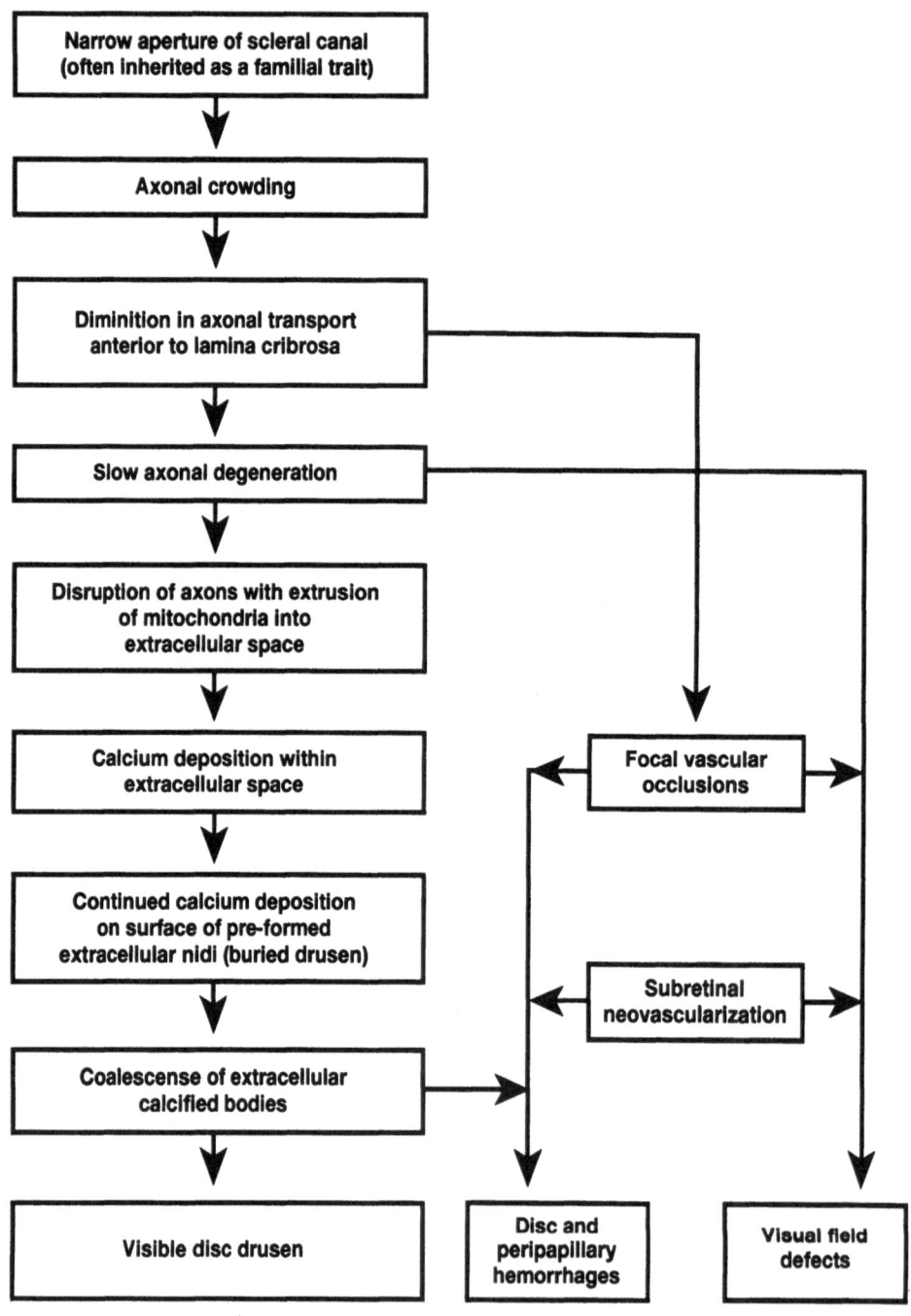

FIGURE 3.17. Pathogenesis of optic disc drusen. (Modified from Tso.[269])

of good visual function, rare patients may experience acquired progressive loss of visual field or visual acuity via a number of different mechanisms. Acquired visual loss in eyes with drusen is rare in childhood but may afflict young adults. As such, it is appropriate to inform patients that, while disc drusen rarely cause blindness, there is a remote possibility that affected patients may develop visual symptoms later in life.

Visual field defects have been detected in 71% to 87% of eyes with visible disc drusen and in 21% to 39% of eyes with pseudopapilledema but no visible drusen.[165,193,236] In most cases, the asymptomatic nature of the defects reflect the insidious attrition of optic nerve fibers over decades.[236] Less common but equally recognized is the abrupt visual field loss that may accompany vascular occlusions or hemorrhagic phenomena.[236]

Using Goldmann perimetry, Savino et al found field defects in 71% of patients with visible drusen, as opposed to only 21% with buried drusen.[236] Visual field defects fall into three general categories: (1) nerve fiber bundle defects; (2) enlargement of the blind spot; and (3) concentric field constriction.[82] Several studies noted inferonasal steps to be the most common nerve fiber bundle defect, but both arcuate defects and sector defects are not uncommon.[165,166,236,260] Mustonen found an afferent pupilary defect associated with asymmetrical visual field defects in 14 of 200 patients with optic disc drusen.[191,192] Miller stated that an afferent pupillary defect is the rule rather than the exception in the setting of unilateral or asymmetrical visual field loss from optic disc drusen without visual acuity loss.[179] Although concentric constriction of the visual field is recognized as a chronic phenomenon, three adults have recently been documented to have sudden severe visual field constriction with preservation of central vision.[181,185] There was no disc swelling or retinal edema to suggest an ischemic process in these patients.

The pathogenesis of visual field loss in eyes with disc drusen could involve one or more of the following: (1) abnormality in axoplasmic flow leading to dysfunction of nerve fibers—the formation of drusen has been postulated to be related to axonal degeneration from altered axoplasmic flow;[258,269] (2) compression of nerve fibers by the drusen, or (3) ischemia within the optic nerve

head.[23] The visual field defects often fail to correspond to the position of the visible drusen on the disc.[234,235] The presence of disc drusen also does not preclude superimposition of field defects from other ocular or intracranial disease.[236]

Transient visual loss was reported in 8.6% of the patients with disc drusen in Lorentzen's study.[165] Episodes of transient visual loss may be a harbinger of vascular occlusions in some patients.[194]

Superficial splinter or flame-shaped hemorrhages on the surface of the disc or peripapillary area may be seen in patients with optic disc drusen.[191,233] Splinter hemorrhages associated with optic disc drusen tend to be single and prepapillary in location, in contrast to the multiple hemorrhages in the nerve fiber layer that characterize papilledema.[124] They are not visually significant, but may cause diagnostic confusion if they arouse suspicion of papilledema.[82] Large superficial hemorrhages can rarely extend into the vitreous.

Deep peripapillary hemorrhages have been documented in children with disc drusen.[69,225] These hemorrhages may be subretinal or subpigment epithelial and are typically circumferentially oriented around the disc. The question of whether these hemorrhages can be caused by compression of thin-walled veins by drusen conglomerates or by erosion of the vessel wall by the sharp edge of the druse remains unsettled.[138] Wise et al postulated that enlarging disc drusen could result in circulatory compromise and local hypoxia, which might then stimulate the growth of new vessels between the RPE and Bruch's membrane which are prone to hemorrhage.[286] Peripapillary pigmentary disruption may remain following resolution of subretinal hemorrhage. Subretinal hemorrhage may also occur in papilledema, but its occurence in early papilledema is rare and should suggest the possibility of disc drusen.[124]

Peripapillary subretinal neovascularization is a recognized complication in eyes with disc drusen (Figure 3.16). Peripapillary subretinal neovascularization may manifest as a peripapillary subpigment epithelial hemorrhage and may be associated with either transient or permanent visual disturbances.[286] In severe cases, this complication may simulate a neuroretinitis (Figure 3.18). Harris found subretinal neovascularization in seven eyes

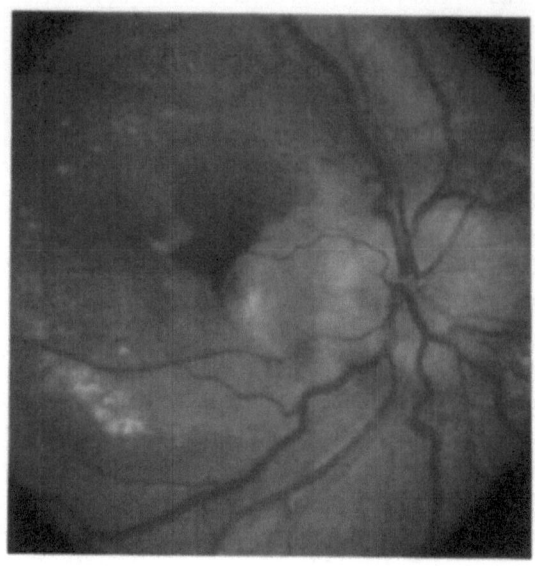

FIGURE 3.18. A 10-year-old child with buried drusen and subretinal neovascular membrane simulating neuroretinitis. (Courtesy of Stephen C. Pollock, MD.)

of 57 patients with optic disc drusen.[113] They also noted that hemorrhages occuring in the absence of choroidal vascularization produced no symptoms and resolved without sequelae, while hemorrhages resulting from choroidal neovascularization commonly produced visual symptoms. In their study, six of seven eyes with neovascular membranes retained visual acuities of 20/40 or better. Based upon their findings, they recommended observation rather than laser photocoagulation for peripapillary choroidal neovascularization associated with disc drusen.

Vascular occlusions have been reported in patients with disc drusen. The most common of these causes ischemic optic neuropathy which may occur as a single episode or as successive episodes of discrete visual loss over years.[234] Karel et al[138] documented ischemic optic neuropathy in three patients (including one 13-year-old boy) with optic disc drusen. Branch retinal artery occlusion, central retinal artery occlusion, and central retinal vein occlusion have also been reported. Retinal vascular occlusions can occur in young adulthood, and rare cases in children have been documented.[194,211]

The mechanism by which disc drusen produce vascular occlusion is uncertain.[194] The following theories have been advanced:

Vascular anomalies are commonly associated with intrapapillary drusen, and it has been suggested that these tortuous vessels with abnormal branching patterns and loops are more susceptible to disrupted hemodynamics.[194]

Disc drusen are associated with small cupless discs that may predispose to crowding of the vasculature and vascular compromise. The association of ischemic optic neuropathy with small cupless discs is well established.[234]

Drusen are hard, unyielding structures that may directly compromise adjacent vessels.[194]

Peripapillary central serous choroidopathy has been described in association with disc drusen.[184] Fluorescein angiography showed a bright hyperflourescent spot superonasal to the disc. The detachment resolved following focal laser photocoagulation of the RPE defect.

Loss of central acuity has been reported as a rare complication of disc drusen. In most cases, this follows a series of episodic, stepwise events that progressively diminish the peripheral visual field.[23,151] Loss of visual acuity should only be attributed to disc drusen after potential intracranial causes have been ruled out.

Systemic Associations

Retinitis Pigmentosa. Globular excrescences of the optic nerve head are occasionally seen in patients with retinitis pigmentosa. They differ in appearance from typical disc drusen in that the disc does not appear elevated and they often lie just off the disc margin in the superficial retina. Some investigators have documented an increase in size, leading to the conjecture that they may be hamartomas rather than drusen.[59,208] More recent histopathological examination has confirmed that the globular excresences of the optic nerve in retinitis pigmentosa are indeed drusen.[210] Children with retinitis pigmentosa and buried drusen may present with optic disc elevation and masquerade as having neurological disease.[121]

The combination of vitreous cells with optic disc elevation may masquerade as uveitis in a child with retinitis pigmentosa. In this setting, the finding of attenuated retinal arterioles provides an important (and easily overlooked) clue to the diagnosis, which is confirmed by electroretinography.[121]

Pseudoexanthoma Elasticum. The incidence of optic disc drusen in pseudoxanthoma elasticum is 20 to 50 times greater than in the general population.[48] Disc drusen may be the earliest clinical manifestation of pseudoxanthoma elasticum.[48] Coleman et al postulated that an abnormal aggregation of macromolecules with a high affinity for calcium (which affects elastin in the dermis, arterial walls, and Bruch's membrane) may also develop at the lamina cribrosa, disrupting axonal transport and leading to disc drusen formation.[48] The association of angioid streaks with disc drusen should suggest the systemic diagnosis of pseudoxanthoma elasticum.

Megalencephaly. Hoover et al found megalencephaly in 3 of 40 children with pseudopapilledema and cautioned that such children can be misdiagnosed as having hydrocephalus.[126]

Migraine Headaches. Migraines are said to occur with increased frequency in patients with disc drusen.[193,273] Some have pointed out that the concurrence of migraine and optic disc drusen probably reflects the frequent and often expedited referral of patients with headache and elevated discs for specialty evaluation.[194]

Pigmented Paravenous Retinochoroidal Atrophy. Disc drusen were recently noted in a patient with pigmented paravenous retinochoroidal atrophy.[289] This association may be fortuitous.

Natural History and Prognosis

The evolution of disc drusen is a dynamic process that continues throughout life. It is rare to see visible drusen or significant optic disc elevation in an infant. During childhood, the involved optic discs begin to appear "full" and acquire a tan, yellow, or straw color.[258] Gradually, buried drusen become apparent as they produce subtle excrescences that impart a scalloped appearance to the margin of the disc. Buried drusen gradually enlarge, calcify, and become visible on the surface of the disc.[180] In adult years, the optic disc elevation diminishes, and the disc slowly becomes pale as the nerve fiber layer thins.[258] It is rare to see optic disc elevation in elderly adults with drusen. This evolution reflects the slow attrition of optic axons over decades. Despite this process, most patients remain asymptomatic and retain normal acuity.

Neuroimaging of Optic Disc Drusen

The distinction between papilledema and pseudopapilledema has been aided by CT scanning and ultrasonography, which readily demonstrate calcification within the elevated optic disc.[20,86] It is not uncommon to see a child referred for possible papilledema arrive for consultation with their "negative" CT scan in hand, only to find undetected calcification of the optic discs upon review of the scan (Figure 3.19).

Ultrasonography appears to be equally sensitive in demonstrating buried disc drusen.[32] It has the advantage of not subjecting the child to radiation; however, it requires skilled personnel and has the relative disadvantage of not simultaneously imaging the brain.

Ocular Disorders Associated with Pseudopapilledema

The small cupless disc associated with optic disc drusen is the most common cause of pseudopapilledema. Other local causes include the following:

A persistent anterior hyaloid artery may produce anterior traction on the optic disc.[149]

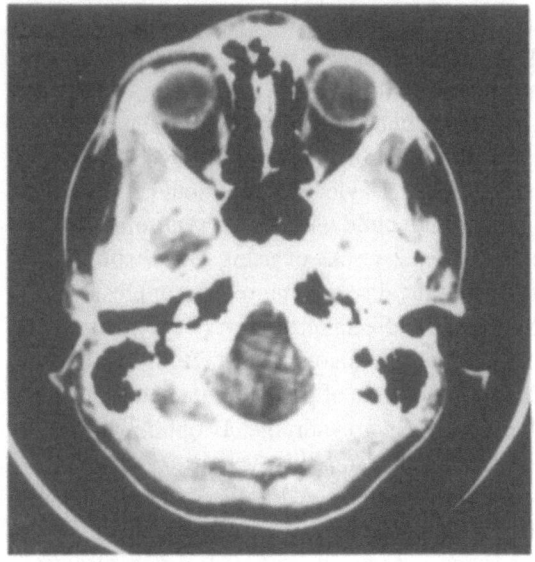

FIGURE 3.19. "Normal" CT scan showing posterior scleral calcification corresponding to optic disc drusen. (Courtesy of Stephan C. Pollock, MD.)

- Epipapillary glial tissue associated with Bergmeister's papilla may produce anterior traction that elevates the disc. Flat opaque epipapillary glial tissue may obscure visualization of the underlying disc margins and thereby simulate disc edema.
- Hypermetropic or nanophthalmic eyes with small scleral canals may have elevated optic discs.[267] Nanophthalmic eyes may also be associated with a solitary retinal fold extending from the disc to the macula.
- Juxtapapillary myelinated nerve fibers are occasionally mistaken for papilledema.[267]

Systemic Disorders Associated with Pseudopapilledema

Down Syndrome

Children with Down syndrome are said to have a characteristic optic disc appearance consisting of a rosy plethoric disc, RPE attenuation surrounding the disc, and an increased number of major vessels emanating from the disc.[2] Catalano and Simon[46] have recently described optic disc elevation without venous engorgement or obscuration of vessels in five children with Down syndrome. Although two of these had congenital cardiac defects that cause right to left shunts which may cause elevated intracranial pressure, the elevated optic discs did not appear to be swollen in these cases. Three children showed partial, complete, or intermittent resolution of the disc elevation.

Children with Down syndrome may also develop true optic disc edema by several different mechanisms. Taylor[267] has noted optic disc swelling in a child with Down syndrome that resolved after 2 weeks of using elbow splints. He attributed the disc edema to the compressive/decompressive effects of the severe eye poking that can be seen in this condition. Additionally, we know of two cases of pseudotumor cerebri in children with Down syndrome. If ophthalmoscopic signs of papilledema (i.e., venous distension, obscuration of vessels at the disc margin, hemorrhages, exudates) are present, children with Down syndrome associated with optic disc elevation should not be relegated to a benign diagnosis until elevated intracranial pressure is ruled out by a lumbar puncture.

Alagille Syndrome

The Alagille syndrome, or arteriohepatic dysplasia, is a well-recognized multiple-malformation syndrome consisting of a paucity of intrahepatic biliary ducts, cholestatic facies, peripheral pulmonary artery hypoplasia or stenosis (often with other cardiac abnormalities), butterfly-like vertebral arch defects, and variable ocular defects, most commonly posterior embryotoxon.[5] Both sporadic and familial cases have been reported, and it has been suggested that Alagille syndrome is inherited as an autosomal dominant trait with variable expressivity and reduced penetrance.[189,249] An interstitial deletion of the short arm of chromosome 20 recently has been found in some patients with the Alagille syndrome.[290] It has been proposed that this condition is a contiguous gene syndrome assigned provisionally to an approximately 8-Mb segment on chromosome 20 (p11.23 to p12.1).[238]

The Alagille syndrome comprises a broad spectrum of ocular anomalies involving the cornea, iris, retina, and optic disc.[36] Characteristic ocular anomalies include posterior embryotoxon, slightly small corneas, a peculiar mosaic pattern of iris stromal hypoplasia, anomalous optic discs, and streaky peripapillary depigmentation.[36] Optic disc elevation has been described in numerous cases of Alagille syndrome (Figure 3.20). The optic disc elevation in Alagille syndrome has been attributed to pseudopapilledema, because previous studies have found no leakage of fluorescein at the optic disc, no evidence of drusen by ultrasonography, and no change in appearance in one patient who was observed over a 10-year period.[89,223] These findings suggest that the optic disc elevation is a genetically determined anomaly that is unrelated to pulmonary vascular compromise or to metabolic imbalance.[36] Patients with Alagille syndrome may also display horizontally elongated or obliquely oriented anomalous optic discs (Figure 3.20).

Kenny Syndrome

Systemic findings in Kenny syndrome include low birth weight, dwarfism, delayed closure of the anterior fontanel, thickened long bone cortex with stenotic medullary cavities, transient hypocalcemia with hyperphosphatemia leading to tetany, and normal mentation.[34] Ocular findings range

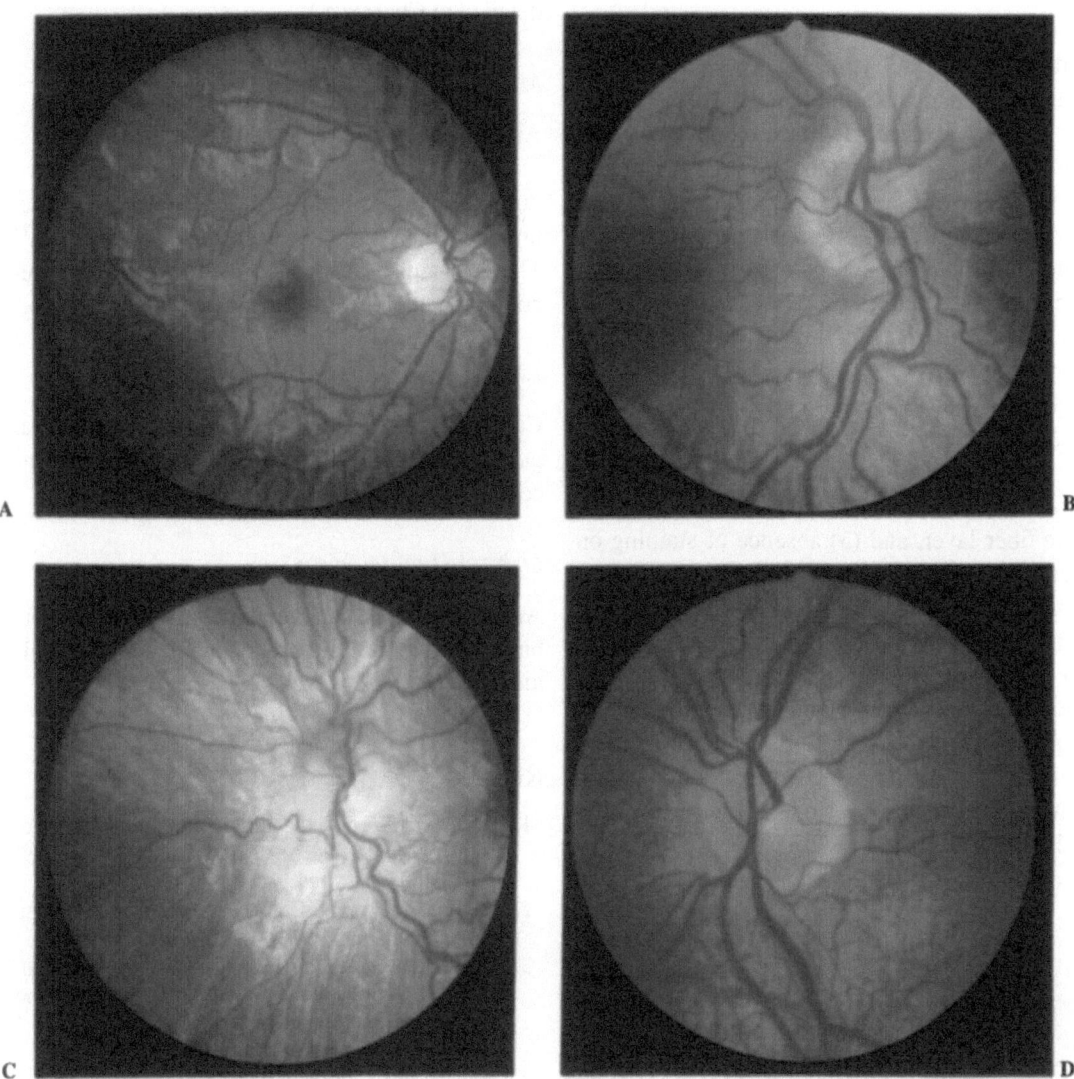

FIGURE 3.20. (A) Characteristic optic disc anomalies in Alagille syndrome including horizontal elongation of the disc, (B, C) pseudopapilledema, and (D) anomalous inferotemporal scleral crescent. Note streaky peripapillary depigmentation characteristic of Alagille syndrome.

from uncomplicated nanophthalmos with high hyperopia to extreme pseudopapilledema, vascular tortuousity, and macular crowding.[34]

Autopsy examination from one patient with Kenny syndrome disclosed narrow scleral apertures with elevation and lateral displacement of disc tissue.[34] This patient also had total absence of parathyroid tissue. Several small, calcified prelaminar drusenlike bodies were noted in one eye. The pseudopapilledema in this condition presumably results from local factors (interruption of axonal transport associated with nanophthalmos and small scleral canals), although the associated metabolic imbalance (i.e., hypocalcemia with or without associated hypoparathyroidism) may also play a role. Kenny syndrome should be suspected when pseudopapilledema and nanophthalmos occur in a child with a history of dwarfism, hypocalcemia, and tetany.

Leber Hereditary Neuroretinopathy

Leber hereditary neuroretinopathy is characterized by acute or subacute loss of vision in both
eyes that can occur simultaneously or can be
seperated by a period of weeks, months, or years.
It is transmitted by mitochondrial inheritance.
Several different mitochondrial mutations that appear to have differing prognosis have heretofore
been identified.[195] There is a definite male predominance. Visual loss usually occurs in the second to fourth decades but may occasionally occur
in childhood.

Patients with this disorder and many asymptomatic carriers display characteristic peripapillary retinal alterations consisting of (1) peripapillary microangiopathy, (2) pseudoedema of the
nerve fiber layer, and (3) absence of staining on
flourescein angiography[197,256] (Figure 3.21).
Retinal vascular tortuousity may also be prominent.[195] When the disease occurs for the first time
in a family, it is often mistaken for papillitis. The
disc often initially appears cupless, although cupping may develop as optic atrophy supervenes.[195]
Central visual loss is permanent, although a subgroup of patients recover one or more small islands of central vision within their central scotoma up to a year or two after vision is lost. (The

genetic and systemic aspects of this disorder are
detailed in Chapter 4.)

Mucopolysaccharidosis

As mentioned earlier, optic disc edema is a common finding in children with mucopolysaccharidosis. Pseudopapilledema may also occur, as documented in a patient with Scheie syndrome.[271]
The mechanisms of optic disc elevation in the mucopolysaccharidosis are summarized in Table 3.6.

Linear Sebaceous Nevus Syndrome

Campbell and Patterson[45] described unilateral
pseudopapilledema in a child with linear sebaceous nevus syndrome.

Orbital Hypotelorism

Awan[12] has described an association between orbital hypotelorism and pseudopapilledema with situs inversus of the vessels.

References

1. Aaberg TM. The expanding ophthalmologic spectrum of Lyme disease. Am J Ophthalmol 1989;
   107:77-80.
2. Ahmad A, Pruett RC: The fundus in mongolism.
   Arch Ophthalmol 1976;94:772-776.
3. Ahmadieh H, Roodpeyma S, Azarmina M, et al.
   Bilateral simultaneous optic neuritis in childhood
   systemic lupus erythematosis: a case report. J
   Neuro-ophthalmol 1994;14:84-86.
4. Ainsworth JR, Bryce IG, Dudgeon J. Visual loss in
   osteopetrosis. J Pediatr Ophthalmol Strabis 1993;
   30:201-203.
5. Alagille D, Estrada A, Hadchouel M, et al. Syndromic paucity of interlobular bile ducts (Alagille
   syndrome or arteriohepatic dysplasia): review of
   80 cases. J Pediatr 1987;110:195-200.
6. Alexandrakis G, Filatov V, Walsh T. Pseudotumor
   cerebri in a 12-year-old boy with Addison's disease. Am J Ophthalmol 1993;116:650-651.
6a. Al-Mefty O, Fox JL, Al-Rodhan N, Dew JH. Optic
   nerve decompression in osteopetrosis. J Neurosurg
   1988;68:80-84.
7. Al-Rodhan NRF, Sundt TM, Piepgras DG. Occlusive hyperemia: a theory for the hemodynamic
   complications following resection of intracerebral
   arteriovenous malformations. J Neurosurg 1993;
   78:167-175.
8. Allen RA, Straatsma BR. Ocular involvement in
   leukemia and allied disorders. Arch Ophthalmol
   1961;66:68-86.

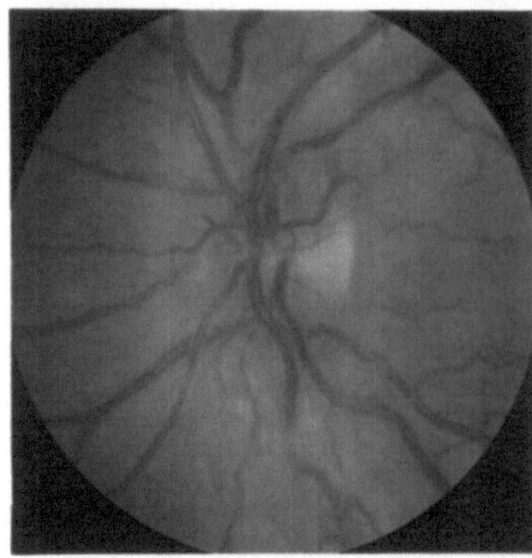

FIGURE 3.21. Pseudopapilledema in Leber hereditary
neuroretinopathy.

9. Alper MG. Management of primary optic nerve meningiomas. J Clin Neuro-ophthalmol 1981; 1:101-117.

10. Atlas SW, Grossman RI, Goldberg HI, et al. MR Diagnosis of acute disseminated encephalomyelitis. J Comput Asst Tomogr 1986;10:798-801.

11. Avery R, Jabs DA, Wingard JR: Optic disc edema after bone marrow transplantation. Ophthalmology 1991;98:1294-1301.

12. Awan KJ. Hypotelorism and optic disc anomalies: an ignored ocular syndrome. Ann Ophthalmol 1977;9:771-777.

13. Babikian P, Corbett J, Bell W. Idiopathic intracranial hypertension in children: the Iowa experience. J Child Neurol 1994;9:144-149.

14. Baker RS, Carter D, Hendrick EB, Buncic JR. Visual loss in pseudotumor cerebri: a follow-up study. Arch Ophthalmol 1985;103:1681-1686.

15. Baker RS, Baumann RJ, Buncic JR. Idiopathic intracranial hypertension (pseudotumor cerebri) in pediatric patients. Pediatr Neurol 1989;5:5-11.

16. Bar S, Segal M, Shapira R, Savir H. Neuroretinitis associated with cat scratch disease. Am J Ophthalmol 1990;110:703-705.

17. Barr CC, Glaser JS, Blankenship G. Acute disc swelling in juvenile diabetes. Arch Ophthalmol 1980;98:2185-2192.

18. Baum PA, Barkovich AJ, Coch TK, Berg BO. Deep gray matter involvement in children with acute disseminated encephalomyelitis. AJNR 1994;15:1275-1283.

19. Beardsley TL, Brown S, Sydnor CF, et al. Eleven cases of sarcoidosis of the optic nerve. Am J Ophthalmol 1984;97:62-77.

20. Bec P, Adam P, Mathis A, et al. Optic nerve head drusen: high resolution computed tomographic approach. Arch Ophthalmol 1984;102:680-682.

21. Beck M. Papilledema in association with Hunter's syndrome. Br J Ophthalmol 1983;67:174-177.

22. Beck M, Cole G. Disc oedema in association with Hunter's syndrome: ocular histopathological findings. Br J Ophthalmol 1984;68:590-594.

23. Beck RW, Corbett JJ, Thompson HS, Sergott RC. Decreased visual acuity from optic disc drusen. Arch Ophthalmol 1985;103:1155-1159.

24. Beck RW, Arrington J, Murtagh FR, et al. Brain MRI in acute optic neuritis: experience of the optic Neuritis Study Group. Arch Neurol 1993;8: 841-846.

25. Beck RW, Cleary PA, Trobe JD, et al. The effect of corticosteroids for acute optic neuritis on the subsequent development of multiple sclerosis. N Engl J Med 1993;329:1764-1769.

26. Beck AD, Newman NJ, Grossniklaus HE, et al. Optic nerve enlargement and chronic visual loss. Surv Ophthalmol 1994;38:555-566.

27. Benson WE. Posterior scleritis. Surv Ophthalmol 1988;32:297-316.

28. Berrios RR, Serrano LA. Bilateral optic neuritis after a bee sting. Am J Ophthalmol 1994;117:677.

29. Bertelsen TI. The premature synostosis of the cranial sutures. Acta Ophthalmol (Copenh) 1980;58 (suppl):733.

30. Bird AC, Smith JL, Curtin VT. Nematode optic neuritis. Am J Ophthalmol 1970;69:72-77.

31. Blaustein A, Caccavo A. Infectious mononucleosis complicated by bilateral papilloretinal edema. Arch Ophtahlmol 1950;43:853-856.

32. Boldt HC, Byrne SF, DiBernardo C. Echographic evaluation of optic disc drusen. J Clin Neuro-ophthalmol 1991;11(2):85-91.

33. Boyce SW, Platia EV, Green WR. Drusen of the optic nerve head. Ann Ophthalmol 1978;10:695-704.

34. Boynton JR, Pheasant TR, Johnson BL, et al. Ocular findings in Kenny's syndrome. Arch Ophthalmol 1979;97:896-900.

35. Brazis PW, Stokes MR, Ervin FR. Optic neuritis in cat scratch disease. J Clin Neuro-ophthalmol 1986;6:172-174.

36. Brodsky MC, Cunniff C. Ocular anomalies in the Alagille syndrome. Ophthalmology 1993;100: 1767-1774.

37. Brodsky MC, Beck RW. The changing role of MR imaging in the evaluation of acute optic neuritis. Editorial. Radiology 1994;192:22-23.

38. Brodsky MC, Glasier CM. Intraocular enhancement of the swollen optic disc on MR imaging. J Clin Neuro-ophthalmol, 1995. In press.

39. Brodsky MC, Wald KJ, Chen S, Weiter JJ. Protracted posttraumatic optic disc swelling. Ophthalmology 1995. In press.

40. Budenz DL, Farber MG, Mirchandani HG, et al. Ocular and optic nerve hemorrhages in abused infants with intracranial injuries. Ophthalmology 1994;101:559-565.

41. Burde RM. Optic disk risk factors for nonarteritic anterior ischemic optic neuropathy. Am J Ophthalmol 1993;116:759-764.

42. Bye A, Dendall B, Wilson J. Multiple sclerosis in childhood: a new look. Dev Med Child Neurol 1985;27:215-222.

43. Byrd SE, Locke GE, Biggers S, Percy AK. The computed tomographic appearance of cerebral cysticercosis in adults and children. Radiology 1982; 144:819-823.

44. Caffey J. On the theory and practice of shaking infants: its potential residual effects of permanent brain damage and mental retardation. Am J Dis Child 1972;124:161-169.

45. Campbell SH, Patterson A. Pseudopapilloedema in the linear naevus syndrome. Br J Ophthalmol 1992;76:372-374.

46. Catalano RA, Simon JW. Optic disc elevation in Down syndrome. Am J Ophthalmol 1990; 110:28-32.

47. Chrousos GA, Drack AV, Young M, et al. Neuroretinitis in cat scratch disease. J Clin Neuro-ophthalmol 1990;10:92-94.

48. Coleman K, Hope Ross M, McCabe M, et al. Disk drusen and angioid streaks in pseudoxanthoma elasticum. Am J Ophthalmol 1991;112:166-170.

49. Collins MLZ, Traboulsi EI, Maumenee IH. Optic nerve head swelling and optic atrophy in the systemic mucopolysaccharidoses. Ophthalmology 1990;97:1445-1449.

50. Connally MB, Farrell K, Hill A, Flodmark O. Magnetic resonance imaging in pseudotumor cerebri. Dev Med Child Neurol 1992;34:1091-1094.

51. Corbett J. neuro-ophthalmologic complications of hydrocephalus and shunting procedures. Semin Neurol 1986;6(2):111-123.

52. Corbett JJ, Jacobson DM, Mauer RC, Thompson HS. Enlargment of the blind spot caused by papilledema. Am J Ophthalmol 1988;105:261-265.

53. Corbett JJ, Thompson HS. The rational management of idiopathic intracranial hypertension. Arch Neurol 1989;46:1049-1051.

54. Corbett JJ. Mechanisms of elevated intracranial pressure in idiopathic intracranial hypertension. Presented at the North American Neuro-Ophthalmology Society Meeting, Rancho Bernardo, CA, February 1992.

55. Couch R, Camfield PR, Tibbles JAR. The changing picture of pseudotumor cerebri in children. Can J Neurol Sci 1985;12:48-50.

56. Cox TA, Haskins GE, Gangitano JL, Antonson DL. Bilateral toxocara optic neuropathy. J Clin Neuroophthalmol 1983;3:267-274.

57. Currie JN, Lessell S, Lessell IM, et al. Optic neuropathy in chronic lymphocytic leukemia. Arch Ophthalmol 1988;106:654-660.

58. Davis LE, Kornfeld M. Neurocysticercosis: Neurologic, pathogenic, diagnostic, and therapeutic aspects. Eur Neurol 1991;31:229-240.

59. De Bustros S, Miller NR, Finkelstein D, et al. Bilateral astrocytic hamartomas of the optic nerveheads in retinitis pigmentosa. Retina 1983;3: 21-23.

60. Donaldson JO. Pathogenesis of pseudotumor cerebri syndromes. Neurology 1981;31:877-880.

61. Dossetor FM, Landau K, Hoyt WF. Optic disk glioma in Neurofibromatosis Type 2. Am J Ophthalmol 1989;108:602-603.

62. Dreyer RF, Hopen G, Gass DM, Smith JL. Leber's stellate idiopathic neuroretinitis. Arch Ophthalmol 1984;102:1140-1145.

63. Dufier JL, Vinurel MC, Renier D, Marchac D. Les complications ophthalmologiques des crâniofaciosténosis. A propos de 224 observations. J Fr Ophtalmol 1986;9:273-280..

64. Duke-Elder S, Dobree JH. Diseases of the retina. In Duke-Elder S, ed. System of Ophthalmology. St Louis, MO: CV Mosby Co; 1967,10:246-248.

65. Dutton JJ. Optic nerve sheath meningioma. Surv Ophthalmol 1992;37:167-183.

66. Ellis W, Little HL. Leukemic infiltration of the optic nerve head. Am J Ophthalmol 1973;75:867-871.

67. Elrazak MA. Brucella optic neuritis. Arch Int Med 1991;151:776-778.

68. Engelken JD, Yuh WTC, Carter KD, Nerad JA. Optic nerve sarcoidosis. MR findings. AJNR 1992;13:228-230.

69. Erkkila H. Optic disc drusen in children. Acta Ophthalmol 1977;129(suppl):7-44.

70. Fanous M, Hamed LM, Margo CE. Pseudotumor cerebri associated with Danazol withdrawal. JAMA 1991;266:1218-1219.

71. Farris BK, Pickard DJ. Bilateral postinfectious optic neuritis and intravenous steroid therapy in children. Ophthalmology 1990;97:339-345.

72. Fewell AG. Unilateral neuroretinitis of syphilitic origin with a striate figure at the macula. Arch Ophthalmol 1932;8:615.

73. Fish RH, Hogan RN, Nightingale SD, Anand R. Peripapillary angiomatosis associated with cat-scratch neuroretinitis. Arch Ophthalmol 1992; 110:323.

74. Fish RH, Hoskins JC, Kline LB. Toxoplasmosis neuroretinitis. Ophthalmology 1993;100: 1177-1182.

75. Fishman MA, Hogan GR, Dodge PR. The concurrence of hydrocephalus and craniosynostosis. J Neurosurg 1971;34:621.

76. Fitz C. Magnetic resonance imaging of pediatric brain tumors. Topics Magnet Reson Imaging 1993;5:174-189.

77. Folk JC, Weingeist TA, Corbett JJ, et al. Syphilitis neuroretinitis. Am J Ophthalmol 1983;95:448-486.

78. Folk JC, Lobes LA. Presumed toxoplasmic papillitis. Ophthalmology 1984;91:64-67.

79. Foster RE, Lowder CY, Meisler DM, et al. Mumps neuroretinitis in an adolescent. Am J Ophthalmol 1990;110:91-93.

80. Francois J. L'hérédité en ophtalmologie. Paris: Masson; 1958,509-602.

81. Frey T. Optic neuritis in children: infectious mononucleosis as an etiology. Doc Ophthalmol 1973;34:183-188.

82. Friedman AH, Beckerman B, Gold DH, et al. Drusen of the optic disc. Surv Ophthalmol 1977; 21:375-390.

83. Friedman DH, Gartner S, Modi SS. Drusen of the optic disc. A retrospective study in cadaver eyes. Br J Ophthalmol 1975;59:413-521.

84. Friedman DH, Henkind P, Gartner S. Drusen of the optic disc: a histopathological study. Trans Ophthalmol Soc UK 1975;95:4-9.

85. Fries PD, Katowitz JA. Congenital craniofacial anomalies of ophthalmic importance. Surv Ophthalmol 1990;35:87-119.

86. Frisen L, Scholdstrom G, Svendsen P. Drusen in the optic nerve head: verification by computerized tomography. Arch Ophthalmol 1978;96: 1611-1614.

87. Frohman LP, Joshi VV, Wagner RS, Bielory L. Pseudotumor cerebri as a cardinal sign of the

polyangiitis overlap syndrome. Neuro-ophthalmology 1991;11:337-345.

88. Gass JMD. Diseases of the optic nerve that may simulate macular disease. Trans Am Acad Ophthalmol Otolaryngol 1977;83:763-770.

89. Gass JMD. *Stereoscopic Atlas of Macular Diseases: Diagnosis and Treatment.* St Louis, MO: CV Mosby; 1987:470-475, 746-751.

90. Gass JDM. *Steroscopic Atlas of Macular Diseases: Diagnosis and Treatment.* 3rd ed. St. Louis, MO: CV Mosby; 1990;2:727-767.

91. Gass JDM, Callanan DG, Bowman B. Oral therapy in diffuse unilateral subacute neuroretinitis. Arch Ophthalmol 1992;110:675-680.

92. Gaynon MW, Koh K, Marmor JF, Frankel LR. Retinal folds in the shaken baby syndrome. Am J Ophthalmol 1988;106:423-425.

93. Ghose S. Optic nerve changes in hydrocephalus. Trans Ophthal Soc UK 1983;103:217-220.

94. Giangiacomo J, Khan JA, Levine C, Thompson VM. Sequential cranial computed tomography in infants with retinal hemorrhages. Ophthalmology 1988;95:295-299.

95. Gittinger JW, Asdourian GK. Macular abnormalities in papilledema from pseudotumor cerebri. Ophthalmology 1989;96:192-194.

96. Glaser JS. Heredofamilial disorders of the optic nerve. In: Renie, WA. *Goldberg's Genetic and Metabolic Eye Disease.* 2nd ed. Boston, MA: Little, Brown; 1986;483-484.

97. Goldberg MA, Kazacos KR, Boyce WM, et al. Diffuse unilateral subacute neuroretinitis. Morphometric, serologic, and epidemiologic support for Baylisascaris as a causative agent. Ophthalmology 1993;100:1695-1701.

98. Goldberg MF, Scott CI, McKusick VA. Hydrocephalus and papilledema in the Maroteaux-Lamy syndrome (Mucopolysaccharidosis Type VI). Am J Ophthalmol 1970;69:969-975.

99. Golnik KC, Marotto ME, Fanous MM, et al. Ophthalmic manifestations of Rochalimaea species. Am J Ophthalmol 1994;118:145-151.

100. Good WV, Brodsky MC, Edwards MS, Hoyt WF. Bilateral retinal hamartomas in neurofibromatosis type 2. Br J Ophthalmol 1991;75:190.

101. Grant DN. Benign intracranial hypertension. Arch Dis Child 1971;46:651-655.

102. Greer M. Benign intracranial hypertension. I: mastoiditis and lateral sinus obstruction. Neurology 1962;12:472-476.

103. Greer M. Benign intracranial hypertension: II: following corticosteroid therapy. Neurology 1963;13:439-441.

104. Greer M. Benign intracranial hypertension: IV: menarche. Neurology 1964;14:569-573.

105. Greer M. Benign intracranial hypertension (pseudotumor cerebri). Pediatr Clin North Am 1967; 14:819-830.

106. Guiseffi V, Wall M, Siegel PZ, Rojas PB. Symptoms and disease associations in idiopathic intracranial hypertension. Neurology 1991; 41:239-244.

107. Guy J, Sherwood M, Day AL. Surgical treatment of progressive visual loss in traumatic optic neuropathy: report of two cases. J Neurosurg 1989; 70:799-801.

108. Hagberg B, Sillanpää M. Benign intracranial hypertension (pseudotumor cerebri). Acta Paediatr Scand 1970;59:328-329.

109. Haller P, Patzgold U. Die Optikusneuritis im Kindesalter. Fortschr Neurol Psychiatr 1979;47: 209-216.

110. Hamed LM, Purvin VP, Rosenberg M. Recurrent anterior ischemic optic neuropathy in young adults. J Clin Neuro-ophthalmol 1988;8:239-246.

111. Hamed LM, Glaser JS, Schatz NJ, Perez TH. Pseudotumor cerebri induced by Danazol. Am J Ophthalmol 1989;107:105-110.

112. Hamed LM, Silbiger J, Guy J, et al. Parainfectious optic neuritis and encephalomyelitis. J Clin Neuro-ophthalmol 1993;1:18-23.

113. Harris MJ, Fine SL, Owens S. Hemorrhagic complications of optic nerve drusen. Am J Ophthalmol 1981;92:70-76.

114. Hayreh SS. Optic disc edema in raised intracranial pressure. V: pathogenesis. Arch Ophthalmol 1977; 95:1553-1565.

115. Hayreh SS. Anterior ischemic optic neuropathy. V. optic disc edema as an early sign. Arch Ophthalmol 1981;99:1030-1040.

116. Hayreh SS, Servais GE, Virdi PS, et al. Fundus lesions in malignant hypertension. III. arterial blood pressure, biochemical and fundus changes. Ophthalmology 1985;92:45-59.

117. Hayreh SS, Servais GE, Virdi PS. Fundus lesions in malignant hypertension. IV: focal intraretinal periarteriolar transudates. Ophthalmology 1985; 92:60-73.

118. Hayreh SS, Servais GE, Virdi PS. Fundus lesions in malignant hypertension. V: hypertensive optic neuropathy. Ophthalmology 1986;93:74-87.

119. Hayreh SS, Servais GE, Virdi PS. Fundus lesions in malignant hypertension. VI: hypertensive choroidopathy. Ophthalmology 1986;93:1383-1400.

120. Hedges TR. Bilateral visual loss in a child with disc swelling. Surv Ophthalmol 1992;36:424-428.

121. Heidemann DG, Beck RW. Retinitis pigmentosa. A mimic of neurological disease. Surv Ophthalmol 1987;32:45-51.

122. Hiatt RL, Grizzard JT, McNeer P, Jabbour JT. Ophthalmologic manifestations of subacute sclerosing panencephalitis. Trans Am Acad Ophthalmol Otolaryngol 1971;75:344-350.

123. Hierons R, Lyle TK. Bilateral retrobulbar optic neuritis. Brain 1959;82:56-67.

124. Hitchings RA, Corbett JJ, Winkleman J, Schatz NJ. Hemorrhages with optic nerve drusen. Arch Neurol 1976;33:675-677.

125. Hoover DL, Khan JA, Giangiacomo J. Pediatric ocular sarcoidosis. Surv Ophthalmol 1986;30: 215-228.

126. Hoover DL, Robb RM, Petersen RA. Optic disc drusen and primary megalencephaly. J Pediatr Ophthalmol Strabis 1989;26:81-85.

127. Horton JC, Garcia EG, Becker EK. Magnetic resonance imaging of leukemic invasion of the optic nerve. Arch Ophthalmol 1992;110:1207-1208.

128. Hoyt WF, Pont ME. Pseudopapilledema. Anomalous elevation of optic disk. Pitfalls in diagnosis and management. JAMA 1962;181:191-196.

129. Hoyt WF, Beeston D. *The Ocular Fundus in Neurologic Disease.* St Louis, MO: CV Mosby; 1966.

130. Hoyt WF, Knight CL. Comparison of congenital disc blurring and incipient papilledema in red-free light-a photographic study. Invest Ophthalmol 1973;12:241-247.

131. Hrisomalos NF, Mansour AM, Jampol LM, et al. "Pseudo"-combined hamartoma following papilledema. Arch Ophthalmol 1987;105:164-165.

132. Hupp SL, Buckley EG, Byrne SF, et al. Posttraumatic venous obstructive retinopathy associated with enlarged optic nerve sheath. Arch Ophthalmol 1984;102:254-256.

133. Ikkala E, Laitinen L. Papilloedema due to iron deficiency anaemia. Acta Haemat 1963;29:368-370.

134. Ireland B, Corbett JJ, Wallace RB. The search for causes of idiopathic intracranial hypertension. A preliminary case-control study. Arch Neurol 1990;47:315-320.

134a. Jeffrey AR, Buncic JR. The visual outcome of Devic's neuromyelitic optica in the pediatric population. Presented at the American Association for Pediatric Ophthalmology and Strabismus. Orlando, Florida, April 5-9, 1995.

135. Johnson RT. The pathogenesis of acute viral encephalitis and postinfectious encephalomyelitis. J Infect Dis 1987;155:359-364.

136. Johnston I, Hawke S, Halmagyi M, Teo C. The Pseudotumor syndrome: disorders of cerebrospinal fluid circulation causing intracranial hypertension without ventriculomegaly. Arch Neurol 1991;48: 740-747.

137. Josef JM, Burde RM. Anterior ischemic optic neuropathy of the young. J Clin Neuro-ophthalmol 1983;3:137.

138. Karel I, Otradovec J, Peleska M. Fluorescein angiography in circulatory disturbances in drusen of the optic disc. Ophthlmologica 1972;164:449-462.

139. Kattah JC, Suski ET, Killen JY, et al. Optic neuritis in systemic lymphoma. Am J Ophthalmol 1980;89: 431-436.

140. Katz B. Swelling in an adult diabetic patient. Surv Ophthalmol 1990;35:158-163.

141. Katz B. Disc edema, transient obscurations of vision, and a temporal fossa mass. Surv Ophthalmol 1991;36:133-140.

141a. Katz B. Central American mesencephalopathy. Surv Ophthalmol 1994;39:253-259.

142. Kaur B, Taylor D. Fundus hemorrhages in infancy. Surv Ophthalmol 1992;37:1-17.

143. Kaye LD, Rothner D, Beauchamp GR, et al. Ocular findings associated with neurofibromatosis type II. Ophthalmology 1992;99:1424-1429.

144. Kazarian E, Gager W. Optic neuritis complicating measles, mumps, and rubella vaccination. Am J Ophthalmol 1978;86:544-567.

145. Keane JR. Cysticercosis: unusual neuro-ophthalmologic signs. J Clin Neuro-ophthalmol 1993; 13:194-199.

146. Kennedy C, Carter S. Relation of optic neuritis to multiple sclerosis in children. Paediatrics 1961; 28:377-387.

147. Kennedy C, Carroll FD. Optic neuritis in children. Arch Ophthalmol 1960;63:747-755.

148. Kesler A, Manor RS. Papilloedema and hydrocephalus in spinal cord ependymoma. Br J Ophthalmol 1994;78:313-315.

149. Kilty LA, Hiles DA. Unilateral posterior lenticonus with posterior hyaloid remnant. Am J Ophthalmol 1993;116:104-106.

150. Klintworth G. The neurologic manifestations of osteopetrosis (Albers-Schönberg's disease). Neurology 1963;13:512.

151. Knight CL, Hoyt WF. Monocular blindness from drusen of the optic disk. Am J Ophthalmol 1972; 73:890-892.

152. Kriss A, Francis DA, Cuendet F, et al. Recovery after optic neuritis in childhood. J Neurol Neurosurg Psychiatry 1988;51:1253.

153. Krumholtz A, Stern BJ, Stern EG. Clinical implications of seizures in neurosarcoidosis. Arch Neurol 1991;48:842-844.

154. Kuroiwa Y. Neuromyelitis optica: Devic's disease, Devic's syndrome. Handbook of clinical neurology In: Koetsier JC, ed. *Demyelinating Diseases.* New York, NY: Elsevier Science Publishers BV; 1985; 3(47):397-408.

155. Lamas E, Lobato RD, Esparza J, Escudero L. Dural posterior fossa AVM producing raised sagittal sinus pressure. J Neurosurg 1977;46:804-810.

156. Lambert SR, Johnson TE, Hoyt CS. Optic nerve sheath and retinal hemorrhages associated with the shaken baby syndrome. Arch Ophthalmol 1986; 104:1509-1512.

157. Landau K, Muci-Mendoza R, Dossetor FM, Hoyt WF. Retinal hamartoma in neurofibromatosis 2. Arch Ophthalmol 1990;108:328-329.

158. Lanesche RK, Rucker CW. Progression of visual field defects produced by hyaline bodies in optic discs. Arch Ophthalmol 1957;58:115-121.

159. Leber T. Die pseudonephritischen Netzhauterkrankungen, die Retinitis stellata; die Purtscher-sche Netzhautaffektion nach schwerer Schädelverletzung. In: Graefe AC, Saemisch T, eds. *Graefe-Saemisch-Hess Handbuch der Gesamten*

Augenheilkunde. 2nd ed. Leipzig, East Germany: Engelmann; 1916,7, (pt 2):1319-1339.

160. Lepore FE. Unilateral and highly asymmetric papilledema in pseudotumor cerebri. Neurology 1992; 42:676-678.

161. Lessell S, Rosman NP. Permanent visual impairment in childhood pseudotumor cerebri. Arch Neurol 1986;43:801-804.

162. Lessell S. Pediatric pseudotumor cerebri (idiopathic intracranial hypertension). Surv Ophthalmol 1992;37:155-166.

163. Lesser RL, Kornmehl EW, Pachner AR. Neuro-ophthalmologic manifestations of Lyme disease. Ophthalmology 1990;97:699-706.

164. Lilley ER, Bruggers CS, Pollack SC. Papilledema in a patient with aplastic anemia. Arch Ophthalmol 1990;108:1674-1675.

165. Lorentzen SE. Drusen of the optic disk. Dan Med Bull 1967;14:293-298.

166. Lorentzen SE. Drusen of the optic disk, an irregular dominant hereditary affectation. Arch Ophthalmol 1961;39:626-643.

167. Lubow M, Makley TA. Pseudopapilledema of juvenile diabetes mellitus. Arch Ophthalmol 1971; 85:417-422.

168. Lubow ML. "Pseudo" pseudotumor cerebri in aplastic anemia. Arch Ophthalmol 1991;109:1638.

169. Lui GT, Kay MD, Bienfang DC. Pseudotumor cerebri associated with inflammatory bowel disease. Am J Ophthalmol 1994;117:352-357.

170. Mandler RN, Davis LE, Jeffery DR, Kornfeld M. Devic's neuromyelitis optica: a clinicopathological study of 8 patients. Ann Neurol 1993;34: 162-168.

171. Mann NP, McLellan NJ, Cartlidge PHT. Transient intracranial hypertension of infancy. Arch Dis Child 1988;63:966-968.

172. Mansour AM. Hamed LM. Racial variation of optic nerve disease. Neuro-ophthalmology 1991;11: 319-323.

173. Marie J, See G. Acute hypervitaminosis A of infant; its clinical manifestations with benign acute hydrocephalus and pronounced bulge of fontanel; clinical and biological study. Am J Dis Child 1954;87:731.

174. Mathew NT, Mayer JS, Ott EO. Increased cerebral blood volume in benign intracranial hypertension. Neurology 1975;25:646-649.

175. Mathur SP. Macular lesion after influenza. Br J Ophthalmol 1958;42:702.

176. Matzkin DC, Slamovits TL, Genis I, Bello J. Disc swelling: a tall tail? Surv Ophthalmol 1992;37: 130-136.

177. McDonald F, Digre K, Yuh WTC, Corbett JJ. The incidence of empty sella and Chiari 1 malformation in pseudotumor cerebri. Presented as a poster at the North American Neuro-Ophthalmology Society Meeting, Durango, CO, February 1994.

178. Meadows SP. Retrobulbar and optic neuritis in childhood and adolescence. Trans Ophthalmol Soc UK 1969;89:603-638.

179. Miller NR, ed. *Walsh and Hoyt's Clinical Neuro-Ophthalmology, I.* Baltimore, MD: Williams & Wilkins Co; 1982

180. Miller NR. Appearance of optic disc drusen in a patient with anomalous elevation of the optic disc. Arch Ophthalmol 1986;104:794-795.

181. Miller NR. Sudden visual field constriction associated with optic disc drusen. J Clin Neuro-ophthalmol 1993;13:14.

182. Minckler DS, Tso MOM, Zimmerman LE. A light microscopic, autoradiographic study of axoplasmic transport in the optic nerve head during ocular hypotony, increased intraocular pressure, and papilledema. Am J Ophthalmol 1976;82:741-757.

183. Minckler DS, Bunt AH. Axoplasmic transport in ocular hypotony and papilledema in the monkey. Arch Ophthalmol 1977;95:1430-1436.

184. Moisseiev J, Cahane M, Treister G. Optic nerve head drusen and peripapillary central serous chorioretinopathy. Am J Ophthalmol 1989;108:202-203.

185. Moody TA, Irvine AR, Cahn PH, et al. Sudden visual field constriction associated with optic disc drusen. J Clin Neuro-ophthalmol 1993;13:8-13.

186. Morris AT, Sanders MD. Macular changes resulting from papilloedema. Br J Ophthalmol 1980; 64:211-216.

187. Morrissey SP, Miller DH, Kendall BE, et al. The significance of brain magnetic resonance imaging abnormalities at presentation with clinically isolated syndromes suggestive of multiple sclerosis. Brain 1993;116:135-146.

188. Moser FG, Hilal SK, Abrams G, et al. MR imaging of pseudotumor cerebri. AJNR 1988;9:39-45.

189. Mueller RF, Pagon RA, Pepin MG, et al. Arteriohepatic dysplasia: phenotypic features and family studies. Clin Genet 1984;25:323-331.

190. Mullie MA. Sanders MD. Scleral canal size and optic nerve head drusen. Am J Ophthalmol 1985; 99:356-359.

191. Mustonen E. Pseudopapilledema with and without verified optic disc drusen: A clinical analysis. II. visual fields. Acta Ophthalmnol 1979;61:1057-1066.

192. Mustonen E. Pseudopapilloedema with and without verified optic disc drusen. A clinical analysis I. Acta Ophthalmol 1983;61:1037-1056.

193. Mustonen E. Pseudopapilloedema with and without verified optic disc drusen. A clinical analysis II: visual fields. Acta Ophthalmol 1983;61:1057-1066.

194. Newman NJ, Lessell S, Brandt EM. Bilateral central retinal artery occlusions, disc drusen, and migraine. Am J Ophthalmol 1989;107:236-240.

195. Newman NJ. Leber's hereditary optic neuropathy. New genetic considerations. Arch Neurol 1993; 50:540-548.

196. Nikaido H, Mishima H, Ono H. Leukemic involvement of the optic nerve. Am J Ophthalmol 1988;105:294-298.

197. Nikoskelainen E, Hoyt WF, Nummelin K. Ophthalmoscopic findings in Leber's hereditary optic neuropathy. II. the fundus findings in the affected family members. Arch Ophthalmol 1983;101:1059-1068.

198. Novakovic P, Kellie SJ, Taylor D. Childhood leukaemia: relapse in the anterior segment of the eye. Br J Ophthalmol 1989;73:354-359.

199. Nyboer JH, Robertson DM, Gomez MR. Retinal lesions in tuberous sclerosis. Arch Ophthalmol 1976;94:1277-1280.

200. Ohkoshi K, Tsiaras WG. Prognostic importance of ophthalmic manifestations in childhood leukaemia. Br J Ophthalmol 1992;76:651-655.

201. Optic Neuritis Study Group: The clinical profile of optic neuritis: experience of the Optic Neuritis Treatment Trial. Arch Ophthalmol 1991;109:1673-1678.

202. Ormerod IEC, McDonald WI, du Boulay GH, et al. Disseminated lesions at presentation in patients with optic neuritis. J Neurol Neurosurg Psychiatr 1986;49:124-127.

203. Parmley VC, Schiffman JS, Maitland CG, et al. Does neuroretinitis rule out multiple sclerosis? Arch Neurol 1987;44:1045-1047.

204. Pavin PR, Aiello LM, Wafai Z, et al. Optic disc edema in juvenile-onset diabetes. Arch Ophthalmol 1980;98:2193-2195.

205. Petersen RA, Rosenthal A. Retinopathy and papilledema in cyanotic congenital heart disease. Pediatrics 1972;49:243-249.

206. Pickens S, Sangster G. Retrobulbar neuritis and infectious mononucleosis. Br Med J 1975;4:729.

207. Piel JJ, Thelander HE, Shaw EB. Infectious mononucleosis of the central nervous system with bilateral papilledema. J Pediatr 1950;37:661-665.

208. Pillai S, Limaye SR, Saimovici LB. Optic disc hamartoma associated with retinitis pigmentosa. Retina 1983;3:24-26.

209. Pollard ZF. Cysticercosis: an unusual cause of papilledema. Ann Ophthalmol 1975;7:110-112.

210. Puck A, Tso MOM, Fishman GA. Drusen of the optic nerve associated with retinitis pigmentosa. Arch Ophthalmol 1985;103:231-234.

211. Purcell JJ, Goldberg RE. Hyaline bodies of the optic papilla and bilateral acute vascular occlusions. Ann Ophthalmol 1974;6:1069-1076.

212. Purvin V, Herr GJ, Myer W. Chiasmal neuritis as a complication of Epstein-Barr virus infection. Arch Neurol 1988;45:458-460.

213. Raichle ME, Grubb RL, Phelps ME, et al. Cerebral hemodynamics and metabolism in pseudotumor cerebri. Ann Neurol 1978;4:104-111.

214. Regnery RL, Olsen JG, Perkins BA, Bibb W. Serological response to "Rochalimaea henselae" antigen in suspected cat-scratch disease. Lancet 1992;339:1443-1445.

215. Rennie I. Ophthalmic manifestations of childhood leukaemia. Br J Ophthalmol 1992;76:641.

216. Ridgeway EW, Jaffe N, Walton DS. Leukemic ophthalmopathy in children. Cancer 1976;38:1744-1749.

217. Riikonen R, Donner M, Errkila H. Optic neuritis in children and its relationship to multiple sclerosis. A clinical study of 21 children. Dev Med Child Neurol 1988;30:349-359.

218. Riikonen R, Ketonen L, Sipponen J. Magnetic resonance imaging, evoked responses and cerebrospinal fluid findings in a follow-up study of children with optic neuritis. Acta Neurol Scand 1988;77:44-49.

219. Riikonen R, von Willebrandt E. Lymphocyte subclasses and function in patients with optic neuritis in childhood with special reference to multiple sclerosis. Acta Neurol Scand 1988;78:58-64.

220. Riikonen R. The role of infection and vaccination in the genesis of optic neuritis and multiple sclerosis in children. Acta Neurol (Scand) 1989;80:425-431.

221. Rizzo JF, Lessell S. Risk of developing multiple sclerosis after uncomplicated optic neuritis. A long-term prospective study. Neurology 1988;38:185-190.

222. Roach ES, Zimmerman CF, Troost BT, Weaver RG. Optic neuritis due to acquired toxoplasmosis. Pediatr Neurol 1985; 1:114-116.

223. Romanchuk KG, Judisch GF, LaBrecque DR. Ocular findings in arteriohepatic dysplasia (Alagille's syndrome). Can J Ophthalmol 1981;16:94-99.

224. Rose A, Matson DD. Benign intracranial hypertension in children. Pediatrics 1967;39:227-232.

225. Rosenberg MA, Savino PJ, Glaser JS. A clinical analysis of pseudopapilledema: I: population, laterality, acuity, refractive error, ophthalmoscopic characteristics, and coincident disease. Arch Ophthalmol 1979;97:65-70.

226. Rosenthal AR. Ophthalmic manifestations of leukemia: a review. Ophthalmology 1983;90: 899-905.

227. Rozot P, Berrod JP, Bracard S, et al. Stase papillaire et fistule durale. J Fr Ophtalmol 1991;14: 13-19.

228. Ruben JB, Morris RJ, Judisch GF. Chorioretinal degeneration in infantile malignant osteoporosis. Am J Ophthalmol 1990;110:1-5.

229. Rush JA. Idiopathic optic neuritis of childhood. J Pediatr Ophthalmol Strabis 1981;18:39-41.

230. Sacks JG, O'Grady RB, Choromokos E, Leestma J. The pathogenesis of optic nerve drusen. A hypothesis. Arch Ophthalmol 1977;95:425-428.

231. Salmon JF, Lee Pan E, Murray ADN. Visual loss with dancing extremities. Surv Ophthalmol 1991; 35:299-306.

232. Sanders MD, Ffytche TJ. Flourescein angiography in the diagnosis of drusen of the disc. Trans Ophthalmol Soc UK 1967;87:457-468.

233. Sanders TE, Gay AJ, Newman M. Hemorrhagic complications of drusen of the optic disk. Am J Ophthalmol 1971;71:204-217.

234. Sarkies NJC, Sanders MD. Optic disc drusen and episodic visual loss. Br J Ophthalmol 1985;71: 537-539.

235. Savage GL, Centaro A, Enoch JM, Newman NM. Drusen of the optic nerve head. Ophthalmology 1985;92:793-799.

236. Savino PJ, Glaser JS, Rosenberg MA. A clinical analysis of pseudopapilledema. II: visual field defects. Arch Ophthlamol 1979;97:71-75.

237. Schachat AP, Markowitz JA, Guyer DR, et al. Ophthalmic manifestations of leukemia. Arch Ophthalmol 1989;107:697-700.

238. Schnittger S, Höfers C, Heidemann P, et al. Molecular and cytogenetic analysis of an interstitial 20p deletion associated with syndromic intrahepatic ductular hypoplasia (Alagille syndrome). Hum Genet 1989;83:239-244.

239. Schoeman JF. Childhood pseudotumor cerebri: clinical and intracranial pressure response to acetazolamide and furosemide treatment in a case series. J Child Neurol 1994;9:1301-1334.

240. Scott TF. Neurosarcoidosis: progress and clinical aspects. Neurology 1993;43:8-12.

241. Sedwick LA, Burde RM. Unilateral and asymmetric optic disk swelling with intracranial abnormalities. Am J Ophthalmol 1983;96:484-487.

242. Seitz R, Kersting G. Die drusen der sehnervenpapille und des pigmentphitels. Klin Monatsbl Augenheilkd 1962;140:75-88.

243. Seitz R. Die intraocular drusen. Klin Monatsbl Augenheilkd 1968;152:203.

244. Selbst RG, Selhorst JB, Harbison JW, Myer EC. Parainfectious optic neuritis: report and review following varicella. Arch Neurol 1983;40:347-350.

245. Selky AK, Dobyns WB, Yee RD. Idiopathic intracranial hypertension and facial diplegia. Neurology 1994;44.

246. Seltzer S, Mark AS, Atlas SW. CNS sarcoidosis: evaluation with contrast-enhanced MR imaging. AJNR 1992;12:1227-1232.

247. Shaked Y, Samra Y. Q fever meningoencephalitis associated with bilateral abducens nerve paralysis, bilateral optic neuritis, and abnormal cerebrospinal fluid findings. Infection 1989;17:394-395.

248. Sharma OP, Sharma AM. Sarcoidosis of the nervous system. A clinical approach. Arch Intern Med 1991;151:1317-1321.

249. Shulman SA, Hyams JS, Gunta R, et al. Arteriohepatic dysplasia (Alagille syndrome): extreme variability among affected family members. Am J Med Genet 1984;19:325-332.

250. Silbergleit R, Junck L, Gebarski SS, Hatfield MK. Idiopathic intracranial hypertension (pseudotumor cerebri): MR imaging. Neuroradiology 1989;170: 207-209.

251. Silbiger J, Guy JR. Lethargy and visual loss in a child. Presented at the 23rd Annual Frank B. Walsh Society meeting, Park City, Utah, 1991.

252. Silverstein A, Steinberg G, Nathanson M. Nervous system involvement in infectious mononucleosis. Arch Neurol 1972;26:353-358.

253. Singleton EM, Kinsbourne M, Anderson WB. Familial pseudopapilledema. South Med J 1973;66: 796-802.

254. Sivalingam A, Augsburger J, Perilongo G, et al. Combined hamartoma of the retina and retinal pigment epithelium in a patient with neurofibromatosis type 2. J Pediatr Ophthalmol Strabis 1991;28: 320-321.

255. Slavin ML. Chronic asymptomatic ischemic optic neuropathy. J Clin Neuro-ophthalmol 1987;7: 198-201.

256. Smith JL, Hoyt WF, Susac JO. Ocular fundus in acute Leber optic neuropathy. Arch Ophthalmol 1973;90:349-354.

257. Sorenson PS, Thomsen C, Gjerris F, et al. Increased brain water content in pseudotumor cerebri measured by magnetic resonance imaging of brain water self-diffusion. Neurol Res 1989;11:160-164.

258. Spencer WH. Drusen of the optic disc and aberrant axoplasmic transport. Am J Ophthalmol 1978; 85:1-12.

259. Steere AC, Taylor E, McHugh GL, Logigian EL. The overdiagnosis of Lyme disease. JAMA 1993; 269:1812-1816.

260. Stevens RA, Newman NM. Abnormal visual-evoked potentials from eyes with optic nerve head drusen. Am J Ophthalmol 1981;92:857-862.

261. Straussberg R, Amir J, Cohen HA, et al. Epstein-Barr virus infection associated with encephalitis and optic neuritis. J Pediatr Ophthalmol Strabis 1993;30:262-263.

262. Strong LE, Henderson JW, Gangitano JL. Bilateral retrobulbar neuritis secondary to mumps. Am J Ophthalmol 1974;78:331-335.

263. Suh DC, Chang KH, Han MH, et al. Unusual MR manifestations of neurocysticercosis. Neuroradiology 1989;31:396-402.

264. Symonds CP. Otitic hydrocephalus. Brain 1931; 54:55.

265. Taha JM, Crone KR, Berger TS, et al. Sigmoid sinus thrombosis after closed head injury in children. Neurosurgery 1993;32:541-546.

266. Taylor D, Cuendet F. Optic neuritis in childhood. In: Hess RF, Plant GT, eds. Optic Neuritis. Cambridge: Cambridge University Press; 1986:73-85.

267. Taylor D. Pediatric Ophthalmology. Boston, MA: Blackwell Scientific Publications; 1990:213-222.

268. Tso MOM, Fine BS. Electron microscopic study of human papilledema. Am J Ophthalmol 1976;82: 424-434.

269. Tso MOM. Pathology and pathogenesis of drusen of the optic nervehead. Ophthalmology 1981;88: 1066-1080.

270. Ulrich GG, Waecker NJ, Meister SJ, et al. Cat scratch disease associated with neuroretinitis in a 6-year-old girl. Ophthalmology 1992;99:246-249.

271. Usai T, Shirakashi M, Takagi M, et al. Macular edema-like change and pseudopapilledema in a case of Scheie syndrome. J Clin Neuro-ophthalmol 1991;11:183-185.

272. Wang XJ, Chang WM, Lee HL, Chang RF, Xu YZ. Fundus changes in 120 cases of aplastic anemia. Chung-Hua Yen Kotsa Chih 1985;21:344-346.

273. Webb NR, McCrary JA. Hyaline bodies of the optic disc and migraine. In: Smith JL, ed. *Neuro-Ophthalmology Update*. New York, NY: Masson Publishing USA, Inc; 1977:155-162.

274. Weisberg JA, Chutorian AM. Pseudotumor cerebri of childhood. Am J Dis Child. 1977;131: 1243-1248.

275. Weisberg LA, Pierce JF, Jabbari B. Intracranial hypertension resulting from a cerebrovascular malformation. South Med J 1977;70:624-626.

276. Weiss AH, Beck RW. Neuroretinitis in childhood. J Pediatr Ophthalmol Strabis 1989;26:198-203.

277. Welch DF, Pickett DA, Slater LN, et al. Rochalimaea henselae sp. nov., a cause of septicemia, bacillary angiomatosis, and parenchymal bacillary peliosis. J Clin Microbiol 1992;30:275-280.

278. Wilkinson WS, Han DP, Rappley MD, Owings CL. Retinal hemorrhages predicts neurological injury in the shaken baby syndrome. Arch Ophthalmol 1989;197:1472-1474.

279. Williams R, Taylor D. Tuberous sclerosis. Surv Ophthalmol 1985;30:143-154.

280. Wilson CB, Hieshima G. Occlusive hyperemia: a new way to think about an old problem. J Neurosurg 1993;78:165-166.

281. Winrow AP, Supramaniam G. Benign intracranial hypertension after ciprofloxacin. Arch Dis Child 1990;65:1165-1166.

282. Winterkorn JMS. Lyme disease: neurological and ophthalmic manifestations. Surv Ophthalmology 1990;35:191-204.

283. Winterkorn J. High Pressure Diagnosis. Presented at the Frank B. Walsh Society Meeting, New York, NY, March 1993.

284. Winward KE, Smith JL, Culbertson WW, Paris-Hamelin A. Ocular lyme borreliosis. Am J Ophthalmol 1989;108:651-657.

285. Wirtschafter JD. Osteopetrosis-A rare disease: a new treatment. Presented to the North American Neuro-Ophthalmology Society, Steamboat Springs, CO, February 1990.

286. Wise GN, Henkind P, Alterman GM. Optic disc drusen and subretinal hemorrhage. Trans Am Acad Ophthalmol Otolaryngol 1974;78:212-219.

287. Wright JE, McNab AA, McDonald WI. Primary optic nerve sheath meningioma. Br J Ophthalmol 1989;73:960-966.

288. Yohai RA, Bullock JD, Margolis JH. Unilateral optic disc edema and a contralateral temporal fossa mass. Am J Ophthalmol 1993;155:262-264.

289. Young WO, Small KW. Pigmented paravenous retinochoroidal atrophy (PPRCA) with optic disc drusen. Ophthal Pediatr Genet 1993;1:23-29.

290. Zhang F, Deleuze JR, Aurias A, et al. Interstitial deletion of the short arm of chromosome 20 in arteriohepatic dysplasia (Alagille syndrome). J Pediatr 1990;116:73-77.

291. Zouaoui A, Maillard J-C, Dormaont D, et al. Apport de l'irm dans la neurosarcoïdose: MRI in neurosarcoidosis. J Neuroradiol 1992;19:271-284.

4

Optic Atrophy in Children

Introduction

Optic atrophy is a morphologic sequelae to a multitude of anterior visual pathway insults that culminate in loss of retinal ganglion cell axons.[153,185,200] Histopathologically, it is characterized by a variable reduction of nerve diameter with loss of axons and little or no gliosis. Ophthalmoscopically, the disc retains its normal size and shows diffuse or segmental pallor. The pallor in optic atrophy has been attributed to thinning of the neural tissue of the optic disc and resulting changes in cytoarchitecture and decreased transmission of light , rather than to loss of optic disc capillaries or astrocytic proliferation.[184,186] The ophthalmoscopic appearance of the atrophic disc alone only occasionally suggests a specific mechanism of injury.[237]

In adults and older children with optic atrophy, results of the sensory visual examination (visual acuity, color vision, pupillary responses, visual field examination, and optic disc examination) often suggest certain mechanisms of optic nerve injury and definitively rule out others. In infants and toddlers, however, accurate subjective visual testing is often impossible, and clues to the underlying etiology must be sought in the associated systemic, neurological, and neuroimaging findings in addition to the information obtained in the family and medical history.

Infants and children may present with optic atrophy with a known underlying diagnosis (e.g., hydrocephalus, optic glioma) or may require a complete evaluation to establish such diagnosis. Referral may be initiated due to poor vision in one or both eyes or due to presence of other disorders that require neuro-ophthalmologic consultation as a part of a multidisciplinary workup. A thorough gestational, prenatal, birth, and neonatal history is essential. A history of perinatal head trauma, prematurity, perinatal asphyxia, meningitis, encephalitis, hydrocephalus, and related disorders should be specifically sought. A family history should be obtained with appropriate examination of family members and pedigree analysis to establish the diagnosis and the mode of transmission of suspected heritable cases.

A thorough ophthalmologic examination should then be undertaken. Attention to the appearance of the optic discs, pupillary examination, visual field testing, color vision performance, and any related physical findings may provide clues to the diagnosis. Long-standing cases with a relatively stable course are often found in children with a history of hypoxia, meningoencephalitis, congenital hydrocephalus, microcephaly, craniostenosis, or previous head trauma. The clinical identification of such cases usually obviates the need for any further diagnostic workup. In contrast, a previously normal child who develops progressive optic atrophy poses an entirely different diagnostic problem. Such a patient should undergo a thorough neurologic evaluation, and if deemed appropriate, neuroimaging studies with specific views of the anterior visual pathways and posterior fossa should be obtained. Other investigations for neurodegenerative, genetic, and metabolic disorders are customized to fit the overall clinical picture.

Optic atrophy is initially evaluated by observing the color of the discs. The disc will appear pale, either in a diffuse or in a segmental pattern, and will typically show fewer-than-normal fine vessels on its surface. The optic discs of young infants may ordinarily appear gray and slightly pale in appearance, even when excessive pressure on the globe while prying the eyelids open (which may cause vascular blanching and apparent pallor) is avoided.[116] The examiner must be cautious when concluding that optic atrophy is present in a young infant and should reconsider the diagnosis if it is incompatible with other clinical findings. Similarly, the finding of normal visual acuity in an older child does not exclude the possibility of optic nerve damage, since the degree of optic atrophy is not tightly correlated with visual acuity. Certain parameters may impart a misleading appearance of pallor to a normal disc. These include a large optic disc size, a deep physiologic cup, and axial myopia.

Ophthalmoscopic inspection of the atrophic disc should be accompanied by an attempt to evaluate the peripapillary nerve fiber layer if examination conditions permit.[181] Generalized thinning, sectoral atrophy, wedge-shaped or slitlike defects, or other patterns of nerve fiber layer dropout may be found in children with optic atrophy who are sufficiently cooperative or sedated. Abnormalities in the peripapillary nerve fiber layer often provide early clues regarding axonal loss in equivocal cases of optic atrophy. For instance, selective dropout of the nasal nerve fiber layer is a helpful diagnostic sign of band atrophy. Other ophthalmoscopic correlates of nerve fiber layer loss include a more distinct appearance of the peripapillary retinal vessels, variable attenuation of retinal arterioles,[65] loss of Gunn dots, and blunting of the macular reflex in children with optic atrophy.[201]

Although the appearance of the optic disc is usually unhelpful in localizing the site of visual system injury or defining its mechanism, important exceptions exist. Band atrophy is an important localizing sign in children because it signifies selective injury to those axons that decussate in the chiasm to the contralateral hemisphere. Recognition of band atrophy is especially important in infants and young children, who commonly present with congenital suprasellar tumors and in whom accurate visual field testing is often impossible. Band atrophy appears as a horizontal stripe of pallor extending from the nasal to the temporal disc margin. Examination of the peripapillary

nerve fiber layer shows selective dropout of the nasal sector. (The temporal sector is also absent; however, because the temporal nerve fiber layer is normally difficult to visualize, it cannot be used as a reliable gauge of nerve fiber dropout.)

Bilateral band atrophy occurs exclusively in the setting of chiasmal injury (usually compression from a suprasellar tumor) and is accompanied by bitemporal hemianopia[150] (Figure 4.1). Unilateral band atrophy usually signifies intrauterine retrogeniculate injury with transsynaptic degeneration,[97,98] but may occasionally reflect a pregeniculate abnormality[139]. The most common causes of congenital band atrophy in children are unilateral porencephaly, arteriovenous malformation, and ganglioneuroma, which involve the occipital lobe and lead to transsynaptic degeneration. A congenital optic tract syndrome may be a rare cause of congenital homonymous hemianopia and contralateral band atrophy[139] (Figure 4.3). Acquired band atrophy of one optic disc necessitates injury to the contralateral optic tract.[169] The histology associated with band atrophy was discussed by Unsold and Hoyt.[240] In cases purporting to show bilateral diffuse transsynaptic degeneration of the optic nerves due to bilateral cerebral lesions, coexisting primary damage to the optic nerves should be excluded.[199]

A congenital lesion involving the optic radiations may produce secondary neuronal loss in the lateral geniculate nucleus through the process of transsynaptic degeneration. This leads to a disorder termed homonymous hemioptic hypoplasia characterized by homonymous hemianopia, contralateral band atrophy of the optic disc, and corresponding changes in the nerve fiber layer bilaterally (Figure 4.2).[97,98] Transsynaptic degeneration of the retinogeniculate pathways is well documented to occur in nonhuman primates when the cerebral lesion occurs even during adulthood.[47] In the case of humans, retrograde transsynaptic degeneration of the retinogeniculate pathways has been shown to occur following prenatal or perinatal lesions, but its occurrence after cerebral lesions in adult life is considered rare.[82, 123,151] It is, however, well established that retrograde transsynaptic degeneration affects other neural systems in humans even when the injury occurs during adulthood.[12,23,104,125,143] Some histopathological evidence points to the possibility of transsynaptic

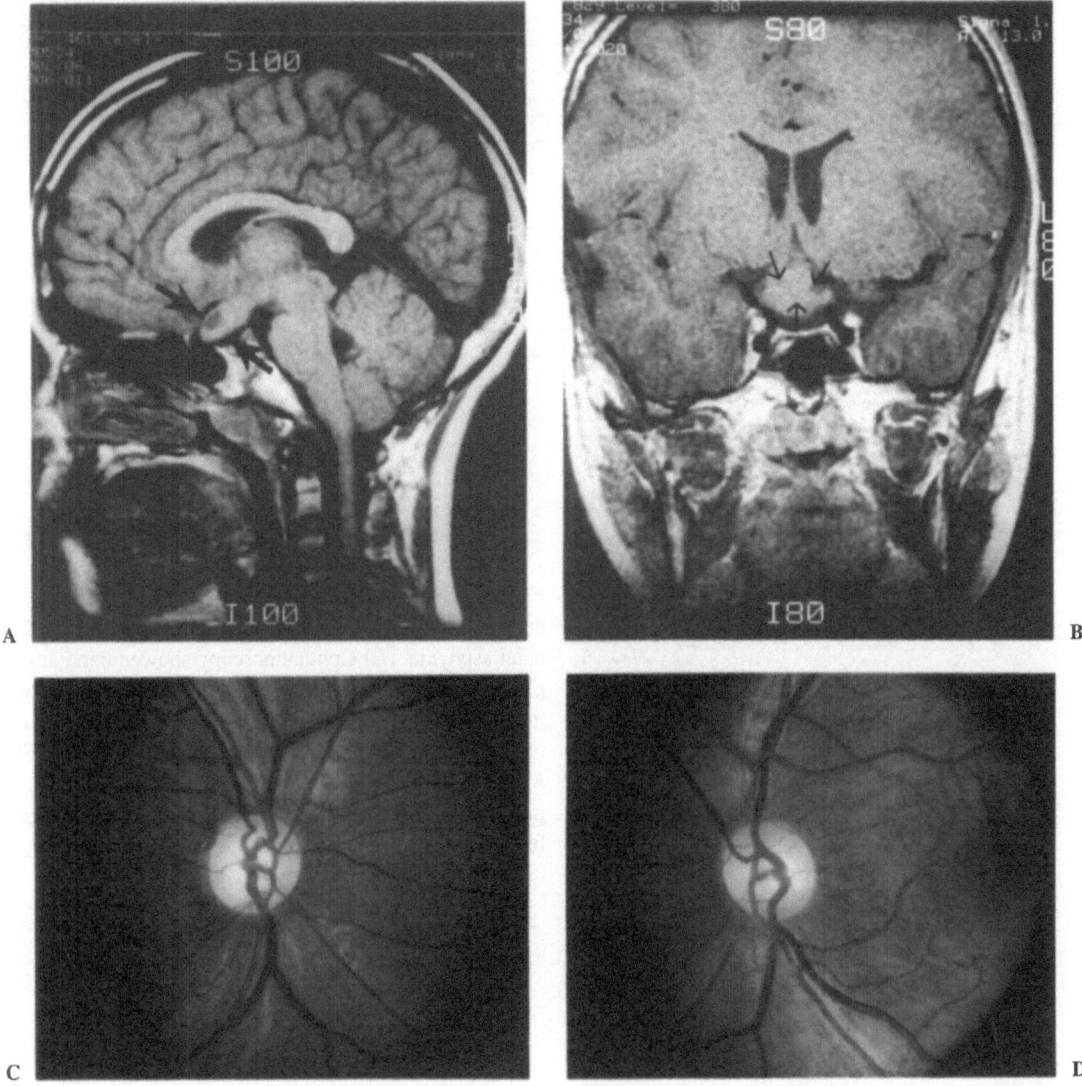

FIGURE 4.1. Chiasmal glioma. (A) Sagittal and (B) coronal MR images show diffuse enlargement of the optic chiasm in a 9-year-old boy who did not have neurofibro-matosis. His optic discs (C, D) showed band atrophy more conspicuous on the left disc (D).

degeneration of the retinogeniculate pathway in humans even when the lesion occurs in adults, but the clinical significance of this is unknown.[10]

Congenital optic atrophy is uncommon. In infants, congenital disc anomalies are a much more frequent cause of optic nerve dysfunction than is optic atrophy.[107] Hypoplastic nerves also frequently appear pale and may be misconstrued as atrophic. In this setting, the optic disc is confused with the peripapillary region, a yellowish rim ap-proximating normal disc diameter which arises from extension of the retinal pigment epithelium over the border of the scleral canal. Many patients with clearly hypoplastic optic nerves show significant associated disc pallor. Neuroimaging studies of the optic nerves are of limited usefulness in differentiating equivocal optic nerve hypoplasia from optic atrophy, since the dimensions of the optic nerves may be either normal or reduced in optic atrophy.[20,175]

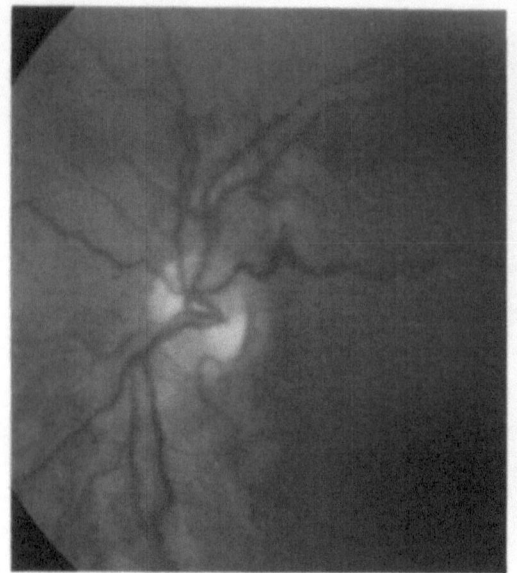
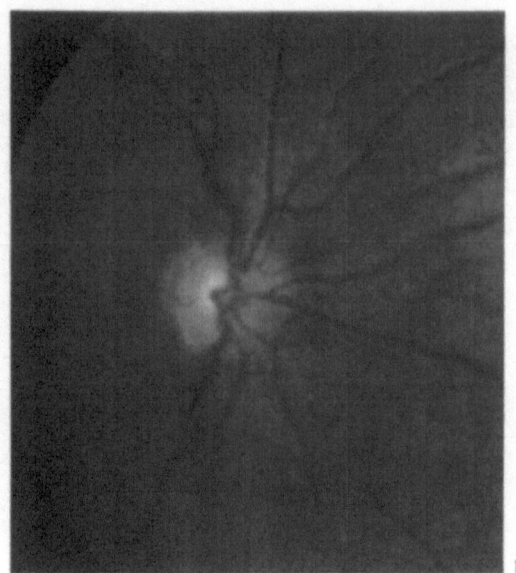

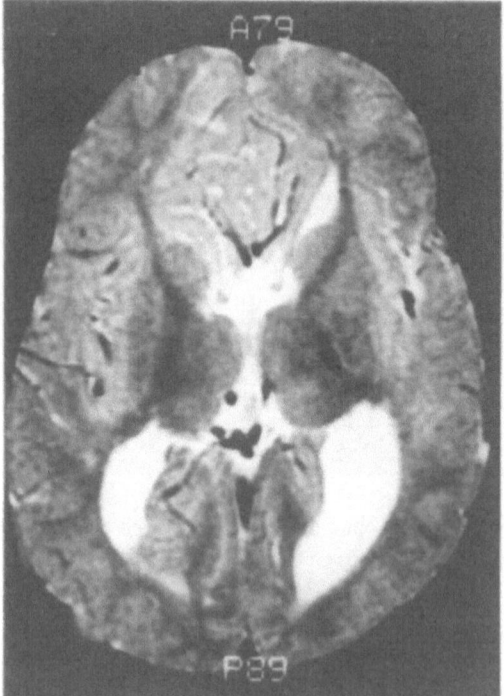

FIGURE 4.2. Homonymous hemioptic hypoplasia. This is an 8-year-old girl with history of prematurity and perinatal asphyxia. (A) Ophthalmoscopy showed band atrophy of the left optic disc with associated thinning of the nasal nerve fiber layer; (B) both optic discs were relatively hypoplastic, the left one appearing more so. (C) MR scans showed periventricular leukomalacia with preferential involvement of the parieto-occipital region bilaterally.

Epidemiology

Optic atrophy is a major cause of visual disability in children. In a recent study, optic atrophy was found to be the leading cause of severe visual impairment among 2527 Nordic children, followed by retinopathy of prematurity and amblyopia.[85] It is also probably the leading cause of visual impairment in mentally handicapped children.[18] The increasing survival rate of premature children in recent decades has resulted in increased incidence of both cortical visual impairment and optic atrophy in infants, the latter largely explained on the basis of their greater predisposition to hydro-

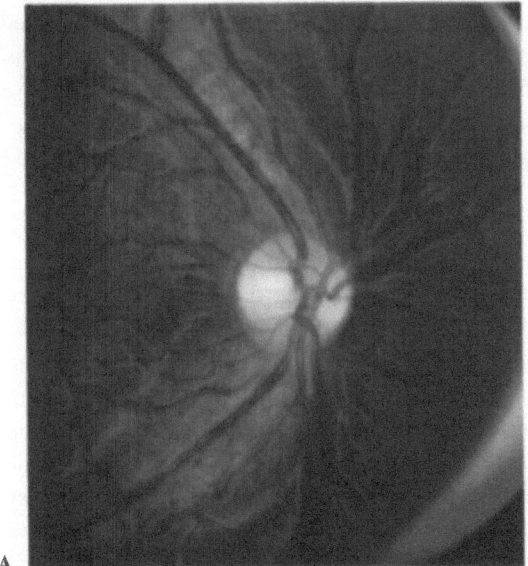

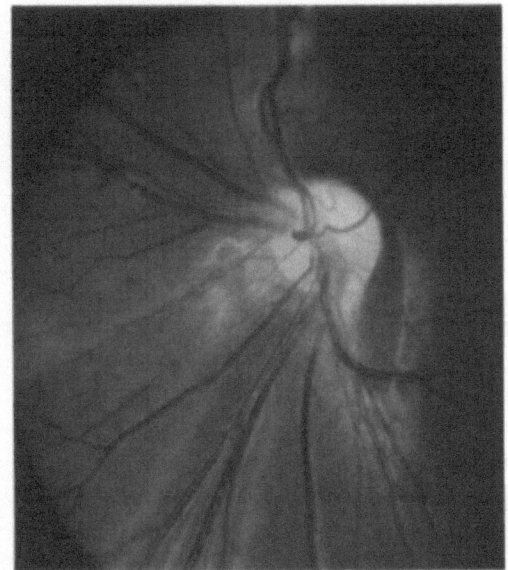

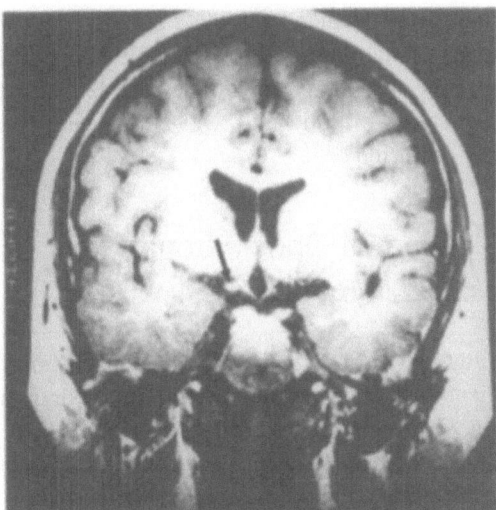

FIGURE 4.3. Congenital optic tract syndrome. This 11-year-old boy was found to have right homonymous hemianopia on routine testing. His optic discs revealed (**A**) band atrophy and (**B**) mild diffuse pallor. (**C**) MR imaging showed intact optic tract on the right (arrow) but an absent tract on the left.

cephalus and, to a lesser extent, due to associated perinatal hypoxia-ischemia. Disorders that are rarely encountered in the United States, such as onchocerciasis and intracranial hydatid cysts, may also cause optic atrophy.[58]

The reported incidence of diseases associated with optic atrophy differs according to series. Referral bias plays an important role, with large neurosurgical referral centers more likely to report higher incidences of compressive or postpapilledema optic atrophy in children who have intracranial tumors or shunt failure and with neurological referral centers more likely to accumulate

neurometabolic cases. Not all cases of optic atrophy in children are readily classifiable. The availability of high resolution neuroimaging modalities, such as magnetic resonance (MR) imaging, and the increased availability of blood tests to identify genetic mutations and metabolic products of enzymatic defects have increased the diagnostic yield.[148,190] In 1968, Costenbader and O'Rourk[42] were able to determine the cause of optic atrophy in a series of children so affected in only 50%, in contrast to 89% of children in the series by Repka and Miller.[190] In the latter study of 218 children with optic atrophy, the underlying causes included tumors (29%), postinflammatory (meningitis, optic neuritis) (17%), trauma (11%), undetermined (11%), hereditary (9%), perinatal disease (9%), hydrocephalus (6%), neurodegenerative disease (5%), toxic/metabolic disease (1%), and miscellaneous (3%). They found that in 13 children less than 1 year of age with optic atrophy, five had a history of intrauterine infection, prematurity, or perinatal trauma; three had tumors; and five had optic atrophy of undetermined etiology. In patients without history of prematurity, perinatal or postnatal trauma, meningitis, optic neuritis, or evidence of familial optic atrophy, the chance of an underlying tumor or hydrocephalus was 45%. The causative tumors included anterior visual pathway gliomas, craniopharyngiomas, other supratentorial tumors, pituitary adenomas, posterior fossa neoplasms, and orbital mass lesions. Rarely, optic atrophy may occur in children with autoimmune and collagen vascular disease.[13] Optic atrophy in children is therefore commonly accompanied by other neurological or systemic abnormalities. In this setting, intracranial, genetic, and neurometabolic diseases need to be ruled out.

The natural history of visual loss in children, due to optic atrophy or other causes, can be difficult to ascertain due to the child's limited ability to provide an accurate history and greater capacity to compensate for handicaps. Children are probably more likely than adults to ignore unilateral visual loss. Many unclassifiable cases of childhood optic atrophy are undoubtedly caused by remote trauma, optic neuritis, neuroretinitis, or other disorders that went unrecognized during the acute phase. The majority of such cases are unilateral.

Optic Atrophy Associated with Retinal Disease

Primary retinal disorders that involve the nerve fiber layer eventually lead to optic atrophy, and optic atrophy is a late finding in many diffuse degenerative retinal disorders. It is often possible to recognize optic atrophy associated with retinal disease by noting the concurrent retinal findings, especially marked arteriolar narrowing. An electroretinogram (ERG) is indicated in the setting of optic atrophy with marked arteriolar constriction. Retinal disorders associated with optic atrophy

include the various congenital retinal dystrophies, tapetoretinal degenerations, neuronal ceroid lipofuscinosis (e.g., Batten disease), infectious/inflammatory retinopathies (e.g., diffuse unilateral subacute neuroretinitis, cytomegalovirus (CMV) retinitis, toxoplasmosis), and central retinal or ophthalmic artery occlusion. It should be emphasized, however, that optic atrophy is not a typical feature of Leber congenital amaurosis, even in older patients.[227] Optic atrophy, especially of the temporal aspect of the disc, may be the sole funduscopic finding in some patients with cone dystrophy.[166,249] Disproportionate involvement of color vision, photophobia, and hemeralopia should increase suspicion for cone dysfunction. Cases of old central retinal artery occlusion may be difficult to distinguish from primary optic atrophy since some cases of central retinal artery occlusion show eventual recanalization of the occluded vasculature, after permanent inner retinal damage occurs. The two conditions may be distinguished with electroretinography that shows diminished b waves in cases of arterial occlusion.

Congenital Optic Atrophy Versus Hypoplasia

Although most prenatal injuries to the developing visual system eventuate in optic nerve hypoplasia, some infants are born with atrophic-appearing discs that are normal in size. Histologically, optic nerve hypoplasia is characterized by a diminution in the number of axons with normal blood vessels and glial tissue. Optic atrophy is characterized by a similar histopathology, except that the diameter of the optic nerve may be mildly diminished in some cases and preserved in others. While we have grown accustomed to interpreting optic atrophy as a clinical marker for postnatal visual system injury and hypoplasia as a marker for prenatal injury, the notion that term birth can demarcate these outcomes is simplistic and contrary to clinical experience.[94] For example, a congenital hemispheric lesion may be associated with either homonymous hemioptic hypoplasia with no pallor or band atrophy of the optic nerve that is contralateral to the side of the lesion (Figure 4.2). Why should some prenatal visual system injuries lead to a hypoplasia and others lead to pallor?

It is our speculation that the timing of injury is probably the critical determinant of whether the injured optic nerve involutes or becomes pale. As gestation proceeds, the optic nerve may become "hard-wired," so that its size and structural integrity are relatively maintained despite a marked diminution of axons. An analogy may be drawn between this scenario and the brain's ability to mount a glial reaction to injury that seems to begin sometime in the late second or early third trimester.[9] In the fetal brain, there is limited capacity for glial reaction; therefore, necrotic tissue is completely reabsorbed (liquefaction necrosis), resulting in a porencephalic cyst.[9] The mature brain, on the other hand, reacts to injury with significant gliosis; the resulting cavity contains glial septations and an irregular glial wall (multicystic encephalomalacia). Similarly, preservation of the structural integrity of the optic nerve in the face of exaggerated dying out (apostosis) of supernumerary axons (see Chapter 2) may require a certain degree of developmental maturation of the glial system and other supporting structures. This notion is consistent with the observations that optic nerve hypoplasia is often associated with other central nervous system (CNS) malformations that occur early in gestation and are not associated with gliosis (e.g., schizencephaly). Prenatal visual system injury may exist as a spectrum ranging from optic nerve hypoplasia (signifying early gestational injury) to atrophy (signifying late gestational injury), with a mixture of atrophy and hypoplasia occurring with midgestational injuries. The critical periods for developing hypoplasia versus atrophy in response to prenatal injury have not been defined. The role of other factors such as the nature of injury (e.g., ischemic versus toxic) and its duration (acute versus sustained) is also unclear.

Causes of Optic Atrophy in Children

Compressive/Infiltrative Intracranial Lesions

Bilateral optic atrophy that is diagnosed within the first 2 years of life is an ominous sign that may portend recurrent shunt dysfunction in a hydrocephalic child or anterior visual pathway compression from a congenital suprasellar tumor. These tumors include craniopharyngiomas, nonfunctional pituitary tumors, gliomas, meningiomas, metastatic tumors, and arachnoid cysts. Rarely, optic atrophy may be associated with suprasellar tumors of maldevelopmental origin such as lipomas or lipodermoids.[80] Bilateral band atrophy may be recognized when compression primarily involves the chiasm. In addition to optic atrophy, children with congenital suprasellar tumors may display congenital nystagmus (from bilateral sensory visual loss), nystagmus simulating spasmus nutans, see-saw nystagmus, or signs of dorsal midbrain syndrome. Systemic examination may provide some clues to the diagnosis in the form of café au lait spots or signs of emaciation in children with suprasellar glioma, signs of hypopituitarism in craniopharyngioma, and an abnormally large head size in hydrocephalus. Ipsilateral proptosis in a child with unilateral optic atrophy is highly suggestive of orbital optic glioma.

The finding of nystagmus in an *older* child with bilateral optic atrophy is an important diagnostic sign that confirms that visual loss was present within the first 2 years of life. A suprasellar lesion should be excluded in this setting. Unilateral optic nerve compression generally presents with proptosis or with sensory esotropia in the preschool years. Optic tract lesions (compressive or otherwise) produce homonymous hemianopia with contralateral band atrophy but no associated nystagmus. Noncompressive retrogeniculate lesions that are congenital in origin can also produce this constellation of findings.

In compressive lesions of the anterior visual pathways, the degree of optic atrophy is a good predictive sign of the potential restoration of vision following neurosurgical decompression.

Optic Glioma

Optic glioma is largely a tumor of childhood, with a mean age at presentation of 9 years (range: birth to old age).[52] No gender predilection appears to exist. Seventy-five percent of cases present during the first decade of life and 90% within the first two decades.

Patients with neurofibromatosis type 1 have a predilection to develop CNS astrocytomas and to show a frequency of optic pathway gliomas of about 15%[132] (Figure 4.4). Most of these tumors

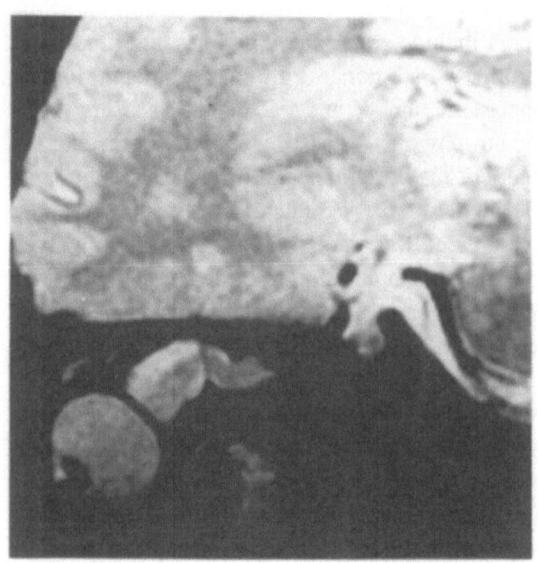

FIGURE 4.4. Optic nerve glioma in neurofibromatosis. Sagittal oblique MR shows characteristic fusiform enlargement and superior kinking of the nerve. An area of high signal intensity (corresponding to perineural arachnoidal gliomatosis) surrounds a core of low signal intensity (optic nerve).

are asymptomatic, with visual impairment in only about 20% of affected individuals. The frequency of neurofibromatosis type 1 in patients with optic pathway glioma varies in different series from 10% to 70%. Approximately one-half of the tumors are intraorbital, and the other half are intracranial. Café au lait spots are often absent or less conspicuous in young children. In patients with neurofibromatosis type 1, optic glioma is more often multifocal, occasionally affecting both optic nerves without apparent connection at the chiasm.[52]

Optic pathway glioma may exist in the absence of anterior visual pathway dysfunction. The absence of optic atrophy or papilledema, therefore, does not rule out chiasmal glioma in the child with neurofibromatosis. Lewis et al[131] reviewed the ocular and intracranial features of neurofibromatosis in 217 patients, 15% of whom had tumors of the anterior visual pathways. In two-thirds of these, the tumors were not detected by ophthalmologic examination, underscoring the importance of neuroimaging studies in these patients.

Due to the heterogeneity of optic pathway gliomas and their varying locations along the ante-

rior visual pathway, a variety of clinical presentations have been noted. However, regardless of location, most patients eventually develop some degree of visual loss. The visual loss is usually due to astrocytic proliferation, separation of longitudinal axonal bundles, axonal compression with subsequent demyelination, and mechanical disruption of axons.[71] There is generally poor correlation between tumor growth and visual acuity.[95]

Optic nerve tumors commonly present as an orbital mass lesion with axial proptosis, painless unilateral proptosis associated with disc edema, neoplastic infiltration of the disc, or optic atrophy. Optic atrophy is eventually noted in most, if not all, cases.

Rarely, a congenital suprasellar glioma may be associated with optic disc dysplasia.[232] An afferent pupillary defect is usually noted in unilateral or asymmetric cases. Visual field examination usually reveals a central scotoma or, with chiasmal involvement, temporal field defects. Temporal field defects are associated with loss of ganglion cells and nerve fiber layer nasal to the fovea. Optic atrophy is thus noted on the nasal and temporal sides of the disc in the classic "band" or "bowtie" distribution (Figure 4.1). Proptosis is generally absent in chiasmal and hypothalamic tumors.

Chiasmal gliomas usually present in childhood with unilateral or bilateral (often asymmetric) optic atrophy and visual loss. Hypothalamic or endocrine dysfunction from hypothalamic involvement is also frequently present. This includes precocious puberty, obesity, panhypopituitarism, and dwarfism. Children with early invasion of the hypothalamus present within the first several years of life with the diencephalic syndrome. Less commonly, hydrocephalus, seizures, cerebrospinal fluid (CSF) rhinorrhea, increased CSF protein, and tumocells in the CSF have been reported with chiasmal gliomas. Occasionally, untreated patients with chiasmal gliomas may show spontaneous visual improvement despite absence of tumor shrinkage on neuroimaging studies.[133] If the chiasmal lesion expands to involve the nearby third ventricle, obstructive hydrocephalus may result. Spasmus nutans may occur, which may be distinguishable clinically from the benign variety by the presence of an afferent pupillary defect and/or optic atrophy. Seesaw nystagmus may also occur.

Plain skull X-rays show classic enlargement of the optic foramen and a J-shaped sella turcica. Computed tomography (CT) shows isodense enlargement of the optic nerve or chiasm, with variable enhancement (Figure 4.1). Fusiform enlargement of the optic nerve is characteristic. The MR studies are preferable in young children, in order to avoid exposure to ionizing radiation, and may be superior for imaging the intracanalicular and intracranial spaces.[103]

Optic nerve gliomas arise from astrocytes surrounding optic nerve axons. Histopathology of optic glioma usually reveals juvenile pilocytic astrocytoma with a benign cytologic appearance, although mixed and malignant cases occur. An exuberant reactive proliferation of the surrounding meningeal tissues (termed arachnoidal gliomatosis) may accompany those gliomas associated with neurofibromatosis, occasionally causing diagnostic confusion with optic nerve sheath meningioma (Figure 4.4). In addition to neoplastic growth and arachnoidal gliomatosis, the tumor mass may show enlargement as a result of intralesional hemorrhage, cyst formation, or accumulation of extracellular Periodic Acid Shiff (PAS)-positive mucosubstance secreted by the glial cell.[52] The malignant form of glioma occurs primarily in adults.

Alvord and Lofton[2] recently provided an extensive review of the topic of optic glioma. In a review of optic pathway gliomas in neurofibromatosis type 1, Hoyt and Imes[96] conclude that "It is agreed that the main bulk of an optic pathway glioma is a low grade neoplasm with unpredictable growth potential. . . . It is not possible to demonstrate clear histological differences between tumors with limited growth and tumors that will grow."

Since most gliomas are benign and enlarge slowly, affected children generally show long-term survival[102] and treatment is controversial. Surgical amputation is considered when there is disfiguring proptosis in a blind eye. When the tumor is confined to the optic nerve, complete surgical excision with clear margin is curative, but many such children have sufficiently useful vision to suggest that conservative management with simple observation is a viable option. Removal or debulking of the orbital portion of the glioma is usually possible while leaving the globe in place.

In this setting, the orbital portion of the tumor can be resected without adverse effect even when the tumor involves the intracranial optic nerves or chiasm.

In 1980, Stern and coworkers[223] reviewed the histopathologic results of 34 tissue specimens from orbital optic gliomas. In 17 of 18 gliomas from patients with neurofibromatosis, a circumferential perineural pattern of growth in the subarachnoid space with minimal involvement of the intraneural compartment was found. They termed this pattern *arachnoidal gliomatosis* to signify that there was a marked proliferation of astrocytes over meningoepithelial cells and fibroblasts. In 14 of 16 gliomas from patients without neurofibromatosis, astrocytic proliferation was strictly intraneural with intact pial boundaries. The authors concluded that the perineural pattern of astrocytic proliferation was highly characteristic of neurofibromatosis-associated gliomas.

Magnetic resonance imaging can often predict tumor histopathology in vivo, since gliomatosis tissue has a long T1 and T2 relaxation time due to its high water content, causing it to appear bright on T2-weighted images and dark on T1-weighted images. Since gliomatosis tissue is primarily perineural (confined to the subarachnoid space surrounding the optic nerve) in neurofibromatosis, MR imaging imparts a double signal to the contents of the expanded dural sheath, with an outer signal that is indistinguishable from CSF and a sharply demarcated inner signal corresponding to optic nerve (Figure 4.4). The peripheral CSF intensity signal in orbital optic glioma correlates with the histopathological finding of peripheral arachnoidal gliomatosis and serves as a neuroimaging marker for neurofibromatosis.[19,208]

When the tumor involves the optic chiasm, the overall prognosis for life diminishes due to hypothalamic or third ventricular involvement. Surgical intervention at this point does not appear to improve survival. Neurosurgical debulking of the tumor and/or ventriculoperotineal shunting procedures are necessary in children with large diencephalic tumors that produce obstructive hydrocephalus. The efficacy of radiation and chemotherapy in these tumors is a subject of debate. Any potential benefit of radiation should be weighed against the potential risks of irradiation to the developing brain. Reported complications after cranial irradiation in children include volume loss and atrophy of normal brain parenchyma, progressive calcification, white matter abnormalities,[45,62] abnormalities in behavior, cognitive dysfunction, hypothalamic-pituitary dysfunction, growth retardation, acute lymphoblastic leukemia and other neoplasms,[194] visual loss, ocular motor nerve palsy, neuromyotonia, and Moyamoya syndrome.[171]

Following surgical resection of an orbital optic glioma, several poorly understood phenomena may be observed. Ophthalmoscopic examination and fluorescein angiography may show a normal central retinal arterial circulation[130] and CT scanning and MR imaging may show an optic nerve–like structure that is normal in size and configuration (termed the "phantom" optic nerve).[21,212]

Craniopharyngioma

Craniopharyngioma is by far the most common supratentorial tumor as well as the most common nonglial intracranial tumor of childhood. It affects primarily children and young adults, but the age range extends from the neonatal period to the eighth decade of life.[35] Craniopharyngioma is a histologically benign epithelial neoplasm thought to arise from epithelial vestiges found at the junction of the lower infundibular stem and the pars distalis. These tumors bear resemblance to Rathke's pouch cysts and epidermoid cysts of the region, and the three tumors may be related. They frequently exhibit invasive and aggressive local growth. Despite the histological appearance of craniopharyngioma, its intimate association with the visual apparatus, the hypothalamus, and the ventricular system frequently predisposes children with these tumors to anterior visual pathway compression and endocrine dysfunction.[247]

These tumors grow slowly and rarely present before 3 to 4 years of age. Craniopharyngioma is a particularly devastating tumor with respect to its long-term effects upon the visual system. Children with craniopharyngioma develop gradual, progressive visual loss from compression of one or both optic nerves, chiasm, tract, or less commonly, as a result of chronic papilledema. Occasionally, visual loss may be rapid, and the child may be thought to have retrobulbar neuritis. It is not unusual for children with craniopharyngioma to complain of non-specific symptoms and be assigned the diagnosis of psychogenic visual loss prior to the developing optic atrophy.[152]

By the time they are examined, many children with craniopharyngioma already have profound optic atrophy.[152] Optic atrophy occurred in 47% of eyes in one series.[241] In another series, optic atrophy was found in 12 of 24 eyes of patients younger than 18 years and in 11 of 36 eyes of patients older than 18 years.[189] Band atrophy is commonly seen. Papilledema, secondary to extension of the tumor into the third ventricle, may also occur in children and young adults with craniopharyngioma.[142] The rare association of anomalous optic discs with craniopharyngioma and other congenital suprasellar tumors[232] is attributed to the tumor's proximity to the anterior visual pathways and its potential for disrupting optic axonal migration during embryogenesis. Children and adolescents with craniopharyngioma may present with signs of hypopituitarism (e.g., short stature, retarded sexual development, obesity, infantilism), signs of hypothalamic involvement (e.g., thermolability), elevated intracranial pressure, or visual disturbances. Some children develop seesaw nystagmus. Diabetes insipidus is rare as a presenting sign, but it commonly develops following tumor resection.

Craniopharyngiomas are uniformly located, at least partially, in the suprasellar cistern. The symptoms and signs produced depend on the age of the patient, the size of the tumor, the direction of its growth, and the location of the optic chiasm (i.e., prefixed, fixed, and postfixed). The location of the chiasm determines whether the tumor compresses the optic nerves, the anterior chiasm (junctional syndrome), the chiasm, or the optic tract, each with its attendant-visual consequences. The tumor may project into the third ventricle causing hydrocephalus. Although craniopharyngioma usually occupies the suprasellar cistern in location, it may rarely originate beneath the sella, within the third ventricle or even within the chiasm.[22] Posterior extension of the tumor may compress the ventral brainstem and cerebellum.

Craniopharyngioma is a congenital tumor which may be solid, cystic, or both. The cyst is often filled with fluid that resembles machine oil, but the fluid may be straw colored. The fluid contains cholesterol crystals. Characteristic calcification within the tumor is readily demonstrated with plain skull films. Computed tomography is excellent for demonstrating the characteristic areas of calcification and cyst formation. On MR imaging, the calcification can be indirectly inferred (Figure 4.5).

The treatment of craniopharyngioma remains somewhat controversial. Surgical resection remains the treatment of choice for craniopharyngioma, but the issue of whether to attempt complete removal with its potential morbidity and mortality, or subtotal resection followed by radiotherapy, is not completely resolved. In a recent clinicopathological analysis of 56 patients operated on for craniopharyngioma, Weiner et al[247] found that gross total resection was associated with a lower recurrence rate (17%) than subtotal resection with or without radiation therapy (58%). In this study, the histopathological subtype did not significantly influence the surgical outcome. Some tumors are extremely difficult to eradicate,

because of their adherence to the optic nerves, hypothalamus, and the vessels of the circle of Willis, necessitating local irradiation therapy. Interstitial irradiation (interstitial brachytherapy) is an additional option.[241]

Many patients enjoy a significant return of vision after treatment. Repka and colleagues[189] assessed 30 patients with craniopharyngioma preoperatively and postoperatively to evaluate the degree of visual recovery. At the time of presentation, visual acuity was reduced in 42% of eyes; 20% of eyes had normal visual fields. One week postoperatively, acuity was reduced in 23% of eyes; 48% of eyes had normal fields with a slight decrease to 44% upon long-term follow-up. Patients with visual defects that were present after the first postoperative month showed no long-term improvement in acuity or field.

The differential diagnosis of craniopharyngioma in children includes meningioma, pituitary aden-

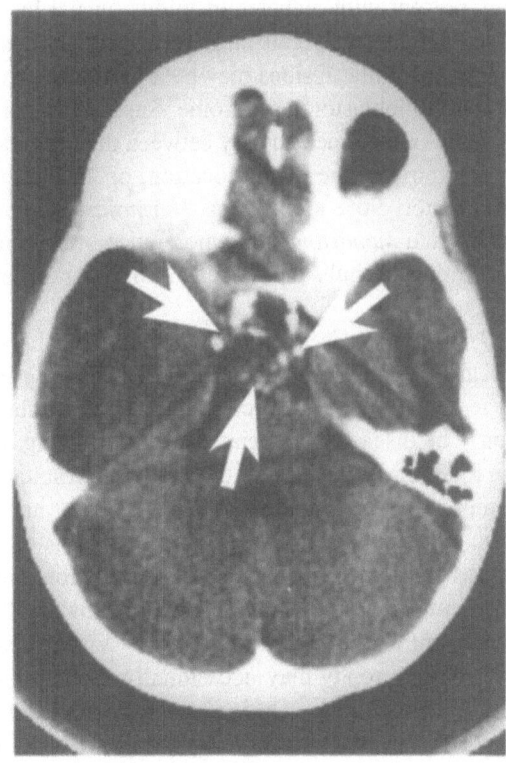
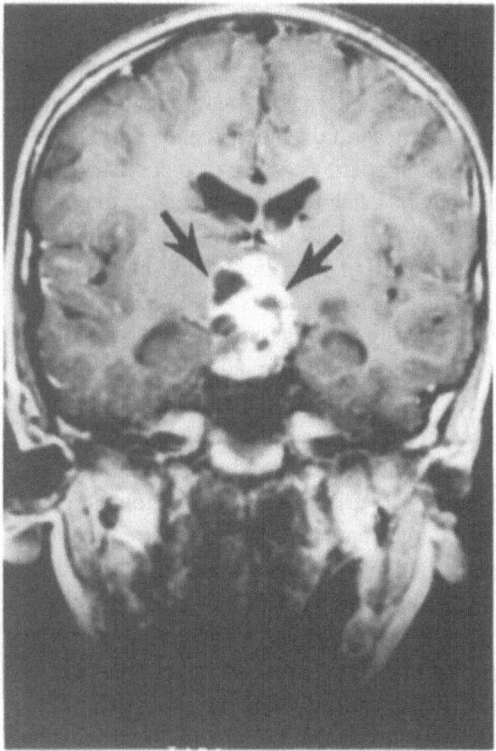

FIGURE 4.5. Craniopharyngioma. (A) Axial CT scan shows low density suprasellar mass with calcification. (B) Coronal MR image of the same lesion shows an in-homogeneous signal, reflecting both solid and cystic components of the suprasellar mass. The calcification cannot be directly demonstrated on MR images.

oma,[157] dysgerminoma, Rathke's pouch cyst, and suprasellar epidermoid cyst.

Rare Compressive Lesions Causing Optic Atrophy in Children

Pituitary adenoma is uncommon in childhood and adolescence.[68,157] In these age groups, the most common presenting complaint is failure of sexual maturation. Similarly to adults, 70% of children have evidence of pituitary hypersecretion at presentation.[191] Visual symptoms and signs appear less commonly in children than in adults with pituitary adenomas. In a series of 25 children with pituitary adenomas, three showed optic atrophy, with two of these having visual failure as a part of the presenting symptoms.[191]

Optic nerve sheath meningioma is rare in children.[44] The diagnosis is suggested by the triad of optociliary shunt vessels, optic atrophy, and visual loss, although this triad may less commonly be encountered in optic nerve glioma.[152] Other features common to both glioma and sheath meningioma include proptosis, afferent pupillary defect, strabismus, limitations of eye movements, and visual field defects.[106] These overlapping features and the purported rarity of optic nerve sheath meningioma in children may lead to diagnostic confusion with optic nerve glioma. The presence of optociliary shunt vessels may be a helpful diagnostic sign; they were present in only 1 of 22 patients with optic nerve glioma but in 10 of 47 patients with nerve sheath meningioma in a recent series.[106]

Neuroimaging findings may help differentiate optic nerve glioma from sheath meningioma. Computed tomographic scans of orbital gliomas reveal fusiform enlargement and kinking of the optic nerve with erosion and enlargement of the optic canal. The CT scans of meningiomas reveal diffuse enlargement, shaggy borders, frequent calcification, and hyperostotic thickening of the optic canalicular bone along with intraorbital "railroad tract sign" on axial images, representing abnormal enhancement of the periphery of the nerve. Gadolinium-enhanced MR may be particularly suited to delineate the extent of intracranial involvement of nerve sheath meningioma.[256] In equivocal cases, a direct biopsy may be needed to establish the diagnosis. It is important to biopsy both the sheaths and the nerve itself to avoid a false-positive diagnosis on the basis of finding arachnoid hyperplasia that may surround a glioma, imparting a histological appearance of a meningioma.

It is particularly important to establish the correct diagnosis of optic nerve sheath meningioma in children, as many authors consider this lesion to be more malignant in the younger age group than in adults.[44,253,254] There is some evidence that the childhood tumors have a higher propensity to show intracranial, intraneural, intraorbital, and intraocular spread than their adult counterparts. The treatment of optic nerve sheath meningioma is controversial.[44]

Dysgerminoma should be suspected in a child who presents with diabetes insipidus and who is found to have bitemporal hemianopia. With the exception of histiocytosis X, it is rare for other compressive lesions in this location to present with diabetes insipidus. These usually solid tumors show similar histological features to pinealomas but present in the perichiasmatic region. They occur within the first or second decade of life and may present with diabetes insipidus, visual loss, visual field defects, optic atrophy, or pituitary dysfunction. Similar lesions may be a part of the trilateral retinoblastoma syndrome. Suprasellar germinomas are divided equally between the genders, unlike those in the pineal location, of which approximately 90% are in boys. *Dermoids, epidermoids,* and *hamartomas* are more uncommon and constitute the bulk of the remaining suprasellar masses.

Osteopetrosis is an inherited metabolic bone disease characterized by generalized increase in bone density due to reduction in osteoclast function. The disease is associated with narrowing of the foramina of the base of the skull with resultant compressive neuropathy. Visual loss may arise from either optic nerve or retinal dysfunction. Optic atrophy may result secondarily either from papilledema or from compressive neuropathy due to narrowing of the optic foramen.[78,91] Visual loss with optic atrophy may occasionally be the presenting symptom.[173] Optic nerve decompression may result in stabilization or even improvement of vision.[146] It is important to perform electroretinography to exclude an associated retinal degeneration before undertaking optic nerve decompression.[91,173]

Craniosynostoses (e.g., Crouzon syndrome, Pfeiffer syndrome, Apert syndrome, plagiocephaly) are not uncommonly associated with visual failure due to optic atrophy.[7,74,168] The pathogenesis of optic atrophy in craniosynostosis may be related to (1) increased intracranial pressure and papilledema, (2) kinking and stretching of the optic nerve due to abnormal cranial and brain growth, (3) narrowed optic canals, or (4) a complication of craniofacial surgery.[25] One recently described disorder associated with premature fusion of cranial sutures is the GAPO syndrome.[206,207,246] GAPO is an acronym for the manifestations of growth retardation, alopecia, pseudoanodontia, and progressive optic atrophy. It is a rare autosomal recessive disorder that also shows a peculiar geriatric facial appearance, short stature resembling rhizomelic dwarfism, muscular habitus, and large fontanel in infancy. The hair is lost within the first few years of life, and the teeth are normal but unerupted. Optic atrophy has been reported in 30% of affected children. The nature of the optic atrophy is unclear, with possible contributions by concurrent glaucoma or intracranial hypertension. Patients appear to have a shortened life expectancy, with death occurring in midlife.

Fibrous dysplasia is an abnormal fibro-osseous disorder of bone of unknown etiology. The disorder is considered to be a maturational arrest at the woven bone stage, with abnormal development of bony tissue, resulting in fibrous tissue proliferation and defective osteogenesis. Normal bone is gradually replaced with fibrous tissue. The process occurs primarily during childhood but may continue into adulthood. Histological analysis shows areas of fibrous tissue interwoven with newly formed bone.[156] The disorder more commonly involves a single bone (monostotic) or may be disseminated throughout the body (polyostotic). Polyostotic fibrous dysplasia occurs in association with café au lait spots and precocious puberty in girls with Albright syndrome.

In most patients, the lesions in fibrous dysplasia tend to grow slowly and then stabilize in early adulthood. The most commonly affected calvarial bone is the frontal, then the sphenoid, temporal, parietal, and occipital bones in that order. The most common presentation is a painless enlargement of the involved bone, causing facial asymmetry, orbital dystopia, or unilateral proptosis. In-

volvement of the bones at the base of the skull may cause narrowing of the neural foramina with compression of cranial nerves, causing hearing loss, tinnitus, and cranial nerve palsies. If the disorder affects the lesser wing of the sphenoid bone, the optic canal may become narrowed with compression of the optic nerve with subsequent optic atrophy.[156,182] Initially, such patients may be misdiagnosed as having retrobulbar optic neuritis, with the correct diagnosis subsequently suggested by neuroimaging studies obtained when spontaneous visual improvement fails to occur.[248] Involvement of the sella turcica may compress the optic chiasm, leading to chiasmal syndrome and optic atrophy.[251] Trigeminal neuralgia and increased intracranial pressure have also been described.

Prompt surgical decompression of the optic canal in patients with compressive neuropathy may restore some optic nerve function and halt progression of the optic atrophy.

Noncompressive Causes of Optic Atrophy in Children with Brain Tumors

In addition to the direct effect of the tumor itself, optic neuropathies may be seen in children with brain tumors due to several other potential etiologies: (1) Toxic effect of chemotherapy (e.g., vincristine).[214] Vincristine has been implicated in various ophthalmological disturbances including optic atrophy,[214] transient cortical visual impairment, ptosis, and ophthalmoplegia. Disruption of the blood-brain barrier by both radiation and surgical manipulation may increase its toxic potential.[214] (2) Paraneoplastic optic neuropathy. (3) Radiation optic neuropathy. Toxic optic neuropathy will be discussed later in this chapter.

Postpapilledema Optic Atrophy in Children

Postpapilledema optic atrophy is often associated with specific ophthalmoscopic findings that suggest the underlying mechanism of injury (Figure 4.6). Any of the following findings in association with optic atrophy suggest previous optic disc swelling: (1) A fine fibrous sheathing of the retinal vessels as they emanate from the disc. (2) Opaque fibrous tissue overlying the disc and obscuring the peripapillary retina. (3) Circumpapillary pigment changes ("high water marks"). (4) Optociliary shunt vessels.

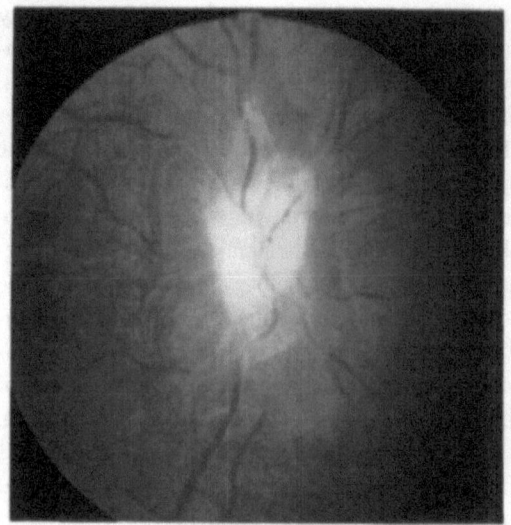 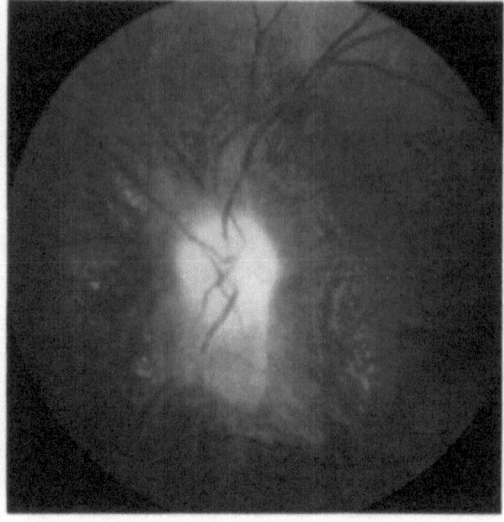

FIGURE 4.6. Postpapilledema optic atrophy in a patient with chronic pseudotumor cerebri. Note bilateral disc pallor with indistinct margins and circumpapillary 'high-water' marks. There is prepapillary and peripapillary glial proliferation which produces a wispy vascular sheathing and radial peripapillary striae.

In addition to brain tumors (especially posterior fossa tumors, but also craniopharyngioma), major causes of postpapilledema optic atrophy in children include shunt failure, pseudotumor cerebri, craniosynostosis, among others. These entities are detailed in Chapter 3. The efficacy of optic nerve sheath fenestration in preventing visual loss in patients with severe or intractable papilledema is now well established. While the indications for optic nerve sheath fenestration in children have yet to be established, many cases of postpapilledema optic atrophy in children are now preventable with early intervention.

Paraneoplastic Syndromes

Optic atrophy may rarely result from paraneoplastic axonal degeneration. Paraneoplastic retinal degeneration is much more common in adults than in children. By contrast, paraneoplastic ocular motility disorders (e.g., opsoclonus-myoclonus in neuroblastoma) are more common in children.[6,207] Presumed paraneoplastic retinal degeneration and optic atrophy was recently described in a 6-year-old boy who had an embryonal rhabdomyosarcoma of the thorax.[83] A few cases of presumed paraneoplastic optic neuropathy have been described in adult patients. In some such cases, retinal pigmentary abnormalities may be absent, and marked arteriolar narrowing may be the only sign of underlying retinal dysfunction. The diagnosis is established by finding an attenuated or extinguished ERG signal.

Paraneoplastic syndromes often have an autoimmune basis. Sera from patients with visual paraneoplastic syndromes have been shown to contain immunoglobulins that are reactive with both the tumor and with various retinal elements (e.g., photoreceptors, large ganglion cells, bipolar cells).

Radiation Optic Neuropathy

Radiation therapy is not infrequently administered for the treatment of various ocular (e.g., retinoblastoma) and intracranial (e.g., craniopharyngioma, dysgerminoma) tumors of childhood. Shielding the globes and the optic nerves from the field of radiation is not always possible. Cases receiving a cumulative dose of radiation of greater than 50 to 60 Gy or dose fractions greater than 200 cGy/day are particularly at risk of developing radiation retinopathy or optic neuropathy, depending upon the path of administered radiation.

Radiation retinopathy reveals findings similar to those seen in diabetes. Radiation optic neuropathy presents 1 to 6 years (peak: 18 months) after radiotherapy. Acute loss of vision occurs along with visual field changes that localize to various parts of the anterior visual pathways, depending upon the site of involvement. Patients are often misdiagnosed as having optic neuritis or recurrent tumor compressing the visual pathways. The MR imaging in the acute phase of visual loss shows intense Gadolinium enhancement of the affected segments of the anterior visual pathway.[76] Functional neuroimaging modalities (PET, SPECT) may help delineate either metabolically active tumor or inactive necrotic neural tissue.

The primary site of pathogenesis is the vascular endothelium, and the underlying pathologic changes are those of radiation-induced occlusive vascular disease: endothelial proliferation, fibrinoid necrosis, and reactive astrocytosis.

Therapeutic trials of corticosteroids and hyperbaric oxygenation have been, with a few exceptions,[17] unsuccessful.

Hydrocephalus

Hydrocephalus is a common cause of optic atrophy in children.[39,66,69,140,239] It is difficult to determine with certainty which, if any, of the various types of hydrocephalus is more likely to result in optic atrophy. In contrast to optic atrophy arising from increased intracranial pressure in older patients, the childhood variety may or may not pass through a stage of papilledema. Optic atrophy and/or cortical

visual impairment are the usual causes of bilateral visual defects in hydrocephalic children.

The following mechanisms have been proposed as possible causes of optic atrophy in hydrocephalus: (1) Long-term papilledema or acute severe papilledema with subsequent atrophy. This typically arises after shunt placement with subsequent failure(s) since hydrocephalic infants tend not to develop significant papilledema due to their expansile cranium. (2) Stretching of the chiasm and its blood supply as a result of intracranial displacement of the brainstem in an effort to accommodate increasing cerebral volume. (3) Optic nerve stretching by an expanding skull. (4) Chiasmal compression by a dilated third ventricle. In such cases, bulging of the third ventricle anteriorly into the sella turcica can be demonstrated on CT or MR imaging (Figure 4.7). Most cases of

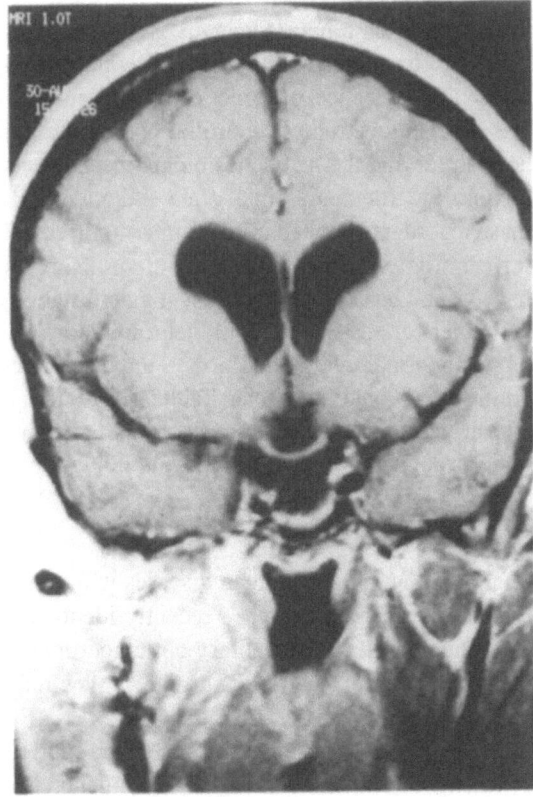

FIGURE 4.7. Chiasmal compression by a dilated third ventricle. Dilation of the third ventricle in a child with hydrocephalus may lead to stretching and ballooning of the optic chiasm.

optic atrophy associated with hydrocephalus are bilateral, although asymmetric and even unilateral cases do occur. Compression of one optic nerve, presumably against the internal carotid artery, with unilateral visual loss, has been reported in a child with an obstructed shunt.[29] (5) Transsynaptic degeneration of the retinogeniculate pathway after cortical damage. (6) Optic tract damage by shunt placement.[66,69,239]

The major mechanism appears to be postpapilledema optic atrophy that occurs in children with poorly controlled hydrocephalus and repeated shunt failure. In our experience, children with hydrocephalus secondary to intraventricular hemorrhage are at particularly high risk of developing severe optic atrophy early in life. The specific mechanism of afferent visual system injury in these infants has not been determined.

Hereditary Optic Atrophy

These represent a heterogeneous group of disorders that generally manifest with bilateral optic atrophy and evidence of genetic transmission.[161] The precise location of the initial pathologic abnormalities and the pathophysiologic mechanisms responsible for neural injury are unknown. All these disorders show significant interfamilial and intrafamilial variability. Some of these disorders have visual loss as the only clinical manifestation, and others are associated with neurologic or systemic abnormalities. In addition to the discussion within the text of this chapter, Table 4.1 provides a partial listing of the genetic disorders that have optic atrophy as a part of the clinical findings.[99]

Leber Hereditary Optic Neuropathy

A growing number of human diseases with a mitochondrial origin have been recently identified. These include Leber hereditary optic neuropathy (LHON), Kearns–Sayre syndrome, myoclonic epilepsy and ragged-red fiber disease (MERRF), infantile lactic acidosis, and a recently reported syndrome of diabetes and deafness. Mitochondria contain their own genetic material consisting of 2 to 10 copies of double-stranded DNA that differs from nuclear DNA in several ways. Mitochondrial DNA is a circular molecule, with few noncoding sequences, and a slightly different genetic code

that is transmitted exclusively by mothers. Mitochondrial DNA is transmitted via the egg cytoplasm and encodes for a number of protein components of the mitochondrial respiratory chain and oxidative phosphorylation system, as well as some 20 transfer RNAs and two ribosomal RNAs. Women transmit the disease to their sons and the carrier state to their daughters; however, carrier females are occasionally affected.

The disease LHON is a maternally inherited form of optic neuropathy that is associated with several mitochondrial DNA (mtDNA) mutations.[89,101,165,245] To date, five such mutations have been identified (nucleotide positions 11778, 3460, 14482, 15257, 4160).[109,111,113,159] It manifests typically within the second or third decade of life, but the age of onset may vary widely. The gender predilection varies in different geographic areas: The male-to-female ratio in the United States is 9:1, but in Japan it is approximately 6:4. Based on reported cases, 50% to 80% of males and 8% to 32% of females at risk experience significant visual loss. About 50% of the males and 10% of the females with the genetic defect develop optic neuropathy. The condition presents initially between the ages of 15 and 35 years (range 1 to 72 years) as unilateral blurred vision that progresses rapidly with sequential involvement of the other eye within days to a few months. Infrequently, the second eye involvement may occur simultaneously, (after many years) or, rarely, not at all. The visual acuity commonly stabilizes at or below 20/200, but this varies widely with a range of 20/40 to no light perception. Color vision is severely diminished. The time course of visual loss differs from that of optic neuritis in that it continues to evolve over several months. The characteristic visual field defect is a central or cecocentral scotoma that may extend superiorly in some patients. The visual loss is permanent in most cases, but an occasional patient may show variable recovery of vision even years after the acute episode. This recovery is typically restricted to a few central degrees and appears to be more likely in patients with the 11778 deletion.[224]

Prior to and during the acute stages, the retinal examination usually shows a characteristic triad of signs: circumpapillary telangiectatic microangiopathy, pseudoedema of the disc and surrounding

TABLE 4.1. Genetic syndromes associated with optic atrophy in children.

Name of syndrome	Reference
Dominant optic atrophy	92, 138, 56
Leber hereditary optic neuropathy	89, 101, 165
Behr optic atrophy	213
Simple recessive optic atrophy	155
DIDMOAD syndrome (Table 4.3)	203, 242, 252
Optic atrophy +/- deafness +/- diabetes mellitus (Table 4.2)	
Biotinidase deficiency (AR)	30, 187, 202
Marshall–Smith syndrome	222
Myoclonus epilepsy with ragged-red fibers	170
Craniosynostosis	74
Acromesomelic-spondyloepiphyseal dysplasia (AD)	211
Familial agenesis of the corpus callosum	32
Osteopetrosis	98
PEHO syndrome (progressive encephalopathy, edema, hypsarrhythmia, optic atrophy)	219, 220
X-linked ataxia, weakness, deafness, early loss of vision, fatal course	5
X-linked severe mental retardation, blindness, deafness, epilepsy, spasticity, early death	75
Early onset spinocerebellar ataxia, optic atrophy, internuclear ophthalmoplegia, dementia, startle myoclonus	210
Dysosteosclerosis	36
X-linked seizures, acquired micrencephaly, agenesis of corpus callosum	183
Kenny syndrome	60
Bilateral striatal necrosis, dystonia, and optic atrophy	129
Heredodegenerative neurological disorders with optic atrophy (Table 4.4)	
Oculocerebral hypopigmentation syndrome (Cross syndrome)	174
Craniosynostosis (Crouzon, Apert, Pfeiffer syndromes)	168
N-Acetylaspartic aciduria (AR)	67
Maple syrup urine disease (AR)	26
Familial dysautonomia (Riley–Day syndrome)	192
Mucopolysaccharidoses	38
GAPO syndrome (growth retardation, alopecia, pseudoanodontia, optic atrophy (AR)	246
Fukuyama-type congenital muscular dystrophy	255
Gait ataxia, dysarthria, dysmetria, adiadochokinesia, cramps, tremor, hypotonia, limited eye movements	172
Spinocerebellar degenerations	134, 146
Familial syndrome of infantile optic atrophy, movement disorder, and spastic paraplegia	41
Homocystinuria	27
Mitochondrial encephalomyopathy, lactic acidosis, strokelike episodes (MELAS)	87
Menkes Kinky hair disease (XLR)	160
Cockayne syndrome	234
Marinesco–Sjogren syndrome	48
Late onset autosomal recessive optic atrophy	179
Familial optic atrophy with negative ERG	250
Neuronal storage disease (e.g., Batten disease) (Table 4.5)	
3-Methylglutaconic aciduria	57, 213
Combined methylmalonic aciduria and homocystinuria	235
N-Acetylaspartic aciduria	67
Neuraminidase deficiency (sialidosis)	233
Marble brain disease (AR)	215
Motor and sensory neuropathy, mental retardation, pyramidal signs, optic atrophy	135
Primary oxalosis	216
Chondrodysplasia punctata	59
Childhood lactic acidosis	87
Neurofibromatosis type I	131
Numerous chromosomal abnormalities	

nerve fiber layer, and absence of leakage on fluo-rescein angiography (Figure 4.8).[217] The discs are typically relatively cupless and crowded looking, and with late branching vessels. These funduscopic changes may also be seen in presymptomatic cases and in asymptomatic maternal relatives. However, some patients with LHON never display these clas-sic findings.[167] Affected patients eventually show optic atrophy with nerve fiber layer dropout, most notably in the papillomacular bundle. Several pa-tients with the 15257 mutation have been recently reported to show a macular degeneration resem-bling Stargardt disease.[88]

Since LHON may be associated with a cardiac myopathy and a preexcitation syndrome, an EKG or a 24 Holter monitor should be performed. His-tological changes in skeletal musculature, without clinical myopathy, may also occur.

Some controversy still exists with regards to the existence of an X-chromosome-encoded modify-ing gene that is invoked to explain the male predominance.[164,243] The commonly observed in-trafamilial phenotypic variability may be explica-ble on the basis of mtDNA heteroplasmy (the co-existence of normal and mutant mtDNA in variable combinations in different patients).[218] Only when the percentage of affected mitochon-dria is high does the disorder become clinically manifested. However, epigenetic factors appear to play a role in the pathogenesis, as attested to by identical twins who are discordant for the disease.[110] The preeminent epigenetic factors that

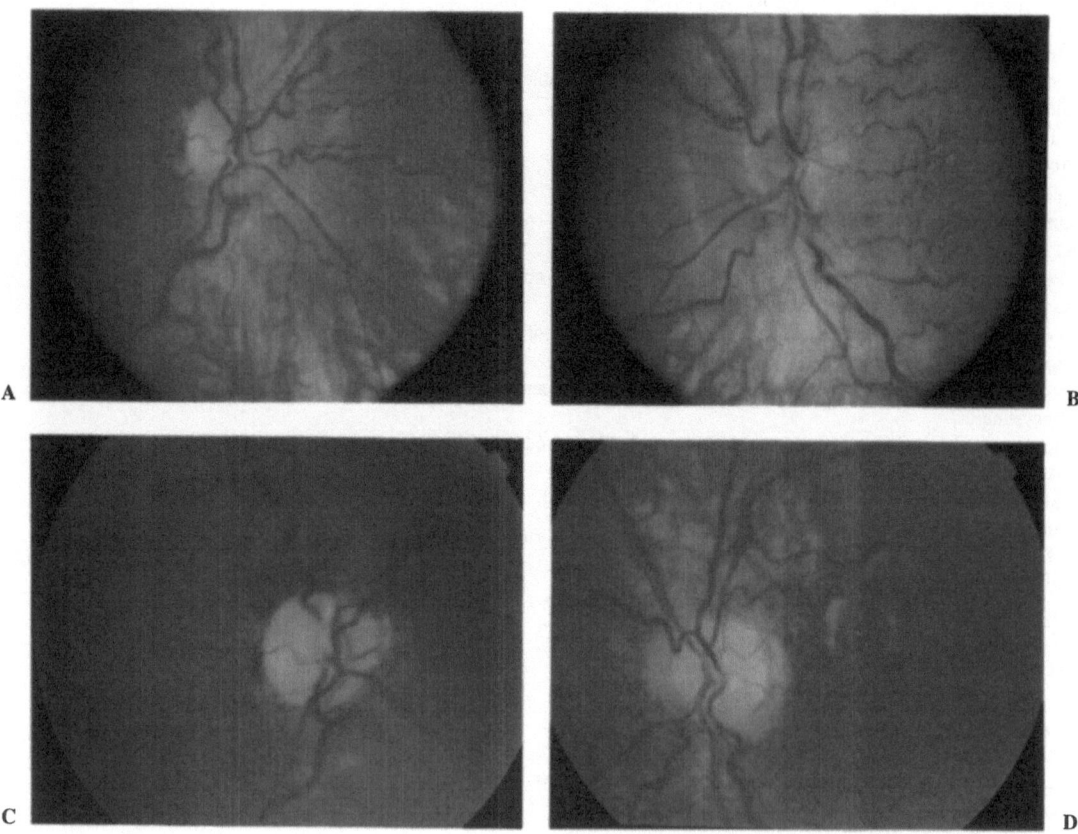

FIGURE 4.8. Leber hereditary optic neuropathy. This 10-year-old boy developed bilateral loss of vision in both eyes to the level of counting fingers. The optic discs ap-peared somewhat swollen ((A) right disc; (B) left disc) with peripapillary telangiectatic microangiopathy most apparent in the inferotemporal arcade below the left disc (B). His mother showed a similar optic disc appearance but was normally sighted. Four months later, his optic discs appeared diffusely pale; the telangiectasia and swollen appearance were absent ((C) right disc; (D) left disc).

are suspected at this time appear to be consumption of tobacco and alcohol.[43] There is also some evidence that systemic illnesses may trigger the clinical disorder in a predisposed individual.[51] The toxic/nutritional modulation of the clinical manifestation of LHON may, in a general sense, be bidirectional. Sadun et al[200] investigated an epidemic of optic neuropathy in Cuba and found that nutritional and toxic factors were producing an acquired mitochondrial injury, with a resulting clinical syndrome that resembles LHON.

LHON is often misdiagnosed.[90,112] In adults, it may be mistaken for anterior ischemic optic neuropathy[16] or tobacco-alcohol amblyopia.[43] In children and adolescents, it may be misdiagnosed as optic neuritis, a possibility made more likely if CNS involvement exists.[176] Such associated neurologic involvement, if it occurs, is usually mild. Unusual cases may be associated with severe neurologic disease, making them difficult to differentiate from multiple sclerosis or Devic disease, especially if the characteristic fundus changes are absent. In that setting, other tests such as mitochondrial DNA studies, visual evoked potentials, or spinal fluid examination may be needed to make the distinction.

No treatment for LHON has been shown to be effective to date.

Dominant Optic Atrophy (Kjer Type)

Dominant optic atrophy is the most common hereditary optic atrophy, with a disease frequency in the range of 1:50 000. It is transmitted as a dominant Mendelian trait with nearly complete penetrance (0.98) and a highly variable clinical expression. The visual loss has an insidious onset within the first decade of life, typically between the ages of 4 and 8 years. Affected children are often unaware of the visual disorder until it is uncovered during routine visual screening. Visual acuity typically ranges from 20/70 to 20/100 but may be as good as 20/20 or as poor as counting fingers.[92,121,162,230] The degree of vision loss varies considerably among members of the same family and may be asymmetric between fellow eyes in an affected individual. A mild degree of photophobia is often present. Affected children usually do not display nystagmus, even when the vision is reduced beyond the 20/200 level. It may

thus be inferred that the acuity of such children must have been considerably better during early visual development. A characteristic blue-yellow color vision defect (tritanopia), best elicited with the Farnsworth–Munsell 100-hue test, is often seen but is not necessary to make the diagnosis. Many patients show generalized nonspecific dyschromatopsia, and some patients may even show a deutan defect.[138] There is usually no correlation between the severity of the dyschromatopsia and the visual acuity. Visual field testing typically shows central or cecocentral scotoma and, because of the characteristic tritanopia, may show inversion of the peripheral field so that it is more constricted to blue than to red targets.[127] The peripheral visual field is full to white targets.

The appearance of the optic disc ranges from mild but definite temporal pallor to complete atrophy. A "characteristic" focal temporal excavation of the disc is seen in some but not all patients (Figure 4.9). An associated loss of the nerve fiber layer in the papillomacular bundle is present and is frequently dramatic. A few patients may show subtle macular pigmentary changes. The severity of disc pallor does not correlate with visual acuity, fields, or color vision.

The visual prognosis is generally good.[56] These children function surprisingly well given the degree of their measured visual deficits. Some patients are even unaware of the visual deficit before the initial examination. Rarely do affected children attend schools for the blind. Long-term follow-up reveals either stabilization of visual function after the middle teens or minimal deterioration of vision (by one to three lines) that is rather gradual and typically unnoticed by the patient. Kjer et al[120] reported that all of his patients younger than 15 years of age had visual acuity better than 20/200, whereas 20% of patients beyond 45 years of age had acuities reduced to this level. In another study, 11 of 40 eyes (27.5%) showed loss of vision between two and four Snellen lines over a 16-year follow-up period.

Visual evoked cortical potentials reveal reduced amplitudes and, in some patients, delayed latencies. The amplitude of the negative component of the pattern ERG is markedly reduced while the positive component is normal.[100] In some patients with normal electrophysiological studies, standard visual fields, and color vision (FM 100 hue), static

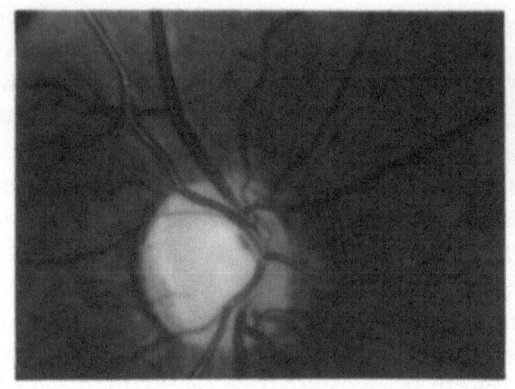
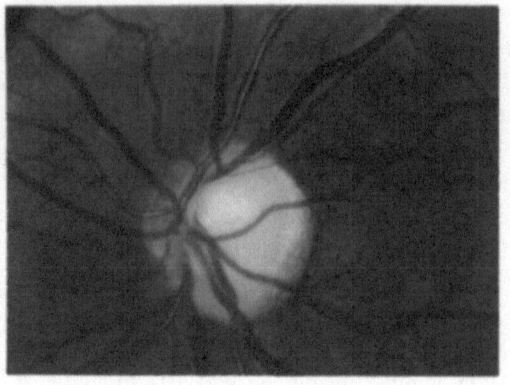

A   B

FIGURE 4.9. Dominant optic atrophy. This 7-year-old girl had failed the vision screening examination at school, with acuities of 20/50 bilaterally. Note pro-

nounced temporal pallor and excavation ((**A**) right eye; (**B**) left eye).

perimetry with blue test spots may show enlarged central scotomas, indicative of subclinical dominant optic atrophy.[14]

Histopathologic studies have shown primary degeneration of the retinal ganglion cell layer, accompanied by loss of myelin and ascending optic atrophy, with intact cerebral hemispheres.[120] Suggestions that there are at least two genetic types of autosomal dominant optic atrophy, one congenital and one manifesting postnatally, are unproven,[193] with some support for the notion that these two types are probably a result of a single genetic defect, representing the variable expressivity so common in autosomal dominant disorders.[177]

The majority of cases of dominant optic atrophy are monosymptomatic. Affected patients are typically entirely healthy with the exception of sight. Rare exceptions have included the association of mental retardation,[114] hearing loss,[149] and chronic progressive external ophthalmoplegia.[147] It is probable that these entities represent genetic defects that are different from the isolated variety. Two families with an autosomal dominant optic atrophy, hearing loss, and peripheral neuropathy have been described.[77] This triad (optic atrophy +/ – hearing loss +/ – polyneuropathy) has been described as an autosomal dominant, autosomal recessive, and X-linked disorder; the various forms have been recently compared by Hagemoser et al.[77] Also, a large family with an autosomal dominant disorder manifesting with progressive optic atrophy, abnormal ERGs without retinal pigmentary changes, and progressive sensorineu-

ral hearing loss has been reported. The disorder appears in the first or second decade of life, followed by the emergence of ptosis, ophthalmoplegia, ataxia, and a nonspecific myopathy in midlife.[236] Table 4.2 lists the various genetic syndromes encompassing the findings of hearing loss and optic atrophy.

It may be difficult sometimes to differentiate dominant optic atrophy from other conditions such as Leber optic neuropathy in patients with remote visual loss.[105] Differentiation of mild cases of dominant optic atrophy from congenital tritanopia, also an autosomal dominant disorder, requires blue cone ERG.[154] In some cases, automated perimetry may show pseudobitemporal hemianopia.

The management of dominant optic atrophy is essentially limited to genetic counseling. Dominant optic atrophy has been recently mapped to chromosome 3 (3q28-qter).[55]

Recessive Optic Atrophy

Recessively inherited optic atrophies are a heterogeneous group of disorders. One end of the spectrum is represented by complex conditions such as "Behr's optic atrophy" as well as various recessively inherited neurologic disorders that show optic atrophy as one of their manifestations. The other end of the spectrum is represented by a monosymptomatic, isolated, rare form of hereditary optic atrophy that occurs as an autosomal recessive disorder.

TABLE 4.2. Hereditary syndromes with association of optic atrophy and deafness.

Reference	Syndrome	Inheritance	Age of onset of vision loss	Degree of vision loss	Hearing loss	Associated findings
3	Progressive optic atrophy, congenital sensorineural deafness	Autosomal dominant	Childhood or midlife	Moderate loss	Moderate, severe	None
50	DIDMOAD (Wolfram) syndrome	Autosomal recessive, ? mitochondrial	First decade	Moderate to severe	Progressive	Diabetes mellitus, diabetes insipidus
229	Optic atrophy, ataxia, progressive hearing loss (Sylvester syndrome)	Autosomal dominant	First decade	Progressive loss	Progressive, moderate to severe	Weakness, muscle wasting
61	Optico-cochleo-dentate degeneration	Autosomal recessive	Infancy	? progressive	Progressive, severe	Progressive spastic quadriplegia, mental deterioration, death
195	Optic atrophy, peripheral neuropathy, hearing loss (Rosenberg–Choturran syndrome)	X-linked or autosomal recessive	Second decade	Moderate loss	Progressive, deafness by age 6 yrs	
117	Optic atrophy, peripheral neuropathy, hearing loss	Autosomal recessive	First decade		Second decade	
77	Optic atrophy, peripheral neuropathy, hearing loss	Autosomal dominant	First decade	Severe	Mild to severe	
236	Optic atrophy, deafness, ptosis, ophthalmoplegia, dystaxia, myopathy	Autosomal dominant	First decade	Moderate to severe	Mild to severe	
108	Optic atrophy, dementia, sensorineural hearing loss	Probable X-linked	Second or third decade	Moderate to severe loss	Severe	
5	Ataxia, weakness, deafness, blindness, fatal course	X-linked recessive	Early childhood	Severe	Severe	Posterior column lack of myelin, death in first decade
36	Dysosteosclerosis	Autosomal recessive	Early childhood	Moderate to severe	Mild to moderate	Skeletal dysplasia, intracranial calcifications, mental retardation

Simple Recessive Optic Atrophy

The visual deficit in this rare disorder is more pronounced than in dominant optic atrophy, with acuities worse than 2/200 and achromatopsia or severe dyschromatopsia being characteristic. The condition is therefore detected earlier in life than dominant atrophy, usually within the first several years of life, and is usually associated with nystagmus. Occasionally, the condition is noted in the neonatal period and labeled as congenital. Because of the rarity of the condition, other more common disorders must first be excluded with thorough clinical, electrophysiological, and neuroimaging means.

The optic discs show profound diffuse atrophy, often with deep cupping. Attenuation of the peripapillary retinal arteriolar vessels has been described, suggesting that at least some such cases might have represented undiagnosed retinal dystrophies such as Leber congenital amaurosis or autosomal recessive cone dystrophy with associated optic atrophy that went unrecognized in the pre-ERG era. Therefore, a complete retinal evaluation and a normal ERG are essential to make a diagnosis of autosomal recessive optic atrophy. In an *infant* with Leber congenital amaurosis, however, optic atrophy is distinctly unusual[227] and a compressive intracranial etiology should be sought. Also, histopathologic studies of eyes with Leber congenital amaurosis have revealed intact optic nerves, the outer nuclear layer and photoreceptors being the primary site of retinal pathology.[226]

It is, however, worthy of note that some authors cast doubt on the existence of simple, monosymptomatic, recessively inherited optic atrophy as a distinct entity.[155] From the practical standpoint, given the rarity of this disorder, if indeed it exists, the diagnosis should be one of exclusion at least insofar as it carries with it the need for specific genetic counseling to prospective parents.

Behr Optic Atrophy
(Optic Atrophy Plus Infantile Optic Atrophy)

In 1909, Behr[11] described a variant of recessive optic atrophy that also occurs in early childhood (1 to 8 years). It differs from the simple variety described above in that it is associated with other abnormalities including ataxia, pyramidal and extrapyramidal dysfunction, hypertonia, juvenile spastic paresis, mental retardation, urinary incontinence, and pes cavus. The visual disability and the optic atrophy are severe, showing a variable period of progression that does not usually extend beyond childhood. Sensory nystagmus occurs in over half of the patients. The MR neuroimaging in a 6-year-old girl with this syndrome demonstrated diffuse, symmetric white matter abnormalities.[141]

It is debatable whether or not Behr optic atrophy is a distinct entity, with recent evidence suggesting that the syndrome may represent a number of nosologically and genetically separate disorders. Some cases may represent undiagnosed adrenoleukodystrophy or hereditary ataxia during the era when diagnostic testing for these entities was not available. Other cases may represent undiagnosed cases of 3-methylglutaconic aciduria,[41,213] a recently described syndrome with similar clinical features to Behr's syndrome. Sheffer[213] examined

three patients who fulfilled the diagnostic criteria of Behr's syndrome who excreted excessive amounts of 3-methylglutaconic acid and 3-methylglutaric acid in their urine. Costeff[40] performed metabolic studies in 18 Iraqi Jews with this syndrome; all 18 showed abnormally elevated urinary excretion of 3-methylglutaconic acid. They recommended that patients with neurologic disturbances compatible with Behr's syndrome should be screened for optic atrophy and that patients with early-onset optic atrophy should be evaluated for neurologic signs and screened for organic aciduria. The basic underlying enzymatic defect remains unknown but is suspected to reside in the mitochondrial respiratory chain.[57] On the basis of these reports, testing for elevated urinary excretion of 3-methylglutaconic acid must be considered in cases of Behr syndrome since the two disorders may be one and the same.

DIDMOAD (Wolfram Syndrome)

Originally described as an association of diabetes mellitus and optic atrophy by Wolfram,[252] the spectrum of this syndrome was subsequently expanded to include central diabetes insipidus, diabetes mellitus, optic atrophy, and sensorineural deafness (hence, the acronym DIDMOAD).[180,198,203,242] Other less common phenotypic features include ptosis, brachydactyly, anosmia, ataxia, nystagmus, seizures, mental retardation, psychiatric disorders, abnormal ERG, elevated protein and cell count in the spinal fluid, small stature, congenital heart disease, myocarditis, and genitourinary abnormalities (Table 4.3).[128,188] The typical urinary tract abnormalities include muscular atony with bilateral hydronephrosis and hydroureters. The mode of inheritance is generally considered to be autosomal recessive or sporadic, but recently, some cases of Wolfram syndrome have been proposed to represent a mitochondrial-mediated disorder.[22,197] It has been suggested that the constellation of findings in Wolfram syndrome fulfill the criteria for a genetic defect of the mitochondrial energy supply.[24] These criteria include the following: (1) an unexplained association of symptoms and signs, (2) with an early onset and a rapidly progressive course, (3) which involves seemingly unrelated organs that share no common embryological origin or biological function.[158]

TABLE 4.3. Neurologic manifestations of Wolfram (DIDMOAD) syndrome.

Diabetes insipidus
Optic atrophy
Nystagmus
Ptosis
Lacrimal hyposecretion
Pupillary abnormalities (e.g., internal ophthalmoplegia)
Sensorineural deafness
Seizures
Anosmia
Psychiatric disorders
Low IQ
Ataxia
Hypogonadotrophic hypogonadism
Neurogenic bladder

Alternatively, a combination of mitochondrial and nuclear genetic defect have been postulated to explain the pleiotropic features of DIDMOAD syndrome.[24] Some authors have proposed that the DIDMOAD syndrome results from an inherited abnormality of thiamine metabolism.[15]

The optic atrophy initially shows rapid progression then plateaus before complete blindness occurs in the majority of cases. Vision is usually reduced to less than 20/200. Pigmentary retinopathy and abnormal ERGs have been described in some cases, indicating the possibility of a more widespread retinal abnormality.

The ages of most patients described in the literature are under 25 years, with many under 15 years. The onsets of the various manifestations of the syndrome are usually temporally separated from each other by months to years. The mean ages at diagnosis of diabetes mellitus is 9 years, optic atrophy 12 years, diabetes insipidus 15 to 20 years. Hearing loss may be detectable only by audiography before the age of 20 years. The fact that diabetes mellitus occurs first in the majority of patients led to the earlier impression that many of the features of the syndrome represent diabetic microvascular complications. This now seems unlikely.[119] Optic atrophy and other neurologic abnormalities may appear before the diabetes mellitus and usually develop in the absence of any complications related to hyperglycemia.[73] The syndrome may remain unrecognized in many patients since most of the symptoms except diabetes mellitus and optic atrophy occur with varying expressivity.[37,50] The occurrence of optic atrophy

and diabetes mellitus but with no other manifestations of the syndrome makes the diagnosis difficult to establish, especially in sporadic cases. The DIDMOAD syndrome should be suspected in diabetic children with unexplained visual loss or with persistent polyurea and polydipsia (due to unsuspected diabetes insipidus) in the presence of adequate blood sugar control. The associated hearing loss may be subtle, often a mild high-frequency loss, and must be tested for.

Most brain CTs of patients with DIDMOAD syndrome have been unremarkable, but the MR neuroimaging findings in a few cases have been described as highly abnormal with widespread atrophic changes throughout the brain, along with absence of the high intensity signal of the posterior pituitary that is consistent with degeneration of the supraoptic and paraventricular nuclei of the hypothalamus.[188]

Differentiation from simple recessive optic atrophy is made on the basis of the congenital onset and the isolated nature of simple recessive optic atrophy. Complicated recessive optic atrophy (Behr syndrome) is readily made on the basis of the serious CNS dysfunction (mental retardation, spasticity, hypertonia, ataxia) and the early age of onset of Behr syndrome. The disorder should be readily differentiated from other disorders showing a combination of diabetes mellitus and optic atrophy, namely, Friedreich's ataxia, infantile Refsum disease, Alstrom syndrome, and Lawrence–Moon–Biedl syndrome. The DIDMOAD syndrome can be distinguished from other syndromes showing a combination of optic atrophy and hearing loss such as Sylvestor syndrome,[229] Jensen syndrome,[108] or a recently described syndrome showing a triad of optic atrophy, hearing loss, and peripheral neuropathy[77] on the basis of other clinical characteristics, the time course of emergence of the various stigmata, and the modes of transmission.

Toxic/Nutritional Optic Neuropathy

Symmetrical, usually insidious bilateral optic neuropathy may result from nutritional deficiency (e.g., thiamine, vitamin B_{12}, pyridoxine, folic acid, cobalamin, riboflavin). Children with a history of malnutrition, on starvation diets (e.g., teenagers with anorexia), other unusually restrictive diets, or gastrointestinal malabsorption disorders should be particularly suspected of harboring this diagnosis. Hoyt and Billson [93] described two children who developed a symmetrical, bilateral optic neuropathy while being treated with ketogenic diets for seizure control. Both patients recovered normal visual acuity following treatment with thiamine.

Optic atrophy may arise from adverse metabolic effects of certain drugs (e.g., ethambutol, chloramphenicol, rifampin, BCNU, voncristine) and toxins (e.g., methanol, lead, cobalt). Numerous substances have been implicated to cause optic atrophy.[72] Alcohol ingestion and intake of recreational and other drugs should be thoroughly reviewed in the clinical history. Maternal ingestion of alcohol and the fetal alcohol syndrome may cause optic nerve hypoplasia or congenital optic atrophy.[33,225] Some cases of the so-called tobacco-alcohol amblyopia have been shown to represent variants of LHON, and whether tobacco-alcohol amblyopia exists as a separate entity is uncertain.

Cecocentral scotomas are the typical visual field defects in toxic/nutritional optic neuropathies, but these may be difficult to elicit in the early stages of these disorders.

Neurodegenerative Disorders with Optic Atrophy

There is a large and ever-expanding number of neurodegenerative disorders of the central and/or peripheral nervous system that can be associated with ophthalmologic disorders, including optic atrophy (Table 4.4). The distinction between neurodegenerative disorders and other genetic and neurometabolic disorders is becoming increasingly blurred as the responsible gene, its enzyme and protein products, and the specific metabolic defect are identified. Many neurodegenerative disorders show considerable overlap, demonstrating combinations of progressive degeneration of the cerebellum, pyramidal tract, polyneuropathies (sensory neuropathy, motor neuropathy, or both), deafness, and optic atrophy. In some instances, overlapping features preclude separate nosologic classification. Generally, these disorders are diagnosed on the ba-

TABLE 4.4. Neurodegenerative disorders commonly associated with optic atrophy in children.

Pelizaeus–Merzbacher disease
Canavan disease
X-linked adrenoleukodystrophy
Alexander disease
Leigh disease
Metachromatic leukodystrophy
Krabbe disease
Multiple sclerosis
Spinocerebellar degeneration (Friedrich's ataxia, olivopontocerebellar degeneration)
Neuronal ceroid lipofuscinosis
Hallervorden–Spatz disease
MELAS
Congenital lactic acidosis

sis of associated clinical findings and other features rather than by the optic atrophy. In some sense, even isolated optic atrophies such as dominant optic atrophy may be thought of as limited neurodegenerative disorders that preferentially involve the optic nerve.

Degenerative disorders affecting gray matter are less common than those affecting white matter, and generally the two are very difficult to differentiate on clinical grounds. Optic atrophy is common in children with neurodegenerative disease. Because it reflects irreversible injury to the pregeniculate pathways, optic atrophy occurs preferentially in neurodegenerative disorders that primarily affect the white matter. Children with white matter disease tend to present with corticospinal tract dysfunction, peripheral neuropathies, and optic atrophy. By contrast, gray matter disease tends to present with seizure disorders, movement disorders, and dementia. The child with purely gray matter disease (e.g., Tay-Sachs disease) will tend to have seizures without optic atrophy, whereas the child with purely white matter disease may present with optic atrophy without seizures. The development of optic atrophy in a child with seizures may signify a spread of the disease process from gray to white matter (as may occur in the later stages of Leigh disease). Although neurodegenerative and neurometabolic diseases are often classified as gray or white matter disorders, most eventually involve both gray and white matter to some degree. Neurodegenerative disorders that are commonly associated with optic atrophy are summarized in Table 4.4.

Some of the neurodegenerative disorders present in infancy as infantile progressive encephalopathies, and these are exemplified by the first six disorders subsequently discussed. These represent a heterogeneous group of disorders that can be differentiated on the basis of metabolic abnormalities (e.g., Krabbe disease, Menkes' syndrome), typical histopathological findings (e.g., neuronal ceroid lipofuscinosis), additional extracerebral findings (e.g., Aicardi syndrome), or dysmorphic features (e.g., PEHO syndrome).

Krabbe Infantile Leukodystrophy

This is an autosomal recessive disorder of sphingolipid metabolism, due to deficiency of B-galactosidase.[8] Affected children are normal at birth but begin to deteriorate within the first few months of life, developing irritability, restlessness, spasticity, convulsions, hyperacusis, and, in the terminal stages, bulbar signs, deafness, and flaccidity. Optic atrophy and blindness are prominent features. Neuroimaging studies reveal diffuse white matter atrophy. Death usually occurs by the age of 2 years.[244] Autopsy shows loss of myelin in the brain with globoid cells in the area of demyelination. A rare, juvenile-onset form of Krabbe disease has also been reported in association with optic atrophy.[8]

Canavan Disease (Spongiform Leukodystrophy)

This is an autosomal recessive disorder in which the neurological deterioration begins by 3 to 6 months of age and manifests with hypotonia, lack of movements, a large head size without hydrocephalus, optic atrophy and blindness. This disorder occurs almost exclusively in Ashkenazi Jews. The MR imaging reveals diffuse symmetric lesions of the cerebral white matter and, in the later stages, cortical atrophy. Death usually occurs between the ages of 1 and 3 years. Histopathology reveals demyelination and spongy degeneration in the cortex.

Subacute Necrotizing Encephalomyelopathy (Leigh Disease)

This is a progressive autosomal recessive disease with an infantile, juvenile, and an adult form.[122] It is caused by a deficiency of pyruvate carboxylase with increased levels of lactate and pyruvate in the blood. The infantile form begins within the first 6 months of life. A positive family history is present in half of the infantile cases. The course of the disease ranges from weeks to years, with patients developing somnolence, deafness, psychomotor regression, and spasticity, in addition to optic atrophy and blindness. In the infantile form, death occurs between 2 and 10 years of age. Necropsy findings show bilateral, multifocal, subacute necrotic lesions from the thalamus to the pons, and demyelination in the optic nerve.

Childhood lactic acidosis comprises a number of clinically heterogeneous disorders that share increased levels of lactate and pyruvate in the blood.[87] In addition to Leigh disease, disorders showing childhood lactic acidosis include MELAS (mitochondrial myopathy, encephalopathy, lactic acidosis, and strokelike episodes), pyruvate decarboxylase deficiency, pyruvate dehydrogenase deficiency, puruvate dehydrogenase phosphatase deficiency, cytochrome c oxidase deficiency, dietary ketoacidosis, or idiopathic.[28,87] Optic atrophy is a common neuro-opthalmologic finding in children with lactic acidosis due to their propensity for CNS white matter involvement.[87]

Pelizaeus-Merzbacher Disease (Sudanophilic Leukodystrophy)

This is an X-linked recessive disorder that differs from the other leukodystrophies by the presence within the first few months of life of irregular pendular nystagmus and head shaking. Poor head control, cerebellar dysfunction, choreiform movements of the arm, and spasticity develop later. The nystagmus may later disappear. Optic atrophy and retinal degeneration occurs later. Intellectual function is generally preserved despite neurological deterioration. Death ensues between 5 and 7 years of age. Autopsy findings show patchy demyelination.

The PEHO Syndrome

The PEHO syndrome denotes progressive encephalopathy with edema, hypsarrhythmia, and optic atrophy.[79,204,219,220] It is apparently transmitted as an autosomal recessive disorder. Most patients are healthy or only slightly hypotonic at birth. The disorder becomes manifest between 2 weeks and 3 months of life with progressive hypotonia, poor vision, and limb jerks. Affected patients also show infantile spasms, exaggerated deep tendon reflexes, and early arrest of psychomotor development. Subcutaneous edema in the limbs and blindness with optic atrophy and nystagmus are also present.[219,220] Affected infants show typical dysmorphic facial features that include epicanthal folds, midfacial hypoplasia, prominent ear lobes, gingival hypertrophy, small chin, and tapered fingers. The most typical physical finding is subcutaneous nonpitting edema of the limbs and face. A few patients have survived into the teens. Magnetic resonance scans show progressive brain atrophy, especially in the cerebellar and brainstem areas, and abnormal myelination.

Although the progressive course of the disease suggests a metabolic disturbance, no underlying biochemical marker has yet been identified.

Neonatal Adrenoleukodystrophy

This is one of the peroxisomal disorders that includes a wide array of disorders including Zellweger cerebrohepatorenal syndrome, infantile refsum disease, neonatal adrenoleukodystrophy, rhizomelic chondrodysplasia punctata, X-linked adrenoleukodystrophy, primary hyperoxaluria type I, and classical Refsum disease.[63] The various clinical features of these disorders are summarized in Table 4.5. With the exception of X-linked adrenoleukodystrophy, the inheritance of these disorders is autosomal recessive. In cases suspected to harbor peroxisomal disorders, analysis of cultured fibroblasts for very long chain fatty acids (VLCFA), DHAP-AT, and/or plasmalogen are helpful.

Metachromatic Leukodystrophy

Several forms of this autosomal recessive disorder are recognized, including a late infantile and a juvenile form. The various forms are associated with deficiency of arylsulfatase A, an enzyme whose gene is located on chromosome 22. The late infantile form presents between 1 and 2 years of life with gait disorder and strabismus. Speech impairment, spasticity, intellectual deterioration, and op-

tic atrophy follow. Optic atrophy is found in about one-third of cases and is, along with cortical visual impairment, a cause of significant visual loss.[64] Other less common ophthalmological features include a cherry red spot and nystagmus. The ERG is usually normal or mildly abnormal, in contrast to the various juvenile amaurotic idiocies. Deep tendon reflexes are reduced or absent in the lower extremities. The CSF protein is elevated. The patients suffer unexplained episodes of fever or abdominal cramps. Death usually occurs by 6 years of age. Neuroimaging demonstrates white matter disturbances, especially of the periventricular region. The diagnosis is confirmed by demonstration of intracellular metachromatic substances in the urine and assay of arylsulfatase A in leukocytes.

X-Linked Adrenoleukodystrophy (Addison–Schilder Disease)

This is an X-linked recessive disorder that usually presents with visual defects and neurological disturbances within the first decade. Affected boys may present with bizarre visual symptoms and associated behavioral disturbances that may lead to the mistaken diagnosis of hysterical blindness. This is particularly likely in the early stages when the fundus findings are normal.[231] Affected boys develop hormonal disturbances manifesting as Addison disease with skin hyperpigmentation or hypogonadism. The disease is characterized by inexorable neurological deterioration culminating in death within a few years.

The visual impairment early on is of cortical origin. Neuroimaging demonstrates symmetric bilateral involvement of the periventricular white matter, especially posteriorly (hence the cortical visual impairment). Optic atrophy develops later in the disease.

The diagnosis can be confirmed by measurement of long chain fatty acids in skin fibroblasts. Carrier females may occasionally develop a variable degree of neurological impairment and may have symptoms and MR lesions similar to those found in multiple sclerosis.

Hallervorden–Spatz Syndrome

Hallervorden–Spatz syndrome is a rare familial neurodegenerative disorder that presents in childhood or early adolescence with progressive dys-

TABLE 4.5 Clinical features of peroxisomal disorders.

Disorder	Age at onset	Ophthalmologic findings	Other clinical findings
Zellweger syndrome	Neonatal period	Pigmentary retinopathy Attenuated retinal arterioles Optic atrophy Corneal clouding Glaucoma, cataract Extinguished ERG	Craniofacial dysmorphism Seizures Hypotonia Psychomotor retardation Hepatomegaly, renal cysts
Neonatal adrenoleukodystrophy	Neonatal period	Pigmentary retinopathy Attenuated retinal arterioles Pigment epithelial clumping Optic atrophy Extinguished ERG	Adrenal cortical atrophy Seizures Hypotonia Psychomotor retardation
Infantile Refsum disease	First decade	Pigmentary retinopathy Attenuated retinal arterioles Optic atrophy Extinguished ERG	Deafness Psychomotor retardation
Rhizomelic chondrodysplasia punctata	Neonatal period	Cataract Normal ERG	Short proximal extremities Dermatitis Psychomotor retardation Radiographic epiphyseal stippling
X-linked adrenoleukodystrophy	First decade	Optic atrophy Visual pathway demyelination Normal ERG	Adrenal cortical atrophy Darkened skin Emotional lability Hearing loss Incoordination, spasticity Intellectual deterioration
Primary hyperoxaluria type I	First through second decade	Parafoveal pigmentary changes Optic atrophy	Renal failure Osteodystrophy Hydrocephalus
Classical Refsum disease	First through fourth decade	Pigmentary retinopathy Attenuated retinal arterioles Night blindness Optic atrophy Attenuated ERG	Polyneuropathy Ataxia Hearing loss Anosmia Metatarsal/metacarpal abnormalities Ichthyosis-like skin

tonic and sometimes choreoathetotic movements, dysarthria, gait impairment, and dementia. Death occurs after an average of 15 years from onset. There is no known biochemical basis or genetic marker for the disorder yet.[1] Before the advent of MR neuroimaging, confirmation of the diagnosis was done on autopsy. Characteristic MR changes include decreased signal intensity in the globus pallidus, and the substantia nigra on T2-weighted images compatible with iron deposition.[4,228]

A mild degree of visual impairment is frequently described in Hallervorden–Spatz syndrome, typically attributed to optic atrophy, pigmentary retinopathy, or tapetoretinal degeneration. In some children, visual loss due to optic atrophy is the presenting symptom.[31]

Neuronal Ceroid Lipofuscinoses (Batten Disease)

The ceroid lipofuscinoses are autosomal recessive disorders that have been subdivided according to the age at which the neurologic symptoms first appear. The clinical features of these various types are detailed in Table 4.6. These disorders must be considered in the differential diagnosis in the infant or child who develops seizures, loss of acquired milestones, progressive intellectual deterioration, and progressive visual impairment. A definitive diagnosis requires electron microscopic examination of suitable specimens derived from skin, conjunctiva, muscle, or rectal biopsy that demonstrate characteristic storage materials. A brain biopsy may be required if other sites fail to yield a diagnosis. There has been no identified enzymatic deficiency. Neuroimaging studies reveal nonspecific changes but are helpful in distinguishing the lipofuscinoses from the various leukodystrophies in which there are striking abnormalities of the white matter.

Juvenile Batten disease (Spielmeyer–Vogt) is of particular importance to the ophthalmologist since visual impairment is commonly the presenting symptom (Table 4.6).[221] In contrast, the infantile and late infantile forms show a rapidly progressive downhill course and are rarely diagnosed by the ophthalmologist.

Familial Dysautonomia (Riley–Day Syndrome)

This is an autosomal recessive disorder that is confined to Ashkenazi Jews. Although the name suggests that the disorder is strictly one of autonomic dysfunction, the peripheral sensory and motor nerves as well as other neuronal populations are affected.

Children present at birth with poor suck reflex, hypotonia, hypothermia, and nursing difficulties with frequent regurgitation. Patients with this syndrome also show poor temperature control, motor incoordination, reduced deep tendon reflexes, postural hypotension, and emotional lability. The children lack the fungiform papillae on the tongue and have markedly diminished taste sensation.

The most prominent ophthalmological findings are pronounced corneal hypesthesia and absent tears, which in combination lead to corneal ulcerations. Other findings include retinal vascular tortuosity, ptosis, anisocoria, exotropia, and increased

TABLE 4.6. Clinical features of the neuronal ceroid lipofuscinoses.

	Infantile	Late infantile	Juvenile	Variant
Eponym	Santavuori	Batten–Bielschowsky	Spielmeyer–Vogt	Batten
Age at onset	8 to 18 months	2 to 4 years	4 to 10 years	5 to 7 years
Myoclonic seizures	Present	Present (presenting sign)	Occasional	Present
Ataxia	Marked	Marked	Mild and late	Marked
Late features	Microcephaly death by 4 years	Death by 7 years	Dementia Death 2nd to 3rd decade	Dementia Death 2nd decade
Ophthalmologic findings	Macular pigmentary changes	Marked pigmentary changes	Bull's eye maculopathy (early)	Pigmentary changes, retinal pigment aggregation
	Attenuated retinal arterioles	Attenuated retinal arterioles	Diffuse pigmentary changes (late)	Attenuated retinal arterioles
	Optic atrophy	Optic atrophy	Attenuated arterioles	Optic atrophy
	Extinguished or attenuated ERG	Extinguished ERG	Optic atrophy Extinguished ERG	
Blindness	Early	Late	Early (presenting symptom)	Early
Electron microscopy (lymphocytes)	Granular, amorphous inclusions	Curvilinear or fingerprint inclusions	Fingerprint inclusions	Negative, ? fingerprint inclusions

incidence of myopia. Optic atrophy has been rarely reported.[46] Rizzo et al[192] reported three patients with the syndrome who showed visual impairment due to optic atrophy, initially diagnosed after the first decade. The authors suggested that the presence of an optic atrophy demonstrates that there is some degree of CNS involvement in familial dysautonomia.

Spinocerebellar Degenerations

The spinocerebellar degenerations, also referred to as the hereditary ataxias, consist of a group of disorders with clinical manifestations that include ataxia and dysmetria, resulting from the predominant involvement of the cerebellum and its pathways. In addition to the cerebellar dysfunction, patients may show disturbances in the basal ganglia, optic atrophy, retinitis pigmentosa, and peripheral nerve disease. There is a wide spectrum of these disorders that includes pure cerebellar dysfunction, mixed cerebellar and brainstem disorders, cerebellar and basal ganglia syndromes, and spinal syndromes or peripheral nerve disease.[86,134,172,196] Overlapping features may uncommonly occur even within members of the same families.

Friedreich ataxia is an autosomal recessive disorder characterized by the onset of progressive cerebellar ataxia, dorsal root ganglion degeneration, and corticospinal tract involvement, generally associated with muscular wasting. The age of onset is before puberty. Patients show dysarthria, abnormal position and vibration sense and absent deep tendon reflexes in lower extremities, progressive scoliosis and pes cavus, and hypertrophic progressive cardiomyopathy.[134,229] Unlike Charcot–Marie–Tooth syndrome, the motor nerve conduction is normal, and the sensory nerve conduction is abnormal, especially in the lower extremities. Optic atrophy occurs frequently in the disorder.

Charcot–Marie–Tooth syndrome is an autosomal dominant disorder with an age of onset in late childhood. It manifests with a slowly progressive motor neuropathy affecting the lower more than the upper extremities. Affected children show distal wasting of the legs, foot drop, and pes cavus. Optic atrophy rarely complicates the syndrome and is typically detected during the teenage years. The associated oc-

currence of LHON in patients with Charcot–Marie–Tooth disease has been reported.[145]

Olivopontocerebellar atrophy denotes a group of disorders that show progressive cerebellar ataxia, tremor, spasticity, and speech impairment. Some forms show marked extrapyramidal signs, nystagmus, and ophthalmoplegia. Involvement of the inferior olivary nuclei is present. Intellectual deterioration and dementia may occur later in the course of the disease. Both autosomal dominant and recessive inheritance patterns have been described. The majority of cases become evident in adulthood, but a dominantly inherited form that is associated with retinal degeneration can present as early as the first year of life. The optic atrophy seen in some patients with olivopontocerebellar atrophy may be secondary to associated retinal degeneration or may occur primarily as part of the multisystem CNS atrophy seen on MR imaging in this condition.[49,84,126,136,205]

Mucopolysaccaridosis

The mucopolysaccharidoses (MPS) are storage diseases caused by a deficiency of certain lysosomal enzymes, leading to abnormal degradation of one or several mucopolysaccharides (e.g., dermatan, heparan, keratan sulfate). These materials then accumulate in multiple organ systems leading to progressive clinical disorders.[163]

The ophthalmologic findings in the MPS include corneal clouding, retinal pigmentary dystrophy, glaucoma, optic nerve head swelling, or optic atrophy. Collins et al[38] reviewed the ocular findings in 108 patients with MPS with attention to optic disc appearance. They concluded that patients with Hurler, Hurler–Scheie, Maroteaux–Lamy, and Sly syndromes showed a greater than 40% chance of developing optic nerve head swelling, while the chance in those with Hunter's and Sanfilippo's was 19.7% and 4.6%, respectively. Some patients showed optic nerve head swelling in one eye and optic atrophy in the other. In others, the optic atrophy was documented to follow disc swelling. The authors concluded that optic nerve head swelling precedes the development of optic atrophy in patients with systemic MPS. The cause of disc swelling is not always obvious, but hydrocephalus plays a role at least in some cases.[115]

Optic Atrophy due to Hypoxia-Ischemia

Optic atrophy due to perinatal hypoxia-ischemia is more commonly encountered in the setting of prematurity.[238] The parents should be questioned thoroughly about the perinatal and neonatal period of their child, and if available, the related medical records should be reviewed. Cicatricial retinopathy of prematurity, cortical visual impairment, and optic atrophy are the major causes of significant visual loss in patients with a history of premature birth.[118,144] One Danish study found that perinatal stress factors (e.g., prematurity, low birth weight, perinatal asphyxia) accounted for a significant percentage of cases of optic atrophy in children reported to the Danish National Register.[178] Significantly, they found that all children with optic atrophy attributed to perinatal difficulties showed one or more additional handicaps (e.g., cerebral palsy, epilepsy, psychomotor retardation). This is supported by other studies[144] and may attest to the relative resilience of the anterior as compared with the posterior visual pathways to hypoxia. It also argues against attributing perinatal hypoxic damage to solitary cases of optic atrophy in otherwise healthy children.[70]

Despite the frequency of hypoxia-ischemia in the perinatal period, damage to the anterior visual pathway with optic atrophy appears to occur less frequently than damage to the posterior visual pathway. Six of 30 children with hypoxic cortical blindness described by Lambert et al[124] showed mild optic atrophy. In a retrospective study, 28% of all infants who had documented hypoxic encephalopathy showed optic atrophy,[70] and essentially, all of these showed significant neurological dysfunction. The authors considered these findings to indicate a relative resilience of the optic nerve to hypoxia. Besides the possibility that the concurrent optic atrophy described in such cases may represent primary damage to the retinogeniculate pathway, some cases may represent transsynaptic degeneration. It has therefore been concluded that in the presence of normal neurologic findings and neuroimaging results, optic atrophy should not be attributed to perinatal hypoxia.[70]

Patients in cardiovascular shock with hypotension due to acute blood loss are at risk of ischemic damage to the optic nerves. Shock patients who are on positive pressure ventilation may be at an increased risk for such damage. The increased intraocular pressure associated with positive pressure ventilation along with the low systemic perfusion pressure may compromise the perfusion of the optic discs.[34]

A rare idiopathic disorder, termed anterior ischemic optic neuropathy of the young, has been reported to affect teenagers and young adults.[53,81] It is included in this section because of its designation as ischemic, which is adopted due to certain resemblance to the adult variety of ischemic optic neuropathy. Differentiation from optic neuritis, however, cannot be made with certainty. Unlike the variety affecting older patients, the disorder displays a propensity for recurrence in the same eye that may lead to significant visual impairment. Affected patients are otherwise healthy.

Traumatic Optic Atrophy

Trauma is a significant cause of optic nerve damage in children.[137] Damage to one or both optic nerves may result from direct or indirect trauma. Direct trauma is commonly associated with penetrating injuries or severe blunt trauma to the globes and orbit. Indirect trauma occurs without external or ophthalmoscopic evidence of injury to the eye and related structures (e.g., shaken baby syndrome). The possible pathophysiologic mechanisms of traumatic optic neuropathy of childhood is not different from the adult variety and includes tears or avulsion of the optic nerve, laceration of the nerve substance by bone fragments; hemorrhage into the optic nerve sheath spaces or into the dura itself; or contusion, necrosis, or edema of the optic nerve tissue.[137] Traumatic chiasmal syndromes may also occur.

The optic disc appears normal in the typical traumatic cases involving the intracanalicular or intracranial portion of the nerve. Optic atrophy eventually ensues. A 4- to 6-week latent period has been demonstrated in primates between optic nerve disruption and subsequent development of optic atrophy, irrespective of the site of damage.[185]

Cases due to remote trauma that the patient does not specifically recollect may pose a diagnostic quandary. If such trauma had been associated with blunt injury to the globe itself, as well as to the head or orbit, ophthalmologic signs like iris sphincter tears, angle recession, lens subluxation, corneal scarring, chorioretinal scarring, and bony defects of the cranium may provide valuable clues as to the traumatic etiology.

Generally, prognosis for recovery of vision is poor. Therapeutic attempts include administration of high-dose intravenous corticosteroids. Surgical decompression of the optic canal, with or without corticosteroid administration, may be helpful in selected cases.[209]

Summary of the General Approach to the Pediatric Patient with Optic Atrophy

Important clues to the etiology, nature, and location of the lesion underlying optic atrophy are often provided by the age of the patient, best corrected visual acuity, laterality of optic atrophy, funduscopic appearance of the disc and retina, color vision anomalies, the natural history (onset and rate of progression), visual field defects, and other associated ophthalmologic, neurologic, and systemic findings. The combination of a thorough, tailored medical and family history, with physical, neurologic, and ophthalmologic examination should pinpoint at least the general category of optic atrophy in the majority of cases.

The *medical history* is of paramount importance. In infants and children with optic atrophy and poor vision, the answers to certain questions can be very important diagnostically. Are there any identifiable factors in the medical and family history that can help in the diagnosis, specifically, perinatal hypoxia, intracranial hemorrhages, meningitis, encephalitis, hypoxia-ischemia, trauma, poisoning, maternal toxin intake, etc. (e.g., optic atrophy due to hypoxia-ischemia, transsynaptic degeneration, maternal alcohol intake, traumatic optic neuropathy)? Again, optic atrophy due to hypoxia-ischemia is commonly associated with brain damage and generally indicates that such insult had been severe. Is there a family history of blindness or consanguinity (e.g., inherited optic atrophy, neurodegenerative disorders)? Was the child normally-sighted at some point before losing vision (e.g., Leber hereditary optic atrophy, Juvenile

Batten disease), or was the vision always impaired (congenital optic atrophy)? Aside from the visual impairment, is the child otherwise neurologically and systemically normal in all respects? If neurologic or systemic disease exists, are there known causes for these findings, such as perinatal hypoxia, intracranial hemorrhages, trauma, or a family history of similar affliction? This history helps differentiate these disorders from metabolic, neoplastic, and neurodegenerative disorders. If no known cause for the neurologic or systemic disease exists, at what age did these findings present; specifically, was the child normal initially before developing these disorders (e.g., Juvenile Batten disease, X-linked adrenoleukodystrophy), or had these disorders been present within the neonatal period? Has the visual impairment been stable since onset, or has there been any progression in the visual impairment (e.g., compressive intracranial lesions, neurodegenerative disorders)? Has there been any progression in the neurologic and/or systemic disease (neurodegenerative or metabolic disorders), or have these been stationary since onset (static encephalopathy, mental retardation, hydrocephalus)? We recognize that exceptions to these generalizations exist but believe that the general framework is helpful.

The *clinical examination* can further narrow down the diagnostic possibilities raised by the medical and family history. The presence of nystagmus excludes all disorders with onset after the second birthday. The presence of deafness suggests one of the disorders associated with optic atrophy and deafness. Cerebellar signs suggest one of the cerebellar ataxias or spinocerebellar degeneration associated with optic atrophy. Static encephalopathy, most commonly encountered in the setting of prematurity, suggests that the optic atrophy is either due to primary damage to the anterior visual pathways due to hypoxia-ischemia or associated hydrocephalus or due to secondary transsynaptic degeneration following perinatal brain damage. The presence of café au lait spots, emaciation, spasmus nutans, or unilateral proptosis or a family history of neurofibromatosis suggests optic pathway glioma.

Ancillary testing (e.g., neuroimaging, metabolic workup) is not necessary to arrive at the diagnosis in most children with optic atrophy. Any associated ocular abnormalities must be detected, and in infants, it is advisable to consider performing an ERG to rule out retinal disease. Visual evoked potentials may be helpful to assess the integrity of the visual pathways but are generally not helpful in determining a specific diagnosis. Neuroimaging is helpful when neurological signs indicative of intracranial dysfunction are present. Metabolic workup is indicated in selected cases. Ancillary testing is most clearly indicated in a previously healthy child who develops progressive visual loss and optic atrophy, with or without associated neurologic and systemic signs and symptoms, to rule out underlying neurologic, metabolic, and neoplastic disorders.

References

1. Adams RD, Victor M. *Principles of Neurology*. 4th ed. New York, NY: Mc Graw Hill; 1989:804.
2. Alvord EC, Lofton S. Gliomas of optic nerve or chiasm. J Neurosurg 1988;68:85-98.
3. Amemiya T, Honda A. A family with optic atrophy and congenital hearing loss. Ophthalmic Genet 1994;15:87-93.
4. Angelini L, Nardocci V, Rumi C, et al. Hallervorden-Spatz disease: clinical and MRI study of 11 cases diagnosed in life. J Neurol 1992;239: 417-425.
5. Arts WF, Loonen MC, Sengers RC, et al. X-linked ataxia, weakness, deafness, and loss of vision in early childhood with a fatal course. Ann Neurol 1993;33(5):535-539.
6. Aysun S, Topcu M, Gunay M, et al. Neurologic features as the initial presentations of childhood malignancies. Pediatr Neurol 1994;10:40-43.
7. Badea N. Crouzon's disease. Oftalmologia 1991: 63-66.
8. Baker RH, Trautmann JC, Younge BR, et al. Late juvenile-onset Krabbe's disease. Ophthalmology 1990;97:1176-1180.
9. Barkovich AJ. *Pediatric Neuroimaging*. New York, NY: Raven Press; 1990:35-75.
10. Beatty RM, Sadun AA, Smith L, et al. Direct demonstration of transsynaptic degeneration in the human visual system: a comparison of retrograde and anterograde changes. J Neurol Neurosurg Psychiatry 1982;45:143-146.
11. Behr C. Die Komplizieric hereditar-familiare optikusatrophie des kindesalters. Klin Mb Augenheilk 1909;47:318.
12. Benecke R, Berthold A, Conrad B. Denervation activity in the EMG of patients with upper motor neuron lesions: time course, local distribution and pathogenetic aspects. J Neurol 1983;230:143-151.
13. Berman JL, Kashii S, Trachtman MS, et al. Optic neuropathy and central nervous system disease secondary to Sjogren's syndrome in a child. Ophthalmology 1990;1606-1609.
14. Berninger TA, Jaeger W, Krastel H. Electrophysiology and colour perimetry in dominant infantile optic atrophy. Br J Ophthalmol 1991;75:49-52.
15. Borgna-Pignatti C, Marradi P, Pinelli L, et al. Thiamine-responsive anemia in DIDMOAD syndrome. J Pediatr 1989;114:405-410.
16. Borruat FX, et al. Late onset Leber's optic neuropathy: a case confused with ischaemic optic neuropathy. Br J Ophthalmol 1992;76:571-575.
17. Borruat FX, Schatz NJ, Glaser JS, et al. Visual recovery from radiation-induced optic neuropathy. The role of hyperbaric oxygen therapy. J Clin Neuro-Ophthalmol 1993;13:98-101.
18. Bothe N, Lieb B, Schafer WD. Development of impaired vision in mentally handicapped children. Klin Monatsbl Augenheilkd 1991;198;509-514.
19. Brodsky MC. The "pseudo-CSF" signal of orbital optic glioma on magnetic resonance imaging: a signature of neurofibromatosis. Surv Ophthalmol 1993;38(2):213-218
20. Brodsky MC, Glasier CM, Pollock SC, et al. Optic nerve hypoplasia identification by magnetic resonance imaging. Arch Ophthalmol 1990;108: 1562-1567.
21. Brodsky MC, Hout WF, Newton DR. The "phantom" optic nerve: demonstration in CT and MR scans 19 years after resection of optic glioma. J Clin Neuro-Ophthalmol 1988;8:67-68.
22. Brodsky MC, Hoyt WF, Barnwell SL, et al. Intrachiasmatic craniopharyngioma: a rare cause of chiasmal thickening. Case report. J Neurosurg 1988;68(2):300-302.
23. Brown WF, Snow R. Denervation in hemiplegic muscles. Stroke 1990 ; 21:1700-1704.
24. Bu X, Rotter JI. Wolfram syndrome: a mitochondrial-mediated disorder? Lancet 1993;342: 598-600.
25. Buncic JR. Ocular aspects of Apert syndrome. Clin Plast Surg 1991;18:315-319.
26. Burke JP, O'Keefe M, Bowell R, et al. Ocular complications in homocystinuria—early and late treated. Br J Ophthalmol 1989;73(6):427-431.
27. Burke JP, O'Keefe M, Bowell R, et al. Ophthalmic findings in maple syrup urine disease. Metab Pediatr Syst Ophthalmol 1991;14:12-15.
28. Byrd DJ, Krohn HP, Winkler L, et al. Neonatal pyruvate dehydrogenase deficiency with lipoate responsive lactic acidaemia and hyperammonaemia. Eur J Pediatr 1989;148(6):543-547.
29. Calogero JA, Alexander E. Unilateral amaurosis in a hydrocephalic child with an obstructed shunt: case report. J Neurosurg 1971;34:236.
30. Campana G, Valentini G, Legnaioli MI, et al. Ocular aspects in biotinidase deficiency. Clinical and genetic original studies. Ophthal Paediatr Genet 1987;8:125-129.
31. Casteels I, Spileers W, Swinnen T, et al. Optic atrophy as the presenting sign in Hallervorden-

Spatz syndrome. Neuropediatrics 1994; 25:265-267.

32. Castro-Gago M, Rodriguez-Nunez A, Eiris J, et al. Familial agenesis of the corpus callosum: a new form. Arch Fr Pediatr. 1993;50(4):327-330 .

33. Chan T, Bowell R, O'Keefe M, et al. Ocular manifestations in fetal alcohol syndrome. Br J Ophthalmol 1991;75(9):524-526.

34. Chelluri L, Jastremski MS. Bilateral optic atrophy after cardiac arrest in a patient with acute respiratory failure on positive pressure ventilation. Resuscitation 1988;16:45-48.

35. Cherninkova S, Tzekov H, Karakostov V. Comparative ophthalmologic studies on children and adults with craniopharyngiomas. Ophthalmologica 1990;201(4):201-205.

36. Chitayat D, Silver K, Azouz EM. Skeletal dysplasia, intracerebral calcifications, optic atrophy, hearing impairment, and mental retardation: nosology of dysosteosclerosis. Am J Med Genet 1992;43:517-523.

37. Cillino S, Anastasi M, Lodato G. Incomplete Wolfram syndrome: clinical and electrophysiologic study of two familial cases. Graefe's Arch Clin Exp Ophthalmol 1989;227:131-135.

38. Collins ML, Traboulsi EI, Maumenee IH. Optic nerve head swelling and optic atrophy in the systemic mucopolysaccharidoses. Ophthalmology. 1990;97:1445-1449.

39. Corbett JJ. Neuro-ophthalmologic complications of hydrocephalus and shunting procedures. Semin Neurol 1986;6:111-123.

40. Costeff H, Elpeleg O, Apter N, et al. 3-Methylglutaconic aciduria in "optic atrophy plus." Ann Neurol 1993;33(1):103-104.

41. Costeff H, Gadoth N, Apter N, et al. A familial syndrome of infantile optic atrophy, movement disorder, and spastic paraplegia. Neurology 1989;39:595-597.

42. Costenbader FD, O'Rourk TR. Optic atrophy in childhood. J Pediatr Ophthalmol 1968;5:77.

43. Cullom ME, Hehler KL, Miller NR, et al. Leber's hereditary optic neuropathy masquerading as tobacco-alcohol amblyopia. Arch Ophthalmol 1993;111:1482-1485.

44. Dailey RA. Optic nerve sheath meningiomas of childhood. Ophthalmol Clin North Am 1991;4(3):519-529.

45. Davis PC, Hoffman JC Jr, Pearl GS, et al. CT evaluation of effects of cranial radiation therapy in children. Am J Neuro-Radiol 1986;7:639-644.

46. Diamond GA, D'Amico RA, Axelrod FB. Optic nerve dysfunction in familial dysautonomia. Am J Ophthalmol 1987;104:645-649.

47. Dineen J, Hendrickson A, Keating EG. Alterations of retinal inputs following striate cortex removal in adult monkey. Exp Brain Res 1982;47:446-456.

48. Dohi MT, Bardell AM, Stefano N, et al. Optic atrophy in Marinesco-Sjogren syndrome: an additional ocular feature. Ophthal Paediatr Genet 1993;14: 5-7.

49. Drack AV, Traboulsi EI, Maumenee IH. Progression of retinopathy in olivopontocerebellar atrophy with retinal degeneration. Arch Ophthalmol 1992;110:712-713.

50. Dreyer M, Rudiger HW, Bujara K, et al. The syndrome of diabetes insipidus, diabetes mellitus, optic atrophy, deafness, and other abnormalities (DIDMOAD-syndrome). Two affected sibs and a short review of the literature (98 cases). Klin Wochenschr 1982;60:471-475.

51. DuBois LG, Feldon SE. Evidence for a metabolic trigger for Leber's hereditary optic neuropathy. A case report. J Clin Neuro-Ophthalmol 1992;12: 15-16.

52. Dutton JJ. Gliomas of the anterior visual pathway. Surv Ophthalmol 1994;38:427-452.

53. Dutton JJ, Burde RM. Anterior ischemic optic neuropathy of the young. J Clin Neuro-Ophthalmol 1983;3(2):137-146.

54. el-Azazi M, Malm G, Forsgren M. Late ophthalmologic manifestations of neonatal herpes simplex virus infection. Am J Ophthalmol 1990;109:1-7.

55. Elberg H, Kjer B, Kjer P, et al. Dominant optic atrophy (OPAI) mapped to chromosome 3q region. I: linkage analysis. Hum Molecular Genet 1994;3: 977-980.

56. Eliott D, Traboulsi EI, Maumenee IH. Visual prognosis in autosomal dominant optic atrophy (Kjer type). Am J Ophthalmol 1993;115(3):360-367.

57. Elpeleg ON, Costeff H, Joseph A, et al. 3-Methylglutaconic aciduria in the Iraqi-Jewish "optic atrophy plus" (Costeff) syndrome. Dev Med Child Neurol 1994;36:167-172.

58. Ersahin Y, Mutluer S, Guzelbag E. Intracranial hydatid cysts in children. Neurosurgery 1993;33: 219-224; (discussion):224-225.

59. Eustis HS, Yaplee SM, Kogutt M, et al. Microspherophakia in association with the rhizomelic form of chondrodysplasia punctata. J Pediatr Ophthalmol Strabismus 1990;27:237-241.

60. Fernandez RG, Munoz-Negrete FJ, Garcia-Martin B, et al. Bilateral optic atrophy in Kenny's syndrome. Acta Ophthalmol Copenh. 1992;70: 135-138.

61. Ferrer I, Campistol J, Tobena L, et al. Degenerescence systematisee optico-cochleo-dentelee. J Neurol 1987;234(6):416-420.

62. Fletcher WA, Imes RK, Hoyt WF. Chiasmal gliomas: appearance and long-term changes demonstrated by computerized tomography. J Neurosurg 1986;65(2):154-159.

63. Folz SJ, Trobe JD. The peroxisome and the eye. Surv Ophthalmol 1991;35(5):353-368.

64. Francois J. Ocular manifestations in demyelinating disease. Adv Ophthalmol 1979;39:1-36.

65. Frisen L, Claesson M. Narrowing of the retinal arterioles in descending optic atrophy: a quantitative clinical study. Ophthalmology 1984;91:1342.

66. Gaston H. Ophthalmic complications of spina bifida and hydrocephalus. Eye 1991;5(pt 3): 279-290.

67. Gay C, Divry P, Macabeo V, et al. N-acetylaspartic aciduria. Clinical, biological and physiopathological study. Arch Fr Pediatr 1991;48(6):409-413.

68. Gelber SJ, Heffez DS, Donohoue PA. Pituitary gigantism caused by growth hormone excess from infancy. J Pediatr 1992;120:931-934.

69. Ghose S. Optic nerve changes in hydrocephalus. Trans Ophthalmol Soc UK 1983;103(pt 2): 217-220.

69a. Goldberg MF, Custis PH. Retinal and other manifestations of incontinenti pigmenti (Bloch-Sulzberger syndrome). Ophthalmology 1993;100: 1645-1654.

70. Good WV, Hoyt CS, Lambert SR. Optic nerve atrophy in children with hypoxia. Invest Ophthalmol Vis Sci 1987;28(suppl):309.

71. Goodman SJ, Rosenbaum AL, Hasso A, et al. Large optic nerve glioma with normal vision. Arch Ophthalmol 1975;93:991-995.

72. Grant WM. Toxicology of the eye. 3rd ed. Springfield IL: Charles C. Thomas; 1986:1048-1049.

73. Grosse-Aldenhovel HB, Gallenkamp U, et al. Juvenile onset diabetes mellitus, central diabetes insipidus and optic atrophy (Wolfram syndrome)—neurological findings and prognostic implications. Neuropediatrics 1991;22:103-106.

74. Gupta S, Ghose S, Rohatgi M, et al. The optic nerve in children with craniosynostosis. A pre and post surgical evaluation. Doc Ophthalmol 1993; 83:271-278.

75. Gustavson KH, Anneren G, Malmgren H, et al. New X-linked syndrome with severe mental retardation, severely impaired vision, severe hearing defect, epileptic seizures, spasticity, restricted joint mobility, and early death. Am J Med Genet 1993;45:654-658.

76. Guy J, Mancuso A, Beck R, et al. Radiation-induced optic neuropathy: a magnetic resonance imaging study. J Neurosurg 1991;74:426-432.

77. Hagemoser K, Weinstein J, Bresnick G, et al. Optic atrophy, hearing loss, and peripheral neuropathy. Am J Med Genet 1989;33(1):61-65.

78. Haines SJ, Erickson DL, Wirtschafter JD. Optic nerve decompression for osteopetrosis in early childhood. Neurosurgery 1988;23:470-475.

79. Haltia M. Somer M. Infantile cerebello-optic atrophy. Neuropathology of the progressive encephalopathy syndrome with edema, hypsarrhythmia and optic atrophy (the PEHO syndrome). Acta Neuropathol Berl. 1993;85(3):241-247.

80. Hamed LM, Maria B, Quisling R, et al. Suprasellar lesions of maldevelopmental origin in Klinefelter's syndrome. J Clin Neuro-Ophthalmol 1992;12(3): 192-197.

81. Hamed LM, Purvin V, Rosenberg M. Recurrent anterior ischemic optic neuropathy in young adults. J Clin Neuro-Ophthalmol 1988;8:239-246.

82. Hamed LM. Retrograde transsynaptic degeneration of the retinogeniculate pathway after postnatal cerebral damage. Ophthalmology 1994;101(suppl): 134. Abstract.

83. Hammerstein W, Jurgens H, Gobel U. Retinal degeneration and embryonal rhabdomyosarcoma of the thorax. Fortschr Ophthalmol 1991;88:463-465.

84. Hammond EJ, Wilder BJ. Evoked potentials in olivopontocerebellar atrophy. Arch Neurol 1983; 40:366-369.

85. Hansen E, Flage T, Rosenberg T, et al. Visual impairment in Nordic children. III: diagnoses. Acta Ophthalmol Copenh 1992;70:597-604.

86. Harding AE. The Hereditary Ataxias and Related Disorders. London: Churchill Livingstone; 1984.

87. Hayasaka S, Yamaguchi K, Mizuno K, et al. Ocular findings in childhood lactic acidosis. Arch Ophthalmol 1986;104:1656-1658.

88. Heher KL, Johns DR. A maculopathy associated with the 15257 mitochondrial DNA mutation. Arch Ophthalmol 1993;111:1495-1498.

89. Howell N. Mitochondrial gene mutations and human disease: a prolegomenon. Am J Hum Genet 1994;55:219-224.

90. Howell N, Halvorson S, Burns J, et al. When does bilateral optic atrophy become Leber hereditary optic neuropathy? Am J Hum Genet 1993;53: 959-963. Letter.

91. Hoyt CS, Billson FA. Visual loss in osteopetrosis. Am J Dis Child 1979;133:955-958.

92. Hoyt CS. Autosomal dominant optic atrophy: a spectrum of disability. Ophthalmology 1980;87: 245.

93. Hoyt CS, Billson FA. Optic neuropathy in ketogenic diet. Br J Ophthalmol 1979;63(3):191-194.

94. Hoyt CS, Good WV. Do we really understand the difference between optic nerve hypoplasia and atrophy? Eye 1992;6(pt 2):201-204.

95. Hoyt WF, Fletcher WA, Imes RK. Chiasmal gliomas. Appearance and long-term changes demonstrated by computerized tomography. Prog Exp Tumor Res 1987;30:113-121.

96. Hoyt WF, Imes RK. Optic gliomas of neurofibromatosis-1 (NF-1): contemporary perspectives. In: Ishibashi Y, Hori Y, eds. *Tuberous Sclerosis and Neurofibromatosis: Epidemiology, Pathophysiology, Biology and Management.* Amsterdam: Excerpta Medica; 1990:239-246.

97. Hoyt WF, Rios-Montenegro EN, Behrens MM, et al. Homonymous hemioptic hypoplasia. Funduscopic features in standard and red-free illumination in three patients with congenital hemiplegia. Br J Ophthalmol 1972;56:537-545.

98. Hoyt WF. Ophthalmoscopy of the retinal nerve fibre layer in neuro-ophthalmologic diagnosis. Aust J Ophthalmol 1976;4:14.

99. Huber A. Genetic diseases of vision. Curr Opin Neurol 1994;7:65-68.

100. Hull BM, Thompson DA. A review of the clinical applications of the pattern electroretinogram. Ophthalmic Physiol Opt 1989;9:143-152.

101. Huoponen K, Lamminen T, Juvonen V, et al. The spectrum of mitochondrial DNA mutations in families with Leber hereditary optic neuroretinopathy. Hum Genet 1993;92:379-384.
102. Imes RK, Hoyt WF. Childhood chiasmal gliomas: update on the fate of patients in the 1969 study. Br J Ophthalmol 1986;70:179-182.
103. Imes RK, Hoyt WF. Magnetic resonance imaging signs of optic nerve gliomas in neurofibromatosis 1. Am J Ophthalmol 1991;111:729-734.
104. Jacobson DM. Pupillary responses to dilute pilocarpine in preganglionic 3rd nerve disorders. Neurology 1990;40:804-808.
105. Jacobson DM, Stone EM. Difficulty differentiating Leber's from dominant optic neuropathy in a patient with remote visual loss. J Clin Neuro-Ophthalmol 1991;11:152-157.
106. Jakobiec FA, Depot MJ, Kennerdell JS, et al. Combined clinical and computed tomographic diagnosis of orbital glioma and meningioma. Ophthalmology 1984;91:137-155.
107. Jan JE, Robinson GC, Kinnis C, et al. Blindness due to optic nerve atrophy and hypoplasia in children: an epidemiology study (1944-1974). Dev Med Child Neurol 1977;19:353.
108. Jensen PKA, Reske-Nielsen E, Hein-Sorenson O, et al. Syndrome of opticoacoustic nerve atrophy with dementia. Am J Med Genet 1987;28:517-518.
109. Johns DR, Heher KL, Miller NR, et al. Leber's hereditary optic neuropathy: clinical manifestations of the 14484 mutation. Arch Ophthalmol 1993;111:495-498.
110. Johns DR, Smith KH, Miller NR, et al. Identical twins who are discordant for Leber's hereditary optic neuropathy. Arch Ophthalmol 1993;111:1491-1494.
111. Johns DR, Smith KH, Miller NR. Leber's hereditary optic neuropathy. Arch Ophthalmol 1992;110:1577-1581.
112. Johns DR, Neufeld MJ. Pitfalls in the molecular genetic diagnosis of Leber hereditary optic neuropathy (LHON). Am J Hum Genet. 1993;53(4):916-920.
113. Johns DR, Smith KH, Savino PJ, et al. Leber's hereditary optic neuropathy. Clinical manifestations of the 15257 mutation. Ophthalmology 1993;100(7):981-986.
114. Johnston PB, Gastor RN, Smith VC, et al. A clinico-pathologic study of autosomal dominant optic atrophy. Am J Ophthalmol 1975;88:868-875.
115. Kendall BE. Disorders of lysosomes, peroxisomes, and mitochondria. AJNR 1992;13:621-653.
116. Khodadoust AA, Ziai M, Biggs SL. Optic disc in normal newborns. Am J Ophthalmol 1968;66:502-504.
117. Kim I, Ohnishi A, Kuroiwa Y. Three cases of Charcot-Marie-Tooth disease with neural deafness: the classification and sural nerve pathology. Rinsho Shinkeigaku 1980; 20:264-270.
118. King KM, Cronin C. Ocular findings in premature infants with grade IV intraventricular hemorrhage. J Pediatr Ophthalmol Strabismus 1993;30:84-87.
119. Kinsley BT, Firth RG. The Wolfram syndrome: a primary neurodegenerative disorder with lethal potential. Ir Med J 1992;85:34-36.
120. Kjer P, Jensen OA, Klinken L. Histopathology of eye, optic nerve and brain in a case of dominant optic atrophy. Acta Ophthalmol Copenh 1983;61(2):300-312.
121. Kline LB, Glaser JS. Dominant optic atrophy: the clinical profile. Arch Ophthalmol 1979;97: 1680-1686.
122. Krageloh-Mann I, Grodd W, Niemann G, et al. Assessment and therapy monitoring of Leigh disease by MRI and proton spectroscopy. Pediatr Neurol 1992;8:60-64.
123. Lambert SL, Hoyt C. Brain problems. In: Taylor D, ed. Pediatric Ophthalmology. Boston, MA: Blackwell Scientific Publications; 1990:507.
124. Lambert SR, Hoyt CS, Jan JE, et al. Visual recovery from hypoxic cortical blindness during childhood. Computed tomographic and magnetic resonance imaging predictors. Arch Ophthalmol 1987;105:1371-1377.
125. Lapresle J. Palatal myoclonus. Adv Neurol 1986; 43:265-273.
126. Leeuwen MA, van Bogaert L. Hereditary ataxia with optic atrophy of the retrobulbar neuritis type , and latent pallido-Luysian degeneration. Brain 1949;72:340.
127. Leinonen MT, Elenius V. Perimetric testing of tritan deficiency. Ophthalmologica 1992;204: 204-209.
128. Lessell S, Rosman NP. Juvenile diabetes mellitis and optic atrophy. Arch Neurol 1977;34:759.
129. Leuzzi V, Bertini E, De-Negri AM, et al. Bilateral striatal necrosis, dystonia and optic atrophy in two siblings. J Neurol Neurosurg Psychiatry. 1992; 55(1):16-19.
130. Levin ML, O'Conner PS, Aguirre G, et al. Angiographically normal central retinal artery following the total resection of an optic nerve glioma. J Clin Neuro-Ophthalmol 1986;6:1-8.
131. Lewis RA, Gerson LP, Axelson KA, et al. Von Recklinghausen neurofibromatosis. II. incidence of optic gliomata. Ophthalmology 1984;91:929-935.
132. Listernick R, Charrow J, Greenwald MJ, et al. Optic gliomas in children with neurofibromatosis type 1. J Pediatr 1989;114:788-792.
133. Liu GT, Lessell S. Spontaneous visual improvement in chiasmal gliomas. Am J Ophthalmol 1992;114:193-201.
134. Livingstone IR, Mastaglia FL, Edis R, Howe JW. Visual involvement in Friedreich ataxia and hereditary spastic ataxias: a clinical and visual response study. Arch Neurol 1981;38:75-79.
135. Macdermot KD, Walker RWH. Autosomal recessive hereitary motor and sensory neuropathy with

mental retardation, optic atrophy and pyramidal signs. J Neurol Neurosurg Psychiatr 1987;50: 1342-1347.

136. Madreperia SA. Olivopontocerebellar atrophy with retinal degeneration. Fundus characteristics and diagnostic MRI findings. Ophthalmol Ped Genet 1993;14:61-68.

137. Mahapatra AK. Optic nerve injury in children. A prospective study of 35 patients. J Neurol Sci 1992;36:79-84.

138. Mantyjarvi MI, Nerdrum K, Tuppurainen K. Color vision in dominant optic atrophy. J Clin Neuro-Ophthalmol 1992;12:98-103.

139. Margo C, Hamed LM, McCarty J. Congenital optic tract syndrome. Arch Ophthalmol 1991;109: 1120-1122.

140. Maruyama K, Arisaka O, Lee T, et al. Optic atrophy in aqueduct stenosis. Eur J Pediatr 1989; 148(7):682. Letter.

141. Marzan KA, Barron TF. MRI abnormalities in Behr syndrome. Pediatr Neurol 1994;10:247-248.

142. Matson DD, Crigler JF Jr. Management of craniopharyngioma in childhood. J Neurosurg 1969; 30(4):377-390.

143. McComas AJ. Invited review: motor unit estimation: methods, results, and present status. Muscle Nerve 1991;14:585-597.

144. McGinnity FG, Bryars JH. Controlled study of ocular morbidity in school children born preterm. Br J Ophthalmol 1992;76:520-524.

145. McKluskey DJ, O'Connor PS, Sheehy JT. Leber's optic neuropathy and Charcot-Marie-Tooth disease. J Clin Neuro-Ophthalmol 1986;6:76-81.

146. Mefty O, Fox JL, Al-Rodhan N, et al. Optic nerve decompression in osteopetrosis. J Neurosurg 1988; 68:80-84.

147. Meire F, De Laey JJ, de Bie S, et al. Dominant optic nerve atrophy with progressive hearing loss and chronic progressive external ophthalmoplegia (CPEO). Ophthalmic Paediatr Genet. 1985;5(1-2): 91-97.

148. Menon V, Arya AV, Sharma P, et al. An aetiological profile of optic atrophy. Acta Ophthalmol Copenh 1992;70:725-729.

149. Mets MB, Mhoon E. Probable autosomal dominant optic atrophy with hearing loss. Ophthalmic Paediatr Genet 1985;5(1-2):85-89.

150. Mikelberg FS, Yidegiligne HM. Axonal loss in band atrophy of the optic nerve in craniopharyngioma: a quantitative analysis. Can J Ophthalmol 1993;28:69-71.

151. Miller NR, Newman SA. Transsynaptic degeneration. Arch Ophthalmol 1981;99:165. Letter.

152. Miller NR, Solomon S. Retinochoroidal (optociliary) shunt veins, blindness, and optic atrophy: a non-specific sign of chronic optic nerve compression. Aust N Z J Ophthalmol 1991;19:105-109.

153. Miller NR. Optic atrophy. In: Walsh FB, Hoyt WF. Clinical Neuro-Ophthalmology. 4th ed. Baltimore, MD: Williams & Wilkins; 1982:329-342.

154. Miyake Y, Yagasaki K, Ichikawa H. Differential diagnosis of congenital tritanopia and dominantly inherited optic atrophy. Arch Ophthalmol 1985;103: 1496-1501.

155. Moller HU. Recessively inherited, simple optic atrophy—does it exist? Ophthalmic Paediatr Genet 1992;13:31-32. Letter.

156. Moore AT, Buncic JR, Munro IR. Fibrous dysplasia of the orbit in childhood. Clinical features and management. Ophthalmology 1985;92:12-20.

157. Mukai K, Seljeskog EL, Dehner LP. Pituitary adenomas in patients under 20 years old. A clinico-pathological study of 12 cases. J Neuro-Oncol 1986;4:79-89.

158. Munnich A, Rustin P, Rotig D, et al. Clinical aspects of mitochondrial disorders. J Inherited Metab Dis 1992;15:448-455.

159. Nakamura M, Tanigawa M, Yamamoto M. A case of Leber's hereditary optic neuropathy with a mitochondrial DNA mutation at nucleotide position 3460. Jpn J Ophthalmol 1994;38:267-271.

160. Neetens A, Leroy J, Smets RM. Menkes' kinky hair disease. Bull Soc Belge Ophtal 1982;203:75-83.

161. Neetens A, Martin JJ. The hereditary optic atrophies. Neuroophthalmology 1986;6:277.

162. Neetens A, Rubbens MC. Dominant juvenile optic atrophy. Ophthalmic Paediatr Genet 1985;5:79-83.

163. Neufeld EF, Muenzer J. The mucopolysaccharidoses. In: Scriver CR, Beaudet AL, Sly WS, Valle D, eds. The Metabolic Basis of Inherited Disease, 6th ed. New York, NY: McGraw-Hill; 1989;II: 1565-1587.

164. Newman NJ. Leber's hereditary optic neuropathy. New genetic considerations. Arch Neurol 1993; 50:540-548.

165. Newman NJ. Leber's hereditary optic neuropathy. Ophthalmol Clin North Am 1991;4:431-447.

166. Newman NJ. Optic disc pallor: a false localizing sign. Surv Ophthalmol 1993;37:237-282.

167. Newman NJ, Lott MT, Wallace DC. The clinical characteristics of pedigrees of Leber's hereditary optic neuropathy with the 11778 mutation. Am J Ophthalmol 1991;111(6):750-762.

168. Newman SA. Ophthalmic features of craniosynostosis. Neurosurg Clin North Am 1991;2:587-610.

169. Newman SA, Miller NR. Optic tract syndrome. Neuro-ophthalmologic considerations. Arch Ophthalmol 1983;101:1241-1250.

170. Ohtsuka Y, Amano R, Oka E, et al. Myoclonus epilepsy with ragged-red fibers: a clinical and electrophysiologic follow-up study on two sibling cases. J Child Neurol 1993;8(4):366-372.

171. Okuno T, Prensky AL, Gado M. The Moyamoya syndrome associated with irradiation of optic

glioma in children: report of two cases and review of the literature. Pediatr Neurol 1985;1:311-316.

172. Orozco Diaz G, Nodarse Fleites A, Cordoves Sagaz R, et al. Autosomal dominant cerebellar ataxia: clinical analysis of 263 patients from a homogeneous population in Holguin, Cuba. Neurology 1990;40(9):1369-1375.

173. Ouvrier RA. Pallor of the optic disc in children. Aust N Z J Ophthalmol 1990;18:375-379.

174. Ozkan H, Unsal E, Kose G. Oculocerebral hypopigmentation syndrome (Cross syndrome). Turk J Pediatr 1991;33(4):247-252.

175. Parravano JG, Toledo A, Kucharczyk W. Dimensions of the optic nerves, chiasm, and tracts: MR quantitative comparison between patients with optic atrophy and normals. J Comput Assist Tomogr 1993;17:688-690.

176. Paulus W, Straube A, Bauer W, et al. Central nervous system involvement in Leber's optic neuropathy. J Neurol 1993;240:251-253.

177. Pearce WG. Variable severity in autosomal dominant optic atrophy. Ophthalmic Paediatr Genet 1985;5(1-2):99-102.

178. Peterson JR, Rosenberg T, Ibssen KK. Optic atrophy with particular attention to perinatal damage. Ugeskr Laeger 1990;152:3865-3867.

179. Phillips CI, Mackintosh GI, Howe JW, et al. Autosomal recessive "optic atrophy" with late onset and evidence of ganglion cell dysfunction: a sibship of two females. Ophthalmologica 1993;206:89-93.

180. Pilley SF, Thompson HS. Familial syndrome of diabetes insipidus, diabetes mellitus, optic atrophy and deafness (DIDMOAD) in children. Br J Ophthalmol 1976;60:294-298.

181. Pollock SC, Miller NR. The retinal nerve fiber layer. Int Ophthalmol Clin 1986;26:201-221.

182. Posnick JC, Wells MD, Drake JM, et al. Childhood fibrous dysplasia presenting as blindness: a skull base approach for resection and immediate reconstruction. Pediatr Neurosurg 1993;19:260-266.

183. Proud VK, Levine C, Carpenter NJ. New X-linked syndrome with seizures, acquired micrencephaly, and agenesis of the corpus callosum. Am J Med Genet 1992;43(1-2):458-466.

184. Quigley HA, Anderson DR. The histologic basis of optic disk pallor in experimental optic atrophy. Am J Ophthalmol 1977;83(5):709-717.

185. Quigley HA, Davis EB, Anderson DR. Descending optic nerve degeneration in primates. Invest Ophthalmol Vis Sci 1977;16:841-849.

186. Quigley HA, Hohman RM, Addicks EM. Quantitative study of optic nerve head capillaries in experimental optic disc pallor. Am J Ophthalmol 1982;93(6):689-699.

187. Ramaekers VT, Brab M, Rau G, et al. Recovery from neurological deficits following biotin treatment in a biotinidase Km variant. Neuropediatrics 1993;24:98-102.

188. Rando TA, Horton JC, Layzer RB. Wolfram syndrome: evidence of a diffuse neurodegenerative disease by magnetic resonance imaging. Neurology 1992;42:1220-1224.

189. Repka MX, Miller NR, Miller M. Visual outcome after surgical removal of craniopharyngiomas. Ophthalmology 1989;96:195-199.

190. Repka MX, Miller NR. Optic atrophy in children. Am J Ophthalmol 1988;106:191-193.

191. Richmond IL, Wilson CB. Pituitary adenomas in childhood and adolescence. J Neurosurg 1978;49:163-168.

192. Rizzo JF, Lessell S, Liebman S. Optic atrophy in familial dysautonomia. Am J Ophthalmol 1986;102:463-467.

193. Roggeveen HC, de Winter AP, Went LN. Studies in dominant optic atrophy. Ophthalmic Paediatr Genet. 1985;5:103-109.

194. Ron E, Modam B, Boice JD, et al. Tumors of the brain and nervous system after radiotherapy in childhood. N Engl J Med 1988;319:1033.

195. Rosenberg RN, Chutorian A. Familial opticoacoustic nerve degeneration and polyneuropathy. Neurology 1967;17:827-832.

196. Rosenberg RN, Grossman A. Hereditary ataxia. Neurol Clin. 1989;7(1):25-36.

197. Rotig A, Cormier V, Chatelain P, et al. Deletion of mitochondrial DNA in a case of early-onset diabetes mellitus, optic atrophy, and deafness (Wolfram syndrome, MIM 222300). J Clin Invest 1993;91(3):1095-1098.

198. Saatci U, Soylemezoglu O, Ozen S, et al. Diabetes mellitus, diabetes insipidus, optic atrophy and deafness (DIDMOAD syndrome). Turk J Pediatr 1990;32:211-215.

199. Sachdev MS, Kumar H, Jain AK, et al. Transsynaptic neuronal degeneration of optic nerves associated with bilateral occipital lesions. Ind J Ophthalmol 1990;38:151-152.

200. Sadun AA, Martone JF, Muci-Mendoza R, et al. Epidemic optic neuropathy in Cuba. Eye findings. Arch Ophthalmol 1994;112:691-699.

201. Safran AB, Lupolover Y, Berney J. Macular reflexes in optic atrophy. Am J Ophthalmol 1984;98:494.

202. Salbert BA, Astruc J, Wolf B. Ophthalmologic findings in biotinidase deficiency. Ophthalmologica 1993;206(4):177-181.

203. Salih MA, Tuvemo T. Diabetes insipidus, diabetes mellitus, optic atrophy and deafness (DIDMOAD syndrome). A clinical study in two Sudanese families. Acta Paediatr Scand 1991;80:567-572.

204. Salonen R, Somer M, Haltia M, et al. Progressive encephalopathy with edema, hypsarrhythmia, and optic atrophy (PEHO syndrome). Clin Genet 1991;39:287-293.

205. Savoiardo M, Strada L, Girotti F, et al. Olivocerebellar atrophy: MR diagnosis and relationship to

multisystem atrophy. Radiology 1994;174: 693-696.

206. Sayli BS, Gul D. GAPO syndrome in three relatives in a Turkish kindred. Am J Med Genet 1993;47:342-345.

207. Schor NF. Nervous system dysfunction in children with paraneoplastic syndromes. J Child Neurol 1992;7:253-258.

208. Seiff SR, Brodsky MC, McDonald G, et al. Orbital optic glioma in neurofibromatosis: magnetic resonance diagnosis of perineural arachnoidal gliomatosis. Arch Ophthalmol 1987;105: 1689-1692.

209. Seiff SR. Trauma and the optic nerve. Ophthalmol Clin North Am 1992;5:389-394.

210. Senanayake N. A syndrome of early onset spinocerebellar ataxia with optic atrophy, internuclear ophthalmoplegia, dementia, and startle myoclonus in a Sri Lankan family. J Neurol 1992; 239(5):293-294. Letter.

211. Sener RN, Ustun EE, Ozkinay C, et al. Acromesomelic-spondyloepiphyseal dysplasia associated with congenital optic atrophy: report of a family. Pediatr Radiol 1993;23(4):321-324.

212. Shedden AM, Smith JC, O'Conner PS, et al. The "phantom" optic nerve. J Clin Neuro-Ophthalmol 1985;5:209-212.

213. Sheffer RN, Zlotogora J, Elpeleg ON, et al. Behr's syndrome and 3-methylglutaconic aciduria. Am J Ophthalmol 1992;114:494-497.

214. Shurin SB, Rekate HL, Annable W. Optic atrophy induced by vincristine. Pediatrics 1982;70: 288-291.

215. Sly WS, Whyte MP, Sundaram V, et al. Carbonic anhydrase II deficiency in 12 families with the autosomal recessive syndrome of osteopetrosis with renal tubular acidosis and cerebral calcifications. N Engl J Med 1985;313:139-145.

216. Small KW, Pollock S, Scheinman J. Optic atrophy in primary oxalosis. Am J Ophthalmol 1988; 106:96-97.

217. Smith JL, Hoyt WF, Susac JO. Ocular fundus in acute Leber optic neuropathy. Arch Ophthalmol 1973;90:349-354.

218. Smith KH, Johns DR, Heher KL, et al. Heteroplasmy in Leber's hereditary optic neuropathy. Arch Ophthalmol 1993;111:1486-1490.

219. Somer M, Sainio K. Epilepsy and the electroencephalogram in progressive encephalopathy with edema, hypsarrhythmia, and optic atrophy (the PEHO syndrome). Epilepsia 1993;34(4):727-731.

220. Somer M, Salonen O, Pihko H, et al. PEHO syndrome (progressive encephalopathy with edema, hypsarrhythmia, and optic atrophy): neuroradiologic findings. AJNR 1993;14:861-867.

221. Spalton DJ, Taylor DSI, Sanders MD. Juvenile Batten's disease; and ophthalmological assessment of 26 patients. Br J Ophthalmol 1980;64:726-732.

222. Sperli D, Concolino D, Barbato C, et al. Long survival of a patient with Marshall-Smith syndrome

without respiratory complications. J Med Genet 1993;30(10):877-879.

223. Stern J, Jakobiec FA, Housepian EM. The architecture of optic nerve gliomas with and without neurofibromatosis. Arch Ophthalmol 1980;98; 505-511.

224. Stone EM, Newman NJ, Miller NR, et al. Visual recovery in patients with Leber's hereditary optic neuropathy and the 11778 mutation. J Clin Neuro-Ophthalmol 1992;12:10-14.

225. Stromland K. Eyeground malformations in the fetal alcohol syndrome. Birth Defects 1982;18(6): 651-655.

226. Sullivan TJ, Heathcote JG, Brazel SM, et al. The ocular pathology in Leber's congenital amaurosis. Aust N Z J Ophthalmol 1994;22:25-31.

227. Sullivan TJ, Lambert SR, Buncic JR, et al. The optic discs in Leber congenital amaurosis. J Pediatr Ophthalmol Strabismus 1992;29:246-249.

228. Swaiman KF. Hallervorden-Spatz syndrome and brain iron metabolism. Arch Neurol 1991; 48(12):1285-1293.

229. Sylvestor PE. Some unusual findings in a family with Friedreich ataxia. Arch Dis Child 1958; 33:217-221.

230. Szedelyova L, Vaisova Z. Dominant infantile optic nerve atrophy. Cesk Oftalmol 1989;45(6):440-444.

231. Taylor D. Ophthalmological features of some human hereditary disorders with demyelination. Bull Soc Belge Ophtal 1983;208-209:405-413.

232. Taylor DR. Congenital tumors of the anterior visual system with dysplasia of the optic discs. Br J Ophthalmol 1982;66:455.

233. Till JS, Roach ES, Burton BK. Sialidosis (neuraminidase deficiency) types I and II: neuroophthalmic manifestations. J Clin Neuro-Ophthalmol 1987;7(1):40-44.

234. Traboulsi EI, DeBecker I, Maumenee IH. Ocular findings in Cockayne syndrome. Am J Ophthalmol 1992;114:579-583.

235. Traboulsi EI, Silva JC, Geraghty MT, et al. Ocular histopathologic characteristics of cobalamin C type vitamin B_{12} defect with methylmalonic aciduria and homocystinuria. Am J Ophthalmol 1992; 113(3):269-280.

236. Treft RL, Sanborn GE, Carey J, et al. Dominant optic atrophy, deafness, ptosis, ophthalmoplegia, dystaxia, and myopathy. A new syndrome. Ophthalmology 1984;91:908-915.

237. Trobe JD, Glaser JSS, Cassady JC. Optic atrophy: differential diagnosis by fundus observation alone. Arch Ophthalmol 1980;98:1040-1045.

238. Tuppurainen K, Herrgard E, Martikainen A, et al. Ocular findings in prematurely born children at 5 years of age. Graefe's Arch Clin Exp Ophthalmol 1993;231:261-266.

239. Tzekov C, Cherninkova S, Gudeva T. Neuroophthalmological symptoms in children treated for internal hydrocephalus. Pediatr Neurosurg 1991-1992;17(6):317-320.

240. Unsold R, Hoyt WF. Band atrophy of the optic nerve. The histology of temporal hemianopsia. Arch Ophthalmol 1980;98 (Sept):1637-1638.

241. Van-den-Berge JH, Blaauw G, Breeman WA, et al. Intracavitary brachytherapy of cystic craniopharyngiomas. J Neurosurg 1992;77(4):545-550.

242. Van-den-Bergh L, Zeyen T, Verhelst J, et al. Wolfram syndrome: a clinical study of two cases. Doc Ophthalmol 1993;84(2):119-126.

243. Vikki J, Ott J, Savontaus ML, Aula P, et al. Optic atrophy in Leber's hereditary optic neuropathy is probably determined by an X-chromosome gene closely linked to DXS7. Am J Hum Genet 1991; 48:486-491.

244. Volpe JJ. Neurology of the newborn. Philadelphia, PA: WB Saunders; 1987.

245. Volpe NJ, Lessell S. Leber's hereditary optic neuropathy. Int Ophthalmol Clin 1993;33:153-168.

246. Wajntal A, Koiffmann CP, Mendonca BB, et al. GAPO syndrome—a connective tissue disorder: report of two affected sibs and on the pathologic findings in the older. Am J Med Genet 1990; 37:213-223.

247. Weiner HL, Wisoff JH, Rosenberg ME: Craniopharyngiomas: a clinicopathological analysis of factors predictive of recurrence and functional outcome. Neurosurgery 1994;6:1001-1011.

248. Weisman JS, Hepler RS, Vinters HV. Reversible visual loss caused by fibrous dysplasia. Am J Ophthalmol 1990;110:244-249.

249. Weleber RG, Eisner A. Cone degeneration ("bull's eye dystrophies") and color vision defects. In: Newsome DA, ed. Retinal Dystrophies and Degenerations. New York, NY: Raven Press; 1988: 233-256.

250. Weleber RG, Miyake Y. Familial optic atrophy with negative electroretinograms. Arch Ophthalmol 1992;110:640-645.

251. Weyand RD, Criag WM, Rucker CW. Unusual lesions involving the optic chiasm. Proc Staff Meet Mayo Clin 1952;27:505-511.

252. Wolfram DJ. Diabetes mellitus and simple optic atrophy among siblings. Report of 4 cases. Mayo Clin Proc 1938;13:715-718.

253. Wright JE, McNab AA, McDonald WI. Optic nerve glioma and the management of optic nerve tumors in the young. Br J Ophthalmol 1989;73: 967-974.

254. Wright JE, McNab AA, McDonald WI. Primary optic nerve sheath meningioma. Br J Ophthalmol 1989;73:960-966.

255. Yoshioka M, Kuroki S, Kondo T. Ocular manifestations in Fukuyama type congenital muscular dystrophy. Brain Dev 1990;12(4):423-426.

256. Zimmerman CF, Schatz NJ, Glaser JS. Magnetic resonance imaging of optic nerve meningiomas. Ophthalmology 1990;97:585-591.

5

Transient, Unexplained, and Psychogenic Visual Loss in Children

Introduction

Some children have visual disturbances that occur in the absence of, or are out of proportion to, their objective ophthalmological findings. These symptoms reflect a wide range of processes that may be benign or may be a sign of neurological, systemic, or psychiatric disease. This chapter deals with the neuro-ophthalmologic detection of organic and psychogenic disorders that may manifest as transient or unexplained visual loss in childhood.

Transient Visual Disturbances in Children

Most of what is known about transient visual disturbances has come from correlating pathology and pathophysiology from the richly detailed descriptions given by some adults. Formed and unformed visual hallucinations have occurred in artists who have been able to paint or draw what they have seen. Physicians and scientists have experienced and have described many visual disturbances, such as amaurosis fugax and the scintillating scotoma of migraine. Many of the same episodic visual disturbances occur in childhood, but several formidable problems confront the physician trying to reach the correct diagnosis. The descriptions of episodic visual disturbances and hallucinations in children are less complex in detail than those of the adult population, because children have a limited vocabulary and a limited experiential basis of sensory phenomenon to draw upon.

Children share with adults a difficulty in distinguishing homonymous from monocular defects and may insist that a homonymous defect affects only one eye. Children are also less likely than adults to draw a distinction between a positive and a negative visual disturbance. They may simply maintain that something is blocking their vision and may be unable to describe it further. If pressured by the examiner to be more descriptive, a child or even a teenager may attempt to give the examiner what they think is being asked for, even if it does not accurately depict their symptoms. Children with refractive errors or other organic visual problems may describe visual symptoms only in terms of their effect upon a specific activity (such as difficulty reading the blackboard at school or reading textbooks), making it difficult to determine from the history whether the disturbance is indeed episodic.

The commonest cause of episodic visual loss disturbances in childhood is migraine. The visual disturbance of migraine is characterized by episodic visual hallucinations and visual loss, as well as other neurological disturbances, with headache being the most common. However, the characteristic hemicranial throbbing headache is often absent in the pediatric age group, and the diagnosis is based upon a compilation of circumstantial evidence. A personal profile of the child should be explored with specific attention to eliciting a history of extreme fussiness or colic as a baby, night terrors, recurrent abdominal pains, or motion sickness.[40] A family history of migraine must be sought since family members with migraine may never have been diagnosed or may have been misdiagnosed as having tension or sinus headaches. The diagnosis of migraine for the child's visual disturbances and the parent's headaches can often be established in the same interview.

Careful questioning may determine that the child is describing a visual hallucination rather than a visual obscuration. As in adults, visual hallucinations in children may be formed or unformed and may be simple or complex. Unformed hallucinations typically consist of lights, heat wave sensations, or simple geometric patterns that may be spatially stable or move. Formed hallucinations consist of recognizable objects or people. These may be simple, such as visualizing a single animal or an object, such as a table or chair, or they may demonstrate varying degrees of complexity involving the purposeful movement of several people in a scene with appropriate colored backgrounds and facial expressions. If the attacks are repetitive, the hallucination may be stereotyped, or a new scene or object may be visualized with each recurrence.

Visual hallucinations are generally divided into *irritative* and *release* hallucinations.[74] Irritative hallucinations are usually caused by epileptic discharges that occur as part of a seizure.[122,174] Irritative hallucinations emanating from the temporal lobes tend to be complex and stereotyped, while those arising in the occipital lobes tend to be simple and unformed. Other aspects of the seizure disorder are often more prominent, including changes in consciousness and sensory or motor abnormalities due to the spread of the epileptic activity; however, isolated and localized occipital or temporal lobe seizures may produce visual hallucinations as their only manifestation.

Release hallucinations often occur in patients with decreased vision or visual field defects. They may also occur in the setting of monocular or binocular visual loss or homonymous hemianopia and may manifest in patients with relatively mild visual loss.[36] These hallucinations range from unformed phosphenes to formed hallucinations with complex patterns. Release hallucinations presumably occur when normal visual impulses are removed, releasing indigenous cerebral activity within the visual system.[36] They tend to be continuous and can last from minutes to days, in contradistinction to irritative hallucinations that last for seconds to a few minutes.[36] Release hallucinations are neither associated with electroencephalographic abnormalities nor altered by anticonvulsant therapy.

The failure to clearly distinguish the irritative from the release type of hallucination has led to considerable confusion regarding their localizing value. The concept that hallucinations of occipital origin comprise unformed phosphenes applies only to the irritative variety. Unlike irritative hallucinations, which vary in character depending upon their site of origin, release hallucinations have no localizing value and can follow injury to the visual system anywhere from the eye to the occipital cortex.[36,130,237] For example, formed release hallucinations occasionally occur in adults with dense cataracts or macular degeneration.[139] Children can experience "phantom vision" following enucleation of one or both eyes.[37] Patients with visual loss frequently acknowledge experiencing both formed and unformed visual hallucinations when specifically asked.

Migrainous Phenomena

Migraine is not just a headache.[31] It is a disorder that can cause transient sensory, autonomic, motor, visual, and cognitive impairment. Although headache is a prominent feature of migraine, it is not invariably present.[31] Many migraine attacks begin slowly and evolve through sequential stages of neurological dysfunction. Selby[202] described migraine as a "drama in three acts," comprising prodrome (frequently not recognized) and aura, a headache phase, and a post-headache phase. The aura may occur prior to, concurrently, or even after the onset of the headache. It cannot be overemphasized that the diagnosis of pediatric migraine is established on the basis of the personal profile, attack profile, and family history, as well as the absence of physical findings. In the child with transient visual disturbances or unexplained headache, the personal history often provides an important clue to the diagnosis of migraine.[40] Pediatric migraineurs often have a history of migraine equivalents, including colic, recurrent abdominal pain, cyclic vomiting, pavor nocturnus (night terrors), and paroxysmal torticollis within the first few years of life.[15,31] Even between attacks, migraineurs often describe themselves as very reactive to extraneous visual, auditory, gustatory, and thermal stimuli.[6,77] Bright lights (sunlight reflecting from snow or water) or strong smells (e.g., perfume, gasoline) can precipitate a migraine attack. A history of motion sickness is also strongly associated with migraine and considered to be an associated feature of the migraine diathesis.[6,13] In attempting to elicit a family history of migraine, it is useful to ask whether any of the first degree relatives have "sick headaches" or have ever had to go into a dark room, put a damp rag on their head, and go to sleep because of a severe headache. Features of the attack history include the presence or absence of an aura, the characteristics of the headache, and the presence or absence of additional neurological impairment.

The prevalence of migraine is approximately equal in boys and girls under 7 years of age. A female predominance of 3:2 is present from 7 years of age until puberty. After puberty, the relative prevalence becomes further skewed toward girls, with a ratio of 2½ to 1.[21]

Migraine Aura

Although migraine headache is less prevalent in children than in adults, the presenting complaint of transient visual disturbances will result in the diagnosis of migraine with considerable frequency in the pediatric age group.[21,35,56] The stereotypical visual migraine aura lasts 25 to 30 minutes, but occasionally, it may subside in a few minutes or last several hours. The variability in the characteristics and the frequency of migraine aura so common in adults is even greater in children. The examiner must be aware not only of the classic adult migraine aura but also of the variations on this theme that are presented in the pediatric age group.[3,61,103]

Some children are able to describe the classical form of scintillating scotoma with expansion or buildup of the fortification figure. The visual disturbance typically begins as a fog or loss of illumination pericentrally in one hemifield, progressing in a few seconds or minutes to a few degrees of central scotoma lined on the temporal side by a luminous zigzag line, or teichopsia (Greek word meaning *fortification-seeing*). The jagged lines of the fortification specter may be colored or gray

and appear to be varying in brightness in a way that is often described as flashing, jabbing, boiling, or rolling.[126] The visual disturbance expands in the shape of a horseshoe with the open end central. The open end also frequently encompasses a negative scotoma.[103] This sensation usually begins as a small pericentral disturbance encompassing only a few degrees and gradually expands toward the temporal periphery over 20 to 30 minutes to involve a large portion of the hemifield of both eyes (although patients may interpret the visual disturbance as monocular). As the fortification scotoma expands peripherally, it transiently erases the visual field to produce a transient homonymous scotoma. Fortification scotomas are seen with the eyes open or closed and are even perceived in patients with no eyes. This hemifield scotoma frequently precedes the characteristic headache of migraine, but it may also occur alone in the absence of a headache, in which case it is termed an *acephalgic migraine*.[161]

In addition to the typical fortification scotoma, the range of visual disturbances in adult migraine is quite broad and includes positive and negative scotomas,[61] blurred vision, foggy vision, flickering lights, colored lights, zigzag lines, and a heat wave sensation, all presumably of occipital origin. Children with migraines are more likely than adults to describe a variety of other visual disturbances in place of the classic fortification scotoma.[40] The descriptions provided by children tend to be more picturesque, such as "heat waves," "water coming down a window," "lines coming down from the sky like it's raining," "like looking through cellophane," "sparkles," "dancing lights," or "dots and blobs" that gradually enlarge to obliterate the visual field.[87,166]

Migraine with aura (classic migraine) is preceded by or accompanied by a focal disturbance of cerebral or brainstem function.[31] The migraine aura may also be nonvisual. Some patients experience a sensory aura consisting of migratory paresthesias of the tongue, lips, and hand (cheiro-oral migraine). Common migraine may not have a clearly defined visual or sensory prodrome, but autonomic prodromal symptoms may occur, including yawning, hunger, irritability, edema, euphoria, or depression. The premonitory mood changes and skin pallor, which are often noted by parents prior to the onset of childhood migraine, may be other reflections of the same autonomic symptomatology.[155] Mothers learn to recognize their child's migraine attack prior to the onset of headache by observing skin pallor and "goose bumps," with cold, clammy perspiration, and cold extremities.[31] Some children develop periorbital discoloration during or just before a migraine.[208]

Amaurosis Fugax as a Migraine Equivalent in Children

The term *amaurosis fugax* is somewhat arbitrarily applied to transient monocular visual loss of relatively rapid onset and fairly rapid resolution. The episodes characteristically last 2 to 10 minutes and are unaccompanied by significant pain. In adults over 50 years of age, the term amaurosis fugax has come to signify transient visual loss associated with ipsilateral carotid atherosclerosis. The characteristics and duration of transient visual loss have therefore become the critical historical determinants in distinguishing retinal embolization from migrainous visual loss in older adults. In young adults or children, however, migraine is a common cause of amaurosis fugax. Tomsak and Jergens[222] described 24 adults with benign recurrent transient monocular blindness that was presumed to be migrainous in etiology. The visual loss was predominantly one-sided and stereotyped in character, although symptoms varied greatly from patient to patient. Postural change or exercise was a provocative factor in half of the cases. Other neurological symptoms were not present, and only one patient developed permanent visual loss during an attack. Evaluation by computed tomography (CT) scanning, cerebral angiography, echocardiography, and ophthalmodynamometry, when performed, were uniformly normal. Tippin et al[220] reported similar findings in a group of adolescents and young adults with amaurosis fugax. They found that headache or orbital pain accompanied the amaurotic spells in 41% of cases and that an additional 25.3% had severe headaches independent of the visual loss. None of the 11 patients who had angiography had an atherosclerotic lesion of the carotid artery. None of the patients who were reexamined after an average follow-up of 5.8 years had had a stroke. The authors concluded that amaurosis fugax is associated with a more benign clinical course in young patients and that migraine is a likely cause for the visual episodes. They advised that carotid angiography and invasive diagnostic studies are unwarranted in young patients with transient visual loss who are otherwise healthy, since significant and/or systemic diseases are rarely discovered.

O'Sullivan et al[166] found a personal or family history of migraine in 8 of 9 children and young adults with transient monocular visual loss. They noted that, as with migraines, the episodes of visual loss tended to occur in clusters. Investigation revealed no embolic or atheromatous etiology. Appleton et al[8] also attributed atypical forms of transient visual loss in children with acephalgic migraine and found that it carries a benign prognosis in young patients. While the term *migraine* is reassuring to parents and useful to clinicians in connoting a benign prognosis in children with transient monocular visual loss, little is known about the underlying pathophysiology or the site (retinal neurons, retinal vessels, optic disc) of dysfunction.

The term *vasospasm* is often postulated as the mechanism for migrainous transient monocular visual disturbances in both children and adults.[106] However, retinal vasospasm may occur as an independent event or as a component of migraine. Retinal vasospasm has been described, visualized, and photographed in adult patients.[28] During these attacks, the retina appears pale, the arterioles are narrowed, there are focal arteriolar constrictions, the veins are narrowed, and fluorescein angiography shows delayed filling. The retinal veins appear to dilate dramatically as the attack abates. Similar arterial vasospasm may affect other tissues in the same patients (Raynaud phenomenon, Prinzmetal angina). The clinical course is generally benign, but optic nerve or retinal infarction has been documented as an uncommon consequence of retinal vasospasm.[103]

The spreading depression associated with migraine has been demonstrated experimentally in the cortex and retina.[230,231] We suspect that many cases of transient monocular visual loss in children may involve a transient neuronal inhibition or depression at the retinal level rather than focal ischemia and that such cases will eventually be classified as migraine equivalents.

Migraine Headache

Migraine headache in adults may be hemicranial (classic migraine) or holocranial, bifrontal, or frontal in distribution (common migraine). Migraine headache has a gradual onset and builds in intensity over minutes or hours. It can last a few hours to several days.[31] It is described as a dull headache if the pain is not severe, but it becomes throbbing or pulsatile as the pain increases, although the character of the headache in children differs somewhat from that of adults in that a minority of children describe their headache as throbbing.[155] Complaints of bifrontal or bitemporal headaches or central forehead pain are more common in children, and unilaterality is uncommon.[155] Head trauma may be a significant triggering factor. Migraine headache is often associated with nausea or vomiting, and children are often phonophobic and sonophobic during the attack.[10,155] The pain is relieved by vomiting or sleep. In attempting to determine whether headaches are migrainous, we ask the patient what they do when they get an attack. They often give a stereotypical reply such as "I go in my room, close the door, turn off the lights, pull down the shades, pull the covers over my head, and go to sleep." Additional symptoms may include increased urination, diarrhea, and facial pallor or flushing before or during the headache.

Migraineurs may also describe jabs of pain in the scalp or eye when they are not having headaches as well as during a migraine attack.[31] These have been termed "ice-pick headaches" or "the syndrome of jabs and stabs."[185] They may be isolated or occur repetitively over a day or two. Those involving the eye are known as *ophthalmodynia fugax*.[29]

The diagnosis of migraine in an infant or toddler is often made only in retrospect, when the child is older and clear symptoms of pediatric migraine become evident. Barlow found the most common migraine manifestations in the first years of life to be repeated vomiting followed by a behavioral change (irritability or lethargy), vertigo, ataxia, or pallor, and sleep relief.[15,38] Many of these children were also able to communicate that they had a headache either verbally or by holding their head. Headaches that interrupt play are also an important clue to the diagnosis of migraine.

Complicated Migraine

Complicated migraine syndromes are more common in children and adolescents than in adults.

Acute confusional migraine was first reported by Gascon and Barlow[67] in four children ages 8 to 16. It resembles acute toxic psychosis and usually presents as one of the first episodes of migraine in a child.[67] During an attack, the child may display confusion, agitation, an altered sensorium, or withdrawn noncommunicative behavior. The attack usually ends with a period of prolonged sleep. Recurrent 30- to 60-minute episodes of confusion or even psychotic behavior in children should lead one to consider the diagnosis of migraine. These attacks eventually evolve into more typical migraine episodes.[54]

Acute hemiplegic migraine may occur as a manifestation of complicated migraine or as a familial disorder.[75] Familial hemiplegic migraine is characterized by attacks of hemiplegia and hemianesthesia that begin in childhood and may last several days.[34] Recurrent episodes may vary from side to side and may be associated with hallucinations, aphasia, or confusion. The gene for familial hemiplegic migraine has recently been mapped to chromosome 19.[105]

Other disturbances of higher cortical function have also been described with migraine.[119,161] In older children, these disorders include disturbances of color vision (central achromatopsia), abnormal facial recognition (prosopagnosia), difficulty reading (alexia with or without agraphia), and transient global amnesia.[20,57,60,67,87,103] The Alice in Wonderland syndrome, characterized by distortions of time, sense, and body image, has also been described as a manifestation of pediatric migraine.[76,221]

Although the term migraine connotes a benign and fundamentally reversible condition, a subgroup of patients develop *infarction* following a severe episode. Rossi et al[192] described seven children who had at least one episode of CT-documented infarct, possibly during an attack of migraine. Although a causal relationship could not be assured, the epidemiological data suggest that childhood migraine can be a contributing risk factor for childhood stroke.[145] Lewis et al[135] analyzed the Humphrey 30-2 threshold test results in 60 migraine patients and found visual field abnormalities in 35%.

The prevalence of visual field loss was greater with increasing age and duration of disease. The etiology of visual field loss was unclear, since very few patients had homonymous defects, as would be expected with a cortical injury. Whether reports of optic nerve and retinal infarction in patients with retinal vasoconstriction (which are invariably designated as *migraine*) are the result of an underlying migraine diathesis is unknown.

Bickerstaff[19] first described symptoms of *basilar artery migraine* as referable to the very diffuse circulation territory of the basilar artery involving virtually all structures in the posterior fossa and brain stem. This type of migraine has a predilection for children. In one study,[143] 5% of children with migraine in an outpatient clinic were diagnosed with basilar artery migraine. Symptomatology is progressive during an attack, with each attack lasting 2 to 45 minutes. Visual loss is often the initial event, with a disturbance of central vision, which is often described as resembling a bright sun or flashbulb.[31] This visual disturbance may be followed by total loss of vision or large blotches of positive visual scotomas obscuring both hemifields. The visual symptoms are then followed by some combination of vertigo, ataxia, dysarthria, tinnitus, and occasionally tingling of the hands and feet. Headache may be absent, but when it occurs, it is frequently occipital and throbbing. Abrupt loss of consciousness, lasting for a few minutes can also occur.[98,125] Benign recurrent vertigo of childhood may be a precursor of basilar artery migraine.[31] Most children also have common or classic migraine attacks, and the basilar migraines gradually become less frequent and eventually stop altogether. Basilar artery migraine must be distinguished from *benign childhood epilepsy with occipital paroxysms* (discussed later).

Ophthalmoplegic migraine usually manifests as a unilateral third nerve palsy in the wake of a migraine headache.[232] It has a predilection for young children and the first episode may be in infancy.[189,235] Even in children, ophthalmoplegic migraine is rare and has always been considered a diagnosis of exclusion. However, several recent reports of MR imaging in ophthalmoplegic migraine have described focal gadolinium enhancement of the oculomotor nerve in the perimesencephalic cistern,[213] suggesting that there may now be a way to positively establish the diagnosis in some cases.[50,143] The clinical features and differential diagnosis of ophthalmoplegic migraine are detailed in chapter 6.

Pathophysiology of Migraine

Originally, the symptoms of migraine were attributed to abnormal vascular activity. It now seems more likely that most of the visual symptomatology is related to spreading depression and secondary vasoconstriction.[127,164] Olesen et al[163] have used serial cerebral blood-flow measurement by the intracarotid xenon-133 technique to show that patients with classic migraine have localized decreases in blood flow beginning in the occipital lobes that spread continuously along the cerebral cortex and do not follow a vascular pattern. Bilateral cerebral hypoperfusion beginning in the occipital lobes and spreading anteriorly into the temporal and parietal lobes was also recently documented by positron emission tomography (PET) scanning during a classic migraine attack.[252] The region of decrease in cerebral blood flow expands at a rate of 2.2 mm/min. This is similar to the rate of spread of experimentally produced spreading depression through the occipital lobe, as well as the involvement of the visual scotoma reported by many patients with classic migraine.[120,127] The concept of spreading depression was introduced on the basis of experimental data in which changes in intracellular/extracellular potassium ion concentrations were induced to spread across the cortex after a central depolarization.[128] It could be surmised that the reductions in cerebral blood flow and the spread of the reduction in cerebral blood flow at a rate similar to spreading depression could occur because the blood flow to the area decreases in response to the metabolic abnormality. (Spontaneous spreading depression is difficult to record in humans because the slowly varying phenomena of spreading depression cannot be observed in surface electroencephalography, but it has been demonstrated by magnetic encephalography.)[238] It is unknown whether spreading depression can occur spontaneously, and its role in migraine is unproven but remains circumstantially appealing.[127]

There is also evidence for increased extracellular potassium and glutamate and reduced intracellular magnesium levels in the brains of migraine patients.[238,239] Stimulation of the serotonergic pathways from the brainstem to the cortex and cerebral arteries may initiate the migraine. Large quantities of serotonin from neurons and platelets are released during the aura with subsequent depletion of serotonin in the headache stage to follow. The other major physiologic abnormalities described in migraine pathogenesis relate to platelet function. Elevation of the serum content of the platelet factors has been documented during migraine attacks, including beta-thromboglobulin and platelet factor IV.[90] Patients experiencing a migraine attack have been documented to show a decrease in serotonin and a rise in urinary 5-HIAA.[43] It has been postulated that spontaneous platelet aggregation and release of platelet contents in the occipital cortex could trigger spreading depression with a subsequent drop in regional cerebral blood flow following the migration of spreading depression.[103]

As stated previously, the known pathophysiology, clinical manifestations, and treatment of migraine bear little resemblance to those of isolated vasospasm with secondary constriction and dilation of intracranial and extracranial arteries. Migraine seems to be a common inherited diathesis, probably dominantly involving central nervous system (CNS) neuronal excitability,[238] with vascular epiphenomena involving primarily large and medium-sized vessels. The visual aura in migraine may be related to cerebral ion flux and the headache to edema. It is usually treated with vasoconstriction and anti-inflammatory drugs.[250] By contrast, vasospasm denotes a temporary reduction in arterial caliber that is grossly discernible on angiography or retinal examination. It is usually demonstrated in the anterior circulation and best studied at the microvascular level. Vasospasm is rarely accompanied by headache and can be successfully treated with vasodilating agents.[249] While retinal vasospasm may occur idiopathically, affected individuals often may have medical histories that are significant for Raynaud phenomenon, systemic lupus erythematosus, hypercoagulability, autoimmune diseases, and atherosclerosis. Retinal vasospasm may be precipitated by a number of factors, *including* migraine headache or its pharmacological treatment with vasoconstrictors. The preponderance of evidence now suggests that reti-

nal vasoconstriction is an *epiphenomenon* rather than a *cause* of migraine.

Treatment

Reassurance that the migraine symptoms are benign is the mainstay of initial therapy. Most practitioners treating children with migraine have noted that there is a significant reduction in the frequency and intensity of migraine in children once the anxiety is relieved.[176] Parents are understandably concerned that their child may have a brain tumor or some other neurological disorder. The parents are often migraine sufferers who have adapted to the condition and are familiar with the fundamentally benign nature of the diagnosis. On occasion, it is possible to introduce the parents to a therapeutic program for their own migraine headaches at the same time the child is diagnosed and managed.

Symptomatic relief of pain and nausea is the second order of treatment. Aspirin, acetaminophen, propoxyphene, and codeine are all superior to placebo in the treatment of migraine.[88,94,116,171,209,218,240] However, many children who seek medical attention for their headaches either have tried over-the-counter analgesics with minimal relief from pain or there has been a change in the frequency or intensity of their headaches. Pharmacological treatment for pediatric headache can be divided into abortive and prophylactic therapy. The avoidance of medications with addictive potential should be encouraged in any treatment plan.

There are few clinical studies that have evaluated the use of either abortive or prophylactic medications in the pediatric population; in fact, most do not have pediatric indications for treating headache. However, the majority have been used extensively in children and are felt to be safe and effective. Abortive therapy should be considered for those children who experience infrequent headaches (less than two per month), especially if the headaches are preceded by a visual, sensory, or motor aura. Abortive medications are most effective in the preheadache phase. However, new medications are available that have proven effective when administered during any phase of the headache. These medications are more attractive for use in the child, who is less likely to ask for medication until they have significant head pain or are experiencing other symptoms of migraine, such as vomiting.

Abortive medications include Midrin (acetaminophen, isometheptene, and dichloro-phenazone), taken at onset and repeated hourly for 1 to 2 hours; Fioricet (acetaminophen, caffeine, and butalbital), taken 1 or 2 every 6 hours for headache; and Imitrex (sumatriptan), 6 mg given subcutaneously at onset of headache.[144] While there are few clinical studies that prove efficacy, these agents have been widely used and appear to be safe and effective. Ergotamines are rarely used in children due to their propensity to cause vomiting.[70] Compazine and DHE-45 have been used in an emergency room setting for the treatment of acute headache.

Migraine headaches that are frequent or severe enough to require prophylactic therapy are relatively uncommon in childhood.[220] Only 18% of children less than 8 years of age with migraine have more than one attack per month.[156] Prophylactic therapy is warranted when the child has frequent headaches (>4 per month) or if the headaches are infrequent but severe or if the child fails to respond to abortive therapy. Most medications used for adult migraine prophylaxis have been used in pediatrics, some have clinical studies to support their use while others are used based on clinical experience. Some studies have shown propranolol and anticonvulsants to be effective in the treatment of migraine in children;[10,68,141] however, other studies have questioned these results.[64,165] In our experience, these medications frequently have side effects (lethargy, tiredness, apathy, memory problems), and we use them infrequently. Periactin (cyproheptadine) is an effective prophylactic medication, but it causes drowsiness and weight gain.

The most effective prophylactic medications in our experience are the tricyclic antidepressants (particularly amitriptyline) at small doses and the calcium channel blockers (particularly verapamil). If the headache is exclusively migrainous, with no other headache (e.g., tension headache) occurring at regular intervals, we consider verapamil a safe and effective prophylactic medication.[7] The starting dose is generally 20 mg t.i.d. in younger children and 40 mg t.i.d. in older children. This dosage can gradually be increased, with the final daily dosage rarely exceeding 240 mg. Side effects are few, with constipation being the most common. Amitriptyline also appears to be a safe and effective prophylactic medication. It has been proven effective in the treatment of both migraine and tension-type headaches in adults[41,257] and appears to be equally safe and effective in children, at much lower doses than those used to treat depression. For this reason, the prophylactic effect of amitriptyline against migraine is believed to be independent of its antidepressant effect. Once-a-day dosing (bedtime), relative infrequent side effects (transient daytime sedation), and improvement in sleep patterns makes it attractive to use in children. Children younger than 5 years of age are usually given 10 mg as a starting dose, while older children are started at 25 mg. This dose can be gradually increased at 3- to 4-week intervals, with a maximum dose that rarely exceeds 75 mg a day. A baseline EKG should be obtained prior to starting any tricyclic antidepressant to look for a prolonged PR (greater than 0.20 ms) or corrected QT interval, which is greater than 0.45 ms. A follow-up EKG is obtained once a therapeutic level has been reached. Treatment for 2 to 6 months is usually recommended before the child is weaned from the medication. Many children will, at some point, require reinstitution of a prophylactic medication if the headaches become frequent again. Relaxation techniques and biofeedback have been found to have both short- and long-term benefits in migraine.[48] The concentration and effort required to learn these techniques limit their usefulness in children, but these techniques should be considered in children who seem intractable to other therapy.

Epilepsy

Epileptiform Visual Symptoms with Seizure Aura

Gowers,[79] in 1879, described a patient with epilepsy who had "epileptoid attacks with visual aura." The patient described episodes of having a very brilliant image before him "as if he had a polished plate on his breast" or "a flickering light, like a gold serpent." Gowers then examined the records of a thousand of his personal patients with epilepsy and found 84 who exhibited a visual aura.[79] Holmes[99] expanded on the findings of Gowers in his classic studies of gunshot wounds to the occipital region and elaborated on elementary visual hallucinations and temporary blindness as features of epilepsy in these patients. Penfield and Erickson[172] reported the ability to reproduce the visual aura by cortical stimulation of the occipital lobe at the time of surgery. Since that time, elementary visual hallucinations have been reported as the commonest symptom of occipital lobe epilepsy.[142,197,247,248]

Children with a seizure focus may have irritative visual hallucinations associated with a purely focal seizure in which the visual hallucinations are associated with only minimal alterations in consciousness or with a more dramatic seizure with secondary generalization. The degree of organization of the visual hallucinations or images reflects the anatomical area of the visual sensory system that is involved in the abnormal discharge. The most complex visual scenes will be produced by seizure discharge in the temporal lobe, which may take the form of vivid and detailed scenes containing recognizable human and animal forms that move and interact. Some children report autoscopic phenomena (visual reproductions of the self or parts of the body in external space) as part of a temporal lobe aura.[244] Focal seizures in visual association areas may also produce complex imagery, including geometric shapes, such as squares and triangles, or simple animal forms.

Occipital lobe seizure foci are more common in children than adults. Generalized seizures may or may not emanate from this focus. When they do, epileptic photopsias last only seconds or, rarely, minutes before the onset of a seizure. A focal seizure in the occipital cortex produces the simplest form of epileptic visual image consisting of multicolored hallucinations with circular or spherical patterns contralateral to the focus.[169] Some patients also report an unusual sensation that their eyes are moving.[100] In a review of 42 patients with medically refractory occipital lobe epilepsy, 29% of the patients described blacking out of the vision, sometimes lasting for several minutes. In many of these patients, no other manifestation of seizure activity occurred.[197] Visual hallucinations, usually described as flashing, colored lights, stars, wheels, or triangles, were commonly described. Only a small number of patients had formed vi-

sual hallucinations, and of these patients, all had right-sided occipital lesions. In this series, 46% became seizure free, and 21% had a significant reduction in seizure frequency following surgical excision of the epileptic focus. Ludwig and Marsan[142] found simple visual aura to be the most prevalent subjective sensory experience (47%) among 55 epileptic patients with EEG evidence of exclusively or predominantly occipital involvement.[258] Visual field defects are found in 20% of epileptic patients with electroencephalographic evidence of occipital foci.[142] Other estimates of the overall incidence of visual disturbances in epilepsy have ranged from 4% to 10%.[73,173] Visual aura was most common in the reports in which the patients were selected according to the criteria of occipital epileptiform involvement.[258]

Occipital lobe epilepsy has been divided into *symptomatic* and *benign* categories. The benign form (termed *benign childhood epilepsy with occipital paroxysms*) is characterized by a prominent abnormal ERG but no structural lesions or focal neurological signs. The seizures may begin with unformed visual hallucinations followed by a sequence of events that simulate basilar artery migraine.[168] This form of epilepsy tends to be easily controlled with medication and gradually resolves with age.[158] Affected children often have a positive family history of both migraine and epilepsy.[71] The symptomatic variety is caused by structural lesions (e.g., gliotic or inflammatory scarring of brain tissue, porencephalic cysts, glial tumors, or angiomatous lesions) and focal neurological signs. It tends to be more refractory to medical treatment.[142]

Ictal Cortical Blindness

Since occipital epileptiform activity is most common in children, ictal cortical blindness should be considered in the differential diagnosis of intermittent cortical blindness in children.[258] Children with epilepsy limited to the occipital lobe may have acute cortical blindness as the major manifestation of the seizure.[258] Most reports describe cases in which amaurosis was the sole presentation of epileptic activity (i.e., an "ictal equivalent") or cases in which epileptiform activity was documented by EEG during the amaurotic episode. Due to the inherent difficulty involved in obtaining an EEG during these brief attacks (unless they occur frequently), the diagnosis is often made presumptively based upon the presence of interictal occipital epileptiform activity. Strauss[215] described an 11-year-old boy who suffered from attacks of complete blindness lasting 2 to 10 minutes with preservation of consciousness. The postictal EEG showed biooccipital epileptic activity, with similar and often simultaneous activity in the temporal lobes. Zung and Margalith[258] described a 7-year-old boy who experienced several episodes of complete visual loss, accompanied by gastrointestinal symptoms and a sensation of fright, but with preservation of consciousness. These episodes ended abruptly with visual recovery and no postictal phenomena. Computed tomography scanning was normal, and interictal EEG showed biooccipital epileptiform activity.

Postictal Blindness

Cortical blindness is a rare but well-recognized manifestation of epilepsy. Children seem to have transient visual loss following seizures more commonly than adults.[118,195] Similar to the weakness of Todd's paralysis, postictal blindness is usually temporary; but cases of permanent visual loss have been described.[2,117,194] These episodes of permanent visual loss have occurred in patients with pre-existing visual abnormalities.[170] Harris[92] reported several cases of hemianopia following unilateral convulsions. Postictal blindness may range in duration from minutes to days, and in rare cases, it may last several weeks.[118] The mechanisms of postictal visual loss are poorly understood. Perma-

nent neurological damage following seizures has usually been attributed to the effects of hypotension, ischemia, acidosis, and hypoxia. Permanent blindness following generalized seizures has been likewise attributed to the effects of poor oxygenation.[195] However, primate studies have demonstrated that prolonged seizure activity can produce neuronal damage without hypotension, acidosis, or hypoxia.[150] It may be that prolonged seizure activity can directly injure the visual cortex and thereby lead to permanent visual loss.

Distinguishing Epilepsy from Migraine

There is considerable overlap in the symptoms produced by epilepsy and migraine in children.[14] Both disorders are episodic, with sudden onset and recovery. Both may have visual loss or hallucinations, are frequently associated with headache and behavioral changes, and are associated with neuronal hyperexcitability. There is an increased incidence of epilepsy among migraineurs and of migraine among epileptics.[16,45,113,138] Although headaches associated with seizures are usually postictal, ictal headaches may occasionally be the sole expression of a seizure in the limbic system and/or other parts of the cortex.[145,216] The utility of electroencephalography in distinguishing epilepsy from migraine is unfortunately limited since EEG abnormalities, including focal epileptiform changes, have been reported in up to 74% of children with migraine who never develop clinical epilepsy.[14]

The neurological features that can be used to differentiate migraine from epilepsy are summarized in Table 5.1. The major differentiating

Table 5.1. Clinical features useful in differentiating migraine from epilepsy. (Modified from Hanson[91].)

	Migraine	Seizure
Onset	Rapid (minutes)	Acute (seconds)
Duration	Longer (minutes to hours)	Brief (minutes)
Termination	Gradual	Sudden (but may be followed by a more gradual postictal recovery)
Family history of migraine	Positive (+++)	Negative (+/−)
Consciousness	Usually normal	Commonly impaired
Other symptoms of seizures	Usually absent	Usually present
Quality of symptoms	Pain	Ill-defined, not similar to any previous experience (if recurrent, then stereotypical)
EEG	Variable, usually not epileptiform	Usually frankly epileptiform
Response to treatment	Responds to migraine medications or antiepileptic drugs	No response to migraine medications, response to antiepileptic drugs

feature is that consciousness may be lost or substantially altered during a seizure and the transition is relatively abrupt. The most common phenomenon in a complex partial seizure is progression to a state of altered consciousness with an appearance of confusion and bewilderment accompanied by unresponsiveness. This is frequently the result of spread of the ictal discharge into the temporal lobe following occipital origination. Progression to loss of consciousness or secondary generalization with the production of a convulsive seizure may also occur. Loss of consciousness does not occur in most forms of migraine, but it may occur in basilar artery migraine.[19]

The characteristics of the visual hallucinations and their temporal relationship to other symptoms are also useful in distinguishing epilepsy from migraine. The visual hallucinations of migraine are usually present longer (20 to 30 minutes) than the visual aura of a seizure (seconds to a few minutes). The classic fortification specter of migraine has not been reported as a seizure manifestation.[167] Panayiotopoulos[169] recently compared elementary visual hallucinations in 50 patients with migraine and 20 patients with occipital epileptic seizures and found that epileptic seizures are predominantly multicolored with circular or spherical patterns as opposed to the predominantly black and white linear patterns of migraine. Elementary visual hallucinations, particularly when combined with headache, vomiting, or blindness, are more likely to be diagnosed as characteristic of migraine despite the fact that they are also common ictal manifestations of occipital lobe seizures.[169] Other major points of differentiation between epilepsy and migraine are summarized in Table 5.2 (see page 184).

The distinction between migraine and epilepsy becomes critical in the child with photopsias and headaches who harbors an occipital arteriovenous malformation. In the absence of other clinical evidence of seizure activity, the character of the photopsias and their temporal relationship to the headache can often provide a historical clue to the presence of an occipital seizure focus. A history of flickering photopsias that begin abruptly, terminate abruptly, and remain stationary rather than enlarging in a crescendo-like fashion suggests the possibility of an occipital arteriovenous malformation (AVM) or other seizure focus as opposed to mi-

grainous cortical phenomena, and the need for neuroimaging and electroencephalography.[224] Darkening or dimming of the homonymous visual field is also suggestive of seizure activity.[224] In patients with arteriovenous malformations, the visual disturbances start and almost always remain on the same side of the visual field (contralateral to the lesion), and headaches are usually localized to the side of the lesion and often lack the typical pulsatile quality of migraine.[224]

There is some evidence to suggest that occipital mass lesions may also predispose patients to developing classic migraine headaches.[154] Troost et al[225] reported a patient with an occipital AVM who described typical fortification scintillating scotomas lasting less than 30 minutes with "buildup" that preceded a pulsatile, nauseating headache. After removal of the AVM, the migrainous attacks resolved. Riaz et al[186] described a similar patient whose typical migraine headaches resolved following resection of a meningioma. The authors speculated that activation of intradural and extradural arteriovenous shunts by a vascular meningioma could effectively create a migraine diathesis.

Posttraumatic Transient Cerebral Blindness

Occipital head trauma in children may produce a syndrome of transient cerebral blindness. This condition occurs preferentially following occipital head trauma, and there may be a delay of minutes to hours between the trauma and the onset of the blindness. The blindness is often accompanied by other symptoms, including somnolence, confusion, agitation, or vomiting. The duration of blindness may range from several hours to a day, and the prognosis for return to normal vision is excellent. Electroconvulsive discharges are sometimes recorded from the occipital head regions during the first day following the injury. Greenblatt[82] has called attention to the strong migraine and seizure diathesis in children who develop this syndrome and suggested that vasomotor and neuronal instability may be important factors in its pathogenesis. The "ding" injury in football may produce a transient confusional state indistinguishable from transient global amnesia. These patients may have migraine features, and it has been suggested that most cases of transient global amnesia are migrainous.

The possibility of *arterial dissection* should also be considered in children who present with transient visual loss following head or neck trauma.[95] Carotid artery dissection presents with a nonthrobbing headache ipsilateral to the dissection. The pain may be retro-orbital and extend to the face and neck. It is often accompanied by a bad taste in the mouth. The telltale neuro-ophthalmologic sign in carotid dissection is an ipsilateral postganglionic Horner syndrome. Carotid artery dissection may produce transient monocular visual loss or scintillating scotomata with headache, which simulates a migraine headache.[183] Vertebral artery dissection is characterized by posterior headache or neck pain, which may be accompanied by other brainstem signs of vertebrobasilar ischemia. The most common visual symptoms include transient visual symptoms and diplopia. Treatment of arterial dissection usually consists of anticoagulation or anticoagulation followed by an antiplatelet agent.[95] Surgical intervention is an option in patients with progressive neurological deficits.

Cardiogenic Embolism

Heart disease is considered to be the most common cause of stroke in children.[187] Cerebrovascular emboli from the heart have been associated with a number of congenital and acquired disorders. Potential sources of cardiac emboli include left atrial myxoma, vegetative valvular lesions associated with bacterial endocarditis or old rheumatic heart disease, mitral valve prolapse, and atrial septal defects (including patent foramen ovale), which may be associated with right-to-left shunting of "paradoxical emboli."[251] Heart defects with a right-to-left intracardiac shunt can also cause polycythemia, with potential for thrombosis.[187] Most of these conditions can be identified by echocardiography. However, the demonstration of a cardiac abnormality in a child with a previous stroke or with transient neurological disturbances does not constitute proof that the cardiac lesion is causative.

Emboli from the venous circulation are ordinarily unable to enter the systemic arterial circulation since they are filtered by the lungs. A patent foramen ovale provides venous emboli direct access to the systemic circulation and may be a source of "paradoxical" embolism that can cause cerebral and retinal dysfunction in patients of all ages.[251] As with mitral valve prolapse, the subject of patent foramen ovale has generated considerable interest as more sensitive echocardiographic techniques have revealed a higher prevalence of anatomical defects than was previously recognized. Specifically, a number of recent studies have attempted to define the risk of developing neurological dysfunction when a patent foramen ovale is present. Several studies have found a significantly higher prevalence of patent foramen ovale in patients with stroke (40% versus 10%) and transient cerebral ischemic events than in control patients.[129,255] One recent study found that the association of mitral valve prolapse with stroke is not significant when controlled for the presence of a patent foramen ovale.[129]

Transesophageal echocardiography has proven to be more sensitive than routine transthoracic echocardiography for detecting patency of the foramen ovale in older patients.[47,255] In infants and young children, transesophageal echocardiography requires general anesthesia. Many pediatric cardiologists reserve transesophageal echocardiography for cases in which there is a high index of suspicion for intrinsic cardiac disease.

The diagnosis of paradoxical embolism associated with a patent foramen ovale should be considered in children with cerebral or retinal ischemic events who (1) have been at prolonged bedrest, (2) have a history of lower extremity or pelvic fracture (producing the potential for venous stasis), and (3) have symptoms brought on by a Valsalva maneuver (which can reverse the normal intracardiac left-to-right pressure gradient).[23] Associated venous thrombosis may be clinically occult, with no detectable signs of thrombophlebitis.[129] Treatments for patent foramen ovale with paradoxical emboli include anticoagulation, interruption of the vena cava, or surgical closure of the foramen ovale.[129] Many cardiologists are unenthusiastic about closing a patent foramen ovale surgically, even in children who have had cerebral ischemic events.

Nonmigrainous Cerebrovascular Disease

An exhaustive list of systemic vasculopathies and coagulopathies has been associated with stroke in children.[187] Many of these conditions also produce retinal vascular occlusions. These include systemic vascular disease (e.g., hypertension), hemoglobinopathies (e.g., sickle cell disease), coagulopathies (e.g., antiphospholipid antibody syndrome, protein C deficiency, protein S deficiency), collagen vascular diseases (e.g., systemic lupus erythematosus), and structural vasculopathies (e.g., moyamoya disease).[187] Nantowicz and Kelley[159] have summarized the many hereditary disorders that predispose to embolic, thrombotic, or hemorrhagic stroke. Certain rare conditions, especially moyamoya disease, can be present with transient visual loss or scintillating scotoma.[153a] Whether all of these conditions can produce transient visual loss in children is unclear, since children with known cerebrovascular disease are rarely asked about previous visual symptoms. Statistically, children with transient visual loss rarely turn out to have cerebrovascular disease as the underlying cause. Furthermore, a positive laboratory study does not necessarily establish a cause for the visual symptoms. Investigative studies are generally reserved for children who display other systemic signs of vascular disease or who have had a previous stroke or retinal vascular occlusion.

The MELAS syndrome (mitochondrial encephalopathy, lactic acidosis, and strokelike episodes) can frequently present with transient visual loss in early childhood.[58] These children have episodes of vomiting, migrainelike headaches, seizures, and strokelike events. The MELAS syndrome may underlie the "malignant migraine syndrome" in which children with complicated migraine headaches develop intractable seizures and large alternating occipital infarcts.[51] Initially, there may be surprising improvement with partial recovery, but recurrent strokelike episodes leave these children with mental deterioration, hemiparesis, hemianopsia, or blindness. Additional neuro-ophthalmologic findings include chronic progressive external ophthalmoplegia, optic atrophy, and atypical pigmentary retinopathy with macular involvement.[193] Other systemic abnormalities may include short stature, sensorineural deafness, and muscle weakness.[78] Ragged-red fibers and complex I deficiency is usually seen in their muscle biopsies, and serum lactate levels are elevated.[78] Similar features may be found in family members. Magnetic resonance (MR) imaging shows multifocal areas of hyperintense signal confined to the cortex of the cerebrum, cerebellum, and immediately adjacent white matter, with relative sparing of deep white matter.[149] At present, three mitochondrial DNA mutations have been associated with MELAS syndrome.[97]

Miscellaneous Transient Visual Disturbances in Children

Transient Visual Obscurations Associated with Papilledema

Transient visual obscurations associated with increased intracranial pressure may be monocular or binocular. They may be described by the child as a graying out or a blurring out of the vision and usually last only a few seconds at a time. There is usually a buildup in the frequency of the obscurations over time until a diagnosis is made. The child may describe dozens of these episodes over the course of a day. Precipitating factors may include rapid changes in position or Valsalva maneuvers; however, the obscurations may occur with no precipitating event. These transient visual obscurations can be distinguished from migraine by their frequency, lack of any positive visual scotoma, and the rapidity with which they come and go. In our experience, most children with elevated intracranial pressure present initially with complaints of headache, nausea, and vomiting and acknowledge transient visual disturbances only when asked. Transient visual disturbances are rare as a presenting symptom.

Headaches associated with elevated intracranial pressure share a number of similarities with migraine headaches. Like migraine headaches, these headaches are made worse by coughing, sneezing, or changes in posture, and they are not relieved by mild analgesics, such as acetaminophen. Headaches associated with increased intracranial pressure tend to be worse in the reclined position, causing some patients to prop themselves up to sleep in a position that reduces venous pressure. Unlike migraine headaches, they are rarely of sufficient severity to necessitate an emergency room visit (*excruciating* headaches are rarely caused by brain tumors). They are frequently present on awakening, in contradistinction to migraine headaches, which are usually *relieved* by sleep. In a comparison study of headache characteristics in patients with migraine versus brain tumors, Rossi and Vassella[191] found nocturnal headache, headache present on arising, and increased frequency of headache, to be most predictive of brain tumor. The authors noted that progressive neurological symptoms or signs appeared within 4 months of the headache onset in 94% of cases with tumors. However, elevated intracranial pressure headaches cannot always be clinically distinguished from migraine since vascular symptomatology may also accompany the headache of elevated intracranial pressure. Children with preexisting migraine headaches can also develop brain tumors.

Anomalous Optic Discs

Transient visual loss has been documented in eyes with anomalous elevated optic discs, including pseudopapilledema with and without visible drusen, and congenitally tilted discs. Most reported cases are in adults, suggesting that the disc elevation may have to reach some critical degree before visual symptoms develop. Lorentzen[140] reported an 8.6% incidence of visual obscurations (and in some cases amaurosis) in patients with disc drusen. Sadun et al[196] proposed a vascular hypothesis by which both papilledema and anomalous elevation of the optic discs lead to increased interstitial pressure and decreased perfusion pressure in the intraocular portion of the optic nerve so that minor fluctuations in arterial, venous, or cerebrospinal fluid pressure would result in brief but critical decrements in perfusion, leading to transient obscurations of vision. Katz and Hoyt recently described an uncommon disorder associated with anomalous optic discs and posterior vitreous detachment.[111] They described a group of young myopic Asians (ages ranging from 11 to 42) whose optic discs were mildly dysplastic and slightly elevated. These patients manifested

intrapapillary and subretinal peripapillary hemorrhages, with incomplete posterior vitreous detachment. Visual symptoms were mild (blur, spot, smudge) or absent, but abnormalities were detected on visual field testing in most cases. They suggested that elevated anomalous optic discs may have abnormal vitreopapillary adhesions and may be unusually susceptible to vitreous traction.

Transient visual loss can also occur in patients with excavated optic disc anomalies.[80,204] Graether[80] described a young adult who had episodes of amaurosis accompanied by transient dilation of the retinal veins in an eye with a morning glory disc anomaly. Seybold described a young adult who had transient visual obscurations in an eye with a peripapillary staphyloma. In both cases, the amaurosis could be induced by light stimulation.

Entoptic Images

Entoptic images are formed by the reproducible perception of objects within the eye, the anatomical structures of the eye, or the perception of the consequences of nonphotic stimulation of the visual sensory apparatus of the eye. Under normal circumstances, these stimuli are either not perceived or ignored; however, under special viewing circumstances, they may become manifest. Although children are less likely to report them, there is no reason to believe that they are less able to perceive them.

Media Opacities

The common entopic phenomenon of the perception of vitreous floaters seen in adults occurs by similar mechanism in children. Posterior vitreous detachment is only rarely seen in children, but children with vitreous hemorrhages may report the characteristic movement of shadows as the blood clears. Perceptive and articulate children with corneal or lenticular opacities are sometimes able to see the opacity and describe the circumstances in which they become most apparent to them, such as with variability in illumination.

Retinal Circulation

Children may independently report the flying capillary phenomenon that consists of bright dots of light moving away from the blind spot area when looking at a Ganzfeld-like background, such as the sky, or a large uniform surface, such as a ceiling or a light-colored painted wall.

Phosphenes

The production of phosphenes by pressing on the eye is a particularly important phenomenon when dealing with children with low vision, especially of retinal origin. The repetitive finger poking into the eye in order to produce these sensations by the otherwise blind child may result in atrophy of orbital fat and discoloration of the lids and periorbital tissues. Strategies to keep the child otherwise occupied may prevent these disfiguring consequences. However, the determined child will be very difficult to dissuade from this activity. Phosphenes on eye movement and with sudden loud noises have been reported in young adults with optic neuritis, and this has been likened to Lhermitte sign.[44,133]

Uhthoff Symptom

In patients with multiple sclerosis, minor elevation of body temperature by external causes or physical activity increases neural transmission but rapidly leads to electrophysiological blockage through areas of demyelination. This phenomenon, termed Uhthoff symptom, commonly affects the optic nerve, causing visual blurring or amaurosis lasting minutes to an hour. It is less common in children than adults, presumably due to the lower incidence of multiple sclerosis in children. Transient monocular diminution in vision can be brought on by bathing in hot water, hot weather, exercise, consuming hot food or drink, and less frequently, by emotional disturbances, fatigue, menstruation, increased lighting, smoking, or cooking.[131]

Lepore[131] found Uhthoff syndrome in 18 of 100 patients with pregeniculate visual loss; 10 had multiple sclerosis, four had compressive lesions, and four had other lesions. Neither the extent of visual field loss, decreased acuity, or binocular deficits correlated significantly with Uhthoff symptom. Thus, Uhthoff symptom is strongly but not invariably associated with multiple sclerosis. It has been suggested that hyperthermia is not the exclusive cause of Uhthoff symptom and that

changes in metabolic status and ionic channel kinetics that alter the conduction properties of demyelinated fibers can cause this phenomenon.[131, 203,236]

Alice in Wonderland Syndrome

In 1952, Lippman[137] used the term "Alice in Wonderland syndrome" to describe the impairment of time sense and body image in a patient with migraine. Todd[221] later used the term to describe the strange distortions of body size and distance from their surroundings perceived by patients with migraine, epilepsy, hypnotic states, drug intoxication with LSD or marijuana, fever, cerebral lesions, and schizophrenia. Copperman[39] reported the association between infectious mononucleosis and Alice in Wonderland syndrome in three children whose symptoms included macropsia, micropsia, metamorphopsia, teleopsia, xanthopsia, and a detached feeling. Numerous children have since been noted to develop these acute perceptual disturbances, usually during the acute phase of infectious mononucleosis[39,83,136,198] and as an accompaniment of juvenile migraine.[76] The condition is self-limited and requires no specific treatment.

Charles Bonnet Syndrome

Healthy elderly patients with bilaterally decreased vision may experience vivid, formed hallucinations in the absence of a psychiatric disorder (termed the Charles Bonnet syndrome). These vivid images are believed to represent release hallucinations since they occur in the absence of CNS pathology and may cease following improvement in vision.[162] These hallucinations have the following general features: (1) They are exclusively visual, complex, well formed, and often lifelike in their actions, frequently involving people and places. (2) They occur with insight and an otherwise clear consciousness; affected patients know they are hallucinating. (3) The hallucinations are devoid of emotional content (unlike those of peduncular hallucinosis, which is associated with a pleasurable affective reaction). (4) They are superimposed on or occur in combination with normal perceptions. (5) They are brief, lasting a few minutes at most. (6) They are much more common in the elderly. (7) They generally occur in the setting of visual loss, which has been gradual (most commonly cataract formation).[190] The Charles Bonnet syndrome is benign and usually self-limited; however, occasional patients may continue to hallucinate for years with little response to anticonvulsants or other medications.

The rarity of this syndrome in children may reflect the fact that most forms of bilateral visual loss in childhood are congenital and nonprogressive. However, White and Jan recently documented the Charles Bonnet syndrome in a 3½-year-old child who became acutely blind following surgical resection of a chiasmal glioma.[246] The child developed complex visual hallucinations that he believed were real. This child would see his brother, Santa Claus, animals, and other familiar objects in his visual field, when, in fact, he had no light perception. Although the child had had diminished vision prior to surgery, the change to no light perception was acute. Apart from these findings, the child had a normal mental status examination and an electroencephalogram was normal.[246]

The formed and unformed visual hallucinations that occur in the hemianopic field of adults with occipitovascular disease may be of the irritative or release variety.[36] Children with congenital hemianopic defects do not complain of similar hallucinations, probably because they have never experienced vision in the affected hemifield and therefore do not have the visual association area connections that become deafferented in adults.

Lilliputian Hallucinations

The term Lilliputian hallucinations refers to the perception of very small, perfectly formed figures, usually active and mobile, gaily colored, and pleasant to look upon.[199] Despite their unique character, they seem to be a nonspecific finding, since they have been reported in various forms of intoxication, visual deprivation, acute infection, epilepsy, and CNS tumor and infarction. Lilliputian hallucinations have been reported in children with scarlet fever and measles.[199]

Palinopsia

Palinopsia is a rare symptom in which there is visual perseveration beyond the physiological afterimage.[42,102,132] It is experienced as a persistence or reappearance of portions of a recently-viewed scene. Some cases consist of freeze-frame or stroboscopic images of a moving stimulus.[102] Palinopsia is usually accompanied by other visual hallucinations or a hemianopia. When a visual field defect is present, symptoms usually involve the hemianopic field.[152] It is rare for palinopsia to occur as an isolated visual phenomenon. Palinopsia has been noted predominantly with vascular or neoplastic lesions of the posterior portions of the cerebral hemispheres, the majority of which have been right-sided.[17] Less commonly, it has been reported in association with seizures, hallucinogenic drug use, antidepressant therapy (Trazadone), encephalopathy, and migraine.[102] Palinopsia may occasionally respond to anticonvulsant therapy.[26]

Although a number of elaborate theories have been advanced to explain the existence of palinopsia (enhancement of the normal physiological afterimage, release hallucination, sensory seizure, involuntary visual memory), its neuropharmacological mechanism remains unclear.

Peduncular Hallucinosis

Peduncular hallucinosis is a rare phenomenon in which vascular disease of the cerebral peduncles or associated midbrain structures is associated with moving, intensely colorful visual imagery that changes in a kaleidoscopic fashion and is nonthreatening and often pleasurable to the patient.[72,244] The hallucinations may consist of geometric patterns and designs or as more elaborate pictures, such as landscapes, country and mountain scenes, flowers, birds, animals, or human beings.[160] Although formed visual hallucinations do not generally have strong localizing value, peduncular hallucinosis is usually associated with other neuro-ophthalmologic signs of midbrain dysfunction, allowing clinical localization of the lesion.[72] Autopsy studies and neuroimaging have confirmed lesions intrinsic to or compressing the midbrain.[32,49,59,72,157,228]

Peduncular hallucinosis is believed to be a special form of release hallucination caused by diminished activity in the reticular activating system and other ascending brainstem pathways leading to abnormal activity in the temporal lobes. Sleep disturbances often coexist, and it has been suggested that peduncular hallucinosis may be due to a dissociation of the sleep mechanism causing dream activity to be released while consciousness remains normal or nearly so.[160]

Hypnagogic Hallucinations

Hypnagogic hallucinations are fragments of rapid eye movement (REM) sleep that occur during entry into sleep. They may be visual or auditory. The visual ones consist of vivid scenes, objects, animals, or people that may be frightening to the child or elementary hallucinations, such as flashes or patterns.[133] Hypnagogic visual hallucinations may occur in normal children,[244] but the child should be evaluated for narcolepsy if there is also a history of sleep attacks, cataplexy, or sleep paralysis.[85,86]

Hypertensive Encephalopathy

Transient cortical blindness may be the presenting manifestation of hypertensive encephalopathy in children, which is usually associated with severe renal disease.[93,147] In this setting, T2-weighted MR imaging demonstrates focal, symmetrical areas of increased signal intensity involving both gray and white matter, with no significant mass effect or cortical effacement. Vision normalizes and the associated MR abnormalities resolve following successful lowering of blood pressure, suggesting that the MR abnormalities are caused by extravasation of fluid and protein across the blood brain barrier rather than infarction.

Neurodegenerative Disease

As in adults with Alzheimer's disease, transient visual disturbances may occur as early symptoms in a variety of neurodegenerative diseases that eventually involve the optic nerves or higher cortical centers. Examples include episodic visual loss in the early stages of ornithine decarboxylase deficiency (a hyperammonemia syndrome),[207] transient homonymous hemianopia in subacute sclerosing panencephalitis,[112] and formed visual hallucinations in juvenile ceroid lipofuscinosis.[124,210,254]

Multiple Sclerosis

Transient visual disturbances may occur in children with multiple sclerosis. Recognized causes of transient visual disturbances include mild or sub-

clinical episodes of optic neuritis, Uhthoff phenomenon, phosphenes induced by ocular motion, and the Pulfrich phenomenon. (The Pulfrich effect is a well-known visual illusion in which a pendulum swinging in a frontal plane in front of a subject is perceived as moving in an oval trajectory, with the plane of the oval being parallel to the floor. It is noted most commonly in patients who have recovered from optic neuritis in one eye.)[245]

Miscellaneous

Schizophrenia

Schizophrenic hallucinations are more often auditory in nature but they may also be visual.[244] The visual hallucinations are usually of frightening objects, such as skeletons or ghosts, or may represent a recently deceased relative or friend.[65] Schizophrenic hallucinations are not influenced by eye closure or opening, as opposed to drug-induced visual disturbances that tend to exacerbate with the eyes closed.[244] Visual hallucinations have also been described in children with reactive psychosis, depressive syndromes and organic brain syndromes[65] and are reported more frequently in psychoses of late childhood.[53] Differential diagnosis from temporal lobe epilepsy is sometimes difficult due to overlap in symptomatology.

Children with less severe psychiatric disorders, such as emotional and behavior problems, also experience hallucinations in the form of fantasies and "pretend companions" that may possibly aid them in coping with their situational disturbances.[53] Such children do not appear to be at increased risk for psychosis, depressive illness, organic brain damage, or other psychiatric disorders.[66]

Hallucinogenic Drug Use

While lysergic acid diethylamide (LSD), mescaline, and psilocybin ingestion can all produce visual hallucinations, the hallucinatory phenomena associated with LSD have been studied most extensively. Ingestion of LSD can produce several organic mental disorders causing hallucinations. The first is an acute dose-related reaction involving complex formed and unformed visual hallucinations, often with auditory-visual synesthesia (the transformation of a sound stimulus into a visual experience).[244] Individuals ingesting LSD often report that they can see music or that they can hear pictures translated into sound. In some individuals, sounds of different frequencies evoke different visual hallucinations.[133,233]

A second perceptual abnormality is a delayed phenomenon involving visual flashbacks. Visual flashbacks have been estimated to occur in 5% of hallucinogenic drug users.[134] Symptoms include alterations of color perception, positive and negative afterimages, illusions of movement, halos around objects, shimmering of images, micropsia, macropsia, teleopsia, and palinopsia.[179a] These phenomena are not dose related. They may occur after only one exposure to LSD or may begin long after cessation of the drug. Flashbacks are usually episodic but, in some cases persist indefinitely.[1,4,107,134]

Cannabinoid Use

Abnormal visual perceptions may be described by patients who are using marijuana or hashish or who have recently discontinued their use. Symptoms include the following: (1) black and white spots flickering at high frequency similar to interference on a television screen, (2) a perceived reduction in depth perception, (3) visual perseveration after looking at bright objects, and (4) the perception of moving objects as a series of still pictures.[121,134] These symptoms are made worse by physical exertion or staring at bright objects. Because chronic marijuana and hashish consumption is widespread in our society and common in teenagers, a history of illicit drug use should be suspected in teenagers with these symptoms.

Toxic and Nontoxic Drug Effects

Antimetabolites and Cancer Therapy

Seizure activity, complex visual hallucinations, and cortical blindness have all been described in patients with cyclosporin neurotoxicity.[96,205,211,229] Transient or permanent visual loss has been reported among other neurological complications in patients receiving a variety of anticancer agents, including L-asparaginase and vinca alkaloids, methotrexate, FK506, methylprednisolone, and tiazofurin.[29,104,177–179,184,188,205] The mechanisms for these neurological complications are multiple. The vinca alkaloids may cause direct damage to neuronal cells by interfering with microtubule function.[29] Alternatively, arterial spasm in arteritis has been postulated as a cause in some patients.[188] Some authors have noted a pattern of lesions demonstrated by CT and MR imaging that are more characteristic of intravascular venous thrombosis rather than direct neural toxicity or arterial disease. It is well known that coagulation abnormalities are a complication of cancer, including the commonly encountered myeloproliferative disorders of childhood.[153,175] It has also been postulated that there may be direct myelin toxicity in those patients whose neuroimaging shows mainly white matter abnormalities.[205]

Digitalis

Digitalis has been known for many years to cause xanthopsia (yellow vision) in toxic dosages. Other visual abnormalities associated with digitalis toxicity include scintillating scotomas, defects in the yellow/blue color vision, and paracentral scotomas. Electroretinograms obtained in patients with digitalis toxicity have shown decreased cone-mediated wave forms and increased photopic b-wave implicit times. Symptoms of digitalis toxicity may be the result of abnormalities of sodium and potassium metabolism of the cellular membrane leading to abnormal photoreceptor polarization.[241]

Erythropoietin

Recombinant human erythropoietin is widely used in patients on dialysis to treat the anemia of chronic renal failure. Steinberg[212] described moving formed visual hallucinations without delirium or psychosis in patients who were being treated with erythropoietin.

Atropine (Anticholinergic Drugs)

Atropine can serve as a model drug for the toxicity of all anticholinergics. Visual system toxicity may be produced by overadministration of these drugs therapeutically or by encountering these in the form of belladonna, jimson weed, and stramonium. The neuropsychiatric features specifically include agitated behavior with formed visual hallucinations frequently involving seeing insects and small animals on clothing or blankets as well as disorientation to person, time, and place. Treatment is usually supportive, but cholinergic agonist therapy that penetrates the blood brain barrier, such as physostigmine, may hasten recovery.[81]

Carbon Monoxide

Carbon monoxide poisoning causes hypoxia of neural tissue due to reduced oxygen carrying capacity of blood that has had a portion of its hemoglobin converted to carboxyhemoglobin. The principle complication is CNS dysfunction. Transient visual loss of cortical origin is frequently encountered, and vision may wax and wane for several days during recovery. Visual hallucinations and agnosia have also been reported. Optic nerve damage has also been reported, but the retina is unaffected.[81]

Summary of Clinical Approach to the Child with Transient Visual Disturbances

Our approach to the child with transient visual disturbances is summarized in Figure 5.1. It includes

1. Obtaining a detailed attack history, personal profile, and family history to determine the likelihood of migrainous phenomena and to rule out other readily identifiable causes, such as drug ingestion, entoptic phenomena, transient visual obscurations, or Uhthoff phenomenon. Inquire about congenital heart disease, rheumatic fever, or cardiac symptoms, such as palpitations or shortness of breath unrelated to vigorous activity. Ask whether the child has had previous epileptic events and specifically inquire about contraversive eye movements, blinking, automatisms, or other evidence of seizure activity coincident with the visual disturbance. Has there been recent head trauma to suggest the possibility of transient posttraumatic cerebral blindness or arterial dissection? Inquire about a personal or family history of thromboembolic events and look for nail bed splinter hemorrhages that would suggest the rare possibility of antiphospholipid antibody syndrome or a protein S or C deficiency.[46]
2. Performing a complete neuro-ophthalmologic examination to look for papilledema, pseudopapilledema or other optic disc anomalies,

optic disc pallor (possibly suggesting old optic neuritis), homonymous hemianopia, or other neurological deficits. If a child is examined during an episode of monocular visual loss, look for retinal vasospasm. Carefully examine the retina for detachments, tears, signs of vitreous traction (which are easily overlooked when they overlie the disc), or retinal whitening to suggest recent infarction. When transient visual disturbances are unilateral, look for an ipsilateral Horner syndrome, which would suggest carotid artery dissection.
3. Obtaining a pediatric examination to rule out clinical signs or symptoms of cardiac disease, collagen vascular disease, hypertensive encephalopathy, or other systemic disease.

Laboratory Evaluation of Transient Visual Disturbances in Children

The laboratory investigations ordered depend upon the examiner's clinical impressions that are based on the history and physical findings (Figure 5.1). If a clear-cut clinical picture of migraine is obtained, then no investigations are indicated. If the description of the visual disturbance is reminiscent of a seizure disorder or there are other abnormalities suggestive of a CNS disorder, then MR imaging and electroencephalography should be undertaken.

Children in whom the pathophysiology of the transient visual disturbance is not clearly migrainous or epileptic pose the greatest diagnostic dilemma. Cardiac disease is more frequently recognized as a cause of permanent neurologic impairment in children now that advanced noninvasive cardiac imaging techniques such as transesophageal echography are available.[187,255] Children with a history suggestive of intrinsic cardiac disease should be referred to a pediatric cardiologist for clinical and echocardiographic evaluation. A serum hemoglobin electrophoresis is indicated in black children to rule out sickle cell disease. A complete hemogram, erythrocyte sedimentation rate, platelet count, antinuclear antibody, and partial thromboplastin time (to screen for antiphospholipid antibodies) should be obtained when there are other systemic signs to suggest a vasculopathy. In the rare cases that are particularly suspicious for thromboembolic disease, anticardiolipin antibodies,

APPROACH TO THE CHILD WITH TRANSIENT VISUAL DISTURBANCES

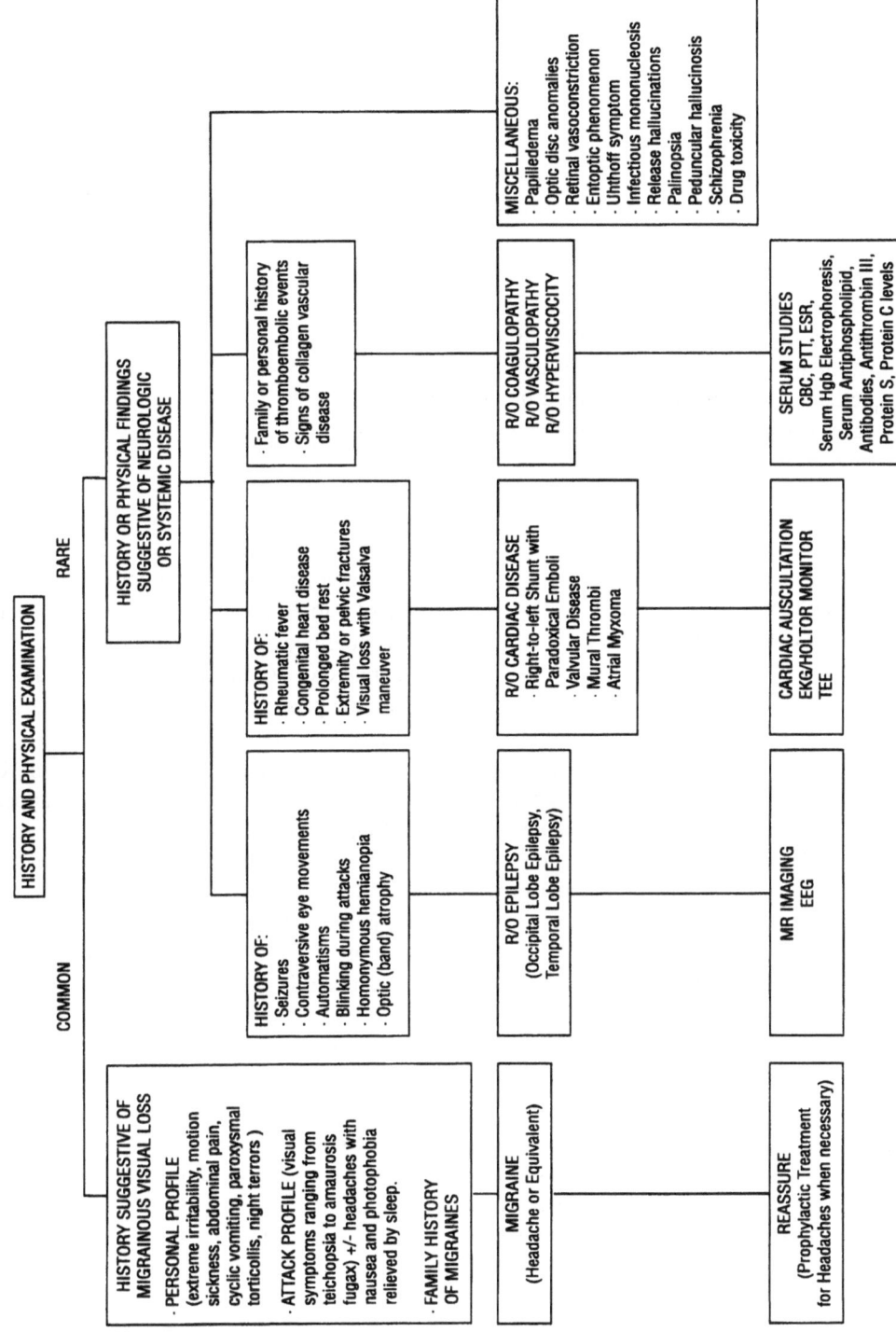

FIGURE 5.1. Approach to the child with transient visual disturbances.

antithrombin III, and protein C and S levels can be obtained to rule out a coagulopathy.

The diagnostic yield for these tests is low, but they are more likely to be abnormal when they are applied only in suspicious cases.

Unexplained Visual Loss in Children

Many children who have decreased vision are referred for neuro-ophthalmologic evaluation after ocular abnormalities have been ruled out. The subspecialist must be familiar with common as well as rare causes of unexplained visual loss in childhood so that the neuro-ophthalmologic examination and ancillary work-up can be directed in an expedient fashion (Table 5.2). Underlying conditions can range from refractive errors to retinal or intracranial disorders that can reduce vision before visible signs of disease become evident.

Causes of Unexplained Visual Loss in Childhood

Transient Amblyogenic Factors

Occasionally, a child is found consistently to have decreased vision in an eye that is otherwise normal. In such cases, it is assumed that transient amblyogenic factors must have led to amblyopia and subsequently resolved.[234] Such factors may include neonatal lid swelling, early anisometropia, transient strabismus, macular hemorrhage, and vitreous hemorrhage. Suppression on sensory testing (Bagolini striated lens, Worth Four Dot) of an eye with no structural abnormality is suggestive of amblyopia.

There is a unique disorder that may present as a deficit of stereopsis, despite relatively normal monocular visual acuity in either eye. This disorder, labeled the *monofixation syndrome,* is characterized by the presence of a facultative central scotoma in one eye under binocular viewing conditions, which is absent under monocular conditions. As a result, central fusion and fine stereopsis are lacking, but peripheral fusion (which provides fusional vergence amplitudes and gross stereopsis) is retained. While the presence of strabismus is not a prerequisite for this condition,

Table 5.2. Causes of unexplained visual loss in children.

Refractive abnormalities
  Bilateral high hyperopia
  Bilateral meridional amblyopia
Cornea
  Early keratoconus
Retina
  Stargardt disease
  Cone dystrophies (congenital cone dystrophy, early
    progressive cone dystrophy, blue-cone monochromatism)
  Acute idiopathic blind spot enlargement, MEWDS, and
    related disorders
Optic nerve
  Early bilateral optic neuritis
  Mild or segmental optic nerve hypoplasia
  Mild optic atrophy
Central nervous system
Structural abnormalities
  Suprasellar tumors (craniopharyngioma, chiasmal glioma)
  Cortical visual loss
Nonstructural deficits
  Amblyopia (due to transient amblyogenic factors)
  Monofixation syndrome
  Posttraumatic blindness

it is common for affected children to have an esotropia of 8 to 10 prism diopters or less on simultaneous prism cover testing and a larger esotropia (in the range of 16 diopters to 25 prism diopters) on alternate prism cover testing. The smaller deviation on simultaneous prism cover testing reflects the preservation of peripheral fusion. Children with monofixation syndrome may appear to have straight eyes and be found to have a surprisingly large deviation on prism alternate cover testing.

Children with monofixation syndrome often show some degree of superimposed amblyopia. The diagnosis is established by placing a four-prism diopter base-out prism sequentially in front of one eye then the other eye while the child fixates a distant target binocularly. A rapid horizontal refixation movement is observed in one eye but not in the opposite eye with the central scotoma. The absence of central fusion with preservation of peripheral fusion is also confirmed by performing the Worth Four Dot test using the handheld flashlight at near and at distance. In the monofixation syndrome, this test reveals the presence of fusion for near targets (which subtend a large angle and thereby stimulate peripheral fusion) and suppression of the involved eye for small distant targets (for which images fall within the scotoma).

Refractive Abnormalities

Children with bilateral hyperopia of 6 diopters or more can present with bilaterally decreased vision in the range of 20/100. When given their full cycloplegic refraction, their vision initially improves to 20/40 to 20/70 and in some cases may approach normal. The subnormal vision is presumed to represent a bilateral form of ametropic (form deprivation) amblyopia. Because the optic discs appear small in high hyperopes, the diagnosis of optic nerve hypoplasia may be entertained, but close examination reveals a normal peripapillary nerve fiber layer. Children with corrected bilateral meridional amblyopia may present with unexplained visual loss when the increased visual demands of school work brings attention to their visual difficulty.

One should inquire about recent ingestion of medications with anticholinergic side effects in any child who complains of blurred vision that is worse for near tasks. If accommodative amplitudes are found to be decreased, other systemic disorders associated with hypoaccommodation, such as botulism, dorsal midbrain syndrome, diabetes, head and neck trauma, diphtheria, and familial forms of hypoaccommodation, must be considered in the differential diagnosis.[217,223]

Cornea

Keratoconus in children can reduce vision in the absence of any biomicroscopic findings. Keratoconus is a progressive, noninflammatory ectasia in which the cornea assumes a progressively conical shape secondary to central thinning and protrusion. Its incidence has been estimated at 50 to 230 per 100,000. It is usually bilateral but may be unilateral or highly asymmetrical. Most patients have no family history of keratoconus, but a few autosomal dominant and recessive pedigrees have been described. Keratoconus is generally an isolated finding but may occasionally be associated with systemic disease, most notably atopic disease and Down syndrome.[9]

In children with unexplained visual loss, retinoscopy through an *undilated* pupil is a sensitive office screening test, since the earliest changes may be confined to the central cornea, and the bright reflex obtained from dilated retinoscopy may obscure these changes. The diag-

nosis of early keratoconus can be confirmed by keratoscopy.[9] Slit lamp biomicroscopic signs may be absent early on in the disorder. Corneal topography is a sensitive means of diagnosing keratoconus, although expense and availability limits its general application.

Retina

Stargardt macular dystrophy should be a major diagnostic consideration in the child who presents with unexplained or psychogenic visual loss in both eyes. Stargardt macular dystrophy is a hereditary condition (usually autosomal recessive but rarely autosomal dominant) in which central vision decreases in childhood. Occasional patients become symptomatic in adulthood.[69] Over time, there is development of atrophic macular degeneration, surrounded by yellow pisiform flecks that increase in size and number and may subsequently disappear.[24] A bull's eye maculopathy may be seen as an intermediate stage. Peripheral pigmentary clumping is also occasionally seen.

Although children with Stargardt disease eventually develop distinct retinal abnormalities, the retina may appear normal until visual acuity approaches 20/200. Some children with Stargardt disease experience significant visual loss over the course of weeks to months.[62] Once vision decreases to 20/40, it usually deteriorates rapidly to 20/200. The final visual acuity usually stabilizes in the range of 20/200 to 20/400.[62,243] Despite their diffuse retinal involvement, children with Stargardt disease have mild dyschromatopsia, mildly constricted visual fields, and no symptoms of night blindness.

The diagnosis of Stargardt disease should be suspected in a child whose "psychogenic" visual loss fails to improve with reassurance and whose color vision is relatively preserved despite poor acuity. Electroretinograms and electro-oculograms are generally unhelpful in establishing the diagnosis, since they are normal early in the disease and become only mildly abnormal in advanced disease. Fluorescein angiography shows the characteristic absence of choroidal fluorescence (termed a *silent choroid*), which is often the earliest sign of Stargardt disease.[62,226] This angiographic finding correlates with the histopathological finding of increased retinal pigment epithelial lipofuscin content.[24] Over the past few years, mutations in at least five different genes (including chromosomal regions 6q, 13q34, and 1p) have been associated with Stargardt-like phenotypes.[214,242,243,256]

Other retinal disorders can also manifest as unexplained visual loss in children. In the child with bilateral central visual loss, a normal retinal appearance, and a normal fluorescein angiogram, electroretinography may be useful to rule out a progressive cone dystrophy. In this condition, the attenuated photopic electroretinogram may provide the only clue to the diagnosis. Other congenital retinal dystrophies such as blue-cone monochromatism can also present as acquired visual loss in the absence of visible retinal abnormalities. The diagnosis of blue-cone monochromatism must be established by electroretinography.

Teenagers and adults may develop acute idiopathic blind spot enlargement (AIBSE) without optic disc edema or retinal abnormalities.[63] In some cases, this disorder appears to be a variant of several inflammatory retinal disorders, including multiple evanescent white dot syndrome (MEWDS), multifocal choroiditis, and acute macular neuroretinopathy.[30,89] In other cases, however, the retina appears normal. Acute idiopathic blind spot enlargement is usually unilateral and characterized symptomatically by a paracentral dark spot near fixation that may enlarge to eclipse fixation. The patient may report swirling photopsias within the confines of the spot. Although MEWDS may produce the same constellation of symptoms, a subgroup of patients have no visible retinal abnormalities, and it is unclear whether these patients had retinal lesions early in their course. The diagnosis of AIBSE relies upon the ability to use kinetic perimetry to demonstrate a disc-oriented, steep enlargement of the blind spot with geographic borders but no other visual field abnormalities. The young child's inability to maintain fixation and to provide accurate and consistent responses may make it impossible to establish the diagnosis. These perimetric findings establish that the blind spot enlargement is due to a circumscribed dysfunction of the peripapillary retina rather than an optic neuropathy (which would have smooth borders and a sloping margin). Acute idiopathic blind spot enlargement is believed to be a postviral retinopathy. In some cases, the scotoma resolves, while in others, it persists or shows only minimal improvement.

Optic Nerve

Optic neuritis in children is usually associated with acute bilateral visual loss and bilateral optic disc swelling. In some children, however, the visual loss may precede the development of optic disc swelling by several days. We have examined children who were initially thought to be feigning blindness, only to develop bilateral optic disc edema over several days. In this context, the dilated, poorly reactive pupils may be falsely attributed to the effects of recent mydriatic administration.

Dominant optic atrophy may also present with unexplained visual loss in the pediatric population. Dominant optic atrophy is a disorder in which segmental optic disc pallor is associated with decreased visual acuity in both eyes. Many children are unaware of any visual disability until they undergo routine visual screening. They typically complain of difficulty seeing the blackboard but do well when placed at the front of the class. They are often mildly photophobic but do not have nystagmus. Visual acuity is usually in the 20/70 to 20/80 range but may vary from 20/25 to 20/400.[115] Asymmetry in vision between the two eyes is not unusual. The temporal optic discs show marked focal pallor that may appear triangular, wedge-shaped, or excavated, with absence of the corresponding nerve fiber layer.[115] The severity of visual loss can vary considerably between family members, and it is common to find affected siblings who are visually asymptomatic. Affected patients are systemically normal, although sensorineural hearing loss may occasionally coexist.[101]

Patients with dominant optic atrophy display a psychophysical profile that differs from other forms of optic atrophy. Goldmann or tangent screen perimetry demonstrates a central or centrocecal scotoma that may require considerable effort to identify. Patients with dominant optic atrophy are usually tritanopic when tested with Farnsworth-Munsell hue 100 but show diffuse dyschromatopsia when tested with color plates. This finding distinguishes them from patients with compressive, inflammatory, ischemic or other forms of acquired optic atrophy, which are preferentially associated with red-green or global color deficits. Color perimetry in dominant optic atrophy demonstrates a characteristic inversion of color isopters with the yellow or blue isopters smaller than the red and green isopters.

The major differential diagnostic consideration in dominant optic atrophy is a cone dystrophy, which may also be associated with temporal pallor of the disc and which may show minimal macular changes. Although most children with congenital cone dystrophies have nystagmus and photophobia, exceptions exist. In some cases, electroretinography may be necessary to distinguish these two conditions. Bilateral temporal disc pallor may also be seen as a familial condition in Leber optic neuropathy. These patients initially have normal acuity and experience severe consecutive visual loss over weeks to months. By contrast, visual acuity in dominant optic atrophy remains stable or gradually diminishes by only a few lines over years of observation.[55]

Mild optic atrophy or hypoplasia of any cause can elude detection when close examination of the peripapillary nerve fiber layer is not possible. Segmental optic nerve hypoplasia involving the papillomacular bundle may cause sensory esotropia in the preschool population and present as strabismic amblyopia that is refractory to treatment.

Central Nervous System

A child who seems to have psychogenic visual loss will rarely be found to have a suprasellar tumor infiltrating or compressing the visual pathways. The early diagnosis of functional visual loss is common in children who harbor a craniopharyngioma.[152] Compressive or infiltrative suprasellar lesions often produce bitemporal hemianopia; however, reliable visual fields may be unobtainable in young children, and early visual symptoms may precede optic atrophy or other objective signs of anterior visual pathway dysfunction. It is inevitable that the diagnosis of craniopharyngioma or other suprasellar tumors will be delayed in children who present with early isolated visual symptoms with no objective neuroophthalmologic findings to support an organic basis for their complaints. Close follow-up, neurologic consultation, and neuroimaging are all viable options in suspicious cases.

Neuroimaging is obtained when (1) the pupils are abnormally large or poorly reactive with light-near dissociation, (2) confrontation visual fields show a bitemporal or homonymous hemianopia, (3) examination of the peripapillary nerve fiber layer shows dropout of the nasal nerve fiber layer consistent with band atrophy, and (4) neurologic or systemic signs are found (severe headaches, macrocephaly, café au lait spots, diabetes insipidus, short stature), which suggest that the child may harbor a suprasellar tumor. These cases remind us of the need for caution and humility when diagnosing psychogenic visual loss in a child.

Rarely, occipital dysfunction that is long-standing or recently acquired can present as unexplained visual loss when a child confronts the increased visual demands of the school setting. A history of seizures, developmental delay, or perinatal hypoxia suggests that the child may have unrecognized cortical visual loss. A history of antecedent trauma to the occiput suggests the possibility of transient posttraumatic cerebral blindness. This condition usually resolves within 24 hours but can occasionally last for weeks.

Psychogenic Visual Loss in Children

Psychogenic or "functional" visual loss is surprisingly common in children. Eames[52] found that 9% of 193 unselected school children exhibit tubular visual fields. Bahn[12] stated that "functional nervous disorders . . . are more frequently manifested in the visual mechanism than in any other of the special senses." Psychogenic or functional visual loss in children has a clinical profile that differs from nonorganic visual loss in adults. It should be suspected when a discrepancy exists between the purported visual deficit and the objective findings or when a review of records shows that the level of acuity has varied considerably from one examination to the next. Psychogenic visual loss in children remains a diagnosis of exclusion, and some children who exhibit signs of psychogenic visual loss are later found to have an underlying organic disease.[181] Although the natural history is one of spontaneous resolution, long-term follow-up is important to rule out coexistent organic disease and to adequately treat those children whose psychogenic symptoms persist.[181]

Children and adults are differentially sensitive to their vision, as they are to health in general.

Some tolerate substantial alterations in function without noticing them. Others are so sensitive that any floater or discomfort is perceived as disabling. Children who tend to dwell on their health, or whose parents closely monitor their physical well-being, are more apt to become concerned about subtle visual variations. Children can be viewed as existing along a spectrum with regard to their threshold for feeling visually intact. At one extreme is the intelligent child who needs glasses and is unaware that he or she cannot see well. The child with psychogenic visual loss may represent the opposite extreme.

Clinical Profile of Psychogenic Visual Loss in Children

Psychogenic visual loss is most commonly seen in prepubescent girls in the 9 to 11 year age range.[146] Mäntyjärvi[146] estimated the incidence at 1.4/1000/year. Psychogenic visual loss is often said to preferentially affect children who are of above average intelligence and who are high achievers at school,[180] but this information is largely anecdotal and has never been verified by careful studies. When true, it is unclear whether such children have high self-expectations or whether psychogenic visual loss occurs when the child's psyche eventually "yields" in some way to the high expectations imposed upon them by others.

Systematic psychological evaluation data of children with psychogenic visual loss are generally lacking, and many published opinions represent impressions of ophthalmologists. Mäntyjärvi[146] referred to psychogenic visual loss as the "amblyopic schoolgirl syndrome," which he attributed to the stress of puberty and prepuberty. Rabinowicz[180] believed that psychogenic visual loss usually represents a cry for help and particularly for parental attention. Rada, a psychiatrist, observed that inadequately understood feelings of being threatened, usually because of strife within the family, tend to predominate in young children with psychogenic visual loss.[181] He concluded that information obtained from psychological tests and parental interviews suggests a neurotic conflict between the wish to express feelings of hostility and the wish not to lose the love of the parents.[181] Psychological testing of affected children usually shows a significantly high "neurosomatic" score.[227]

Many afflicted children report that school is the source of their stress. However, these school anxieties sometimes represent a displacement from the real source of the problem, which is often the home,[180,182] as evidenced by the fact that the temporal distribution of psychogenic visual loss in children is virtually even throughout the school year rather than skewed toward the beginning.[146] Decreased acuity is often noted initially as teachers report that the child complains of difficulty seeing the blackboard and doing schoolwork, while parents note that there seems to be no difficulty watching television or playing games.[182] The child is moved closer to the blackboard with little symptomatic improvement. Vision testing at school reveals bilaterally decreased acuity, and the child is referred for ophthalmologic examination.

The child's affliction can have considerable secondary gain. According to Rabinowicz, "the deterioration of grades when an 'A' student begins to perform at a 'B' or 'C' level is certainly something that will immediately focus parental and school attention on the child, and the deteriorated vision brings forth sympathy, of which many of these children feel deprived. The child's visual symptoms may bring about a temporary cease-fire in an ongoing interparental war."[180] While such explanations sound plausible and may indeed be applicable in some cases, it is reasonable to assume that the intricate psychological details of each case are difficult to uncover.

Neuro-ophthalmologic Findings That Support the Diagnosis of Psychogenic Visual Loss in Children

The primary goal of the neuro-ophthalmologic examination is to rule out organic causes of unexplained visual loss. This process requires the examiner to be familiar with organic conditions that may masquerade as psychogenic visual loss in children and to have the necessary clinical and ancillary tests to diagnose them. Major inconsistencies between the current test results and those of previous examinations often provide an early clue to the psychogenic nature of the child's symptoms. The next goal is to determine whether the child's vision is better than he or she reports.

Unlike adults, children with nonorganic visual loss are rarely malingering (i.e., deliberately feigning a visual problem in order to obtain some desired goal) (Table 5.3). When they complain of visual difficulties, they generally believe they are afflicted. They often display genuine bafflement regarding the nature of their visual problems, and they try very hard to cooperate and please the examiner.[146,180]

Ophthalmologic examination usually reveals defective distance acuity in the range of 20/30 to 20/100.[180] The Snellen chart is often read in a hesitating manner with wrinkling of the forehead and facial grimacing, even when the line falls well within the range of the child's purported acuity.[200] Some letters are read quickly, while similar-sized letters seem to present insurmountable difficulty.[180] Attempts to guess at the letters are often inappropriate (the child will call an O an E rather than a D). Some children complain of headaches prior to or during the examination.[180]

Both children and adults with nonorganic visual loss display visual field constriction when tested with Goldmann or automated perimetry.[18,206] Goldmann or tangent screen testing may show the characteristic spiraling of isopters. However, it has been our experience that, with encouragement, most prepubescent children with psychogenic visual loss demonstrate normal confrontation visual fields. Older teenagers, like adults, may display functional visual field constriction when tested with confrontation techniques.[18,206] Bourke and Gole[25] have noted that children with psychogenic visual loss are unable to see the Ishihara numbers while maintaining perfect color vision to shapes (which subtend the same visual angle).

Unlike malingering adults who may have to be *tricked* into seeing, one can often *persuade* the suggestible child with psychogenic visual loss to improve his or her performance on a visual test. Titmus stereoacuity is often initially poor, but many children can be persuaded to identify all Titmus circles with encouragement. Normal Titmus stereoacuity is a valuable finding as it demonstrates that visual acuity is at least 20/30 in each eye, and it demonstrates that the child's visual loss, at least in part, is psychogenic.

In attempting to determine the child's actual visual acuity, it is helpful to place a negligible corrective lens in the phoropter (plano + 0.50 x 90°) and urge the child to read an isolated 20/10 letter on the Snellen line. When the child is unable to read the letter, the examiner can make use of suggestion by offering an isolated 20/15 letter as a major concession, thereby implying that the child's failure to read the letter represents a major visual loss.[219] When an "enormous" letter from the 20/25 line appears on the screen, the child will often readily identify it. In performing this exercise, it is important to use a single letter viewed through a phoropter in a dark room, which removes external cues as to the size of the letter. If the vision fails to improve, it is helpful to repeat the process after dilation, with the suggestion that the pupils are "huge" so that "extra light" can enter the eyes. The ability of the examiner to use negligible refractive lenses to improve acuity is further evidence of psychogenic visual loss.

Visoscopy is a valuable and underutilized diagnostic tool in the evaluation of psychogenic visual loss in children.[151] In this test, the child is instructed to follow the star from the visoscope as the examiner observes the position of the star on the macula. Children with early Stargardt disease will display eccentric (nonfoveal) fixation of the star while those with psychogenic visual loss will

Table 5.3. Different clinical profiles between psychogenic visual loss in children versus adults.

Children	Adults
Malingering uncommon	Malingering common
Strong predilection toward girls	Affects men or women
Clusters around the puberty period	Occurs at any age
Visual loss usually bilateral	Visual loss unilateral or bilateral
Normal confrontation visual fields except in older teenagers	Tubular visual field constriction
Usually resolves with reassurance	Variable response to reassurance
Recurrences rare	Recurrences common

"lock on" to the star and maintain foveal fixation as the star is moved.

In a child with monocular visual loss that is suspected to be nonorganic, a useful test for nonorganic monocular visual loss is to place red-green glasses on the child, with the green filter over the eye with decreased vision. The red-green colored filter bar in the projector is placed over the Snellen line with the red filter over the first three letters and the green filter over the last three. The glasses allow the child to see only the red letters through the red filter, while all letters are visible through the green filter. The child with psychogenic monocular visual loss may demonstrate the nonorganic nature of his or her visual loss by reading the entire line. As an optional second test, the examiner can place the green filter in front of the normal eye. Some children will read only half the letters, despite the fact that all letters can be seen through the green filter.

Categories of Psychogenic Visual Loss in Children

We have found it useful to conceptualize children with psychogenic visual loss as falling into one of four groups.

Group 1: The Visually Preoccupied Child

The majority of children with psychogenic visual loss have, for unknown reasons, become preoccupied with their vision and concerned about their visual health. They start to believe their visual function has changed for the worse. These children can be compared to adults who become concerned about their cardiac function and find that their pulse rate is high whenever they measure it.

Aside from their concern about their vision and the anxiety it engenders, these children seem to have no serious personality disorder that interferes with their day-to-day functioning. Simple reassurance leads to gradual resolution of their symptoms and normalization of their acuity. One might speculate that such cases represent a physiological adjustment period (reminiscent of the general physical awkwardness one sees during puberty) during which hormonal/physiological alterations may somehow underlie this phenomenon in predisposed individuals. It is likely that the psychodynamics differ in these children from those whose visual symptomatology lingers for years despite reassurance.[109,110]

Occasionally, we examine children who are concerned about their ability to function visually and have become convinced that glasses are the solution. These are usually younger children with friends who have recently received glasses. If asked, these children will volunteer that they would like to wear glasses. Although such children may have negligible refractive errors, we sometimes prescribe glasses for them after a frank discussion with the parents and after reaffirming to the child that he or she seems to see normally without glasses. It is difficult to know what symbolic value wearing glasses may have for a given child. If one assumes that this child is expressing some kind of need and that glasses will not harm the child, then one may decide to give glasses and reevaluate the situation after several months.

Group 2: Conversion Disorder

Conversion disorder is a psychiatric term that indicates an unconscious loss of neurologic function (e.g., vision loss) for secondary gain, which is also unconscious. For example, a child may believe that he or she cannot see. The gain is that the child no longer has to go to school where he or she may be experiencing intolerable conflict with the teacher or harassment by students. Children with conversion reactions are more likely to be girls.

A conversion symptom manifests as a disturbance of bodily functioning that does not correspond to concepts of the anatomy of the pathways of the central or peripheral nervous system.[84] Generally, it occurs in the setting of psychological stress and produces considerable impairment. Although conversion reactions may simulate neurological disease, they are not associated with the usual pathological neurodiagnostic signs, but instead, the signs and symptoms correspond to the child's concept of the medical condition. A conversion reaction transforms psychic energy from the turmoil of an acute conflict into somatic symptoms and sometimes leaves the child calm (la belle indifference).

Some forms of psychogenic visual loss may represent a conversion reaction to a previous experience of sexual abuse,[18] in which the visual loss may a signal that the child has seen something inadmissible or unacceptable. Sexual abuse as a cause of psychogenic visual loss has only rarely been reported,[18] and the prevalence of sexual abuse as a precipitant of psychogenic visual loss has not been studied. If a history of sexual abuse is elicited, psychiatric evaluation is warranted.

Group 3: Possible Factitious Disorder

Parents of children with psychogenic visual loss occasionally display behavior that is reminiscent of a *factitious disorder by proxy.* This disorder (sometimes called *Munchausen by proxy*) refers to the intentional production or feigning of physical or psychiatric signs or symptoms in another person who is under the individual's care for the purpose of indirectly assuming the sick role.[5] This possibility should be considered when one or both parents seem overly invested in the child's disability and appear to be actively driving the symptom. At an unconscious level, the child cooperates with the parents and may come to share in the belief.[201] The parents may become hostile and sometimes violent when the physician suggests that the visual loss is nonorganic, and "sabotage" the physician's reassurances by telling the child that the doctor does not believe the symptoms are real. These parents often refuse psychiatric consultation and fail to return for follow-up appointments.

Group 4: Psychogenic Visual Loss Superimposed upon True Organic Disease

Some have noted that approximately one-fourth of children with conversion symptoms have true organic disease.[181] In these children, the psychogenic component can conceal or distract from a true organic visual loss. Such children have organically decreased vision as the cause of their symptoms, and in trying to bring attention to the problem, they exaggerate it to the point where the symptoms appear nonorganic. Visual symptoms that are long-standing, progressive, and relatively nonfluctuating should arouse suspicion of organicity.[181] An organic etiology is also suggested if the child complains of symptoms while engaged in activities he particularly enjoys (e.g., sports). Several investigators have emphasized the importance of long-term follow-up in children with psychogenic visual loss, to detect the subgroup with true organic disorders.[108,181]

Management of Psychogenic Visual Loss in Children

Interview with the Parents

Many children with psychogenic visual loss see several ophthalmologists and/or neurologists before the psychogenic nature of the symptoms becomes evident. The parents have frequently consulted numerous health care professionals and incurred a large medical bill. Parental anxiety induced by the child whose vision seems to be declining intensifies with successive consultations and tests.[180] In this context, the process of informing the parents that there is no organic basis for the symptoms becomes a delicate matter.

Prior to discussing the psychogenic nature of the visual symptoms with the parents, we read the hospital chart for social work notes pertaining to previous psychologically traumatic events, such as sexual abuse. The child is then asked to sit outside, and the parents are invited into the examining room. The parents are informed that the eyes are physically normal and that we believe the child's vision is decreased on a psychological rather than a physical basis. The parents are reassured that psychogenic visual loss is common in children who have high self-expectations. It is emphasized that the child is concerned about his or her vision and that this concern is interfering with the child's ability to see normally. It is explained that the child's vision is truly impaired on a psychological basis. In explaining this, it is helpful to draw an analogy to the adult who develops real headaches or muscle tension from stress. One should inquire about the child's previous school performance and whether it has deteriorated since the symptoms began. One should also inquire about possible stressors, such as family discord, divorce, or a death in the family, and attempt to determine whether other psychologically traumatic events have taken place. Parents can be told their child's visual impairment can be expected to resolve with time. We generally advise parents to de-emphasize the symptomatology by not discussing the child's visual difficulties and by urging the child's relatives and teachers to do the same, although some have questioned the efficacy of this approach.[33]

Interview with the Child

It is counterproductive to tell a child with psychogenic visual loss that his or her vision is normal. The child has teachers, relatives, and friends who are concerned about his or her visual difficulties. If one "confronts" the child about the absence of evidence of a visual disorder, he or she has little choice but to claim that the symptoms are real.

Notwithstanding whatever secondary gains are present, the child may be searching unconsciously for a path to recovery. According to Rabinowicz,[180] "The purpose of the apparent visual loss may have already been served, and the child is often more than ready for a recovery. However, a rapid and 'miraculous' cure in the physician's office is likely to provoke rage from the parents, dismay from the school authorities, and sadness, disappointment, and resentment, together with a feeling of having been deceived from the child's own teacher and friends," thus stigmatizing the child.

Because children are suggestible, psychogenic visual loss in children is usually a "curable" condition.[148] Since these children rarely have serious psychopathology, some authorities feel justified in using placebo therapy to take advantage of the child's suggestibility.[180] This approach may be efficacious, but we believe it is possible to achieve equally good results with patience and reassurance.

In most cases, the child is well-oriented, has normal thought processes (i.e., no hallucinations or delusions), and has a normal affective state. One can then reassure the child that he or she is having a minor visual disturbance but that the eyes are healthy. One can state that visual disturbances are common in children but that the vision will recover over several weeks. This reassurance permits the child to gradually experience improved vision while maintaining esteem with parents, teachers, and friends. A return appointment is scheduled for 2 months (which underscores the notion that there is no urgent physical disorder). On follow-up examination, the child usually claims to be relieved of symptoms and cheerfully

demonstrates normal acuity. We object to the use of placebo therapy for the treatment of psychogenic visual loss in children because it reinforces the notion that a physical illness is the cause, and most mental health professionals oppose reinforcing the patient's misperceptions.[27]

When to Refer Children with Psychogenic Visual Loss for Psychiatric Treatment

The issue of when to obtain psychiatric consultation for the child with psychogenic visual loss is controversial. Advocates for early psychiatric intervention believe that psychogenic visual loss should be viewed as a cry for help or a signal that indicates the child has seen or has experienced something disturbing or unacceptable,[253] and that there is a possibility of sexual abuse.[18] Other stressful events (marital discord, divorce, illness or death in the family, or a poorly kept parental secret that allows the child to sense that something is terribly wrong) may also produce this reaction and be detrimental to the general well-being of the child. They stress that the child may be coping with a deep-rooted emotional conflict and may benefit from professional assistance. Given lack of formal psychiatric training and the time constraints of most ophthalmologists and neurologists, it may be difficult for such physicians to accurately determine which children need psychiatric counseling.

Proponents of limiting initial intervention to reassurance[33,108,146,182] argue that it is counterproductive to react to psychogenic visual loss in children and point to the consistent efficacy of reassurance, the natural history of resolution, and the infrequent recurrence of such symptoms in children. Others stress that psychiatric intervention could stigmatize the child at school and make it difficult to face friends and teachers.[180] Kathol et al point out that there is no hard evidence that a psychiatric referral would substantially hasten the child's visual (or psychological) recovery.[108]

In our experience, most children with psychogenic visual loss do not require psychiatric consultation since most fall into the benign group of visually preoccupied children that respond well to reassurance. Those who desire but do not need glasses and those who are found to have organically decreased vision with a psychogenic overlay do not generally require additional psychiatric intervention. We reserve psychiatric consultation for children who have (1) a history of previous psychogenic disturbances, (2) signs of a frank mental disorder, (3) significant impairment in daily functioning at school or at home, (4) a history of psychic trauma (i.e., sexual abuse or otherwise), (5) a grossly dysfunctional family, (6) signs suspicious for factitious disorder by proxy (Munchausen by proxy), or (7) a history of *chronic* visual loss (i.e., longer than 3 months with no evidence of organic disease).

In such cases, a child psychiatrist can determine the nature of any specific traumatic experience that may have preceded the symptoms and define any ongoing sources of psychological conflict. The psychiatrist will also interview the parents to determine the stresses to which the child is currently subjected. In some cases, the psychiatrist may uncover a previous episode of sexual abuse or other psychic trauma and determine that the child needs more extensive counseling and social intervention.

Horizons

Although the literature describes a basic clinical profile, the problem of psychogenic visual loss in children continues to be a scantily explored condition. Numerous basic questions have yet to be addressed in controlled studies. These questions include the following:

What are the "risk factors" for developing psychogenic visual loss in children? Why is it more prevalent in prepubescent girls? What is the prevalence of sexual abuse in this disorder? Can psychogenic visual loss be a sign of depression in children? Are the symptoms confined strictly to the visual system or do they affect other aspects of the child's life (e.g. school performance, social interactions)? What is the long-term psychological prognosis (e.g. do these children go on to develop other symptoms of somatoform disease in adulthood)?

Systematic studies to address these controversies will hopefully provide a more integrated understanding of the psychodynamics of this disorder and enable us to treat children with psychogenic visual loss more effectively.

References

1. Abraham HD. Visual phenomenology of the LSD flashback. Arch Gen Psychiatr 1983;40:884-889.
2. Aldrich MS, Vanderzant CW, Alessi AG, et al. Tidal ictal cortical blindness with permanent visual loss. Epilepsy 1989;30:116-120.
3. Alvarez WC. The migrainous scotoma as studied in 618 persons. Am J Ophthalmol 1960;49:489-504.
4. American Psychiatric Association. *Diagnostic and Statistical Manual of Mental Disorders,* 3rd ed. (rev). Washington, DC: American Psychiatric Association; 1987.
5. American Psychiatric Association. *Diagnostic and Statistical Manual of Mental Disorders,* 4th ed. Washington, DC: American Psychiatric Association; 1994.
6. Amery WK, Waelkens J, Vandenbergh V. The sensorium of the migraineur. Ital J Neurol Sci 1988; 9:539-545.
7. Andersson KE, Vinge E. Beta-adrenoreceptor blockers and calcium antagonists in the prophylaxis and treatment of migraine. Drugs 1990;39: 355-373.
8. Appleton R, Farrell K, Buncic JR. Amaurosis fugax in teenagers: a migrainous variant. Am J Dis Child 1988;142:331-333.
9. Arffa RC. *Grayson's Diseases of the Cornea,* 3rd ed. St Louis, MO: C.V. Mosby; 1991:401-416.
10. Artman M, Grayson M, Boerth RC. Propranolol in children: safety-toxicity. Pediatrics 1982;70:30-31.
11. Ashkenazi S, Bellah G, Cleary TG. Hallucinations as an initial manifestation of shigellosis. J Pediatr 1989;114:95-96.
12. Bahn CA. The psychoneurotic factor in ophthalmic practice. Am J Ophthalmol 1943;26:369-378.
13. Barabas G, Matthews WS, Ferrari M. Childhood migraine and motion sickness. Pediatrics 1983;72: 188-190.
14. Barlow CF. *Headaches and Migraine in Childhood.* London: Spastics International Pubs; 1984.
15. Barlow CF. Migraine in the infant and toddler. J Child Neurol 1994;9:92-94.
16. Basser LS. The relation of migraine and epilepsy. Brain 1969;92:258-300.
17. Bender MB, Feldman M, Sobin AJ. Palinopsia. Brain 1968;91:321-338.
18. Berman RJ. Psychogenic visual disorders in an abused child: a case report. Am J Optom Physiol Opt 1978;55:735-738.
19. Bickerstaff ER. Impairment of consciousness in migraine. Lancet 1961;2:1057-1059.
20. Bigley GK, Sharp FR. Reversible alexia without agraphia due to migraine. Arch Neurol 1983;40: 114-115.
21. Bille B. Migraine in school children. Acta Paediatr Scand 1962;51(suppl 36):1-151.
22. Bille B, Ludvigsson J, Sanner G. Prophylaxis of migraine in children. Headache 1977;17:61-63.

23. Biller J, Johnson MR, Adams HP, et al. Further observations on cerebral or retinal ischemia in patients with right-to-left intracardiac shunts. Arch Neurol 1987;44:740.

24. Birnbach CD, Järveläinen M, Possin DE, Milam AH. Histopathology and immunocytochemistry of the neurosensory retina in fundus flavimaculatus. Ophthalmology 1994;101:1211-1219.

25. Bourke RD, Gole GA. Detection of functional vision loss using the Ishihara plates. Aust NZ J Ophthalmol 1994;22(2):116-118.

26. Brust JCM, Behrens MM. "Release hallucinations" as the major symptom of posterior cerebral artery occlusion: a report of 2 cases. Ann Neurol 1977;2:432-436.

27. Burch EP. Psychoneurotic reaction patterns in ophthalmology. Am Ophthalmol Soc 1950;48:370-394.

28. Burger SK, Saul RF, Selhorst JB, Thurston SE. Transient monocular blindness caused by vasospasm. N Engl J Med 1991;325:870-873.

28. Byrd RL, Rohrbaugh TM, Raney RB Jr, Norris DG. Transient cortical blindness secondary to vincristine therapy in childhood malignancies. Cancer 1981;47:37-40.

30. Callanan D, Gass DM. Multifocal choroiditis and choroidal neovascularization associated with the multiple evanescent white dot syndrome and acute idiopathic blind spot enlargement. Ophthalmology 1992;99:1678-1685.

31. Campbell JK. Manifestations of migraine. Neurol Clin 1990;8:841-855.

32. Caplan LR. Top of the basilar syndrome. Neurology 1980;30:72-79.

33. Catalano RA, Simon JW, Krohel GB, Rosenberg PN. Functional visual loss in children. Ophthalmology 1986;93:385-390.

34. Chou YH, Wang PJ, Lin MY, et al. Acute hemiplegia in infancy and childhood. Acta Ped Sin 1994;35:45-56.

35. Chu ML, Shinnar S. Headaches in children under 7 years of age. Arch Neurol 1992;49:79-82.

36. Cogan DJ. Visual hallucinations as release phenomena. Graefe's Arch Clin Exp Ophthalmol 1973;188:139-150.

37. Cohn R. Phantom vision. Arch Neurol (Chic) 1971;25:468.

38. Congdon PJ, Forsythe WI. Migraine in childhood: a study of 300 children. Dev Med Child Neurol 1979;21:209-216.

39. Copperman SM. "Alice in Wonderland" syndrome as a presenting symptom of infectious mononucleosis in children: a description of three affected young people. Clin Pediatr 1977;16:143-146.

40. Corbett JJ. Neuroophthalmic complications of migraine and cluster headaches. Neurol Clin 1983;4:973-995.

41. Couch JR, Hassanein RS. Amitriptyline in migraine prophylaxis. Arch Neurol 1979;36:695-699.

42. Critchley M. Types of visual perseveration: "palinopsia" and "illusory visual spread." Brain 1951;74:267-299.

43. D'Andrea G, Toldo M, Cortelazzo S, et al. Platelet activity in migraine. Headache 1982;22:207-212.

44. Davis FA, Bergen D, Schauf C, et al. Movement phosphenes in optic neuritis: a new clinical sign. Neurology 1976;26:1100-1104.

45. Deonna T, Ziegler A, Despland PA. Paroxysmal visual disturbances of epileptic origin and occipital epilepsy in children. Neuro-pediatric 1984;15:131-135.

46. Digre KB, Durcan FJ, Branch DW, et al. Amaurosis fugax associated with antiphospholipid antibodies. Ann Neurol 1989;25:228-232.

47. Drexel M, Harnoncourt K, Meyer J. Transesophageal two-dimensional echocardiography in young patients with cerebral ischemic events. Stroke 1988;19:345.

48. Duckro PN, Cantwell-Simmons EL. A review of studies evaluating biofeedback and relaxation training in the management of pediatric headache. Headache 1989;29:428-433.

49. Dunn DW, Weissberg LA. Peduncular hallucinosis caused by brainstem compression. Neurology 1983;33:1360-1361.

50. Durkan GP, Troost BT, Slamovits TL. Recurrent painless oculomotor palsy in children. A variant of ophthalmoplegic migraine? Headache 1981;21:58-62.

51. Dvorkin G, Andermann F, Melancond, et al. Malignant migraine syndrome: classical migraine, occipital seizures, and alternating strokes. Neurology 1984;34:245. Abstract.

52. Eames TA. A study of tubular and spiral central fields in hysteria. Am J Ophthalmol 1947;30:610-611.

53. Edgell HG, Kolvin I. Childhood hallucinations. J Child Psychol Psychiatr 1972;13:279-287.

54. Ehyai AB, Fenichel GM. The natural history of acute confusional migraine. Arch Neurol 1978;35:368-369.

55. Elliot D, Traboulsi EI, Maumenee IH. Visual prognosis in autosomal dominant optic atrophy (Kjer type). Am J Ophthalmol 1993;115:360-367.

56. Elser JM, Woody RC. Migraine headache in the infant and young child. Headache 1990;30:366-368.

57. Emery ES. Acute confusional state in children with migraine. Pediatrics 1977;60:110-114.

58. Fang W, Huang C-C, Lee C-C, et al. Ophthalmologic manifestations in MELAS syndrome. Arch Neurol 1993;50:977-980.

59. Feinberg WM, Rapcsak SZ. "Peduncular hallucinosis" following paramedian thalamic infarction. Neurology 1989;39:1535-1536.

60. Fisher CM, Adams RD. Transient global amnesia. Trans Am Neurol Assoc 1958;83:143-145.

61. Fisher CM. Late in life migraine accompaniments as a cause of unexplained transient ischemic attacks. Can J Neurol Sci 1980;7:9-17.

62. Fishman GA, Farber M, Patel BS, Derlacki DJ. Visual acuity loss in Stargardt's macular dystrophy. Ophthalmology 1987;94:809-814.

63. Fletcher WA, Imes RK, Goodman D, Hoyt WF. Acute idiopathic blind spot enlargement. A big blind spot syndrome without optic disc edema. Arch Ophthalmol 1988;106:44-49.

64. Forsyth WI, Gillies D, Sills M. Propranolol ("Inderal") in the treatment of childhood migraine. Dev Med Child Neurol 1984;26:737-741.

65. Garralda ME. Hallucinations in children with conduct and emotional disorders. I: the clinical phenomena. Psychol Med 1984;14:589-596.

66. Garralda ME. Hallucinations in children with conduct and emotional disorders. II: the follow-up study. Psychol Med 1984;14:597-604.

67. Gascon G, Barlow C. Juvenile migraine presenting as an acute confusional state. Pediatrics 1970;45:628-635.

68. Gascon GG. Chronic and recurrent headaches in children and adolescents. Pediatr Clin N Am 1984;31:1027-1051.

69. Gass JDM. Stereoscopic Atlas of Macular Diseases: Diagnosis and Treatment, I. 3rd ed. St Louis, MO: CV Mosby; 1987:256-258.

70. Gastaut H. Clinical Analysis in the Epilepsies: Electro-clinical Correlations. Springfield, IL: Charles C. Thomas; 1954:8-44.

71. Gastaut H. A new type of epilepsy: benign. Partial epilepsy of childhood with occipital spike wave. Clin Electroencephalogr 1982;13:22.

72. Geller TJ, Bellur SN. Peduncular hallucinosis: magnetic resonance imaging confirmation of mesencephalic infarction during life. Ann Neurol 1987;21:602-604.

73. Gibbs FA, Gibbs EL. Atlas of Electroencephalography, II: epilepsy. Cambridge, MA: Addison-Wesley Press; 1952:222-224.

74. Gittinger JW Jr, Miller NR, Keltner JL, Burde RM. Sugarplum fairies: visual hallucinations. Surv Ophthalmol 1982;27:42-48.

75. Glista GG, Mellinger JF, Rooke ED. Familial hemiplegic migraine. Mayo Clin Proc 1975;50:307-311.

76. Golden GS. The Alice in Wonderland syndrome in juvenile migraine. Pediatrics 1979;63:517-519.

77. Good PA, Taylor RH, Mortimer MJ. The use of tinted glasses in childhood migraine. Headache 1991;31:533-536.

78. Goto Y, Horai S, Matsuoka T, et al. Mitochondrial myopathy, encephalopathy, lactic acidosis, and stroke-like episodes (MELAS: A correlative study of the clinical features and mitochondrial DNA mutation). Neurology 1992;42:545-550.

79. Gowers WR. Cases of cerebral tumor illustrating diagnosis and localization. Lancet 1879;1:363-365.

80. Graether JM. Transient dilation of one eye with simultaneous dilation of retinal veins. Arch Ophthalmol 1963;70:342-345.

81. Grant WM. Toxicology of the Eye. Springfield, IL: Charles C. Thomas; 1974:55-56.

82. Greenblatt SH. Post-traumatic cerebral blindness. Association with migraine and seizure diathesis. JAMA 1973;225:1073-1076.

83. Gross C. The many faces of infectious mononucleosis: the spectrum of Epstein-Barre virus infection in children. Pediatr Rev 1985;7:35-44.

84. Guggenheim FG. Somatoform disorders. In: Comprehensive Textbook of Psychiatry, VI. 6th ed. Kaplan and Saddock; 1995. In press.

85. Guilleminault C, ed. Sleep and Its Disorders in Children. New York: Raven Press; 1987:181-183.

86. Guilleminault C. Narcolepsy. In: Chokroverty S, ed. Sleep Disorders Medicine. Basic Science, Technical Considerations, and Clinical Aspects. Boston, MA: Butterworth Heinemann; 1994:241-243.

87. Hachinski VC, Porchawka J, Steele JC. Visual symptomatology of the migraine syndrome. Neurology 1973;23:570-579.

88. Hakkarainen J, Quiding H, Stockman O. Mild analgesics as an alternative to ergotamine in migraine: a comparative trial with acetylsalicylic acid, ergotamine tartrate, and dextro-propoxyphene compound. J Clin Pharmacol 1980;20:590-595.

89. Hamed LM, Glaser JS, Gass JDM, Schatz NJ. Protracted enlargement of the blind spot in multiple evanescent white dot syndrome. Arch Ophthalmol 1989;107:194-198.

90. Hanington E. Migraine: a blood disorder? Lancet 1978;1:501-502.

91. Hanson RR. Headaches in childhood. Semin Neurol 1988;8:51-60.

92. Harris W. Hemianopsia with special reference to its transient varieties. Brain 1897;20:308-364.

93. Hauser RA, Lacey M, Knight R. Hypertensive encephalopathy. Magnetic resonance imaging demonstration of reversible cortical and white matter lesions. Arch Neurol 1988;45:1078-1083.

94. Havanka-Kanniainen H. Treatment of acute migraine attack: ibuprofen and placebo compared. Headache 1989;29:507-509.

95. Hicks PA, Leavitt JA, Mokris B. Ophthalmic manifestations of vertebral artery dissection: patients seen at the Mayo Clinic from 1976-1992. Ophthalmology 1994;101:1786-1792.

96. Highley M, Meller ST, Pinkerton CR. Seizures and cortical dysfunction following high-dose cisplatin administration in children. Med Pediatr Oncol 1992;20:143-148.

97. Hirano M, Pavlakis SG. Mitochondrial myopathy, encephalopathy, lactic acidosis, and strokelike episodes (MELAS): current concepts. J Child Neurol 1994;9:4-13.

98. Hockaday JM. Basilar migraine in childhood. Dev Med Child Neurol 1979;21:455-463.

99. Holmes G. Sabill memorial oration on local epilepsy. Lancet 1927;1:957-962.

100. Holtzman RN, Goldensohn ES. Sensations of ocular movement in seizures originating in occipital lobe. Neurology 1977;27:554-556.
101. Hoyt CS. Autosomal dominant optic atrophy. A spectrum of disability. Ophthalmology 1980;87: 245-251.
102. Hughes MS, Lessell S. Trazadone-induced palinopsia. Arch Ophthalmol 1990;108:399-400.
103. Hupp SL, Kline LB, Corbett JJ. Visual disturbances of migraine. Surv Ophthalmol 1989;33:221-236.
104. Jorgensen KA, Sorensen P, Freund L. Effective leuko-chortico steroids on some coagulation tests. Acta Hematolog [Basel] 1982;68:39-42.
105. Joutel A, Bousser MG, Biousse V, et al. A gene for familial hemiplegic migraine maps to chromosome 19. Nat Genet 1993;5:40-45.
106. Kaiser HJ, Flammer J, Gasser P. Ocular vasospasm in children. Neuroophthalmology 1993;13:263-267.
107. Kaminer Y, Hrecznyj B. Lysergic acid diethylamide induced chronic visual disturbances in an adolescent. J Nerv Ment Dis 1991;179:173-174.
108. Kathol RG, Cox TA, Corbett JJ, et al. Functional visual loss. I: a true psychiatric disorder? Psychol Med 1983;13:307-314.
109. Kathol RG, Cox TA, Corbett JJ, et al. Functional visual loss. II: psychiatric aspects in 42 patients followed for 4 years. Psychol Med 1983;13:315-324.
110. Kathol RG, Cox TA, Corbett JJ, Thompson HS. Functional visual loss. Follow-up of 42 cases. Arch Ophthalmol 1983;101:729-735.
111. Katz B, Hoyt WF. Intrapapillary and peripapillary hemorrhage in young patients with uncomplicated post vitreous detachment: signs of vitreopapillary traction. Ophthalmology 1995;102:340-352.
112. Kennedy PGE, Gardner-Thorpe C, Kocen RS. Subacute sclerosing panencephalitis presenting as transient homonymous hemianopia. J Neurol Neurosurg Psychiatr 1983;46:186-187.
113. Kinast M, Lueders H, Rothner AD, Erenberg G. Benign focal epileptiform discharges in childhood migraine (BFEDC). Neurology 1982;32:1309-1311.
114. King RA. Ocular signs and symptoms in children. Pediatr Clin North Am 1993;40:753-766.
115. Kline LB, Glaser JS. Dominant optic atrophy. The clinical profile. Arch Ophthalmol 1979;97:1680-1686.
116. Kloster R, Nestvold K, Vilming ST. A double-blind study of ibuprofen versus placebo in the treatment of acute migraine attacks. Cephalalgia 1992;12: 169-171.
117. Kooi KA. Episodic blindness as a late effect of head trauma. Electrophysiological study of three cases. Neurology 1970;20:569-573.
118. Kosnik E, Paulson GW, Laguna JF. Postictal blindness. Neurology 1976;26-248-250.
119. Kupersmith MJ, Warren FA, Hass WK. The nonbenign aspects of migraine. Neuroophthalmology 1987;7:1-10.
120. Kupersmith MJ. *Neurovascular Neuroophthalmology.* New York: Springer Verlag; 1993:452-453.
121. Laffi GL, Safran AB. Persistent visual hallucinations following hashish consumption. Br J Ophthalmol 1993;77:601-603.
122. Lance JW. Simple formed hallucinations confined to the area of a specific visual field defect. Brain 1976;99:719-734.
123. Lanska DJ, Lanska MJ, Mendez MM. Brainstem auditory hallucinosis. Neurology 1987;37:1685.
124. Lanska DJ, Lanska MJ. Visual release hallucinations in juvenile neuronal ceroid lipofuscinosis. Pediatr Neurol 1993;9:316-317.
125. Lapkin ML, Golden GS. Basilar artery migraine. Am J Dis Child 1978;132:278-281.
126. Lashley KS. Patterns of cerebral integration indicated by the scotomas of migraine. Arch Neurol Psychiatr 1941;46:331-339.
127. Lauritzen M. Cortical spreading depression as a putative migraine mechanism. Trends Neurosci 1987;10:8-13.
128. Leão KAP. Spreading depression of activity in cerebral cortex. J Neurophysiol 1944;7:359-390.
129. Lechat P, Mas JL, Lascault G, et al. Prevalence of patent foramen ovale in patients with stroke. N Engl J Med 1988;318:1148.
130. Lepore FE. Spontaneous visual phenomenon with visual loss: 104 patients with lesions of the retinal and neuro-afferent pathways. Neurology 1990;44: 444-447.
131. Lepore FE. Uhthoff's symptoms in disorders of the anterior visual pathways. Neurology 1994;44: 1036-1038.
132. Lessell S. Higher disorders of visual function: positive phenomenon. In: Glaser JS, Smith JL, eds. *Neuroophthalmology: Symposium of the University of Miami in the Bascom Palmer Eye Institute, VIII.* St. Louis, MO: C.V. Mosby; 1975:27-44.
133. Lessell S, Cohen MM. Phosphenes induced by sound. Neurology 1979;38:1524-1527.
134. Levi L, Miller NR. Visual illusions associated with previous drug abuse. J Clin Neuroophthalmol 1990;10:103-110.
135. Lewis RA, Vijayan N, Watson C, et al. Visual field loss in migraine. Ophthalmology 1989;96:321-326.
136. Liaw SB, Shen EY. Alice in Wonderland syndrome as a presenting symptom of EBV infection. Pediatr Neurol 1991;7:464-466.
137. Lippman CW. Certain hallucinations peculiar to migraine. J Nerv Ment Dis 1952;116:3466.
138. Lipton RB, Ottman R, Ehrenberg BL, Hauser A. Co-morbidity of migraine: the connection between migraine and epilepsy. Neurology 1994;44(suppl 7):528-532.
139. Loewenstein JI. Visual hallucinations in patients with choroidal neovascularization. JAMA 1994; 272:243.
140. Lorentzen SE. Drusen of the optic disk. Dan Med Bull 1967;14:293-298.

141. Ludvigsson J. Propranolol used in prophylaxis of migraine in children. Acta Neurol Scand 1974;50: 109-115.

142. Ludwig BI, Marsan CA. Clinical ictal patterns in epileptic patients with occipital electro-encephalographic foci. Neurology 1975;25:463-471.

143. MacDonald JT. Childhood migraine: differential diagnosis and treatment. Postgrad Med 1986;80: 301-4, 306.

144. MacDonald JT. Treatment of juvenile migraine with subcutaneous sumatriptan. Headache 1994; 34:581-582.

145. Maitland CG. Ocular motility in childhood migraine. Presented at the North American Neuro-Ophthalmological Society Meeting, Rancho Bernardo, CA, February 23-27, 1992.

146. Mäntyjärvi MI. The amblyopic schoolgirl syndrome. J Pediatr Ophthalmol Strabismus 1981; 18:6.

147. Marra TR, Shah M, Mikus MA. Transient cortical blindness due to hypertensive encephalopathy. Magnetic resonance imaging correlation. J Clin Neuroophthalmol 1993;13:35-37.

148. Martyn LJ. Discussion of Catalano et al: Functional visual loss in children. Ophthalmology 1986;93:390.

149. Matthews PM, Tampieri D, Berkovic SF, et al. Magnetic resonance imaging shows specific abnormalities in the MELAS syndrome. Neurology 1991;41:1043-1046.

150. Meldrum BS, Brierly JB. Prolonged epileptic seizures in primates. Arch Neurol 1973;28:10-17.

151. Miller BW. A review of practical tests for ocular malingering and hysteria. Surv Ophthalmol 1973; 17:241-246.

152. Miller NR. *Walsh and Hoyt's Clinical Neuro-ophthalmology, III.* 4th ed. Baltimore, MD: Williams and Wilkins; 1988:1398.

153. Miller SP, Sanchez-Avalos J, Stefanski T, Zukerman L. Coagulation disorders in cancer. I: clinical and laboratory studies. Cancer 1967;20:1452-1465.

153a. Miyamoto S, Kikuchi H, Karasawa J et al. Study of the posterior circulation in moyamoya disease. Part 2: Visual disturbances and surgical treatment. J Neurosurg 1986;65:454-460.

154. Monteiro JMP, Rosas MJ, Correia AP, Vaz AR. Migraine and intracranial vascular malformations. Headache 1993;33:563-565.

155. Mortimer MJ, Kay J, Jaron A. Childhood migraine in general practice: clinical features and characteristics. Cephalalgia 1992;12:238-243.

156. Mortimer MJ, Kay J, Jaron A. Epidemiology of headache and childhood migraine in an urban general practice using Ad Hoc, Vahlquist and IHS criteria. Dev Med Child Neurol 1992;34:1096-1101.

157. Nadvi SS, van Dellen JR. Transient peduncular hallucinations secondary to brainstem compression by a medulloblastoma. Surg Neurol 1994;41:250-252.

158. Nagendran K, Prior PF, Rossiter MA. Benign occipital epilepsy of childhood: a family study. J R Soc Med 1989;82:684-685.

159. Natowicz M, Kelley RI. Mendelian etiologies of stroke. Ann Neurol 1987;22:175-192.

160. Newmark ME. Visual hallucinations. JAMA 1987;257:82. Letter.

161. O'Connor PJ, Tredici TJ. Acephalgic migraine. Fifteen years experience. Ophthalmology 1981;88: 999-1003.

161a.O'Hara MA, Anderson RT, Brown D. MR imaging in ophthalmoplegic migraine of children. Presented as a poster at the American Association of Pediatric Ophthalmology and Strabismus. Orlando, FL, April 5-9, 1995.

162. Olbrich H, Engelmeier MP, Pauleikhoff D, Waubke T. Visual hallucinations in ophthalmology. Graefe's Arch Clin Exp Ophthalmol 1987;225: 217-220.

163. Olesen J, Larsen B, Lauritzen M. Focal hyperemia followed by spreading oligemia and impaired activation of rCBF in classic migraine. Ann Neurol 1981;9:344-352.

164. Olesen J. Migraine and regional cerebral blood flow. Trends Neurosci 1985;8:318-322.

165. Olness K, McDonald JT, Uden DL. Comparison of self-hypnosis and propranolol in the treatment of juvenile classic migraine. Pediatrics 1987;79:593-597.

166. O' Sullivan F, Rossor M, Elston JS. Amaurosis fugax in young people. Br J Ophthalmol 1992;76: 660-662.

167. Panayiotopoulos CP. Difficulties in differentiating migraine in epilepsy based on clinical and EEG findings. In: Anderman F, Lugaressi E, eds. *Migraine in Epilepsy.* Boston, MA: Butterworth; 1987.

168. Panayiotopoulos CP. Benign childhood epilepsy with occipital paroxysms: a 15-year prospective clinical and electroencephalographic study. Ann Neurol 1989;26:51-56.

169. Panayiotopoulos CP. Elementary visual hallucinations in migraine and epilepsy. J Neurol Neurosurg Psychiatr 1994;57:1371-1374.

170. Pavlakis SG, Phillips PC, DiMauro S, et al. Mitochondrial myopathy, encephalopathy, lactic acidosis, and strokelike episodes: a distinctive clinical syndrome. Ann Neurol 1984;16:481-488.

171. Peatfield RC, Petty RG, Rose FC. Double blind comparison of mefenamic acid and acetaminophen (paracetamol) in migraine. Cephalalgia 1983;3: 129-134.

172. Penfield W, Erickson TC. *Epilepsy and Cerebral Localization.* Baltimore, MD: Charles C. Thomas; 1941:101-103.

173. Penfield W, Kristiansen K. Seizure patterns. In: *Epileptic Seizure Patterns.* Springfield, IL: Charles C. Thomas; 1951:16-84.

174. Penfield W, Parot P. The brain's record of auditory and visual experience. Brain 1963;86:595-696.

175. Pochedly C, Miller SP, Mehta A. "Hypercoagulable state" in children with acute leukemia or disseminated solid tumors. Oncology 1973;28:517-522.

176. Prensky AL, Sommer D. Diagnosis and treatment of migraine in children. Neurology 1979;29:506-510.

177. Priest JR, Ramsay NKC, Latchaw RE, et al. Thrombotic and hemorrhagic strokes complicating early therapy for childhood Acute Lymphoblastic Leukemia. Cancer 1980;46:1548-1554.

178. Priest JR, Ramsay NKC, Bennett AK, Krivit W, Edson JR. The effect of L-asparaginase on antithrombin, plasminogen, and plasma-coagulation during therapy for acute lymphoblastic leukemia. J Pediatr 1982;100:990-995.

179. Pui C-H, Jackson CW, Chesney C, et al. Sequential changes in platelet function in coagulation in leukemic children treated with L-asparaginase prednisone of vincristine. J Clin Oncol 1983;1:380-385.

179a.Purvin V, Selky AK. Palinopsia following LSD ingestion. Presented as a poster at the North American Neuro-ophthalmology Society Meeting. Tucson, AZ, February 19-23, 1995.

180. Rabinowicz IM. Amblyopia: In: Harley RD, ed. *Pediatric Ophthalmology, I.* 2nd ed. Philadelphia, PA: WB Saunders;1983:293-348.

181. Rada RT, Krill AE, Meyer GG, Armstrong D. Visual conversion reaction in children. II. follow-up. Psychosomatics 1973;14:271-276.

182. Rada RT, Meyer GG, Kellner R. Visual conversion reaction in children and adults. J Nerv Ment Dis 1978;166:580-587.

183. Ramadan NM, Tietjen GE, Levine SR, Welch KMA. Scintillating scotomata associated with internal carotid artery dissection: report of three cases. Neurology 1991;41:1084-1087.

184. Ramsay NKC, Coccia PF, Krivit W, et al. The effect of L-asparaginase on plasma coagulation factors in acute lymphoblastic leukemia. J Cancer 1977;40:1398-1401.

185. Raskin NH, Schwartz RK. Ice-pick like pain. Neurology 1980;30:203.

186. Riaz G, Selhorst JB, Hennessey JJ. Meningeal lesions mimicking migraine. Neuroophthalmology 1991;11:41-48.

187. Riela AR, Roach ES. Etiology of strokes in children. J Child Neurol 1993;8:201-220.

188. Rippe DJ, Edwards MK, Schrodt JF, et al. Reversible cerebral lesions associated with tiazofurin usage: MR demonstration. JCAT 1988;12:1078-1081.

189. Robertson WC, Schnitzier ER. Ophthalmoplegic migraine in infancy. Pediatrics 1978;61:886-888.

190. Rolak AL, Baram TZ. Visual hallucinations: more diagnosis. JAMA 1987;257:2036. Letter to the editor.

191. Rossi LN, Vassella F. Headache in children with brain tumors. Child Nerv Syst 1989;5:307-309.

192. Rossi LN, Penzien JM, Deonna T, et al. Does migraine-related stroke occur in childhood? Dev Med Child Neurol 1990;32:1016-1021.

193. Rummelt V, Folberg R, Ionasescu V, et al. Ocular pathology of MELAS syndrome with mitochondrial DNA nucleotide 3243 point mutation. Ophthalmology 1993;100:1757-1766.

194. Russell WR, Whitty CWM. Studies in traumatic epilepsy. 3: visual fits. J Neurol Neurosurg Psychiatr 1955;18:79-96.

195. Sadeh M, Goldhammer Y, Kuritsky A. Postictal blindness in adults. J Neurol Neurosurg Psychiatr 1983;46:566-569.

196. Sadun AA, Currie JN, Lessell S. Transient visual obscurations with elevated optic discs. Ann Neurol 1984;16:489-494.

197. Salanova V, Andermann F, Olivier A, et al. Occipital lobe epilepsy: electroclinical manifestations, electrocorticography, cortical stimulation and outcome in 42 patients treated between 1930 and 1991. Brain 1992;115:1655-1680.

198. Sanguineti B, Crovato F, De Marchi R, Desirello G. Alice in Wonderland syndrome in a patient with infectious mononucleosis. J Infect Dis 1983;147:782.

199. Savitsky N, Tarachow S. Lilliputian hallucinations during convalescence from scarlet fever in a child. J Nerv Ment Dis 1941;93:310-312.

200. Schlaegel TF Jr, Quilala FV. Hysterical amblyopia. Arch Ophthalmol 1955;54:875-884.

201. Schreier HA, Libow JA. Munchausen by proxy syndrome: a modern pediatric challenge. J Pediatr 1994;125:S110-S115.

202. Selby G. *Migraine and Its Variants.* Sydney: Adis Health Science Press; 1983:33.

203. Selhorst JB, Saul RF, Waybright EA. Optic nerve conduction: opposing effects of exercise and hyperventilation. Trans Am Neurol Assoc 1981;106:101-105.

204. Seybold ME, Rosen PN. Peripapillary staphyloma and amaurosis fugax. Ann Ophthalmol 1977;9:1139-1141.

205. Shutter LA, Green JP, Newman NJ, et al. Cortical blindness and white matter lesions in a patient receiving FK506 after liver transplantation. Neurology 1993;43:2417-2418.

206. Smith TJ, Baker RS. Perimetric findings in functional disorders using automated techniques. Ophthalmology 1987;94:1562-1566.

207. Snebold NG, Rizzo JF, Lessell S, Pruett RC. Transient visual loss in ornithine transcarbamoylase deficiency. Am J Ophthalmol 1987;104:407-412.

208. Solomon GD. Migrainous periorbital ecchymosis. Headache 1989;29:328. Abstract.

209. Somerville BW. Treatment of migraine attacks with an analgesic combination (Mersyndol). Med J Aust 1976;1:865-866.

210. Sorensen JB, Parnas J. A clinical study of 44 patients with juvenile amaurotic familial idiocy. Acta Psychiatr Scand 1979;59:449-461.
211. Steg RE, Garcia EG. Complex visual hallucinations and cyclosporine neurotoxicity. Neurology 1991;141:1156.
212. Steinberg H. Erythropoietin and visual hallucinations. N Engl J Med 1991;325:285.
213. Stommel JEW, Ward TN, Harris RD. MRI findings in a case of ophthalmoplegic migraine. Headache 1993;33:234-237.
214. Stone EM, Nichols BE, Kimura AE, et al. Clinical features of a Stargardt-like dominant progressive macular dystrophy with genetic linkage to chromosome 6q. Arch Ophthalmol 1994;112:765-772.
215. Strauss H. Paroxysmal blindness. Electroencephalogr Clin Neurophysiol 1963;15:921. Abstract.
216. Swainmann KF, Yizchak F. Seizure headaches in children. Dev Med Child Neurol 1978;20:580-585.
217. Taylor D. *Pediatric Ophthalmology.* Boston, MA: Blackwell Publications; 1990:568-569.
218. Tfelt-Hansen P, Olesen J. Effervescent metoclopramide and aspirin (Migraves) versus effervescent aspirin or placebo for migraine attacks: a double-blind study. Cephalalgia 1984;4:107-111.
219. Thompson HS. Functional visual loss. Am J Ophthalmol 1985;100:209-213.
220. Tippin J, Corbett JJ, Kerber RE, et al. Amaurosis fugax and ocular infarction in adolescents and young adults. Ann Neurol 1989;26:69-77.
221. Todd J. The syndrome of Alice in Wonderland. Can Med Assoc J 1955;73:701-704.
222. Tomsak RL, Jergens PB. Benign recurrent transient monocular blindness: a possible variant of acephalgic migraine. Headache 1987;27:66-69.
223. Tornqvist G. Paralysis of accommodation. Acta Ophthalmol 1971;49:702-706.
224. Troost BT, Newton TH. Occipital lobe arteriovenous malformations. Arch Ophthalmol 1975;93:250-265.
225. Troost BT, Mark LE, Maroon JC. Resolution of classic migraine after removal of an occipital lobe AVM. Ann Neurol 1979;5:199-201.
226. Uliss AE, Moore AT, Bird AC. The dark choroid in posterior retinal dystrophies. Ophthalmology 1987; 94:1423-1427.
227. van Balen AT, Slijper FEM. Psychogenic amblyopia in children. J Pediatr Ophthalmol Strabismus 1978;15(3):164-167.
228. van Bogaert L. L'hallucinose pedunculaire. Rev Neurol 1927;43:608-617.
229. van Gelder P, Geurs Ph, Kho GS, et al. Cortical blindness and seizures following Cisplatin treatment: both of epileptic origin? Eur J Cancer 1993; 29:1497-1498.
230. van Harreveld A. Two mechanisms for spreading depression in the chick retina. J Neurobiol 1978; 6:419-431.
231. van Harreveld A. The nature of chick's magnesium sensitive retinal spreading depression. J Neurobiol 1984;15:333-344.
232. Vijayan N. Ophthalmoplegic migraine: ischemic or compressive neuropathy? Headache 1980;20:300-304.
233. Vike J, Jabbari B, Maitland CG. Auditory-visual synesthesia: report of a case with intact visual pathways. Arch Neurol 1984;41:680-681.
234. von Noorden GK. Idiopathic amblyopia. Am J Ophthalmol 1985;100:214-217.
235. Walsh JP, O'Doherty DS. A possible explanation of the mechanism of ophthalmoplegic migraine. Neurology 1960;10:1079-1084.
236. Waxman SG. Clinical course and electrophysiology of multiple sclerosis. In: Waxman SG, ed. *Functional Recovery in Neurological Disease.* New York: Raven Press; 1988:157-184.
237. Weinberger LM, Grant FC. Visual hallucinations and their neuro-optical correlates. Arch Ophthalmol 1940;23:166-199.
238. Welch KMA, D'Andrea G, Tepley N, et al. The concept of migraine as a state of central neuronal hyperexcitability. Neurol Clin 1990;8:817-828.
239. Welch KMA, Barkley GL, Tepley N, Ramadan NM, et al. Central neurogenic mechanisms of migraine. Neurology 1993;43(suppl 3):S21-S25.
240. Welch KMA. Drug therapy of migraine. N Engl J Med 1993;329:1476-1483.
241. Weleber RG, Shults WT. Digoxin retinal toxicity. Clinical and electrophysiological evaluation of a cone dysfunction syndrome. Arch Ophthalmol 1981;99:1568-1572.
242. Weleber RG, Carr RE, Murphey WH, Sheffield VC, et al. Phenotypic variation including retinitis pigmentosa, pattern dystrophy, and fundus flavimaculatus in a single family with a deletion of codon 153 or 154 of the peripherin/RDS gene. Arch Ophthalmol 1993;11:1531-1542.
243. Weleber RG. Stargardt's macular dystrophy. Arch Ophthalmol 1994;112:752-753. Editorial.
244. Weller M, Wiedemann P. Visual hallucinations. An outline of etiological and pathogenetic concepts. Int Ophthalmol Clin 1989;13:193-199.
245. Wertenbaker C, Gutman I. Unusual visual symptoms. Surv Ophthalmol 1985;29:297-299.
246. White CP, Jan JE. Visual hallucinations after acute visual loss in a young child. Dev Med Child Neurol 1992;34:252-265.
247. Williamson PD, Boone PA, Spencer DD, et al. Occipital and parietal epilepsy. Epilepsy 1988;29:682.
248. Williamson PD, Thadani VM, Darcy TM, et al. Occipital lobe epilepsy: clinical characteristics, seizure spread patterns, and results of surgery. Ann Neurol 1992;31:3-13.
249. Winterkorn JMS, Kupersmith MJ, Wirtschafter JD, Forman S. Treatment of vasospastic amaurosis fugax with calcium channel blockers. N Engl J Med 1993;329:396-398.

250. Winterkorn JMS. Vasospasm or migraine? Presented at the American Academy of Ophthalmology, San Francisco, CA, November 1994.
251. Wisotsky BJ, Engel HM. Transesophageal echocardiography in the diagnosis of branch retinal artery obstruction. Am J Ophthalmol 1993;115:653-656.
252. Woods RP, Iacoboni M, Mazziotta JC. Bilateral spreading cerebral hypoperfusion during spontaneous migraine headache. N Engl J Med 1994;331: 1689-1692.
253. Yasuna ER. Hysterical amblyopia in children. Am J Dis Child 1963;106:505.
254. Zemen W, Donahue S, Dyken P, Green J. The neuronal ceroid lipofuscinosis (Batten-Vogt syndrome). In: Vinken PJ, Bruyn GW, eds. *Leukodystrophies and Polio Dystrophies. Handbook of Clinical Neurology, X.* New York: American Elsevier;1970:588-679.
255. Zenker G, Erbel R, Kramer G, Mohr-Kahaly S, Drexler M, Hernoncort K, Meyer J. Transesophageal two-dimensional echocardiography in young patients with cerebral ischemic events. Stroke 1988;19:345-348.
256. Zhang K, Bither PP, Park R, et al. A dominant Stargardt's macular dystrophy locus maps to chromosome 13q34. Arch Ophthalmol 1994;112:759-764.
257. Ziegler DK, Hurwitz A, Hassanein RS, et al. Migraine prophylaxis: a comparison of propranolol and amitriptyline. Arch Neurol 1987;44:486-489.
258. Zung A, Margalith D. Ictal cortical blindness: a case report and review of the literature. Dev Med Child Neurol 1993;35:917-926.

6

Ocular Motor Nerve Palsies in Children

Introduction

Ocular motor nerve palsies in children pose a different clinical paradigm than in adults and require a specialized knowledge base for proper evaluation and treatment. Children with acute ocular motor nerve palsies come to medical attention because of diplopia, abnormal head posture, ptosis, ocular misalignment, or systemic disease. Those with chronic ocular motor nerve palsies are often referred because of strabismic amblyopia.

Neurologically impaired children have a predilection for developing comitant as well as incomitant forms of strabismus. In strabismic children with a history of neurological disease (brain tumors, congenital hydrocephalus, meningitis), signs of ocular motor nerve palsy (incomitance, pupillary abnormalities, torticollis, etc.) should be carefully sought. Conversely, in children with diagnosed cranial nerve palsies, other signs of neurological disease should be ruled out with a thorough neurological evaluation. Coexistent neurological signs frequently assist the examiner in clinically localizing the lesion or determining its pathophysiology. For example, signs of fever and nuchal rigidity raise the possibility of meningitis while coexistent signs of dorsal midbrain syndrome suggest hydrocephalus or shunt failure.

As with other neuro-ophthalmologic disorders, there is little overlap in the differential diagnosis of ocular motor nerve palsies in children versus adults. This disparity reflects the relative preponderance of congenital ocular motor nerve palsies in children and the unique predisposition of children to develop certain disorders (benign recurrent sixth nerve palsy, ophthalmoplegic migraine, bacterial meningitis), as well as the rarity of aneurysms and vasculopathic palsies in children as compared to adults.[153]

An initial impression can be gained by observing a child's head posture prior to any formal evaluation. A large face turn in an esotropic child is suggestive of an acute sixth nerve palsy, while a head tilt in the absence of obvious strabismus is suggestive of fourth nerve palsy. Although the abrupt, recent onset of torticollis associated with acquired cranial nerve palsy is rarely overlooked by parents, it is not uncommon for torticollis associated with congenital palsies to go unnoticed.

When a cranial nerve palsy is suspected, one must rule out masquerading restrictive disorders or neuromuscular disease. This process begins with a careful history, which includes the following questions:

1. *Is there a history of antecedent head trauma?*
   Traumatic cranial nerve palsies may be single or multiple and may involve any of the ocular motor nerves. Usually, a history of recent head trauma is well established, and there is little question as to the traumatic nature of the palsy. However, cranial nerve palsies due to parasellar tumors may occasionally be precipitated by mild head trauma. In a child with a cranial nerve palsy, the coexistence of a blowout fracture or a skew deviation can complicate the diagnostic task. Perinatal cranial trauma should also be considered, with inquiry about difficult forceps delivery, breech presentation, cephalohematoma, and cranial molding in the perinatal

period. Photographs taken in the perinatal period may be informative in this regard.

2. *Is there a history of variability throughout the day?* Diplopia or ptosis that is minimal upon awakening and becomes worse as the day progresses suggests myasthenia gravis.

3. *Is there a history of headache?* A history of headache suggests the possibilities of elevated intracranial pressure, meningitis, or ophthalmoplegic migraine.

4. *Is the child otherwise neurologically normal (by history)?* Coexistent neurological signs often suggest a specific mechanism or site of ocular motor nerve injury.

5. *Are the symptoms relating to the condition old or of recent onset?* The diagnosis of a congenital ocular motor nerve palsy should be considered in any child with long-standing signs and no diplopia. The ocular motility deficits associated with congenital third nerve palsy or Duane syndrome are often noticed by the parents, in contrast to congenital fourth nerve palsy that may escape detection because of the absence of obvious strabismus. However, observing old family photographs confirms the presence of a long-standing head tilt. It is not unusual for a congenital fourth nerve palsy to first become symptomatic during the teenage years due to a gradual increase in the size of the deviation or a decompensation in fusional control. The facial asymmetry associated with a congenital fourth nerve palsy is frequently overlooked by inexperienced observers. This finding also takes time to develop and may not be sufficiently advanced to be diagnostically helpful in early childhood.

6. *If a head tilt is present, at what age was it first noted?* Does it normalize when the child is reclined? A head tilt associated with congenital fourth nerve palsy is first noted around 6 months of age when the child acquires head and neck control, while a head tilt due to congenital muscular torticollis is noted within the first few months of life. A head tilt associated with superior oblique palsy resolves when the child reclines, while one associated with congenital muscular torticollis persists. Resolution of torticollis in a child with an ocular motor palsy may signal either recovery of the palsy or development of amblyopia and suppression. It

's not established how much stereopsis or binocularity is lost prior to the disappearance of an abnormal head posture. Therefore, the finding of an abnormal head posture in a young child is no guarantee that the child is maintaining normal binocularity and stereopsis. Close monitoring of vision and early institution of amblyopia therapy is recommended in such children.

While fourth nerve palsy is the major cause of vertical diplopia in children, other causes must also be considered. The physical examination of the child with incomitant strabismus consists of gross inspection, examination of versions, ductions, field measurements, sensory and acuity testing, as well as ancillary testing (Double Maddox Rod, Lancaster red-green, Lees screen, forced duction test, active force generation test), as indicated. The details of these techniques are described elsewhere.[281]

The diagnosis of a long-standing cranial nerve palsy is often confounded by the secondary development of extraocular muscle contractures. The term *muscle contracture* refers to a muscle that has been structurally altered by remaining in a shortened position for a prolonged period of time. This results in an increased, nonlinear resistance to stretch that is greater at longer muscle lengths. Early investigations attributed muscle contracture to fiber atrophy and hyalinization, but it is now known that the number of muscle fiber sarcomeres actually decreases.[250]

In a long-standing sixth nerve palsy, a medial rectus contracture may develop. To some degree, the clinician can distinguish residual lateral rectus weakness from medial rectus contracture by observing the saccadic velocity during attempted abduction of the eye and by performing active force generation and forced duction testing. In the case of true lateral rectus weakness, the saccadic velocity will be slow throughout the refixation movement, whereas with medial rectus contracture, the saccadic velocity will be normal until the saccade is abruptly terminated by the leash. A medial rectus contracture with no residual lateral rectus weakness will produce some degree of forced duction limitation, but if the eye is grasped with forceps and the patient is instructed to look away from the contractured muscle, a normal "pull" on the forceps will be felt by the examiner. The phenomenon of muscle contracture renders a superior oblique palsy more horizontally comitant over time. Children with long-standing superior oblique palsies may develop a contracture of the superior rectus muscle in the hypertropic eye if they chronically fixate with their nonparetic eye, or a contralateral inferior rectus contracture if they habitually fixate with the paretic eye. These secondary contractures may confound the diagnosis and alter the surgical strategies to restore normal ocular alignment. The role of medial rectus contracture in the development of horizontal spread of comitance in patients with longstanding sixth nerve palsy, if any, has not been established.

The forced duction test and force generation test play an important role in the neuro-ophthalmologic evaluation of incomitant strabismus in children and in the differentiation of muscle paresis from restrictive strabismus. These tests are most important in the setting of (1) *previous orbital trauma,* when there is a question of muscle entrapment (as in a blowout fracture); (2) *previous ocular surgery,* when there is a possibility of iatrogenic peribulbar scarring (as may occur following a scleral buckling procedure); (3) *incomitant congenital strabismus with ptosis,* when congenital fibrosis syndrome remains a diagnostic consideration; (4) *coexistent signs of orbital inflammation or muscle enlargement on neuroimaging studies,* when the diagnosis of rectus muscle inflammation with secondary restriction must be ruled out;[139,140] and (5) *long-standing muscle paresis,* when the antagonist of a paretic muscle may have undergone contracture secondary to long-term malpositioning of the eye (as in a contracture of the medial rectus muscle following lateral rectus muscle palsy).

In young children, the *forced duction test* must be performed in the operating room under general anesthesia, whereas teenagers may tolerate the necessary manipulation with topical anesthesia. When general anesthesia is used, it is important to avoid succinylcholine or other depolarizing agents that produce prolonged extraocular muscle contracture for up to 20 minutes.[89] In an outpatient setting, careful anesthesia should be obtained by using topical anesthetic drops combined with placement of an anesthetic soaked cotton swab over the area of perilimbal sclera to be grasped by the forceps. Attention should be paid to maintaining the eye in its usual arc of rotation. If the eye is pushed into the orbit, tension is relieved from the rectus muscles and the examiner may erroneously conclude that the muscle in question is not tight. Conversely, a tight oblique muscle may become slack when the eye is proptosed during rotation. The forced duction test is considered positive when an abnormal limitation of movement is demonstrated and negative when the examiner is able to fully rotate the eye.

In the case of an orbital floor fracture, the location of the fracture is an important determinant of the degree of restriction and paresis that develop. When an orbital floor fracture is posteriorly located, then the main contractile portion of the muscle (the midbelly) may be entrapped, but enough elastic muscle will exist anterior to the entrapment site to allow ocular rotation. A posterior orbital floor fracture may result in a combination of mechanical paresis from muscle injury and/or adhesions, and neurogenic paresis from damage to its neural input as it enters the muscle in the posterior orbit.[238] By contrast, anterior entrapment may severely restrict elevation of the globe while the contractility of the muscle is preserved.

A positive forced duction test can also result from anterior scarring of periocular tissue to the globe. In children who have sustained orbital trauma or had previous ophthalmic surgery, it is important to determine whether a positive forced duction test represents a "leash" or a "reverse leash." Jampolsky[135] has described the technique of retropulsing or proptosing the globe during forced duction testing to gain additional information regarding the nature of the restriction. In the case of a leash caused by a tight rectus muscle, the rotational excursion of the globe will increase as the globe is retroplaced during rotation with the forceps and decrease as it is proptosed. In the case of a reverse leash caused by scarring of conjunctiva or peribulbar tissue to the anterior aspect of the globe, the opposite will occur. In Brown syndrome, a congenitally restricted superior oblique tendon also produces a reverse leash that also becomes more restricted as the globe is manually retroplaced.

The *active force generation test* is used to estimate contractile power in the setting of entrapment or recovering muscle paresis. This is an important determination as the antagonist of an entrapped muscle (the superior rectus muscle in the case of a blowout fracture) may appear paretic, or the entrapped muscle itself (the inferior rectus muscle) may be restricted. The eye is grasped with forceps near the limbus and held in a direction opposite the deficient movement while the child attempts to look in the direction of limitation. Forces developed by the contracting muscle can be felt. Attempts have also been made to quantify the force generation test,[244] but valuable clinical information can be obtained from the examiner's subjective assessment.

A saccade produced by a paretic muscle is visibly slower than a normal saccade, causing the eye to appear to drift toward the premature termination of its rotation. Although decreased saccadic velocity is usually seen in the setting of isolated ocular motor paresis, it is not specific to this condition and may also be seen in disease that primarily involves the extraocular muscles (e.g., orbital pseudotumor), the neuromuscular junction (e.g., myasthenia gravis), and the central nervous system (CNS) (e.g., olivopontocerebellar degeneration, chronic progressive external ophthalmoplegia). Nevertheless, the clinical finding of slowed saccadic velocities allows the examiner to quickly tease out the above-mentioned paretic disorders from a mixed bag of conditions including contracture, restriction, and comitant strabismus.

Oculomotor Nerve Palsy

In a study of 30 children with isolated oculomotor palsy, Miller[186] found the differential diagnosis to include congenital palsy (43%), trauma (20%), infection and inflammation (13%), tumor (10%), aneurysm (7%), and ophthalmoplegic migraine (7%). Subsequent series reflect a similar distribution,[120,145] although a recent series by Ing et al[132] included a higher percentage with traumatic cases.

Clinical Anatomy

Nucleus

The oculomotor nerves arise from nuclei in the tectum of the midbrain just anterior to the cerebral aqueduct. The nucleus has a midline opthalmo-

logicpaired portion and lateral paired portions. The currently accepted anatomic scheme was described by Warwick in rhesus monkeys[290] and is supported by neuroimaging correlations in humans.[45] The paired superior rectus subnuclei are unique in providing innervation to the *contralateral* superior rectus muscles. The cells that supply the levator palpebrae superioris muscle of both eyes lie in a single midline structure located dorsally in the caudal portion of the nucleus. Medial rectus neurons are distributed in multiple areas within the nucleus, making an isolated nuclear medial rectus palsy unlikely.[73] Pupillary involvement in nuclear third nerve palsy indicates dorsal, rostral damage that is usually bilateral and is generally associated with additional infranuclear or supranuclear vertical gaze palsies.[188]

Nuclear third nerve palsies are rare. A nuclear lesion is *certain* in the presence of (1) a unilateral third nerve palsy with contralateral superior rectus palsy and bilateral ptosis or (2) a bilateral third nerve palsy with normal levator function.[73] A nuclear lesion is *possible* if there is complete bilateral third nerve palsy, bilateral ptosis, or a selective deficit of one muscle innervated by the oculomotor nerve (except the levator muscle).[73] A complete unilateral third nerve palsy with no involvement of the other eye cannot be nuclear, nor can an isolated unilateral levator weakness. Since medial rectus neurons are distributed in multiple areas within the nucleus, some believe that isolated medial rectus paresis is incompatible with a nuclear lesion.[73]

Fascicle

As the fascicular oculomotor fibers exit from the nucleus, they are separated in both a mediolateral and a rostrocaudal fashion.[159] Fascicular fibers designed for the superior rectus and inferior oblique muscles lie within the lateral fascicle, while those corresponding to the inferior rectus, medial rectus, and pupil are segregated medially. Consequently, brain stem lesions involving the lateral oculomotor fascicle will produce a monocular elevation deficit and ptosis,[128] while those involving the medial fascicle will produce an inferior divisional oculomotor palsy.[159]

The presence of coexistent neurological signs may enable the examiner to specifically localize the site of a fascicular oculomotor injury. A midbrain lesion in the region of the brachium conjunctivum may produce an oculomotor palsy and cerebellar ataxia (Nothnagel syndrome). A dorsal fascicular lesion involving the red nucleus may produce oculomotor palsy combined with contralateral hemidyskinesia (Benedikt syndrome). A ventral fascicular lesion involving the oculomotor nerve may also damage the cerebral peduncle, producing contralateral hemiplegia (Weber syndrome).[188] As it exits the midbrain in the interpeduncular cistern, the oculomotor nerve passes between the posterior cerebral and superior cerebellar arteries. An extra-axial lesion in this location can compress, infarct, inflame, or infiltrate the adjacent cerebral peduncle and produce a Weber syndrome,[61,188] while an intra-axial lesion is usually necessary to produce a Benedikt syndrome.

The nerve then traverses the subarachnoid space in a long course between the midbrain and the posterior aspect of the cavernous sinus. Here it is vulnerable to compression by an internal carotid-posterior communicating artery aneurysm and to injury from basilar skull fracture or contiguous arachnoiditis. The oculomotor nerve passes medial to and slightly inferior to the ridge of the free edge of the tentorium. The tentorial edge may form a deep groove in the oculomotor nerve, indicating the susceptibility of the nerve to pressure with transtentorial herniation at this site. Within the subarachnoid space, the pupilloconstrictor fibers are located superficially in the superior portion of the nerve.

Within the cavernous sinus, the oculomotor nerve is located dorsal to the trochlear nerve, and both nerves lie within the deep layer of the lateral wall of the sinus. In the anterior cavernous sinus, the nerve divides into superior and inferior trunks, which become distinct near the orbital apex. The superior division is smaller and supplies the superior rectus and the levator palpebrae superioris. The inferior division sends branches to the medial rectus, inferior rectus, inferior oblique, and ciliary ganglion. Although divisional palsies are usually caused by superior orbital fissure or orbital lesions, it is now well established that more proximal fascicular lesions can also produce divisional paralysis, since the segregation of oculomotor fibers is maintained at the fascicular level.[108,189] The only location in which a divisional palsy *cannot* occur is in the nucleus.[188]

Clinical Features

Injury to the oculomotor nerve may result in complete or partial weakness of any or all of the muscles it innervates. In complete oculomotor palsy, the eye is markedly exotropic and mildly hypotropic, with complete ptosis and pupillary dilation. There is no elevation, depression, or adduction, and a characteristic intorsion on attempted downgaze reveals the residual presence of superior oblique function. Ptosis is often the most prominent clinical sign and the first to resolve. Loss of tone in all the extraocular muscles except the superior oblique and lateral rectus muscle may cause up to 2 mm of proptosis, which may lead the examiner to incorrectly suspect an orbital mass lesion.

The vertical rectus muscles are the primary elevators and depressors and remain so even in adduction. A pathological process that is uniformly distributed across the fibers of the third cranial nerve will cause little vertical deviation of the affected eye in its exotropic position since the superior oblique muscle has primarily torsional power in this position. A significant hypotropia in this position suggests that the inferior divisional fibers are preferentially affected. As the eye moves into adduction, the depression vector of the superior oblique muscle becomes more prominent, and the eye may become increasingly hypotropic. When the inferior division of the third nerve is primarily affected, the eye will lie in an exotropic position due to involvement of the medial rectus muscle and be hypertropic due to inferior rectus paresis (Figure 6.1). If the superior division is injured, the eye will be hypotropic in any position of gaze.

Isolated Inferior Rectus Muscle Palsy

Isolated inferior rectus palsy is a well-recognized condition that has a limited differential diagnosis[210,226,262,272,282] (Table 6.1). The child with inferior rectus palsy usually complains of vertical diplopia that increases in downgaze. On examination, the child manifests an incomitant hypertropia that increases in downgaze. Although some children show a classic three-step test (Figure 6.2), von Noorden and Hansell[282] have stressed that the three-step test should not be relied upon to

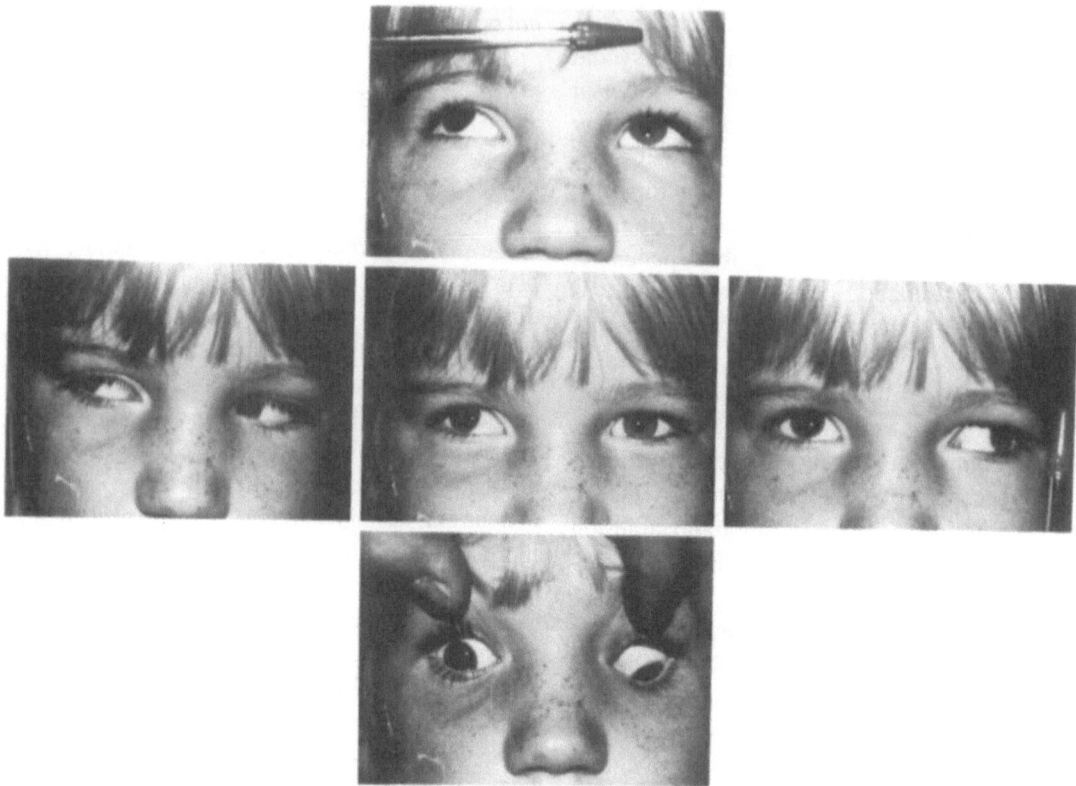

FIGURE 6.1. Inferior divisional paresis of the right oculomotor nerve.

confirm the diagnosis of inferior rectus palsy. Children with acquired inferior rectus palsy may show either incyclotropia of the involved eye or excyclotropia of the opposite eye when tested with the Double Maddox Rod, while children with congenital inferior rectus palsy may have absence of subjective cyclotropia.[282]

The infrequent occurrence of isolated inferior rectus palsy reflects the complex neuroanatomy of the oculomotor nerve.[226] Most compressive, is-

chemic, or inflammatory third nerve lesions affect the portion of the nerve located between the oculomotor nucleus in the dorsal midbrain and its bifurcation into superior and inferior divisions in the anterior cavernous sinus, where axons destined to innervate all extraocular muscles served by the oculomotor nerve are closely bundled. Such injuries generally produce divisional or incomplete palsies.

Neuroanatomically, there are two sites where a third nerve injury can produce an isolated paralysis of the inferior rectus muscle.[261] One site is the oculomotor nucleus, where cell bodies of neurons for each muscle are segregated into distinct subnuclei. A focal vascular, demyelinating, or metastatic lesion involving the inferior rectus subnucleus can result in isolated inferior rectus palsy. The orbit is the second site where an injury or disease process, involving either the branch of the inferior oculomotor division destined for the inferior rectus muscle, the myoneural junction, or the muscle itself,

TABLE 6.1. Differential diagnosis of unilateral inferior rectus palsy in childhood.

Myasthenia gravis
Orbital disease (blowout fracture, orbital inflammation, or tumor)
Iatrogenic (following retrobulbar injection, inferior oblique myectomy, blepharoplasty)
Nuclear third nerve palsy
Congenital
Idiopathic

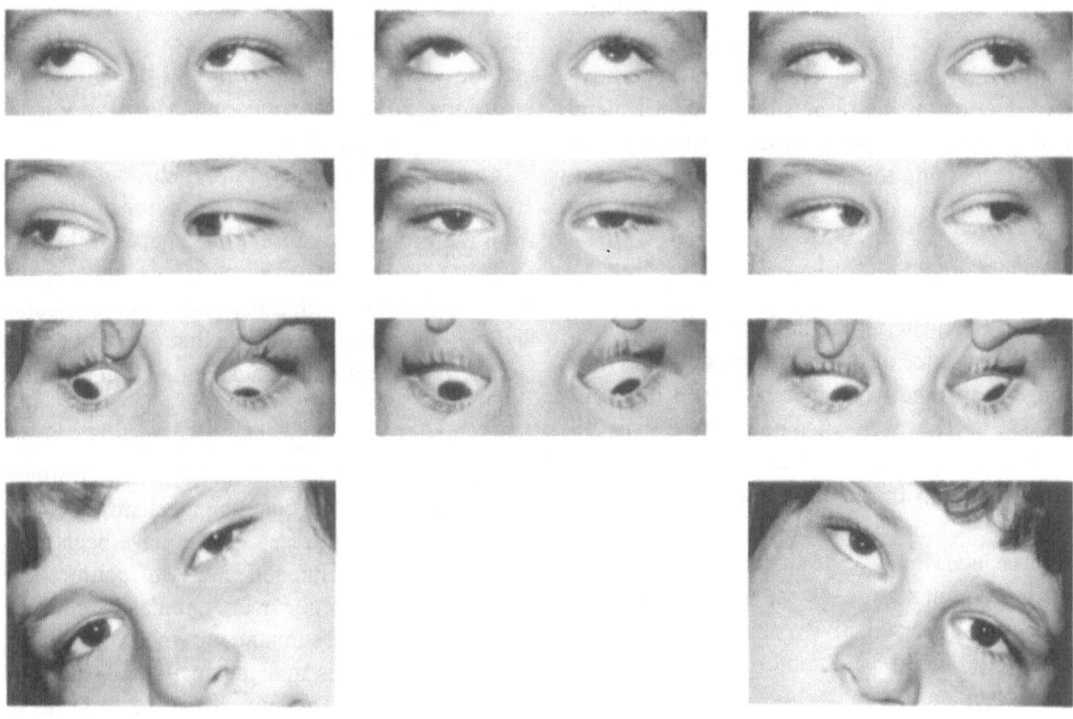

FIGURE 6.2. Child with right inferior rectus palsy and positive three-step test. (From Brodsky MC, Fritz KJ, Carney SH. J Pediatr Ophthalmol of Strabis 1992;29:113–115. With permission.)

could produce an isolated inferior rectus palsy.[261] Myasthenia gravis is the primary diagnostic consideration in a child with unilateral inferior rectus palsy and no history of orbital trauma.

Isolated Inferior Oblique Muscle Palsy

Isolated inferior oblique palsy is rare. Most children who present with a limitation of elevation in adduction have a congenital restriction involving the superior oblique tendon (Brown syndrome). The distinction between inferior oblique palsy and Brown syndrome is primarily based upon three features: (1) In inferior oblique palsy, there is marked overaction of the antagonist superior oblique muscle while in Brown syndrome, there is little, if any, superior oblique muscle overaction. (2) In inferior oblique palsy, there is a large A pattern, while in Brown syndrome, the eyes remain horizontally aligned until the patient looks into far upgaze, where a large exotropia develops (Y pattern). (3) Inferior oblique palsy is usually associated with a negative forced duction test, whereas a positive forced duction test is considered the sine qua non of Brown syndrome.

The three-step test in a right inferior oblique palsy would show a right hypotropia that is worse in left gaze and worse when the head is tilted to the left. Jampolsky contends that a tight superior rectus muscle is a common cause of a positive forced head tilt test.[136a] An isolated tight left superior rectus muscle would produce a pattern on the three-step test that is indistinguishable from a right inferior oblique palsy. However, it may be impossible to determine whether the tight contralateral superior rectus muscle is the primary problem or a secondary consequence of inferior oblique palsy. Inferior adhesions following trauma or surgery can also produce restrictive changes that simulate inferior oblique palsy.[134]

Pollard[208] reported on a series of 25 cases of presumed inferior oblique palsy seen over a 17-year period. No systemic cause was identified, and the majority underwent successful surgery. Most patients with inferior oblique palsy can be successfully treated with a weakening procedure (tenotomy or recession) of the antagonist superior oblique muscle with a low risk of postoperative superior oblique palsy.[13,214] If intraoperative forced duction testing reveals a tight contralateral superior rectus muscle, consideration should be given to recessing this tight muscle in lieu of superior oblique weakening.

Isolated Internal Ophthalmoplegia

Intermittent unilateral pupillary mydriasis can occur in the absence of other motility deficits in the setting of an otherwise uncomplicated migraine headache.[188] However, when headache and mydriasis are accompanied by extraocular muscle paresis or ptosis, an intracranial aneurysm must be ruled out.[42] Compressive lesions of the oculomotor nerve occasionally produce unilaterally impaired accommodation as the initial symptom. Cholinergic supersensitivity of the iris sphincter may develop in any oculomotor palsy with pupillary involvement.[133]

Oculomotor Nerve Synkinesis

Oculomotor synkinesis or aberrant reinnervation can arise a few weeks to months following an oculomotor nerve injury. Oculomotor synkinesis is particularly prominent in traumatic and compressive cases, which involve the physical disruption of axons, as well as many congenital cases. It is not a feature of ischemic oculomotor palsy. Forrester et al[88] summarized the signs of aberrant regeneration of the oculomoter nerve as follows:

Pseudo–von-Graefe sign: retraction of the eyelid on attempted downgaze;

Horizontal gaze eyelid synkinesis: elevation of the eyelid on attempted adduction of the affected eye;

Limitation of elevation and depression of the eye with occasional retraction of the globe on attempted vertical movements;

Adduction of the affected eye on attempted elevation or depression;

Pseudo–Argyll Robertson pupil: the affected pupil will react poorly and irregularly to light stimulation but will constrict on adduction;

Monocular vertical optokinetic responses: the normal eye responds normally, but the involved eye shows poor vertical responses.

Three mechanisms have been proposed to explain abnormal muscular synkinesis.[25,166] These include *peripheral misdirection* at the site of injury, *ephaptic transmission,* and *central reorganization* of motoneurons and their inputs.

In peripheral misdirection, neuronal sprouts grow indiscriminately from the motor nucleus or from the proximal portion of the nerve following an acute injury. These nerve fibers make erroneous alignments within peripheral nerve sheaths and thereby arrive at a muscle that does not correspond to the musculotopic localization of their cell bodies. Bielschowsky[32] suggested that peripheral misdirection may cause oculomotor synkinesis, and contemporary investigators continue to consider it the most common mechanism.

Neuroanatomical tracer studies have been conducted in an experimental model of oculomotor nerve injury, which document anomalous connections between the somatic motoneurons of the oculomotor nucleus and the ipsilateral superior rectus muscle.[258] The superior rectus muscle in this model (cat) is normally 98% innervated by the contralateral nucleus, as is the case in primates. These studies show that after oculomotor injury and partial recovery, neurons terminating in the superior rectus muscle originate from regions of the ipsilateral oculomotor nucleus that previously innervated the inferior rectus, medial rectus, and inferior oblique muscles, thus supporting the peripheral misdirection hypothesis. Similar studies have been conducted on skeletal muscle and in facial synkinesis with similar conclusions.[23,44] Naturally occurring facial nerve injury with motor synkinesis in a primate has also been shown to be due to peripheral misdirection by tracer studies.[23]

Ephaptic transmissions denote a propagation of neural impulses between adjacent cells by an electrotonic mechanism, thereby resulting in "cross talk" between adjacent axons that is not dependent on actual synaptic transmission. Lepore and Glaser[166] cited a case of ophthalmoplegic migraine in which signs of aberrant regeneration occurred as a transient phenomenon and argued that ephaptic transmission may offer a possible explanation for such cases, since rewiring of the peripheral nerve would not be compatible with the evanescence of synkinetic movements.[25] Ephaptic transmission has also been implicated in disorders involving the fifth nerve nucleus.[105] However, the potential role of ephaptic transmission in synkinesis is controversial. This phenomenon is seen only as a transient event in the dystrophic mouse model[213] and is not considered likely in the clinical situation where stereotyped and reproducible movements occur over a period of decades following neuronal recovery.

The final potential mechanism for oculomotor synkinesis is that of central reorganization. After motoneuron transection, dendrites acquire the ability to produce autonomous spike potentials.[104] The rearrangement of synaptic input to the motoneuron may unmask existing inputs that usually are weak or suppressed. Such changes in the efficacy of normally weak pathways could theoretically participate in the development of synkinetic movements. In this scheme, ipsilateral monosynaptic input to motoneurons is lost and not re-established and preexisting, but normally suppressed, projections become functionally significant with synaptic reorganization after nerve damage. Histologic studies have documented such alterations in synaptic contacts upon motoneuron cell bodies.[35] However, these changes are present only transiently after injury and a more normal appearance to the synaptic contacts reappears with time. When Lyle[171] sectioned the right oculomotor nerve in eight monkeys, he observed that bilateral pseudo-Graefe's sign occurred 21 days postoperatively. It is difficult to explain the bilaterality of these synkinetic movements resulting from a peripheral nerve injury without invoking at least one central mechanism.[25] Although neuroanatomical studies provide more direct evidence for peripheral misdirection, the potential for the participation of synaptic reorganization in development of synkinesis cannot be dismissed.[121,271] Rather than serving a maladaptive role that contributes to synkinesis, central reorganization might well be expected to function in the suppression of abnormal motor movements generated by aberrant axonal regrowth and reinnervation.

Etiology

The clinical algorithm in Figure 6.3 is useful in facilitating the diagnostic workup of third nerve palsy in childhood.

Congenital Third Nerve Palsy

Congenital third nerve palsies account for a sizable portion of patients in all reported series of childhood ocular motor nerve palsies. These children very frequently exhibit aberrant reinnervation indicating that the mechanism probably involves an interruption and regrowth of axons. In congenital third nerve palsy with aberrant regeneration, the involved pupil may be miotic compared with the normal pupil.[112]

In children who are otherwise normal, birth trauma, either with prolonged labor and molding of the skull or with a difficult forceps delivery, is considered the most likely etiology.[112,132] The presumed mechanism of third nerve damage in this circumstance is compression of the nerve as it crosses the tentorial edge while passing from the posterior to the middle cranial fossa. This compression is probably due either to diffusely increased intracranial pressure or to compression of the temporal lobe uncus over the tentorial edge and into the posterior cranial fossa. Direct injury to the oculomotor nerve during amniocentesis has also been implicated as a cause of third nerve palsy.[205] Neonates with congenital third nerve palsy may recover some degree of function over weeks to months. Although congenital third nerve palsy is frequently an isolated event,[186,276] it may also be accompanied by neurological deficits.[25,112] Some congenital third nerve palsies may be due to a congenital absence of the nerve and/or nucleus.[100] Contralateral hemiplegia accompanies congenital third nerve palsy in some cases, suggesting a ventral mesencephalic injury.[25,132]

A new syndrome of congenital third nerve palsy, cerebellar hypoplasia, and facial capillary hemangioma has been described in two patients.[292] Hypoplasia of the ventral portion of the midbrain has been associated with bilateral complete third nerve paresis without aberrant regeneration.[87]

Amblyopia is common in congenital third nerve paresis.[132,276] Occasionally, preferential fixation with the paretic eye may lead to the development of amblyopia in the nonparetic eye. This finding has been noted in patients with nystagmus, and probably relates to preferential dampening of the nystagmus on the side with oculomotor palsy.[112,132,142]

THIRD NERVE PALSY IN CHILDHOOD

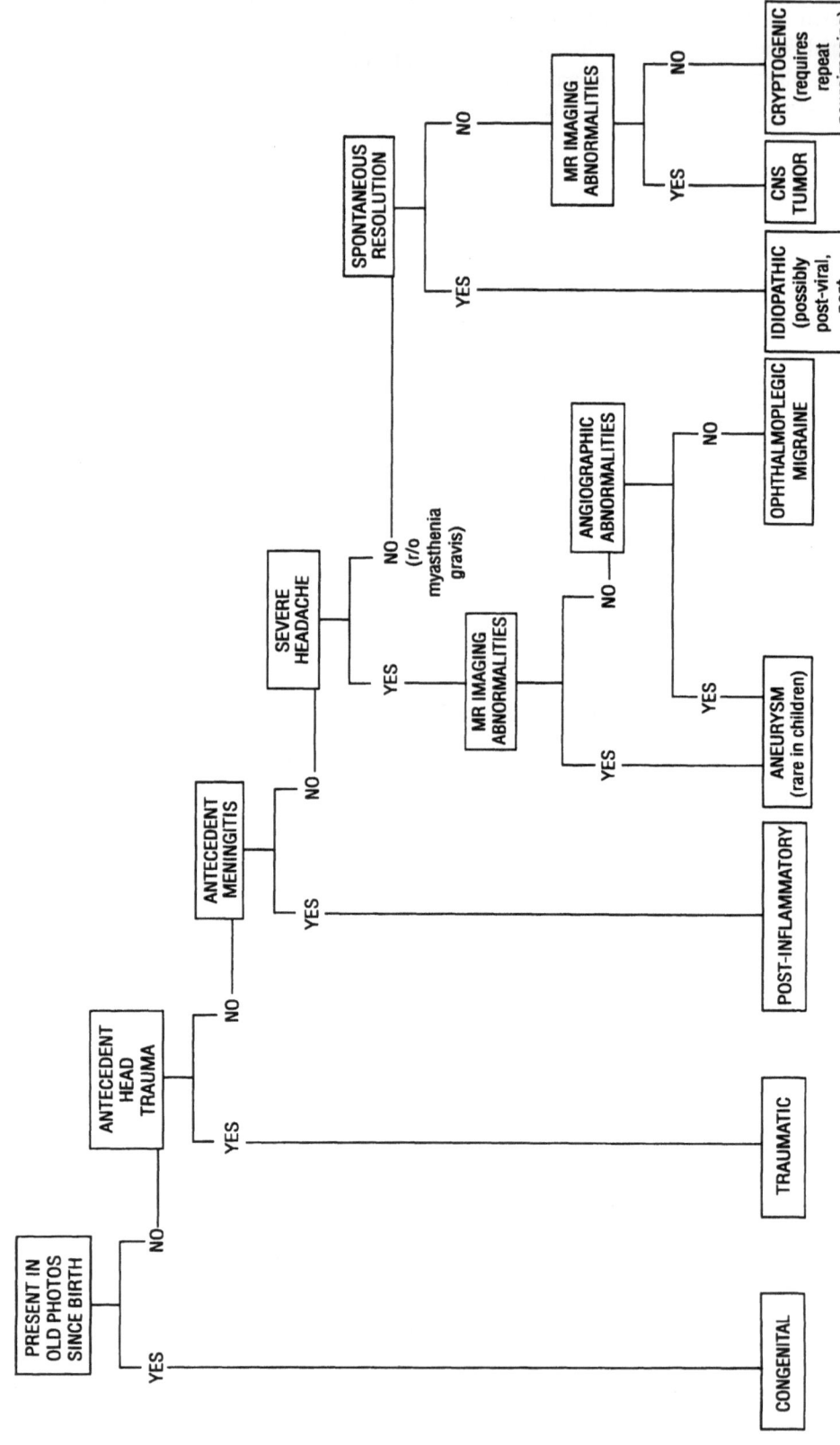

FIGURE 6.3. Clinical algorithm for the evaluation of third nerve palsy in childhood.

Congenital Third Nerve Palsy with Cyclic Spasm

A unique form of oculomotor nerve palsy is associated with cyclic spasm of the affected muscles. This condition is usually noticed during the first year of life and consists of partial or complete third nerve palsy with a dramatic additional feature. Every 1½ to 2 minutes the paretic upper lid elevates, the pupil constricts, the eye adducts, and a myopic shift may occur in the refraction (Figure 6.4). The spastic phase usually lasts less than a minute, giving way to another paretic phase. The cycles continue throughout life and persist during sleep, although they become slower and less extensive than when the patient is awake.

A review of all published cases suggests that the condition is frequently seen in the absence of other neurological abnormalities.[27] A history of birth trauma or a significant intracranial infection may be seen in as many as half of the cases.[85,169] Near fixational effort is noted to increase the extent and duration of the spastic phase in many cases. Abduction efforts shorten and reduce the spasms and accentuate or prolong the paretic phase. The condition is usually fully developed when first noted, but progression to cyclic spasm has been reported in a patient with a partial third nerve palsy.[92]

Cases in which the pupil is the only structure to cycle are probably underrecognized.[92]

Determining the site of the lesion in this condition is an intriguing neurophysiologic problem. The movements resemble oculomotor synkinesis, which is known to be caused primarily by misdirected regrowth of peripheral axons. However, in oculomotor synkinesis, the abnormal involuntary movements are always associated with attempted voluntary movements, whereas in oculomotor paresis with cyclic spasm, the involuntary movements are not reproducible by a particular voluntary effort, although they are influenced by these efforts. The weight of evidence suggests that the primary injury involves the peripheral nerve. However, indirect evidence suggests that reorganization of the central neurons also occurs subsequent to this damage, causing increased susceptibility to supranuclear influences, or recurrent discharges of the neurons themselves due to abnormal supranuclear input. It is known that axotomy leads to changes in central nuclei, predominantly a decrease in synapses on the dendritic tree followed by a hypersensitivity to depolarization when exposed to neurotransmitter from other sources. The observation that the cyclic spasm almost always appears in infancy may reflect a particular sensitivity or predilection of the infant

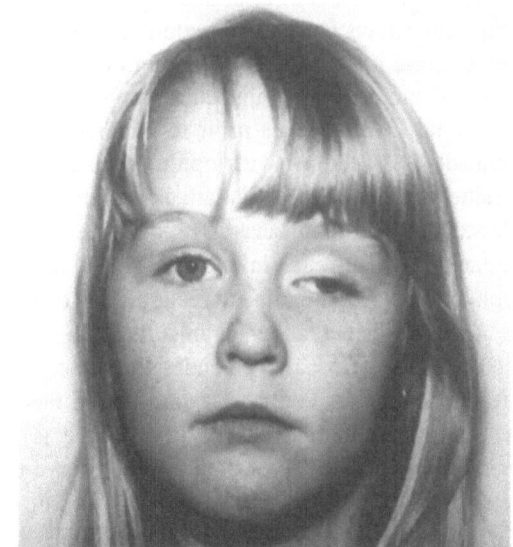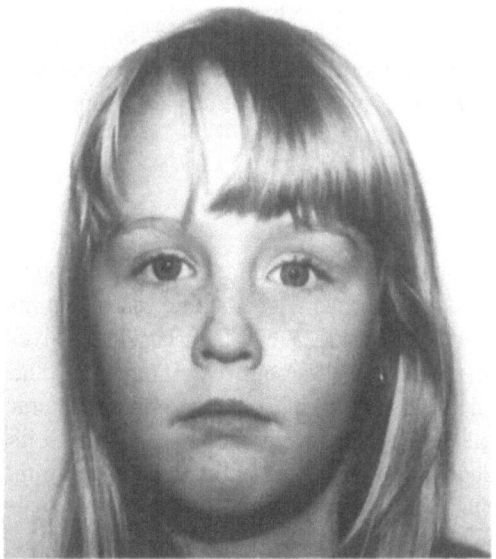

FIGURE 6.4. Cyclic oculomotor palsy: (A) paretic phase and (B) spastic phase (1 minute later).

brain to develop the aforementioned central reorganization.[25,112]

Traumatic Third Nerve Palsy

Head trauma may cause injury to the third cranial nerve anywhere from the nucleus to the orbit. The intra-axial fascicles of the nerve or the nucleus itself may be damaged as part of a diffuse axonal and neuronal injury pattern in severe head trauma, or as part of an ischemic syndrome from temporary occlusion of the perforating branches of the basilar artery as a result of the brain stem movement during rapid acceleration and deceleration of the head. Outside the brain stem, the nerve may be torn at its exit from the midbrain in the interpeduncular fossa, or it may be damaged at the tentorium from elevated intracranial pressure and uncal herniation. A basilar skull fracture may damage the nerve as it courses along the base of the middle cranial fossa and enters the cavernous sinus. Traumatic cavernous sinus thrombosis can cause third nerve palsy alone or in combination with a palsy of cranial nerves IV and VI. The orbital apex and superior orbital fissures syndromes can be the result of penetrating trauma to the orbit or diffuse orbital fractures.

Patients with cranial nerve deficits and a history of trauma will usually have had neuroimaging by the time they arrive for neuro-ophthalmologic consultation. Neuroimaging is usually warranted in traumatic third nerve palsy to rule out the possibility of a subdural hemorrhage[48,297] or an occult intracranial tumor that can compress the oculomotor nerve, predisposing it to injury following relatively minor head trauma.[274,289]

Meningitis

Cranial nerve palsies are more likely to develop in purulent forms of meningitis and in forms that involve the skull base. Due to their basilar involvement, tuberculous, sarcoid, carcinomatous, and fungal meningitis are most likely to injure the cranial nerves, but these are uncommon. Due to its common occurrence, acute bacterial meningitis accounts for most cases of postinflammatory ocular motor nerve palsy.

The possibility of acute bacterial meningitis should be considered when the child with one or more acute ocular motor nerve palsies is febrile or lethargic. Cranial neuropathies in acute bacterial meningitis are often multiple[190] and can sometimes involve all ocular motor nerves bilaterally.[26] Oculomotor palsy is much less common than abducens palsy, but both occur with sufficient frequency to warrant vigilance.[115] The ocular motor nerve palsies that occur in children with acute bacterial meningitis usually result from encasement of the nerves by purulent exudate in the subarachnoid space.[173] Rarely, ocular motor nerve injury in meningitis can result from elevated intracranial pressure or septic cavernous sinus thrombosis.[190]

Acute bacterial meningitis in young children produces nonspecific symptoms and signs, including fever, irritability, drowsiness, failure to feed, and vomiting. Older children present with fever, severe headache, and nuchal rigidity. Other neuro-ophthalmologic complications include cortical blindness and optic atrophy (from the direct effects of the inflammatory process on the optic nerves and chiasm.)[188]

Ophthalmoplegic Migraine

Oculomotor palsy associated with migraine headache is the least common of the migraine syndromes (0.3% of children attending an outpatient neurology practice).[172] Most migraine patients with this finding are in the pediatric age group.[91] Unlike other forms of migraine, ophthalmoplegic migraine shows no female predominance (probably because it is primarily a disorder of childhood, and the incidence of migraine is approximately the same in both sexes prior to puberty).[65] The majority of children with ophthalmoplegic migraine experience their first attack within the first decade of life, and several reports have documented its occurrence in infancy.[190] It is rare for ophthalmoplegic migraine to recur after age 30.

A severe ipsilateral hemicranial headache of the crescendo type usually precedes the attack. The headache may abate hours or days before the onset of ophthalmoplegia. The third nerve is the most frequently involved ocular motor nerve followed in frequency by the sixth nerve and the fourth nerve.[131] Ophthalmoplegic migraine usually involves all branches of the oculomotor nerve, although a case with involvement confined to the superior division has recently been documented.[141] The pupil is usually involved to some degree.[91] The ophthalmoplegia usually lasts three to four days and resolves without any permanent extraocular muscle paralysis.[131] However, repeated or prolonged episodes may last as long as 1 month, and eventually, some degree of permanent ophthalmoplegia and/or pupillary mydriasis may develop. Some patients develop transient or permanent oculomotor synkinesis.[131,166] Nigerians with hemoglobin AS seem to have an especially high incidence of ophthalmoplegic migraine, suggesting that a serum hemoglobin electrophoresis should be obtained in black children who are suspected to have ophthalmoplegic migraine.[202]

Ophthalmoplegic migraine remains a diagnosis of exclusion. Other life-threatening causes of acute painful third nerve palsy must be ruled out by neuroimaging, arteriography, or both.[288] The differential diagnosis of ophthalmoplegic migraine includes aneurysm, pituitary apoplexy, diabetic ophthalmoplegia, and Tolosa-Hunt syndrome.[131] Findings that should call the diagnosis of ophthalmoplegic migraine into question include alteration of consciousness, absence of a history typical for migraine, onset after age 20, signs and symptoms of subarachnoid hemorrhage, and severe or persistent headache with total ophthalmoplegia.[131]

The two theories regarding etiology of ophthalmoplegic migraine invoke either (1) compression of the oculomotor nerve by a dilated intracavernous portion of the carotid artery[288,298] or (2) an ischemic mechanism involving the artery supplying the vasonervosum of the ocular motor nerve. Walsh and O'Doherty[288] suggested that the wall of the intracavernous carotid artery becomes thickened and edematous, causing compression of one or more of the adjacent ocular motor nerves. This mechanism is consistent with the finding that intravenous norepinephrine, which has the capacity to constrict large and small arteries and to reduce edema, has produced resolution of the palsy in several patients. When angiography has been performed during an attack of ophthalmoplegic migraine, changes in the caliber of the intracavernous carotid artery have been observed only occasionally.[277] Some have argued that the partial pupillary sparing in many children with ophthalmoplegic migraine is more consistent with an is-

chemic than a compressive mechanism.[277] Several recent reports demonstrating gadolinium enhancement of the perimesencephalic oculomotor nerve during an attack of ophthalmoplegic migraine support an ischemic mechanism.[198,264]

Recurrent Isolated Third Nerve Palsy

Recurrent isolated third cranial nerve palsy has been described as a rare phenomenon in children.[49,81,85] In such cases, the third nerve palsy resolves without deficit followed by an interval of normal ocular motility and one or more subsequent recurrences. It has been suggested that this condition may represent a variant of ophthalmoplegic migraine since symptoms of migraine become apparent later on in some affected children.[81,202]

Cryptogenic Third Nerve Palsy in Children

Some children may develop an isolated, unremitting, painless, oculomotor palsy with pupillary involvement in the absence of any demonstrable systemic, neurologic, or neuroimaging abnormalities. Mizen et al[192] described two such children who had normal cerebral arteriography and developed no additional signs or symptoms over more than 2 years of follow-up. We have managed similar children. In such cases, neuroimaging studies should be repeated at appropriate intervals before the designation of *cryptogenic* is applied, since some children may harbor intracranial tumors too small to detect on initial imaging studies.[1] Nevertheless, it is important to recognize that acquired isolated oculomotor palsies in children are not always a harbinger of serious disease.

Rare Causes of Third Nerve Palsy in Children

Cerebral aneurysms are rare in children, and posterior communicating artery aneurysms are particularly rare.[39,94] When they do occur, they almost always present with subarachnoid hemorrhage. There have been only a few documented cases of acquired oculomotor palsy in children (ages 11 through 17) from posterior communicating artery aneurysms.[94,186,300] Based upon this information,

Gabianelli et al[94] have recommended that arteriography need not be routinely obtained in children under 10 years of age with acquired oculomotor palsies unless signs and symptoms of subarachnoid hemorrhage are present.

Oculomotor palsy may occasionally develop in children with collagen vascular diseases. Kirkali et al[148] described oculomotor palsies in two children with polyarteritis nodosa that resolved following treatment with cyclophosphamide.

Differential Diagnosis

The differential diagnosis of third nerve palsy in childhood is summarized in Table 6.2. The diagnosis of *myasthenia gravis* should be considered in the child with a painless, pupil-sparing third nerve palsy and no aberrant regeneration (especially when there is prominent inferior rectus or medial rectus weakness).[31] Aberrant regeneration is commonly seen in congenital or acquired third nerve palsies but is never a feature of myasthenia gravis. The improvement of ptosis immediately upon awakening, and a history of fluctuating or ophthalmologic or systemic symptoms (breathing difficulty, choking, drooling, facial palsy) warrant a prostigmine test and an antiacetylcholine receptor antibody test.

Congenital fibrosis syndrome is an autosomal dominant disorder characterized by diffuse replacement of orbital striated muscle by fibrous tissue. Affected children classically present with bilateral upper eyelid ptosis, diffuse ophthalmoplegia, and fixed downgaze with esotropia or exotropia. In some children, the ocular abnormalities are unilateral. The levator is the most common extraocular muscle (EOM) involved, followed by the inferior rectus and the lateral rectus muscles. Children with congenital fibrosis syndrome may therefore present with ptosis, exotropia, and a hypotropia from birth that may simulate a pupil-sparing congenital third

nerve palsy. Aberrant regeneration is now recognized to be a common feature in children with congenital fibrosis syndrome.[43] The diagnosis of congenital fibrosis syndrome is suspected by its hereditary character and confirmed by a markedly positive forced duction test.

The distinction between a third nerve palsy and an *orbital blowout fracture* in the child with head and/or orbital trauma is especially challenging.[299] A blowout fracture may produce limited supraduction, infraduction, ptosis, and pupillary dilation (resulting from paralysis of the parasympathetic pupillomotor fibers from injury to the nerve to the inferior oblique muscle or from traumatic mydriasis). In the acute stage of injury, a forced duction test may not reliably distinguish blowout fracture from third nerve palsy, since a positive forced duction test can result from hemorrhage or edema in and around the fibrous septae that connect the inferior rectus and inferior oblique muscle to the periorbita. Furthermore, it is not uncommon for a blowout fracture and a third nerve palsy to coexist.[299] Coexistent hemorrhage, edema, soft tissue entrapment, and surgical intervention may mask these associated palsies.

Internuclear ophthalmoplegia is rare in children.[148] It may be unilateral or bilateral and is characterized by an isolated adduction deficit with abducting nystagmus in the contralateral eye. The absence of strabismus in primary gaze distinguishes internuclear ophthalmoplegia from isolated medial rectus involvement secondary to a partial third nerve palsy.

Patients with *type II Duane syndrome* can have an isolated adduction deficit that may mimic a third nerve palsy. Duane syndrome can usually be distinguished from third nerve palsy by its normal vertical ductions and by the retraction of the globe during attempted adduction (although rare cases of electromyographically documented type II Duane syndrome show no retraction).[106]

Graves orbitopathy has been reported in children but is exceedingly rare.[278]

TABLE 6.2. Differential diagnosis of third nerve palsy in childhood.

Myasthenia gravis
Blowout fracture
Congenital fibrosis syndrome
Internuclear ophthalmoplegia
Duane syndrome (Type II)

Management

Amblyopia

The ability of children to avoid diplopia and blurred visual images by suppressing one eye renders them prone to develop amblyopia from a third nerve palsy. The main mechanism of amblyopia is ocular misalignment, but occlusion by the ptotic lid and defocusing of the image by loss of accommodative tone also contribute.[10,11] Elston and Timms[83] have shown that children who recover from a third nerve palsy prior to the age of 6 weeks do not develop amblyopia, thus indicating that there may be a latent period of visual development prior to the onset of the sensitive period. Children beyond the age of 4 years are more likely to experience diplopia and less likely to develop amblyopia. Within the remaining sensitive period, the risk of amblyopia must be borne in mind by the physician. Since these children will have a period of normal visual experience, their response to amblyopia therapy, both in the recovery of vision and the redevelopment of stereopsis, is usually good. Ing et al found that amblyopia, although common in children with oculomotor palsy, usually responds readily to treatment.[132] Part-time patching is recommended while conducting clinical investigations or awaiting spontaneous recovery, provided the lid is at a position or level that allows the child to use the eye. If recovery is incomplete, then amblyopia therapy must be continued while awaiting surgical correction.

Ocular Alignment

Of the three ocular motor nerve palsies, the treatment of third nerve palsy presents the most challenging problem to the strabismus surgeon. The only thoroughly satisfactory outcome occurs in children who have enough spontaneous recovery of neural function to regain sensory and motor fusion in all fields of gaze. Those who do not recover spontaneously are left with a complex disorder of static and dynamic ocular motor disturbances in both the horizontal and vertical planes. It is usually impossible to align the eyes in all positions of gaze. The range of outcomes will include diplopia in all gaze positions; single vision with a compensatory head posture, but not with a primary head posture; single binocular vision in primary gaze with a normal head posture but diplopia outside relatively narrow range of eye movements, or a more extensive range of single binocular vision with a normal head position but diplopia on extremes of gaze.[102]

The goals of surgery in treating a third nerve palsy should be (a) to allow single binocular vision in the primary position, (2) to extend single binocular vision into reading position, (3) to maximize the number of degrees around primary position in which single binocular vision can be maintained, and (4) to normalize the appearance of the affected eye. To achieve these goals in children with third nerve palsy, attention will have to be given to both horizontal and vertical misalignment and to the lid position. In addition to the risk of creating new ductional deficits with large recess-resect techniques, the surgery may cause anterior segment ischemia that can occur when simultaneously operating on more than two rectus muscles.[237,241]

If there is some residual medial rectus function and only moderate horizontal misalignment (15 to 30 diopters), then a recession of the lateral rectus muscle and a resection of the medial rectus muscle may be the simplest and most effective procedure. Alternatively, a very large recession of the contralateral rectus muscle will symmetrize ductions and improve postoperative alignment in some cases. If there is no power of adduction remaining in a patient with a third nerve palsy, a maximum recess-resect procedure may initially bring the eye to primary position, but the eye will gradually become exotropic as the lateral rectus muscle undergoes chronic contraction and the resected medial rectus muscle elongates.[102] In this setting, the superior oblique tendon can be severed nasally, and its proximal portion transposed to the insertion of medial rectus muscle to provide a tonic elevation and adduction force that mechanically holds the eye in primary position.[102,246] This procedure is performed in combination with a large lateral rectus recession. This procedure does little to restore adduction, but simply provides an effective mechanical force to prevent recurrent exotropia.[182] We and others have also achieved satisfactory results with primary extirpation of the lateral rectus muscle alone in children who have third nerve palsies and no medial rectus function (Dr. Forrest Ellis, personal communication, 1994).

If exotropia is accompanied by a mild (10 diopter or less) vertical misalignment in primary position, the recess-resect procedure can be combined with a vertical transposition of the horizontal rectus muscles in the direction that one wishes to move the eye.[46] For example, in a patient with a third nerve palsy with partial recovery resulting in a 20 diopter exotropia and an 8 diopter hypertropia, the lateral rectus muscle could be recessed and the medial rectus muscle resected and both transposed a full tendon width inferiorly in an attempt to correct both the vertical and horizontal misalignment. It may ultimately be necessary to do further surgery on the vertical rectus muscles in this situation as would certainly be necessary with larger vertical deviations, but this should be delayed to allow time for anterior segment circulation to be reestablished.

Vertical rectus muscle transposition procedures can also be employed in patients with third nerve palsy and minimal adduction; however, they are less predictable because the vertical rectus muscles are usually weak, limiting their usefulness as candidates for transposition to the medial rectus site. If the lateral rectus muscle has been weakened and transposition of the inferior and superior rectus muscles is contemplated, then it may more safely be done by the technique described by McKeown et al to maintain anterior segment perfusion.[176]

The use of oculinum in the treatment of third nerve palsy is limited to weakening the lateral or inferior rectus muscle. As in the treatment of sixth nerve palsy (discussed later), oculinum injection may be used in an acute setting to prevent antagonist contracture, or in the setting of a residual postoperative deviation, in an attempt to produce a compensatory contracture of the paretic muscle.

In comparing the efficacy of surgical strategies to treat strabismus resulting from ocular motor palsies, it is important to examine all available objective criteria, including (1) residual deviation in primary position, (2) residual face turn, (3) postoperative ductions, and (4) field of single binocular vision (which allows for quantitative comparison of surgical outcomes).[230]

Ptosis

In planning the restoration of function in a patient with an oculomotor palsy, treatment of ptosis is often particularly problematic. A ptotic lid will prevent the patient from having diplopia, and raising it may cause symptoms. However, if any degree of normal binocular vision is to be attained in an affected child, a severe ptosis must be cor-

rected. It is generally preferred to defer ptosis correction until after the eye has been maximally realigned. The degree of residual levator function will largely dictate the ptosis procedure of choice. Patients with minimal or no levator function will require a frontalis suspension procedure. Before a frontalis suspension is performed, the patient should be examined for the presence of Bell's phenomenon and for a normal corneal reflex. If either of these is absent, ptosis surgery may be complicated by postoperative corneal drying and subsequent ulceration. The use of a Silastic sling (which is elastic and allows the lids to close) to produce mild lid elevation, together with frequently applied topical lubricant, will minimize this risk.

Treating ptosis surgically in a child with horizontal-gaze lid dyskinesis presents a unique opportunity to surgically correct ptosis by exploiting the process of aberrant regeneration. If it is noted that the lid of the affected eye elevates during attempted adduction of that eye, then a recess-resect procedure moving the contralateral (unaffected eye) into adduction will create a fixation duress, necessitating increased innervational tone to maintain fixation with the nonparetic eye in primary gaze, which will recruit the paretic medial rectus muscle and thereby elevate the ptotic eyelid.[102]

Trochlear Nerve Palsy

Superior oblique palsy is the most common isolated cranial nerve palsy and the most common cause of acquired vertical diplopia (Figure 6.5).[188] The great majority of superior oblique palsies are traumatic or congenital in origin.[124,279] A vascular, neoplastic, or neurologic etiology is rarely found.[279] Amblyopia is rare in isolated acquired fourth nerve palsy because children can fuse with a compensatory head tilt. The finding of associated amblyopia suggests a congenital origin.

Clinical Anatomy

The trochlear nerve is the smallest and longest of the ocular motor nerves. It is the only cranial nerve to emerge on the dorsal surface of the brainstem and the only one to cross entirely. The

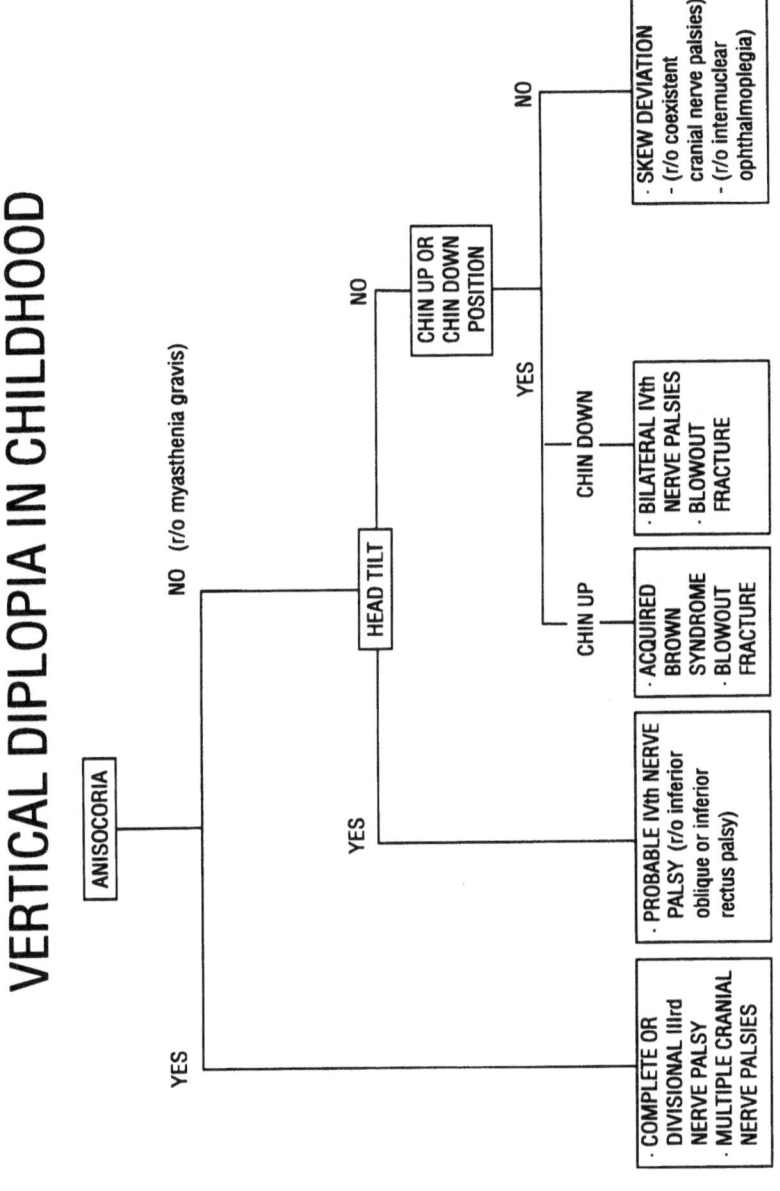

FIGURE 6.5. Clinical algorithm for the evaluation of vertical diplopia in childhood.

trochlear nucleus lies caudal to the oculomotor nuclear complex, dorsal to the medial longitudinal fasciculus, and just ventrolateral to the cerebral aqueduct at the level of the inferior colliculus.[40] The nucleus gives rise to the nerve fascicle that courses posteroinferiorly around the aqueduct to decussate in the anterior medullary velum (the roof of the aqueduct) just caudal to the inferior colliculus. It emerges for the dorsal surface of the lower midbrain as one or more rootlets that leave the midbrain contralateral to their nucleus of origin.[40] The cisternal segment of the trochlear nerve extends anteriorly over the lateral surface of the brain stem. It lies adjacent to the free edge of the tentorium cerebellum and passes between the posterior cerebral and the superior cerebellar arteries. It then travels along the free edge of the tentorium to pierce the dura along the lateral aspect of the clivus to enter the cavernous sinus. The trochlear nerve lies just inferior to the oculomotor nerve in the lateral wall of the cavernous sinus. It enters the orbit through the superior orbital fissure but remains outside the annulus of Zinn along with the lacrimal and frontal nerves. In the orbit, it runs anteriorly and medially beneath the superior periorbita to cross over the superior rectus muscle as a single fascicle just before it enters into the superior nasal portion of the superior oblique muscle.[75]

Clinical Features

Head Posture

Ambulatory children who develop acute fourth nerve palsies will frequently be noted by their parents or teachers to have adopted a head tilt (which is almost always to the side opposite the lesion). Kraft et al found an incidence of compensatory head posture in 71.2% of 139 patients with superior oblique paresis.[157] Similarly, children with a congenital fourth nerve palsy will often tilt their head, but since they do this from infancy, it is more readily overlooked.

Some children with congenital or acquired superior oblique palsy will be brought to medical attention because of vertical diplopia associated with a hypertropia of the affected eye. On testing of versions, the hypertropia will be found to decrease in horizontal gaze toward the affected eye

and increase in horizontal gaze away from the affected eye due to the increasing vertical action of the oblique muscles in adduction. The three-step test will show an increase in the vertical deviation on head tilt toward the side of the affected superior oblique muscle and a decrease in the vertical deviation when tilting away from the affected side.

Even in acute cases of fourth nerve palsy, when there has been insufficient time for an inferior oblique contracture to develop, version testing often shows overaction of the antagonist inferior oblique muscle with little or no underaction of the paretic superior oblique muscle. As the fourth nerve palsy becomes chronic, spread of comitance develops, which leads to vertical measurements that are similar in abduction and adduction. Spread of comitance in long-standing fourth nerve palsy can result from contracture of the superior rectus on the affected side (secondary to a chronic hyperdeviation) or from a contracture of the contralateral inferior rectus muscle (secondary to a contralateral hypotropia in a patient who habitually fixates with the paretic eye). In children who prefer fixation with the paretic eye, overaction of the antagonist inferior oblique muscle will initially produce a "fixation duress" in gaze opposite the palsy, requiring excess downward innervation to fixate in horizontal gaze. This excess innervation may produce the appearance of a paretic superior rectus muscle on the contralateral side when versions are tested. When ductions are tested, however, movement of the eye in the field of action of the underacting superior rectus muscle is found to be normal. The appearance of superior rectus paresis contralateral to a superior oblique palsy when the paretic eye is used for fixation has been termed *inhibitional palsy of the contralateral antagonist*.[280] Over time, the fixation duress produced by fixation with the paretic eye will result in an inferior rectus contracture in the opposite eye, causing hypotropia, restricted elevation, and sometimes enophthalmos (the *fallen eye syndrome*).[77] Such patients may be mistakenly thought to have a blowout fracture or a double elevator palsy in the contralateral eye. Once the appropriate ductions and versions are measured and the three-step test performed, the correct paretic muscles can usually be identified. Children with fourth nerve palsy who habitually fixate with the paretic eye consistently report subjective excyclotropia of the nonparetic eye.[199] This phenomenon results from a sensory adaptation to the cyclodeviation by means of a reordering of the spatial response of retinal elements along new meridians.[199]

Three-Step Test

The three-step test is a diagnostic protocol originating from the work of Bielschowsky and popularized by Parks.[204] The technique has several variations,[117,123] but all address the same three questions: (1) Is there a right or left hypertropia in primary position? (2) Does the deviation increase in right gaze or left gaze? (3) Does it increase with head tilt to the right or to the left? With this test, an isolated paretic cyclovertical muscle can be identified in most cases.

Analysis of the three-step test involves sequential elimination of possible weak muscles responsible for the vertical misalignment until only one choice remains. For example, a patient with a right hypertropia could have weakness of the depressors of the right eye (right inferior rectus or superior oblique muscles) or the elevators of the left eye (left superior rectus or inferior oblique muscles). If the deviation is greater in left gaze and less in right gaze, then the right superior oblique and left superior rectus muscles are the possible culprits because these muscles are responsible for depressing the right eye in left gaze and elevating the left eye in left gaze. If, on head tilt testing, the deviation increases in right head tilt and decreases in left tilt, then the right superior oblique is implicated since the right superior oblique and superior rectus muscles work in concert to incycloduct the right eye during right head tilting. The depression and elevation action of these two muscles is normally offsetting, maintaining the vertical position of the eye. When the superior oblique is weak, the elevating action of the superior rectus muscle is unopposed, and the eye further elevates when the incycloduction is stimulated by right head tilting. The left superior rectus muscle is not innervated in excycloduction of the left eye (the torsional movement stimulated by right head tilt) and therefore is eliminated from consideration in the situation of increased vertical deviation during right head tilting.

A positive three-step test does not necessarily implicate an isolated vertical muscle palsy as the causative factor. Kushner[162] reviewed a group of patients with positive three-step tests who had multiple muscle paresis, dissociated vertical deviation, previous vertical muscle surgery, skew deviation, myasthenia gravis, and small nonparalytic vertical deviations associated with horizontal strabismus. He cautioned that the results of the three-step test must be interpreted in the context of the clinical history and associated neuro-ophthalmologic findings.

Absence of tone in the superior oblique muscle will allow an eye to rotate into an extorted position. Since the amount of torsion in unilateral superior oblique palsy (approximately 5°) falls within a child's sensory cyclofusional range, the majority (77%) of patients with acquired superior oblique palsy do not complain of image tilt under normal-seeing conditions.[279] Furthermore, such children can fuse when a vertical prism is placed before one eye to neutralize the deviation. Subjective torsion is usually measured with the Double Maddox Rod test. Objective torsion is generally evaluated by observing the horizontal position of the optic disc relative to the macula using indirect ophthalmoscopy (in the absence of torsion, the macula should be aligned horizontally with the lower third of the optic disc). In addition to isolated oblique muscle paresis, objective torsion may also be seen in children with primary oblique muscle overaction. The commonly used term "macular torsion" is incorrect, since rotation of the globe in primary gaze occurs around a sagittal axis that goes through the macula. Confirmation of objective torsion is especially important in preverbal children.[34] Discrepancies between subjective and objective tests are common in children with congenital superior oblique palsies (who may deny subjective torsion despite objective torsion)[110,200] and in children who habitually fixate with the paretic eye (who may have objective torsion in the fixating eye but subjective torsion in the opposite eye).[200]

Although most unilateral superior oblique palsies are isolated lesions, a careful search should be made for localizing signs.[40] For example, a lesion that affects the dorsal midbrain might cause upward gaze palsy and other signs of dorsal midbrain syndrome.[40] An intramedullary lesion involving the fascicular portion of the fourth nerve may also involve the descending sympathetic tract to produce a contralateral Horner syndrome or the medial longitudinal fasciculus to produce an internuclear ophthalmoplegia.[40,144] A lesion that affects the trochlear nucleus or fascicle and the adjacent brachium of the superior colliculus will produce a fourth nerve palsy with a contralateral afferent pupillary defect but no associated visual field defect.[82] Associated ocular motor nerve palsies suggest an intracavernous or orbital apical lesion.

Bilateral Superior Oblique Palsy

The incidence of bilateral paresis in a series of trochlear nerve palsies has been estimated at 8%.[155,161] While most cases are traumatic in origin, bilateral fourth nerve palsy secondary to hydrocephalus, tumor, arteriovenous malformation, and multiple sclerosis have been reported.[188] Clinical conjecture, supported by limited pathologic evidence and recent imaging studies, suggests that the trochlear nerve decussation is the usual site of bilateral fourth nerve injuries.[144] In such cases, neuroimaging may reveal ambient cistern hemorrhage which serves as a useful marker for a dorsal midbrain injury.[144]

In contrast to patients with unilateral fourth nerve palsy and a head tilt to the side opposite the paretic eye, children with bilateral fourth nerve palsy usually present with a chin-down head position.[161] They typically display a right hypertropia in left gaze and a left hypertropia in right gaze. The hypertropia increases with head tilt to the same side as the hypertropic eye, and there is a V-pattern esotropia caused by the decreased abducting force of both superior oblique muscles in downgaze.

Difficulties in diagnosis arise when one nerve is damaged more extensively than the other.[51] The child with asymmetrical fourth nerve palsies may display a head tilt rather than a chin-down position, and signs of bilaterality must be carefully sought (Table 6.3). In the child with a severe right fourth nerve palsy and a mild left fourth nerve palsy, a left hypertropia may be present only on left head tilt or on gaze right and up, corresponding to the overacting left inferior oblique muscle. Kushner[161] has termed such cases "almost masked" bilateral superior oblique palsies. To further complicate the issue, there are occasionally

TABLE 6.3. Neuro-ophthalmologic signs of bilaterality in traumatic fourth nerve palsy.

Excyclotropia greater than 10°
Alternating hyperdeviations in lateral gaze or with forced head tilt testing
V pattern with esotropia in down gaze and minimal horizontal deviation in primary and up gaze
Bilateral inferior oblique muscle overaction

children in whom the asymmetry of involvement is sufficient to prevent a reversal of the hypertropia in any position of gaze. These have been termed "true masked" bilateral fourth nerve palsies. Such cases are recognized to be bilateral only after operating on one eye allows the contralateral superior oblique palsy to become clinically manifest.[126] Saunders and Roberts[242] have cautioned that some cases of so-called masked bilateral superior oblique palsy may in fact be surgical overcorrections in which the initial incomitance is maintained. For example, a child with an overcorrected right superior oblique palsy will have a left hypertropia, which is worse in right gaze and worse in left head tilt, simulating an unmasked left superior oblique palsy.

An interesting feature of a bilateral as compared to a unilateral superior oblique palsy is that the absolute difference between the hypertropia on right head tilt and the hypertropia on left head tilt is less in bilateral palsies than in unilateral palsies. For example, a unilateral right fourth nerve palsy may have a right hypertropia of 25 prism diopters on right head tilt and no deviation on left head tilt, giving a difference of 25 prism diopters. A bilateral fourth nerve palsy may have a right hypertropia of 10 prism diopters on right tilt and a left hypertropia of 5 prism diopters on left tilt, giving a total shift of 15 prism diopters. Several explanations have been offered to explain this. Kushner[161] has pointed out that a patient with a unilateral palsy will habitually fixate with the normal eye so that there is no alteration in the resting tone to the antagonistically acting vertical muscles in that eye. In contrast, a patient with a bilateral superior oblique palsy is by definition fixating with a paretic eye which would have a tendency toward hypertropia. Therefore, the innervation to the inferior rectus muscle would be increased and this would be accompanied by a relative inhibitory signal to the superior rectus muscle of the same eye. This inhibitory signal would be presumed to interact with the stimulation of the superior rectus muscle on ipsilateral head tilt, resulting in a smaller deviation than normal.

Torsion can be measured by the Double Maddox Rod test[52,155,161,191,251,252,267,279] or using Bagolini lenses.[179,235,253,278,280] Excyclodeviation of more than 10° should raise the suspicion of bilateral fourth nerve pareses, and that over 15° is highly suggestive of bilaterality. Kraft et al have found that, when the Double Maddox Rod test is performed in 20° of downgaze, the presence of 20° of excyclodeviation has a 90% association with bilateral superior oblique palsy.[158] Recently Simons et al[259] have cautioned that same-color Maddox rods should be placed before both eyes to avoid artifactual localization of the torsion to the eye with the red lens placed before it.

If bilateral superior oblique palsy can be diagnosed preoperatively, then the surgical procedure can usually be directed at correcting both palsies simultaneously.

Etiology of Isolated Superior Oblique Palsy

Traumatic Superior Oblique Palsy

Trauma is the most common cause of acquired unilateral or bilateral trochlear nerve paresis.[47,64,98,118,146,231,232,233,234,302] All traumatic fourth nerve pareses should be assumed to be bilateral until examination proves otherwise. The trochlear nerve may be damaged anywhere along its course by direct orbital trauma, frontal trauma, or an oblique blow to the head.

In severe brain stem damage, trochlear nerve paresis may be obscured by horizontal gaze abnormalities and become apparent only when horizontal gaze begins to recover. As the trochlear nerves emerge from the dorsal surface of the midbrain, they are susceptible to damage from closed head trauma. The neurosurgical trauma involved in resecting a posterior fossa tumor can similarly injure one or both trochlear nerves.[164] More anteriorly, the proximity of the trochlear nerve to the tentorial edge also makes it susceptible to injury in closed head trauma. A blow to the forehead may cause a contrecoup contusion of one or both

nerves by impingement against the rigid tentorium.[22] Traumatic avulsion here has also been described.[122] Damage at this location is often bilateral, and trauma patients must be carefully examined for this possibility.[267]

Lindenberg has described a countrecoup contusion of the midbrain tectum at the caudal edge of the tentorial notch when the forehead or skull vertex strikes a stationary object.[168] Blows to the occiput or even falls on the buttocks may transmit forces that cause the cerebellum to be thrust against the tentorium from below, injuring the trochlear nerve.[168] The fourth cranial nerve may also be injured by contusion or hemorrhage within the substance of the midbrain.[168]

Since the fourth nerve may be injured by remote trauma, reports of coexisting orbital floor fracture and superior oblique palsy are not surprising.[50,52,143,151] The susceptibility of the fourth nerve to trauma that is not severe enough to produce either skull fracture or loss of consciousness may lead one to miss other underlying disease. Neetens has described three cases of basal intracranial tumors associated with trochlear nerve paresis following minor head trauma.[194] It is unusual for the trochlear nerve to be the sole nerve damaged by cavernous sinus lesions, but it can be damaged in combination with other cranial nerves from lesions in the cavernous sinus. When orbital trauma causes superior oblique weakness, it may be impossible to know whether the injury involved the fourth nerve, the trochlea, or the superior oblique tendon.

Direct trauma to the superior-medial orbit can also produce a superior oblique palsy by laceration of the tendon or muscle or by damage to the trochlea.[14] Knapp coined the term "canine tooth syndrome" to describe the association of a mild Brown syndrome and superior oblique palsy caused by orbital trauma (Knapp type VII superior oblique palsy).[150] Blunt trauma to the superior-medial orbit may also produce a Brown syndrome with no superior oblique weakness.[18,24]

Congenital Superior Oblique Palsy

Congenital superior oblique palsy is underdiagnosed, since many children are asymptomatic, and some affected infants may be thought to have congenital muscular torticollis.[119] The vast majority of cases are nonfamilial, but several families with more than one affected member have been documented.[119] Children with congenital superior oblique palsy typically come to medical attention because of a hypertropia in side gaze or an unexplained head tilt. In older children, congenital superior oblique palsy may present as acquired vertical diplopia. The diagnosis is based upon a history of head tilt beginning in late infancy (as demonstrated by examination of family photographs) in a child with no specific inciting event, together with the following findings on examination:

1. Large vertical fusional vergence amplitudes: Normal vertical fusional vergence amplitudes are 2 to 3 prism diopters. Mottier and Mets[193] studied 14 patients with congenital superior oblique palsy and found average vertical vergence amplitudes to be 16 prism diopters. We have seen adults with congenital superior oblique palsy who fuse up to 30 prism diopters of hyperdeviation. On examination, such a patient will initially seem to be orthotropic, but with prolonged occlusion, the measured vertical deviation will slowly increase as the examiner "chases it" with the prism bar. Symptomatically, older children note that once they begin to see double, the images gradually spread apart. It is not unusual for patients with congenital superior oblique palsy to become symptomatic for the first time in their teenage or adult years. Whether such cases result from a gradual increase in the size of the deviation (perhaps related to ipsilateral superior rectus contracture) or from an age-related reduction in fusional vergence amplitudes is unknown.

2. Facial asymmetry: Facial asymmetry is present in most cases of congenital superior oblique palsy, but it may also be seen in acquired cases that are long-standing.[294] Wilson and Hoxie[294] found facial asymmetry to be present in 7 of 9 patients with congenital superior oblique palsy. This facial asymmetry is thought to be secondary to chronic tilting of the head.[294] Patients with facial asymmetry secondary to congenital superior oblique palsy have hemifacial retrusion with an upward slanting of the mouth on the side of the head tilt (Figure 6.6). The recognition of facial asymmetry associated with congenital fourth nerve palsy can be facilitated by drawing one line through the center of

both pupils and another line through the closed lips. In children with facial asymmetry, these lines converge and intersect toward the side of the shallow, more retruded side of the face (Figure 6.6).[294] This form of facial asymmetry must be distinguished from that associated with congenital muscular torticollis, synostotic plagiocephaly, and the nonspecific facial asymmetry that is common in normal individuals. Because facial asymmetry in congenital muscular torticollis has been reported to resolve with continued facial growth, a similar regression is assumed, albeit unproven, to be possible following early treatment for congenital superior oblique palsy. The age of onset of facial asymmetry in congenital superior oblique palsy and the degree of potential resolution relative to the age at corrective surgery are as yet unknown.

Patients with vertical diplopia associated with congenital superior oblique palsy do not complain of associated image tilt, whereas image tilt is noted in approximately 23% of patients with vertical diplopia from acquired superior oblique palsy.[279] The absence of subjective cyclotropia in congenital fourth nerve palsies presumably reflects the gradual development of complex pathophysiological and/or psychological adaptive mechanisms.[279]

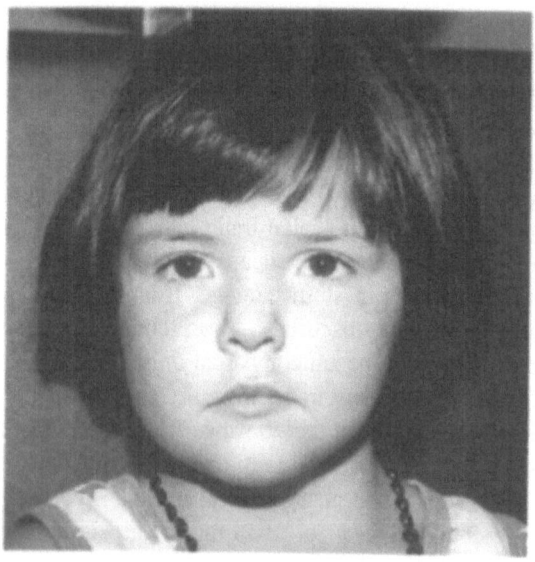

FIGURE 6.6. Residual facial asymmetry in congenital right fourth nerve palsy following surgical correction and resolution of left head tilt. Note the telltale upslanting of the mouth.

The superior oblique traction test is more likely to show tendon laxity in congenital versus acquired cases. Plager[207] used forced duction testing to demonstrate decreased superior oblique muscle resistance to rotation in 14 patients who carried the clinical diagnosis of congenital superior oblique palsy, while all 10 patients with acquired superior oblique palsy had normal resistance to rotation. Helveston et al[124] examined the superior tendon of 89 eyes of patients undergoing surgery for superior oblique palsy and found congenital superior oblique palsy to be associated with an abnormality of the superior oblique tendon in 87% of cases, compared to 8% of cases with acquired superior oblique palsy. Abnormalities of the superior oblique tendon included absence, redundance, misdirection, and insertion into posterior Tenon's capsule. An inherited anomaly confined to the superior oblique tendon could account for reports of familial congenital superior oblique palsy.[119]

Wallace and von Noorden[287] found the following examination findings in the patient with superior oblique palsy to be predictive of a congenitally absent tendon:

1. An associated horizontal deviation.
2. Amblyopia.
3. A large hypertropia in primary position (averaging 20.8 prism diopters).
4. Spread of comitance.
5. Pseudo-overaction of the contralateral superior oblique muscle (due to ipsilateral superior rectus contracture resulting from a long-standing hyperdeviation).

Synostotic Plagiocephaly

Synostotic plagiocephaly caused by stenosis of the ipsilateral coronal suture with subsequent deformation of the orbit has been shown to have a high association of vertical strabismus that mimics a fourth nerve palsy corresponding to the side of the coronal synostosis.[220] One study found an 80% incidence of this vertical ocular misalignment. These patients have apparent overaction of the inferior oblique, and an anatomical deformation of the position of the trochlea has been hypothesized as the cause. In contrast, children with congenital muscular torticollis have an associated torticollis that is not ocular in nature.[90]

Hydrocephalus

Unilateral and bilateral trochlear nerve palsies are not uncommon in children with noncompressive hydrocephalus.[58,66,109] Since the finding of bilateral superior oblique palsy localizes to the superior medullary velum, the associated dilation of the suprapineal recess is assumed to compress the trochlear nerves at their point of decussation.[109] The association of bilateral trochlear nerve paresis with hydrocephalus is easily overlooked because neuro-ophthalmologic signs of rostral midbrain dysfunction usually coexist.[109]

Idiopathic

The diagnosis of idiopathic fourth nerve palsy is assigned to children who develop acute vertical diplopia with signs and symptoms of isolated fourth nerve palsy, no history of recent head trauma, no signs of congenital fourth nerve palsy, and no associated neurological abnormalities.[221] Adults with idiopathic fourth nerve palsies generally show spontaneous recovery over 4 months.[64] This scenario in older adults is often attributed to microvascular infarction of the fourth nerve.[144]

The natural history (persistence versus resolution) of idiopathic fourth nerve palsy in children is unknown. In our experience, the rarity of compressive lesions as a cause of isolated superior oblique palsy in children suggests that clinical observation of persistent fourth nervy palsy may be appropriate and that neuroimaging need only be performed if additional neurological signs develop.

Rare Causes of Fourth Nerve Palsy

Rarely, fourth nerve palsy can occur in patients who have elevated intracranial pressure without ventriculomegaly (pseudotumor cerebri).[17] In this context, trochlear nerve palsy must be distinguished from skew deviation, which can also rarely accompany pseudotumor cerebri.[17] These vertical deviations are usually seen in conjunction with sixth nerve palsy and resolve with normalization of intracranial pressure.

It is rare for a compressive lesion to produce an isolated fourth nerve palsy,[47] although Krohel et al[160] described a 9-year-old child who developed an isolated trochlear nerve palsy as the initial sign of a posterior fossa astrocytoma. Tumor surgery is more likely to cause an isolated trochlear nerve deficit than the tumor itself.[144] The few reports of large aneurysms causing isolated trochlear nerve palsies have been in adults.[4,63,177]

Figure 6.7 provides a clinical algorithm to facilitate the diagnostic work-up in the child with a fourth nerve palsy.

Differential Diagnosis

The differential diagnosis of superior oblique palsy in childhood is listed in Table 6.4. Isolated superior oblique palsies are generally straightforward in older children. In children who have sustained head trauma, however, careful attention should be paid to ruling out *skew deviation.*[114]

The major differential diagnostic considerations in infants with a head tilt are dissociated strabismus and congenital muscular torticollis. *Dissociated vertical deviation* can occasionally present with a hypertropia and a contralateral head tilt and simulate superior oblique palsy.[59] Congenital muscular torticollis is rare. It can be distinguished from congenital superior oblique palsy by (1) the examiner's inability to passively tilt the head in the opposite direction, (2) the palpation of a tight sternocleidomastoid muscle on the side of the tilt, (3) the persistence of the tilt when the infant is reclined, and (4) the persistence of the tilt when either eye is patched. *Synostotic plagiocephaly* can also present with a hypertropia, contralateral head tilt, and facial asymmetry that can resemble a congenital superior oblique palsy. The diagnosis of superior oblique palsy must also be considered in older children who appear to have a monocular *elevation deficiency* ("double elevator palsy"). This situation arises in children who habitually fixate with the paretic, hypertropic eye and develop a contracture in the contralateral inferior rectus muscle (fallen eye syndrome). The *ocular tilt re-*

TABLE 6.4. Differential diagnosis of fourth nerve palsy in childhood.

Dissociated vertical deviation
Congenital muscular torticollis
Synostotic plagiocephaly
Double elevator palsy
Ocular tilt reaction
Incomitant skew deviation

action is a rare ocular motility disturbance of central vestibular origin characterized by vertical divergence of the eyes with a head tilt and bilateral ocular torsion away from the hypertropic eye. The combination of vertical strabismus and a head tilt may initially suggest the diagnosis of superior oblique palsy.

Treatment

Traumatic or other forms of acquired superior oblique palsy should be observed for a minimum of 6 months before considering surgical correction. During this period, occlusion therapy is often unnecessary for unilateral cases since most children can fuse with a compensatory head tilt. The development of amblyopia in this setting suggests a coexistent motility disorder, an associated traumatic disruption of the fusional mechanism, or the inability to obtain fusion by adopting an anomalous head position.

The surgical treatment of unilateral superior oblique palsy should be individualized, but some general guidelines will be summarized. The goal of surgery is to obtain single binocular vision within a functional field of gaze and to normalize the head position. Kraft et al found that patients with fourth nerve palsy who underwent surgery to eliminate a compensatory head posture had a 75.6% incidence of successful restoration of normal head posture.[156]

Using the example of a right superior oblique palsy, the important fields of gaze to consider in planning surgical strategy are *primary gaze, right gaze,* and *downgaze.* (Since there is always a hyperdeviation in left gaze, this finding does not enter into the surgical decision. The following list is a general guideline to surgical strategy:

1. The majority of cases of fourth nerve palsy manifest with isolated overaction of the ipsilateral inferior oblique muscle with little or no underaction of the superior oblique muscle. These cases can be managed by surgically weakening the antagonist inferior oblique muscle (e.g., recession or myectomy). Inferior oblique surgery can neutralize up to 15 prism diopters of hypertropia in primary gaze and has the advantage of being self-titrating.

2. A significant (>10 diopter) right hypertropia in right gaze suggests a secondary right superior

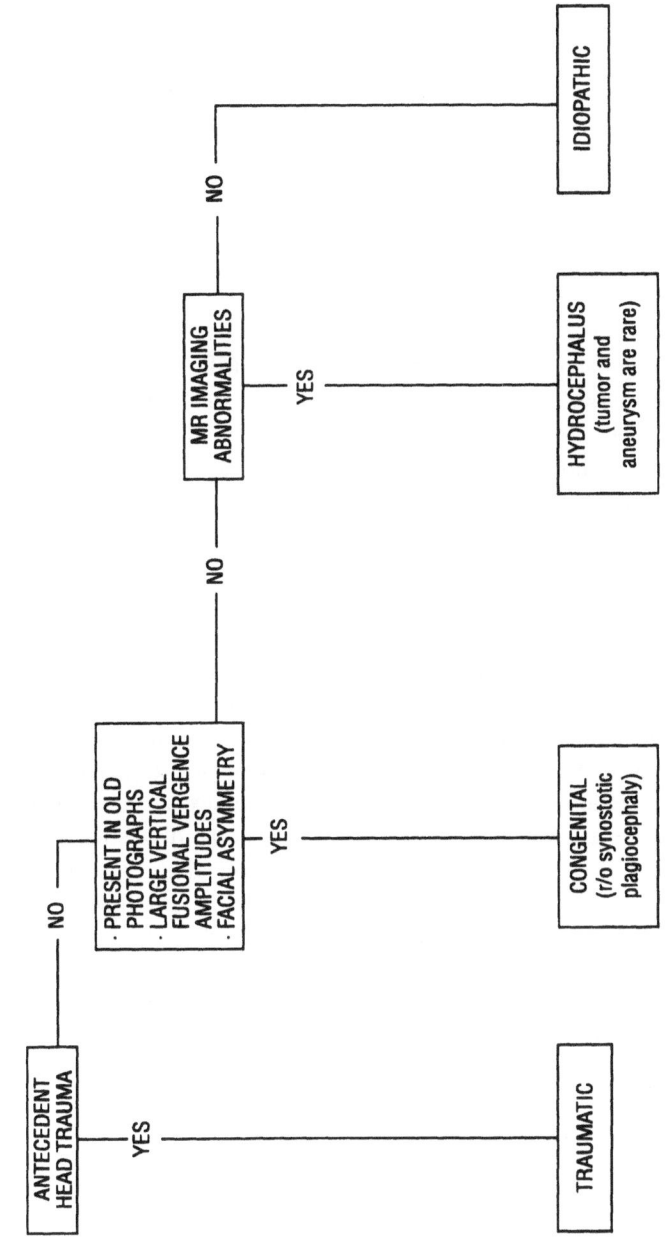

FIGURE 6.7. Clinical algorithm for the evaluation of fourth nerve palsy in childhood.

rectus contracture, which does not respond to inferior oblique weakening alone. In this setting, the ipsilateral superior rectus muscle must also be recessed to eliminate the hyperdeviation in right gaze. Pseudo-overaction of the contralateral superior oblique muscle serves as a useful clinical clue to the presence of a superior rectus contracture.[287,295] Superior rectus contracture can be confirmed by forced duction testing at surgery.

3. A significant (>10 diopter) right hyperdeviation in downgaze suggests a contralateral inferior rectus contracture, as occurs in children who habitually fixate with the paretic eye. Since inferior oblique surgery will not produce a significant effect in downgaze, a contralateral inferior rectus weakening procedure (recession if the deviation is greater than 15 diopters in primary gaze or posterior fixation suture if less than 15 diopters) should be considered.

4. We reserve superior oblique tucks for cases in which there is superior oblique underaction, symptomatic torsion, and minimal ipsilateral inferior oblique overaction. Unlike inferior oblique weakening procedure, a superior oblique tuck must be carefully titrated.[239] A tuck that is too small will produce a negligible treatment effect, while one that is too large will produce a problematic Brown syndrome. Parents must be warned preoperatively that even a successful tuck will produce a mild iatrogenic Brown syndrome that may be associated with vertical diplopia in gaze up and to the opposite side.

Some authors recommend that this surgical strategy be modified for cases of congenital superior oblique palsy, which are often associated with a lax or anomalous superior oblique tendon.[124,207] The absence of normal superior oblique tendon tension can be demonstrated prior to surgical exploration by one of several exaggerated forced duction tests.[110,207] von Noorden[281] has outlined a surgical strategy for treatment of congenital absence of the superior oblique tendon that relies upon inferior oblique weakening as the central procedure with other muscles added with minor modifications to the general rules stated above. Plager[207] has argued that decreased superior oblique tendon tension suggests a lax or absent tendon that should be explored and tucked if present, while a child with normal tendon tension is at high risk of iatrogenic Brown syndrome if the superior oblique tendon is tucked but responds favorably to inferior oblique recession with recession of additional muscles as indicated.

Bilateral superior oblique palsy is more difficult to treat, and parents should be warned preoperatively that comfortable binocular vision in all fields of gaze may not be possible.[116,150,191] In children with alternating hyperdeviations in side gaze and a large esotropia in down gaze, bilateral superior oblique tucks can often restore single binocular vision in primary gaze, but diplopia near the downgaze position usually persists, due to esotropia and residual torsion in this position of gaze. Kushner[163] has utilized a procedure described by Forrest Ellis, MD, and Carlos Souza-Dias, MD, consisting of bilateral inferior rectus recession (5 mm OU) to successfully restore single binocular vision in downgaze. This procedure produces a "fixation duress," requiring excess downgaze innervation that recruits the paretic superior oblique muscles, thereby enhancing abduction and intorsion of the eyes in downgaze. It therefore requires that some residual superior oblique function be present.

Children with bilateral superior oblique palsies may have complaints that are predominantly torsional in nature with minimal alternating hyperdeviations in sidegaze or V pattern in downgaze. In such cases, an alternative to a superior oblique tuck is the dissection and anterior-inferior transposition of the anterior portion of the superior oblique tendon that is primarily involved in torsional movements (Harada–Ito procedure).[116,180] In addition to decreasing or eliminating the excyclodeviation, this procedure will augment abduction in downgaze, thereby reducing the associated V-pattern esotropia.

Abducens Nerve Palsy

Clinical Anatomy

The abducens nucleus lies just lateral to the midline of the pons at its junction with the medulla. The genu of the facial nerve passes close to its dorsal and lateral surface. The medial longitudinal fasciculus is just medial to the nucleus. There are two cell populations in the abducens nucleus: motor neurons of the abducens nerve and interneurons of the contralateral medial longitudinal fasciculus that pass to the medial rectus subnucleus of the contralateral third nerve nucleus. The fascicular portion of the abducens nerve courses ventrally through the pons. Structures near the fascicle include the motor nucleus and fascicle of the facial nerve, the motor nucleus of the trigeminal nerve, the spinal tract and nucleus of the trigeminal nerve, the superior olivary nucleus, the central tegmental tract, and the corticospinal tract.

The extra-axial portion of the sixth nerve turns rostral along the base of the pons lateral to the basilar artery. The nerve ascends through the subarachnoid space along the clivus and penetrates the dura about 1 cm below the crest of the petrous bone. It then passes under the petroclinoid ligament to enter the cavernous sinus. Within the cavernous sinus, the abducens nerve is not situated within the lateral wall as are the oculomotor and trochlear nerves, but it lies in the body of the sinus close to the carotid artery. The sixth nerve enters the orbit through the superior orbital fissure within the annulus of Zinn adjacent to the lateral rectus muscle. The nerve ramifies in the posterior orbit, and its branches enter the lateral rectus muscle diffusely.

A sixth nerve nuclear lesion will paralyze ipsilateral horizontal gaze, because cell bodies of lateral rectus motoneurons and medial longitudinal fasciculus (MLF) interneurons are juxtaposed in the nucleus. Brain stem lesions involving the sixth nerve frequently damage nearby structures, and some localizing syndromes have been named. A large dorsal pontine lesion can produce a horizontal gaze palsy with a variable combination of other signs, including ipsilateral facial palsy, analgesia of the face, peripheral deafness, and loss of taste from the anterior two-thirds of the tongue (Foville syndrome). A ventral pontine lesion involving the pyramidal bundles and tegmentum can produce lateral rectus weakness, with or without ipsilateral facial paralysis, and contralateral hemiplegia (Millard–Gubler syndrome).[188]

The sixth nerve is particularly vulnerable to traumatic, inflammatory, or compressive injury as it leaves the pons and passes vertically through the subarachnoid space to enter the dura overlying the clivus. Blunt trauma may injure the sixth nerve at this point, as may a clivus chordoma or petrous ridge tumor.[68,122,227,243,266,273,303] Basilar meningitis preferentially affects the subarachnoid portion of the abducens nerve. After entering the cavernous sinus, the abducens nerve is especially prone to damage from intracavernous lesions because of its location within the body of the sinus next to the carotid artery, although intracavernous tumors and aneurysms are rare in children, as compared with adults.[147,197] Abducens palsies from cavernous sinus lesions may not be distinguishable from those caused by superior orbital fissure lesions, as associated cranial neuropathies will be similar in both cases. Sympathetic fibers have been demonstrated to leave the carotid plexus and join the abducens nerve in the posterior cavernous sinus.[203] The coexistence of a sixth nerve palsy and an ipsilateral Horner syndrome localizes a lesion to the cavernous sinus.[107]

Clinical Features

Since the sixth nerve innervates only the lateral rectus muscle, the sole action of which is to abduct the eye, the clinical features of a sixth nerve palsy are more straightforward than those of oculomotor or trochlear nerve palsies. Children with an acute sixth nerve palsy will present either with a face turn toward the side of the lesion or with a horizontally noncomitant esotropia that increases in gaze toward the affected eye and decreases or disappears in gaze away from the affected eye. The esodeviation is usually greater at distance than at near fixation. It will also be greater when the child fixates with the paretic eye. Infants and children with a sixth nerve palsy who avoid looking into their diplopic field of gaze may appear to have a gaze palsy.[29] Examining versions with the child's head in its neutral position or spinning an infant to stimulate the vestibulo-ocular reflex should reveal the noncomitancy of the deviation.

A child with an acute complete sixth nerve palsy will have approximately 35 prism diopters of esotropia when fixating with the nonparetic eye at near. In the recovery phase, a significant esotropia may persist despite almost full recovery of abduction. This could result from a residual imbalance in the ratio of phasic to tonic lateral rectus innervation, from secondary medial rectus contracture, or from decompensation of a pre-existing esophoria.

Etiology

Congenital Sixth Nerve Palsy

Congenital sixth nerve palsy is considered to be a rare finding, but it is probably underdiagnosed due to inherent difficulties in identifying abduction deficits in neonates. Such cases are almost always identified in the neonatal nursery and not in the eye clinic. Congenital esotropia has been reported to occur after 6 to 8 weeks of life, since occurrence in the neonatal period has not been documented.[12,196] Therefore, the observation of an esotropia shortly after birth should lead one to consider the possibility of a congenital sixth nerve palsy. Most congenital sixth nerve palsies without peripheral misdirection are transient, probably rising as sequelae to perinatal cranial trauma.

Two forms of transient congenital sixth nerve palsy can be identified. The first presents as a neonatal esotropia with an obvious unilateral abduction deficit that generally improves or resolves over the first month of life.[30,72,216] The incidence has been variously estimated to occur in 1 in 124[216] and 1 in 182[72] neonates. Such cases may be due to perinatal trauma. The second form presents with neonatal esotropia with no obvious abduction deficit.[12] The presence of subtle abduction weakness is, however, very difficult to exclude in such neonates.

Acquired Sixth Nerve Palsy

There are numerous causes of acquired sixth nerve palsy in childhood.[3,95] Robertson et al[223] reviewed 133 cases of isolated acquired sixth nerve palsy in children and found the major diagnostic categories to include neoplasm (39%), trauma (20%), inflammation (17%), and idiopathic (9%), which included cases of benign recurrent sixth nerve palsy. Martonyi[175] reviewed 16 children with sixth nerve palsies and found that eight had benign recurrent sixth nerve palsy, four had elevated intracranial pressure, one had meningitis, one had meningomyelocele, one had ependymoma, and one had idiopathic, and one also had a transient palsy in infancy. The relative prevalence of tumor versus benign recurrent sixth nerve palsy probably reflects the proximity of the investigators to a neurosurgical referral center.

In our experience, the most readily identifiable causes of nontraumatic sixth nerve palsy in childhood are benign recurrent sixth nerve palsy, elevated intracranial pressure, and pontine glioma. When we examine the child with a nontraumatic acquired sixth nerve palsy, our examination is directed toward obtaining historical information and looking for clinical signs that would suggest one of these conditions. We inquire about recent head trauma, antecedent viral illnesses or immunizations, a history of previous episodes, time of onset, symptoms of increased intracranial pressure, or other neurological symptoms. Our initial neuro-ophthalmologic examination is primarily directed toward looking for ipsilateral facial weakness (which would suggest a pontine glioma) and looking for signs of papilledema. We obtain a complete neurological examination and magnetic resonance (MR) imaging in all children with an initial episode of sixth nerve palsy, including cases that are clearly traumatic in origin. The decision whether to perform a lumbar puncture is then predicated upon the results of these studies (Figure 6.8).

Traumatic Sixth Nerve Palsy

Sixth nerve palsies occur frequently in head trauma patients. Blunt trauma is believed to damage the sixth nerve where it is tethered beneath the petroclinoid ligament at its entrance to the dura overlying the clivus.[22] Closed head trauma may also elevate intracranial pressure and secondarily produce unilateral or bilateral sixth nerve paresis. Basilar skull fractures may damage the petrous segment of the abducens nerve after the nerve has penetrated the dura and passed beneath the petroclinoid ligament.[22,41,74,165,222,273] Posttraumatic carotid cavernous fistulas can also be associated with sixth nerve palsy.

Clinical signs of traumatic sixth nerve injury are more readily recognizable than those of fourth nerve injury because the resultant ocular deviation is usually larger in primary gaze position. The occurrence of sixth nerve palsy after apparently trivial head trauma should raise suspicion of an underlying intracranial tumor.[56]

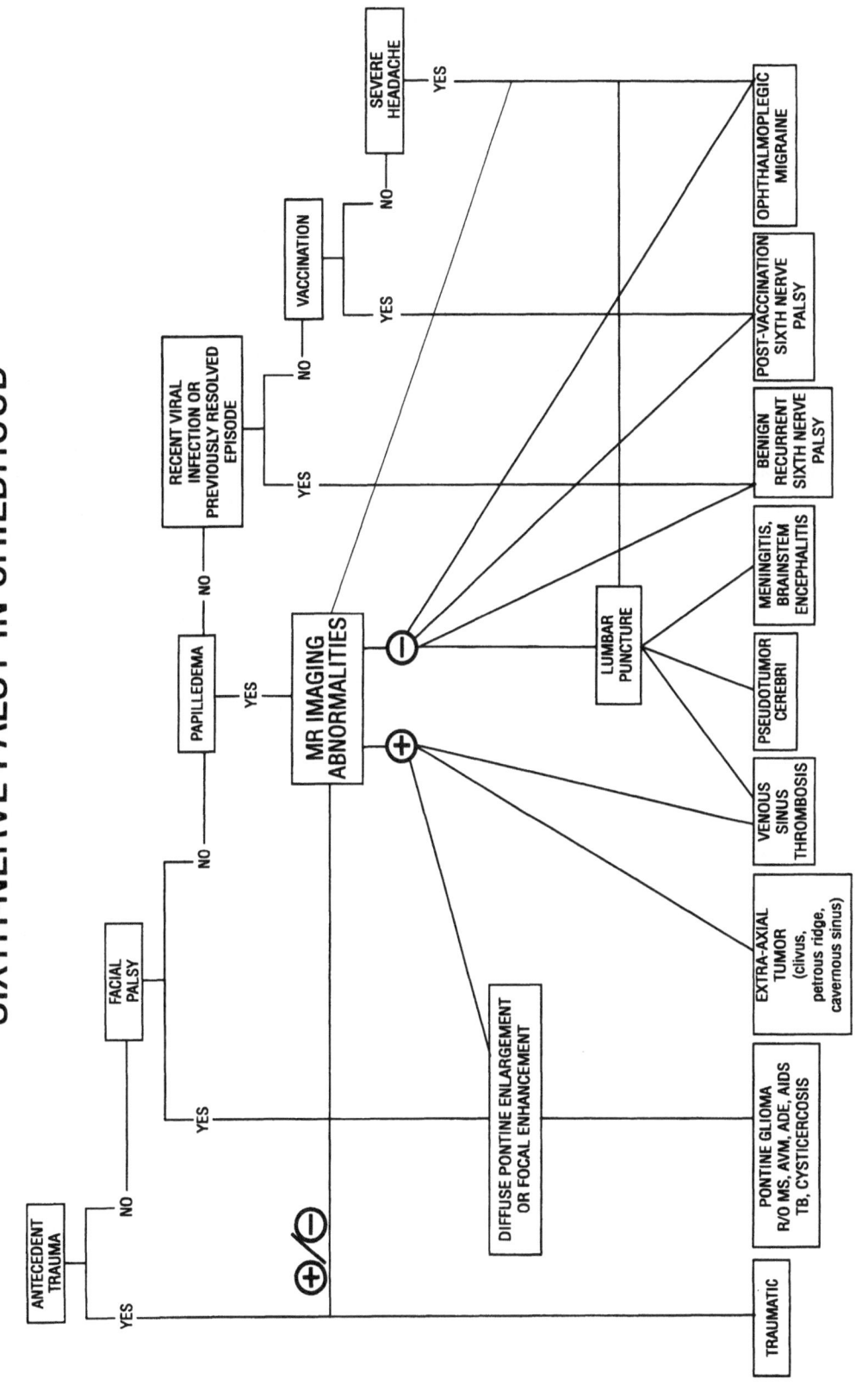

FIGURE 6.8. Clinical algorithm for the evaluation of sixth nerve palsy in childhood.

Benign Recurrent Sixth Nerve Palsy

In 1967, Knox et al[152] described 12 children ranging in age from 18 months to 15 years who developed an acute unilateral sixth nerve palsy after an apparently benign viral illness. Reinecke and Thompson[215] reported five recurrent cases of a similar nature. Werner et al[291] reported several cases of benign recurrent sixth nerve palsy that followed viral illness or immunization (with MMR in one child and DPT in another). Sternberg et al[263] described recurrent attacks of sixth nerve palsy after febrile illness. Afifi et al[2] reviewed the literature and found that this condition had a female and left-sided preponderance. They speculated that possible etiologies could include viral, neurovascular compression by an aberrant artery, and migraine. Isolated reports implicate Epstein-Barr virus infection as the causative agent in some cases.[265] The pathophysiological mechanism and location of injury to the sixth nerve are unclear. It is not known whether the much less common recurrent form of third nerve palsy in childhood represents a variant of the same disorder.

Unlike sixth nerve palsies associated with compression or elevated intracranial pressure, benign recurrent sixth nerve palsies are usually sudden in onset and associated with a severe abduction deficit in the involved eye. Affected children are normal between attacks and have no other intracranial or metabolic abnormalities.[33,37,215,291] Recurrences typically involve the same eye.[175] In most cases, complete resolution occurs over 8 to 12 weeks, however, some children may retain a residual esotropia after numerous recurrences and require surgical correction.[33,215,275] Since strabismic amblyopia may develop prior to resolution,[175] we generally institute part-time occlusion therapy for children in the amblyogenic age range at the initial office visit.

The diagnosis of benign recurrent sixth nerve palsy can be suspected on the initial visit based upon the following information: (1) acute onset, (2) complete absence of abduction, (3) antecedent febrile viral illness, (4) absence of other cranial nerve dysfunction, and (5) absence of signs and symptoms of elevated intracranial pressure. Since there are numerous causes of sixth nerve palsy in children (Figure 6.8), we obtain neuroimaging for all initial episodes of sixth nerve palsy in children, although we rarely repeat these studies for recurrent episodes. However, if an apparently benign sixth nerve palsy in a child with negative neuroimaging studies improves but fails to *completely* resolve, neuroimaging should be repeated since this scenario has been noted in children who are ultimately found to have a pontine glioma on repeat neuroimaging.[296]

Pontine Glioma

Brain stem gliomas are particularly common in children. More than 80% appear to arise from the pons. The peak age of onset is between 5 and 8 years.[174] They characteristically present with an insidious onset of symptoms and signs, including disturbances of gait, sixth and seventh nerve palsies, headaches, nausea, and vomiting. Neuroradiologically, they produce a diffuse, relatively symmetrical expansion of the pons.[174] Larger tumors may elevate the floor of the fourth ventricle to produce obstructive hydrocephalus. Presenting symptoms include ataxia, gait disturbance, and unilateral or bilateral abducens palsy. Esotropia may be the presenting abnormality in some children. Facial palsies, trigeminal deficits, and palsies of cranial nerves IX and X can also develop. Headache, nausea, and vomiting in the absence of hydrocephalus may develop from irritation of the posterior fossa structures. Open biopsy is generally avoided as it commonly worsens the neurological picture and may not result in a positive biopsy due to tissue sampling.[174] Stereotactic biopsy guided by computed tomography (CT) scanning or MR imaging is generally reserved for cases in which there is a major question as to the clinical diagnosis.

The prognosis for pontine glioma remains poor, although it has improved with radiation therapy. Favorable prognostic features include neurofibromatosis, duration of symptoms of 1 year or more before diagnosis, calcification present on neuroimaging studies, focal (versus diffuse infiltrating) tumors, exophytic growth, and histopathological features of a low-grade tumor.[174,188] Chemotherapeutic regimens have not increased survival.

Although the clinical presentation and neuroimaging findings are highly specific for this entity, other conditions can rarely produce similar findings. The differential diagnosis of sixth nerve palsies with a thickened pons on MR imaging includes multiple sclerosis, brain stem vascular malformation, Bickerstaff brain stem encephalitis, tuberculoma, cysticercosis, and AIDS.[174] Since many authors advocate radiotherapy without biopsy, it is important to always consider the possibility of multiple sclerosis (which may improve spontaneously) and to search carefully for other white matter lesions before committing a child with diffuse pontine enlargement to irradiation.[99]

Elevated Intracranial Pressure

Elevated intracranial pressure can result in downward displacement of the brain stem and thereby stretch the sixth nerves which are tethered in Dorello's canal. In children, elevation of intracranial pressure may occur in the setting of posterior fossa tumors, neurosurgical trauma, shunt failure, pseudotumor cerebri, venous sinus thrombosis, meningitis, or Lyme disease.[60,167] In this context, the sixth nerve palsy may be unilateral or bilateral, and it is almost always partial rather than complete. Sixth nerve palsy due to elevated intracranial pressure summarily resolves when the intracranial pressure is normalized.

Other CNS Tumors

As previously discussed, sixth nerve palsy in children may well be the presenting sign of an intracranial tumor. Skull base tumors (chordoma, meningioma, nasopharyngeal carcinoma, metastasis) predominate in adults while posterior fossa tumors (pontine glioma, medulloblastoma, ependymoma, cystic cerebellar astrocytoma) can produce unilateral or bilateral sixth nerve palsies in children. The tempo of onset, associated neurological signs, and the presence or absence of papilledema provide the most important diagnostic clues, but the possibility should be more definitively evaluated with MR imaging. Mechanism of abducens nerve injury include direct infiltration of the pons and elevation of intracranial pressure (with or without hydrocephalus). Sixth nerve palsy is also a common postoperative complication following neurosurgical resection of posterior fossa tumors in children.

Meningitis

Hanna et al[117] found abducens palsy in 16.5% of patients with acute bacterial meningitis, compared with 3% for oculomotor nerve involvement and 3% for facial nerve involvement. The predominance of sixth nerve injury could not be attributed to elevated intracranial pressure, given the low incidence of associated papilledema (3%) in this series. As previously mentioned, cranial neuropathies in the setting of acute bacterial meningitis tend to be multiple and are often bilateral.[57] Transient sixth nerve palsy has been reported as a possible meningitic complication in children with chicken pox.[195,228]

Rare Causes of Sixth Nerve Palsy

Sixth nerve palsy is occasionally seen in children with otherwise typical features of ophthalmoplegic migraine. In this setting, lateral rectus muscle function can be expected to recover. Although intracranial aneurysms are rare in children, Killer et al[147] described an 8-year-old girl who developed an isolated sixth nerve palsy and was found to have an intracavernous carotid aneurysm.

Children with elevated intracranial pressure or hydrocephalus occasionally develop a sixth nerve palsy following lumbar puncture or shunting procedures.[84] Children without elevated intracranial pressure can also develop a sixth nerve palsy following diagnostic lumbar puncture or myelography.[79,206] The mechanism of injury is thought to involve caudal displacement of the brain after loss of cerebrospinal fluid (CSF) support in the basal cisterns.[269] The abducens nerve may be most susceptible to traction as it changes direction at the petrous ridge to pass forward under the petroclinoid ligament.

Gradenigo syndrome is a vanishingly rare condition in which a severe mastoiditis extends from the mastoid air cells to the tip of the petrous bone, producing localized inflammation of the meninges in the epidural space and paresis of the ipsilateral sixth nerve, with very intense pain localized to the temporal and parietal regions.[103] Ipsilateral facial weakness may also develop. More commonly, the association of sixth nerve palsy with mastoiditis in children results from contiguous inflammatory venous sinus thrombosis with elevation of intracranial pressure[60] (Figure 3.4).

Differential Diagnosis

Duane Retraction Syndrome

The differential diagnosis of sixth nerve palsy in childhood is summarized in Table 6.5. *Duane syndrome* is probably the most common pediatric disorder associated with an isolated abduction deficit.[80] Although Duane syndrome is simply a congenital sixth nerve palsy with peripheral misdirection, its clinical features and prognosis differ from other forms of sixth nerve palsy and warrant a more detailed discussion.

Duane syndrome is a common disorder of unknown etiology in which decreased or absent lateral rectus innervation by the sixth nerve occurs in conjunction with misdirected innervation to the lateral rectus muscle from a branch of the third nerve. This neural misdirection leads to cocontraction of the lateral rectus muscle and a characteristic retraction of the globe on attempted adduction. The anomalous recruitment of the paretic lateral rectus muscle in attempted adduction can lead to a variety of bizarre motility disturbances, some of which have only recently been recognized as epiphenomena of Duane syndrome.

Clinically, most children with Duane syndrome exhibit the following common features: (1) limited abduction, (2) widening of the palpebral fissure on attempted abduction, and (3) retraction of the globe with narrowing of the palpebral fissure on attempted adduction.[257] Although adduction is always limited because of lateral rectus cocontraction, it often appears to be full because the globe retracts. Approximately 22% of children with Duane syndrome have significant enophthalmos of the involved eye in primary position, which can occasionally be the most disfiguring aspect of the syndrome.[257] Children with Duane syndrome rarely complain of diplopia, although they can recognize two images when forced to gaze in the

TABLE 6.5. Differential diagnosis of sixth nerve palsy in childhood.

Duane syndrome
Myasthenia gravis
Spasm of the near reflex
Medial orbital fracture with entrapment
Longstanding esotropia with medial rectus muscle contracture
Ocular neuromyotonia
Graves ophthalmopathy

---

direction of the paretic lateral rectus muscle. Most are orthotropic or esotropic in the primary gaze position adapting a small face turn. For this reason, amblyopia is rare in Duane syndrome.[257] Duane syndrome is more common in females and involves the left eye more frequently than the right. It is unilateral in approximately 82% of cases and bilateral in 18%. It occurs as a sporadic condition in approximately 90% of cases and is familial in approximately 10%.[76]

The distinction between Duane syndrome and a sixth nerve palsy can readily be made in a cooperative child but may be difficult in an infant. Jampolsky[136] has cautioned that one cannot rely upon palpebral fissure changes during sidegaze to identify globe retraction, since the palpebral fissure may normally widen in abduction and narrow slightly in adduction. Rather, one must directly observe the globe from a lateral view as the eye is moved from its position of maximal abduction into a position of adduction. The discrepancy between the primary gaze deviation and the degree of abduction deficit often provides an additional clue to the presence of Duane syndrome in an infant. For instance, it is not uncommon for a patient with Duane syndrome to be orthotropic or almost orthotropic despite complete absence of abduction in one eye. By contrast, a complete unilateral sixth nerve palsy produces approximately 35 diopters of esotropia at near fixation. The distinction between Duane syndrome and sixth nerve palsy in infancy is also aided by having the infant view a toy with the affected eye in adduction and performing a quick alternate cover test. The infant with Duane syndrome will be exotropic in this position due to cocontraction of the lateral rectus muscle, whereas the infant with a sixth nerve palsy will be orthotropic or esotropic.

Other Clinical Features of Duane Syndrome

An innervational abnormality of the lateral rectus muscle is the underlying cause of all of the associated ocular motility disorders, which are summarized as follows:

1. *Upshoots and downshoots:* During adduction of the affected eye, the cocontracting lateral rectus muscle overlies the crest of the globe, and there is maximal retraction. When the eye elevates or depresses in adduction, many chil-

dren develop an upshoot or downshoot (or both), which may cause the eye to completely disappear under the upper or lower eyelid (Figure 6.9). Upshoots or downshoots represent a "retraction escape" or "retraction substitute." The finding that these movements in Duane syndrome are associated with electromyographic (EMG) activity in the superior and inferior rectus muscles initially led to the belief that they resulted from anomalous superior rectus recruitment. However, it has since been shown that increased EMG activity will occur with any retraction of the eye.[135] Presumably, these muscles are "taking up the slack" caused by the origins and insertion of the muscle being brought closer together. Since surgically tenotomizing the superior rectus muscle under local anesthesia does not eliminate the upshoot, one must assume that the EMG activity seen in the vertically acting rectus muscles occurs as a result of (rather than causing) the upshoot or downshoot.[136] This supposition is supported by the fact that surgically disinsert-ing the lateral rectus muscle under local anesthesia almost completely eliminates the upshoot or downshoot. The long-standing notion that the cocontracting horizontal rectus muscles slip superiorly or inferiorly over the globe (the "bridal theory" or "leash effect") to produce the upshoot or downshoot has been supported by the improvement or resolution when the lateral rectus muscle is recessed by a large amount, recessed and split, or fixated retroequatorially to the globe. However, recent cinematic MR imaging studies by Bloom et al[36] show little, if any, vertical displacement of the horizontal rectus muscles. von Noorden[282] has argued that these findings confirm (rather than refute) the bridal theory, by providing indirect evidence that it is the center of rotation of the globe that slips beneath the muscles as the eye elevates or depresses, rather than vice versa.

2. *V or Y pattern:* Some children with Duane syndrome display an abrupt splaying of the eyes into exotropia in upgaze[154] (Figure 6.9). This phenomenon results from anomalous recruit-

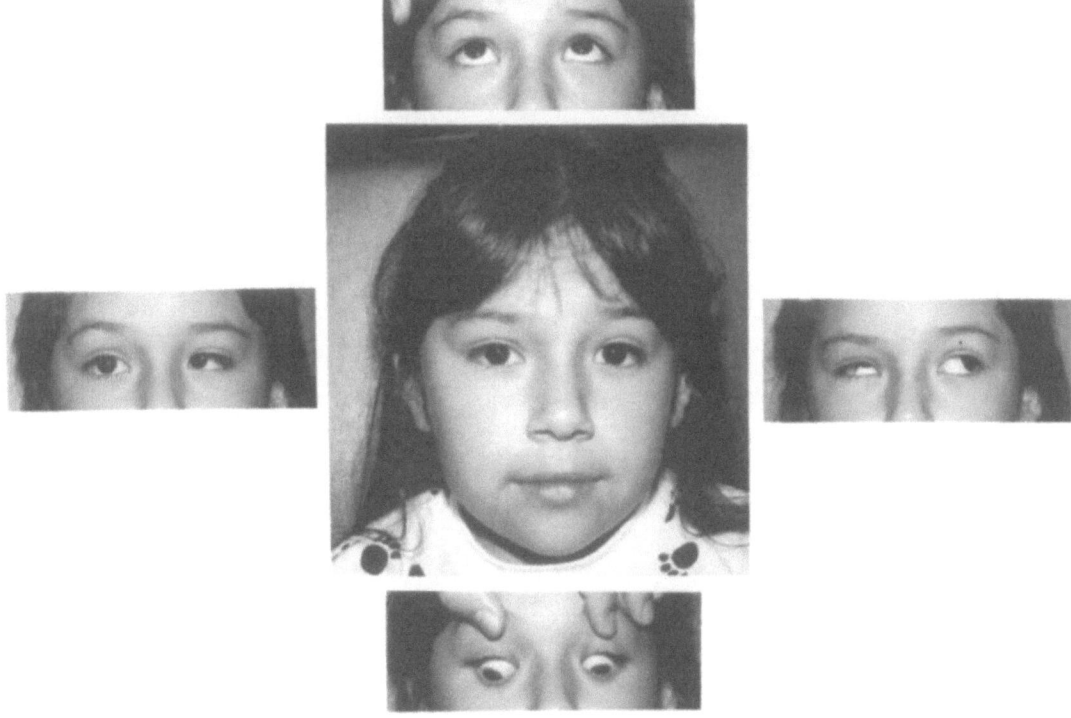

FIGURE 6.9. Child with right Duane syndrome after operation: (1) upshoot in abduction and (2) recruitment of the lateral rectus muscles in down gaze.

ment of the lateral rectus muscle in upgaze. A similar phenomenon is less commonly seen in downgaze (Figure 6.9). The finding of horizontal splaying of the eyes in extreme vertical gaze may cause diagnostic confusion when it occurs in the absence of an abduction deficit (Figure 6.9). Since abduction may be normal or decreased, Kushner[163] has suggested that cases without abduction deficits still fall within the spectrum of Duane syndrome. This rare motility pattern can be distinguished from the more common V pattern associated with inferior oblique muscle overaction by abrupt divergence of the eyes in far upgaze and the absence of alternating hyperdeviations on sidegaze.[163] Kushner[163] has successfully treated this condition with recessions and superior transposition of the lateral rectus muscles. This variant of Duane syndrome shows that the aberrant innervation of lateral rectus muscle need not always

arise from the medial rectus branch of the oculomotor nerve.

3. *Synergistic divergence:* Rarely, recruitment of the lateral rectus muscle in attempted adduction can exceed the force produced by the medial rectus muscle, resulting in a paradoxical abduction of the affected eye (termed synergistic divergence)[284,293] (Figure 6.11). Most patients with this phenomenon have a large exotropia and simultaneous nystagmoid movements on attempted adduction of the affected eye.[76] The condition is usually unilateral, but bilateral cases have been described.[43,69,113,268,293,304] The occurrence of synergistic divergence in several patients with congenital fibrosis syndrome[42,43,111] suggests that a primary failure to establish normal neuronal-extraocular muscle connections may underlie some cases of congenital fibrosis syndrome, since fibrosis in Duane syndrome is only seen

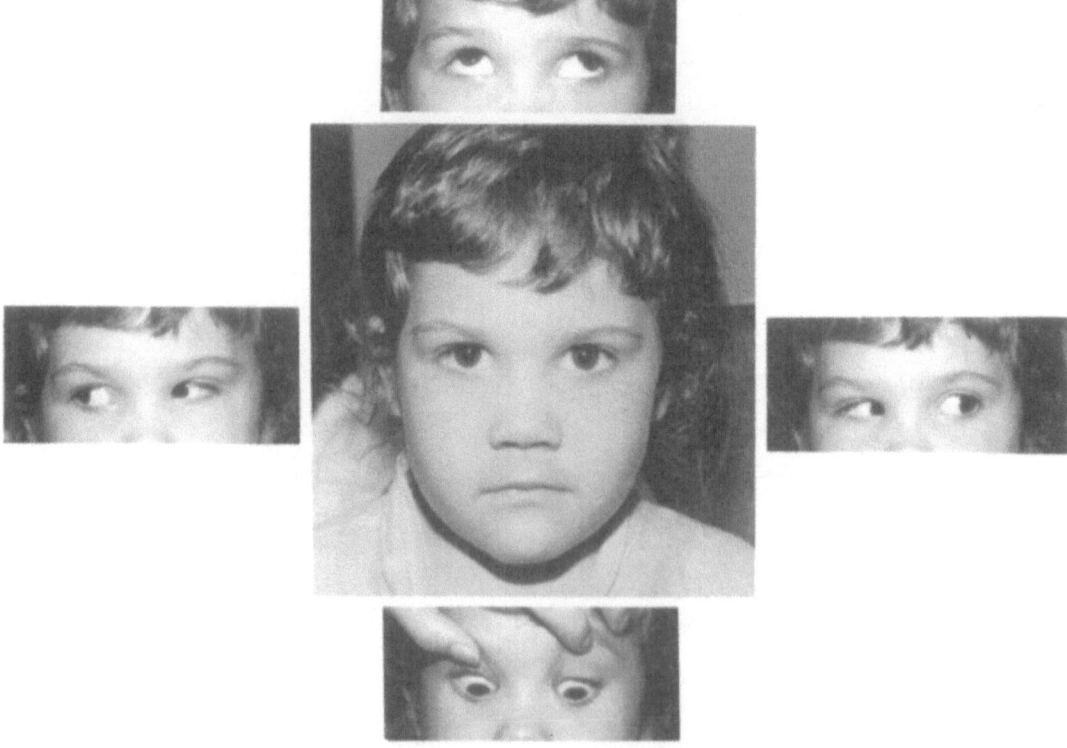

FIGURE 6.10. Child with left Duane syndrome demonstrating a Y pattern secondary to recruitment of the lateral rectus muscles in upgaze. Note minimal abduction limitation despite retraction in adduction. The absence of alternating hypertropia of the adducting eye in sidegaze helps distinguish this condition from primary inferior oblique overaction.

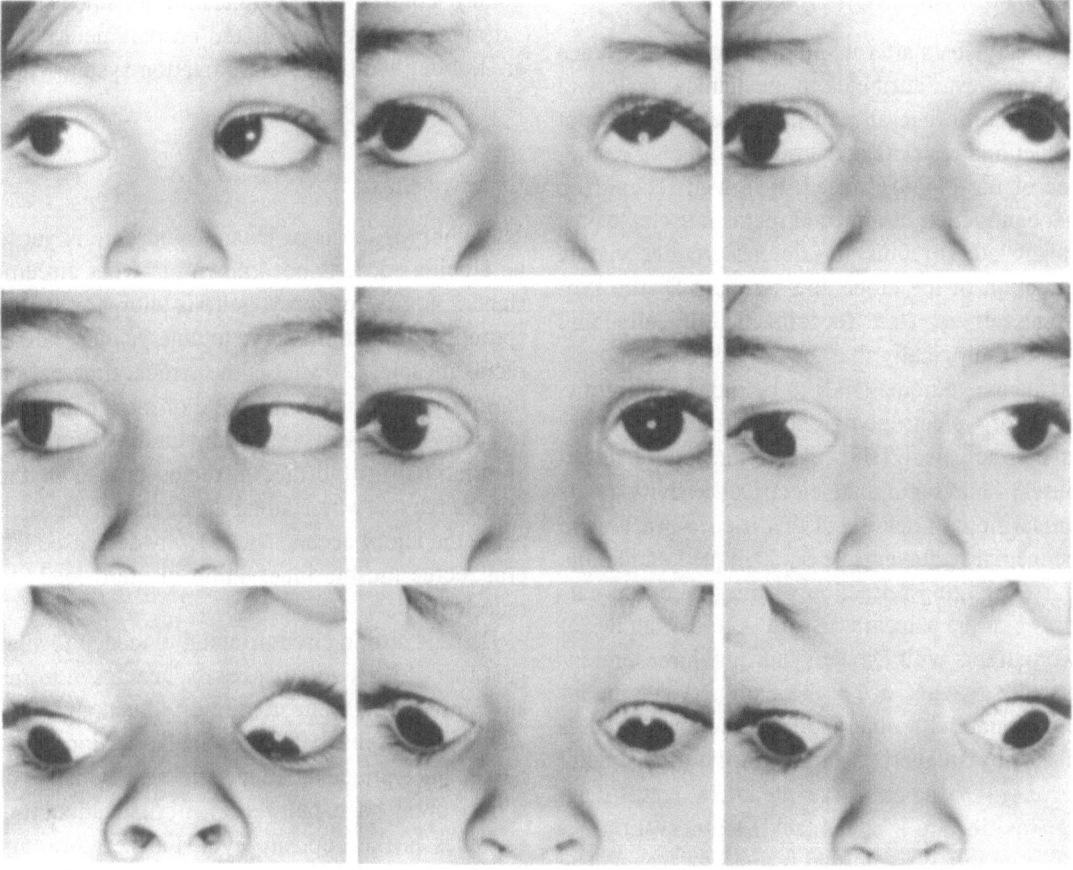

FIGURE 6.11. Child with right Duane syndrome demonstrating synergistic divergence on attempted left gaze. (From Hamed LM, Lingua RW, Fanous MM, et al. J Pediatr Ophthalmol & Strabis 1992;29:30–37. With permission.)

histopathologically in areas of lateral rectus muscle lacking innervation.[127,187] Synergistic divergence may occur as a surgical complication following medial rectus recession in patients with Duane syndrome who have marked lateral rectus cocontraction. The treatment of synergistic divergence is difficult, but extirpation of the ipsilateral lateral rectus muscle has been shown to abolish the phenomenon.[113]

Systemic Associations

Duane syndrome may be associated with one or more additional systemic findings in approximately 33% of cases.[67,201] High-tone hearing loss or sensorineural deafness is found in approximately 10% of patients with Duane syndrome.[149,219,257] Conversely, Duane syndrome was found in 7 of 500 deaf children and a horizon-

tally noncomitant strabismus was found in an additional four.[6] Wilderwanck syndrome (cervico-oculo-acoustic syndrome) comprises Duane syndrome, a cervical malformation known as the Klippel–Feil anomaly, and deafness. Female predominance is much more marked in Wilderwanck syndrome than in Duane syndrome.[76]

Other systemic associations include congenital thenar hypoplasia (Okihiro syndrome), with or without congenital cardiac anomalies (Holt–Oram syndrome).[76] Duane syndrome may also occur as part of the Goldenhar sequence, as well as in arthrogryposis multiplex congenita.[183] The association of familial Duane syndrome and urogenital abnormalities with a defect in chromosome 22 was recently described.[70] Numerous other ocular and systemic anomalies have been described with Duane syndrome, most notably Marcus Gunn jaw winking, crocodile tears, and iris heterochromia.[76,257]

Etiology of Duane Syndrome

For many years after its initial description, Duane syndrome was attributed to mechanical factors (a tight, paretic lateral rectus muscle that does not abduct and restricts adduction, producing retraction of the globe). Indeed, it is well recognized that contraction of a medial rectus muscle against a tight lateral rectus muscle can produce visible retraction of the globe and simulate Duane syndrome. It is also recognized clinically and histopathologically that the lateral rectus muscle in Duane syndrome tends to be tight and fibrotic. However, electromyographic studies[129,236,245] have conclusively shown that the lateral rectus muscle shows minimal electrical activity in its normal field of action but that it cocontracts with the medial rectus muscle on attempted adduction, thus explaining retraction of the globe and narrowing of the palpebral fissure. Autopsy studies of two patients with Duane syndrome have demonstrated a total absence of the sixth nerve on the involved side with innervation of the lateral rectus muscle by an aberrant branch of the third cranial nerve.[127,187] In both cases, the lateral rectus muscle was fibrotic in areas lacking innervation but appeared relatively normal where innervated. The portion of the sixth nerve nucleus corresponding to the abducens cell bodies was also deficient.

Classification of Duane Syndrome Based on Range of Movement

Huber[129] classified Duane syndrome into types I, II, and III, depending on the pattern of horizontal movement abnormality that accompanied the anomalous lateral rectus innervation. Type I Duane syndrome, which is by far the most common form, is characterized by severely limited abduction with mildly limited adduction, with retraction of the globe and narrowing of the lid fissure on attempted adduction. Type II (the rarest) has limited or absent adduction with relatively normal abduction and retraction of the globe with narrowing of the lid fissure on attempted adduction. The adduction deficit in type II Duane syndrome can superficially resemble a partial third nerve palsy (Table 6.2). Patients with type III Duane syndrome demonstrate reduced abduction and adduction and have retraction of the globe and narrowing of the lid fissure on attempted adduction. This classifica-

tion system has limited clinical utility since surgical management is predicted on parameters that are not defined by the classification system (subsequently discussed).

Embryogenesis

The embryogenesis of Duane syndrome is yet to be elucidated. It is not known (1) what circumstances unique to embryogenesis allow for axonal sprouting of the third nerve to innervate the lateral rectus muscle, (2) what is the critical time period in embryogenesis for this type of misinnervation to occur, (3) why neural misdirection occurs preferentially from the medial rectus branch of the third nerve, (4) where along the course of the sixth nerve the injury occurs, and (5) why decreased lateral rectus muscle innervation in utero leads to muscle fibrosis.

There is strong circumstantial evidence to suggest that at least some cases of Duane syndrome are caused by a brain stem injury. Such an injury would have to involve the fascicular portion of the nerve, since affected patients have no evidence of a horizontal gaze palsy (i.e., normal adducting saccades in the opposite eye). Furthermore, autopsy studies have demonstrated selective absence of the cell bodies corresponding to abducens motoneurons, with selective preservation of rostral cell bodies believed to represent internuclear neurons.[187] Jay and Hoyt[137] found a high incidence of abnormal latencies of brain stem auditory evoked responses (BAER) in Duane syndrome. The hearing loss noted in a significant number of patients with Duane syndrome[219] would seem to fit with the abnormalities in BAER. However, auditory function testing and otolaryngologic examination have also implicated associated middle ear disease and cochlear abnormalities in some patients, indicating that thorough auditory evaluation should be undertaken in all children with Duane syndrome.[219] Ramsay and Taylor[212] found a high incidence of Duane syndrome in patients with crocodile tears (which is caused by seventh nerve misdirection). Miller[185] found classic Duane syndrome in 31% of patients with thalidomide embryopathy, while other exposed patients had horizontal gaze palsies, facial weakness, and VIII nerve deficits. The clustering of these effects in patients with early thalidomide exposure suggests teratogenic injury involving the dorsal pons. However, experimental denervation of peripheral cranial nerves in the cavernous sinus of kittens has also led to peripheral misdirection with retraction movements,[295] suggesting that an extra-axial sixth nerve fascicular injury can also eventuate in Duane syndrome.

Two theories exist as to the early events in the ontogenesis of the extraocular muscles. One holds that the anlagen of each muscle condenses from one of three distinct myogenic precursors, separately and at different times.[96,97] The alternative theory[255,256] is that the extraocular muscles develop concurrently from a single mesenchymal condensation that subsequently divides into separate superior and inferior mesodermal complexes. According to this theory, individual extraocular muscles may receive contributions from both mesodermal complexes or may arise from only one complex. During organogenesis, the developing brain stem also is segmented into regions known as rhombomeres that give rise to the cranial nerves.[170] Each of the ocular motor nerves arise from particular rhombomeres, thereby establishing the segmental nature of the cranial nerves. A caudal-to-rostral internuclear gradient for the genesis of oculomotor motoneurons has been described in rats.[7,8] The majority of motoneurons in abducens, trochlear, and oculomotor nuclei are postmitotic by the time the eye muscles are forming. Recent studies suggest that aggregates of myoblasts may be contacted by oculomotor nerves prior to migration and carry their innervation with them into the developing orbit.[19,21,285,286] Whether innervation first occurs in the orbit or while myoblasts are still adjacent to the neural tube, the close proximity of the anlagen of the extraocular muscles may actually facilitate development of anomalous innervation of eye muscles. Taken together, these developmental sequences set the stage for the pattern of malformation of which Duane syndrome is the prototype. Specifically, the muscle anlagen are very close to each other and to the nuclei of the brain stem at the time of their innervation so an oculomotor neural growth cone would have a very short distance to travel to innervate the lateral rectus anlage. Furthermore, the lateral rectus may receive myoblasts from both an upper and a lower anlage, rendering at least partial innervation by the third nerve, which also supplies

upper and lower anlagen, more likely. A similar outcome has been seen in a transgenic mouse model in which the oculomotor and trochlear nuclei are absent and the abducens nerve sprouts to innervate extraocular muscles other than the lateral rectus.[209]

Surgical Treatment of Duane Syndrome

The innervational anomalies in Duane syndrome produce a variety of ocular motility disturbances that dictate the proper surgical management. The fundamental abnormality in Duane syndrome remains the aberrant or inappropriate innervation of the lateral rectus muscle by a branch of the oculomotor nerve. The position of the eye at rest; positions of comfortable binocular vision; and relative amounts of abduction, adduction, and retraction depend upon a continuum of the power of cocontraction of the lateral rectus muscle and, to a lesser extent, the amount of contracture that has developed in the lateral rectus muscle.[211] The general principles that guide the surgical approach to the child with Duane syndrome include the following:

Esotropia in Duane Syndrome

1. Most children with Duane syndrome who require surgical treatment have an esotropia with a compensatory face turn to fuse. In this setting, unilateral recession of the medial rectus muscle in the involved eye is often sufficient to restore ocular alignment in primary gaze. In Duane syndrome, however, the size of the necessary medial rectus recession varies for a given deviation depending upon the *amount of cocontraction* in primary gaze. Surgical treatment of esotropia in Duane syndrome is fraught with pitfalls since a given deviation may be associated with either mild or severe cocontraction of the lateral rectus muscle.

   From a surgical point of view, it is useful to view Duane syndrome with esotropia as existing on a continuum from congenital sixth nerve palsy (i.e., cases with only minimal lateral rectus cocontraction) to cases with severe cocontraction, which tend to manifest with upshoots and downshoots. The most important (and overlooked) step in the preoperative evaluation of Duane syndrome with esotropia is to attempt to assess the amount of cocontraction based upon clinical findings. In a child with minimal cocontraction, even a large medial rectus recession (e.g., 7 mm) may be insufficient to restore ocular alignment (as would be the case with a sixth nerve palsy). In a child with marked cocontraction, even a moderate medial rectus recession may *unleash* the cocontracting lateral rectus muscle and produce postoperative exotropia, limited adduction, and iatrogenic synergistic divergence.

In addition to observing the degree of retraction of the globe in attempted adduction, the amount of lateral rectus cocontraction can be judged by observing the degree of face turn relative to the degree of esotropia. A large face turn relative to the degree of esotropia (as would be seen in a sixth nerve palsy), suggests that there is *minimal* lateral rectus cocontraction and that a large medial rectus recession is therefore required to realign the eyes. A smaller-than-expected face turn in the presence of a large esotropic deviation suggests the presence of *marked* lateral rectus cocontraction in primary position since even mild adduction produces sufficient cocontraction to realign the eyes. In this circumstance, a large medial rectus muscle recession to improve the primary position alignment of the eye will leave the strongly cocontracting lateral rectus muscle unopposed in primary position, resulting in a consecutive exotropia. In gaze away from the affected eye, the cocontracting lateral rectus muscle, which is now unopposed, may now abduct (rather than adduct) the affected eye, resulting in postoperative synergistic divergence. If this complication can be anticipated by preoperative examination, it can be avoided by performing only a small recession of the medial rectus of the affected eye (e.g., 3 mm) along with a large (e.g., 8 mm) recession of the medial rectus muscle in the unaffected eye.[240] This will lead to a mild limitation of adduction of that eye but will serve the purpose of aligning the eye in primary position without allowing the lateral muscle of the affected eye to overwhelm its antagonist when it cocontracts. It will also minimize the risk of postoperative synergistic divergence.[181] Marked enophthalmos in the Duane eye also suggests a large amount of cocontraction is present. The finding

of normal saccadic velocities of adducting saccades in Duane syndrome is also suggestive of minimal contraction, while a decreased adducting saccadic velocity suggests significant cocontraction.[301]

2. Lateral rectus muscle resections are to be avoided. The lateral rectus muscle is already short, tight, and innervationally abnormal in Duane syndrome. Resection of this muscle creates the risk of producing disfiguring enophthalmos, severely limiting adduction and producing iatrogenic synergistic divergence.

3. Although transposition procedures of the vertical rectus muscles can increase abduction, they have the potential to induce a vertical deviation and disrupt fusion, especially in patients with marked cocontraction. Most strabismus surgeons therefore favor the inherent simplicity of unilateral or bilateral medial rectus recessions.

Duane Syndrome with Exotropia

Primary gaze position exotropia is rare in children with Duane syndrome. It is a progressive condition that becomes symptomatic in older adults when the degree of exotropia cannot be comfortably compensated by a face turn. In the setting of a large-angle exotropia, Duane syndrome often goes unrecognized because the adduction limitation may be attributed to a secondary lateral rectus muscle contracture. The clue to the diagnosis lies in the seemingly paradoxical finding of limited abduction in a patient with large-angle exotropia. This scenario exemplifies the importance of distinguishing the *position* of the globe (which may merely reflect muscle tightness) from the *contractility* of the muscles. Surgery usually consists of large (as much as 15 mm from the insertion) unilateral or bilateral lateral rectus recessions. The usual dose response curve of millimeters of surgery to diopters of correction will not apply to Duane syndrome due to the combination of contracture and cocontraction. Patients must be forewarned that although the position of the eye will be transferred to primary gaze, the eye will be unable to move laterally following surgery. Due to the propensity of the lateral rectus muscle to undergo progressive contracture in all exotropic patients, recurrences and undercorrections are common.

There are several options in the surgical management of upshoot or downshoot on adduction. The lateral and medial rectus muscles can both be recessed, decreasing the amount of force on the eye in adduction, allowing the muscle to stay on the main arc of the eye.[283] The distal lateral rectus muscle can be longitudinally split, with the upper and lower segments reattached above and below the horizontal main arc of the eye, making it impossible for the globe to slip over or under the lateral muscle when it cocontracts. Alternatively, a posterior fixation suture of the lateral rectus muscle may be used to prevent the eye from slipping above or below the cocontracting horizontal rectus muscles.[283]

Bilateral Duane Syndrome

Surgical repair of bilateral Duane syndrome with esotropia is especially problematic because of the presence of bilateral cocontraction. In this setting, even moderate (5 mm) bimedial recessions may produce a medial rectus "fixation duress" in the fixating eye while at the same time *unleashing* the cocontracting lateral rectus muscle in the nonfixating eye, leading to a large consecutive exotropia.[136] It is usually necessary to decrease the size of the medial rectus recession from those provided by standard dose-response formulas.

Management of Sixth Nerve Palsy

Children with sixth nerve palsy from head trauma should be observed for a period of 6 months prior to surgical intervention since the majority will recover spontaneously. For children in the amblyogenic age range, we utilize part-time occlusion of the fixating (usually nonparetic) eye to prevent amblyopia or treat it if it has already developed. This therapy also stimulates abduction of the paretic eye and thereby minimizes the chance of contracture formation. Patching the unaffected eye will also stimulate maximal inhibition of the medial rectus muscle in order to establish the most appropriate head position possible, thus minimizing the potential for a secondary medial rectus contracture to develop.[249] Prisms are rarely helpful in the recovery phase, due to the horizontal incomitancy of the deviation. The indications for oculinum injection for acute sixth nerve palsy in children are controversial.[181] We reserve medial rectus oculinum injection for children with a severe palsy who would have to assume an uncomfortably large face turn to fixate with the paretic eye. Its long-term superiority as compared to simple observation has not been documented.

Residual esodeviations in children with sixth nerve palsy can result from incomplete neural recovery, from a medial rectus contracture, or both. Children who show incomplete recovery after 6 months with residual esodeviations in primary gaze are generally treated with strabismus surgery. Surgical treatment in sixth nerve palsy is predicated on the degree of lateral rectus function. Visible abduction past the midline demonstrates the presence of residual lateral rectus function and suggests that a recess-resect procedure will be sufficient to restore ocular alignment. As in Duane syndrome, it is often helpful to perform an additional medial rectus recession and/or a medial rectus posterior fixation suture of the contralateral medial rectus muscle to create a fixation duress that will "drive the palsy." This procedure improves abduction of the paretic eye and leads to a larger postoperative field of single binocular vision.

Absence of abduction past midline indicates either a lateral rectus paralysis or severe medial rectus contracture with some lateral rectus function. In this circumstance, the surgical decision is predicated on the clinical estimation or measurement of saccadic velocity, the forced duction test, and the forced generation test. In the child with no abduction past midline, the finding of a "floating saccade" as the eye moves from a position of adduction toward primary gaze is a useful clue that the lateral rectus muscle is completely paralyzed.[230] By contrast, a rapid saccade from adduction to midline is evidence that the lateral rectus muscle is functioning and that the abduction limitation results from a medial rectus contracture. In cooperative children, a forced generation test is also useful in clinically confirming presence or absence of lateral rectus function, which can be estimated or felt as a "pull" on the forceps when the child attempts to abduct the paretic eye. These clinical tests can be supplemented by a forced duction test (performed either in clinic or under anesthesia prior to strabismus surgery) to further assess the degree of medial rectus contracture.

Those with little or no recovery of sixth nerve function require a transposition procedure of the vertical rectus muscles to the lateral rectus muscle to create a new abduction force.[93,138,254] A large resection of a completely paralytic rectus muscle accomplishes little and sacrifices a portion of the anterior ciliary circulation. Vertical rectus muscle transposition can be performed in conjunction with a recession of the antagonist medial rectus muscle[229]; however, this procedure creates a risk of anterior segment ischemia in adult patients. A large recession (>7 mm) of the *contralateral* medial rectus muscle also works well and does not risk anterior segment ischemia. Most centers currently utilize transposition in conjunction with preoperative or intraoperative injection of botulinum toxin into the ipsilateral medial rectus muscle. Botulinum functions as a "chemical traction suture" by creating a temporary medial rectus paralysis and thereby positioning the eye in abduction for several months.[86,178,247] Parents must be warned that this procedure creates an initial postoperative exotropia and that continued part-time occlusion therapy will be necessary until the paretic medial rectus recovers. Kraft and Clarke found that patients with isolated lateral rectus palsy with a compensatory head posture undergoing surgery to eliminate the head position had a 75.6% incidence of success from the surgery.[156] A therapeutic dilemma arises in the child who is undercorrected after a recess-resect procedure for a complete sixth nerve palsy. In such a case, vertical rectus muscle transposition would disrupt the remaining anterior ciliary circulation, raising the risk of anterior segment ischemia.[230,237,241] In this setting, microdissection of the anterior ciliary vessels of the vertical recti prior to transposition reduces the risk of anterior segment ischemia.[176]

Multiple Cranial Nerve Palsies in Children

There have been no epidemiological studies to examine the causes of multiple cranial nerve palsies in children. Harley[118] described nine children with multiple acquired cranial nerve palsies and found orbital inflammation in four, trauma in three, and a neoplasm in two. Any infectious, inflammatory, or neoplastic disease process confined to the brain stem, skull base, cavernous sinus, or orbital apex can involve multiple cranial

nerves.[130] Intrinsic orbital disorders such as Graves ophthalmopathy[270] and a newly described syndrome of unilaterally congenitally enlarged extraocular muscles[78] are extremely rare but should also be included in the differential diagnosis.

Table 6.6 summarizes the neurological and systemic disorders that, in our experience, warrant consideration in the child with multiple cranial nerve palsies. Most of these conditions are discussed elsewhere.[188]

Möbius Syndrome

Möbius syndrome is a sporadic multiple-malformation complex that affects the face and horizontal gaze mechanisms bilaterally.[188] Some affected children have a deletion of chromosome 13.[268] Affected children have masklike facies with the mouth constantly held open. The upper facial nerves are affected more than the lower facial nerves, and facial asymmetry is common due to asymmetric facial strength. The eyes may be straight, esotropic, or rarely exotropic.[184] A subset of children with straight eyes will utilize convergence substitution to look to the side. Such chil-

TABLE 6.6. Causes of multiple cranial nerve palsies in children.

1. Trauma
   Basilar skull fractures
   Closed head trauma without fractures
2. Neoplasm
   Pontine glioma and other structural brain stem lesions
   Lymphoma
   Pituitary apoplexy
   Metastasis (rhabdomyosarcoma, neuroblastoma, leukemia)
   Gliomatosis cerebri
3. Inflammation
   Guillan-Barre disease
   Multiple sclerosis
   Acute disseminated encephalomyelitis
   Neurosarcoidosis
   Graves ophthalmopathy
4. Infection
   Acute bacterial meningitis
   Septic cavernous sinus thrombosis
   Brain stem cysticercosis
5. Congenital
   Möbius syndrome
   Unilateral congenitally enlarged extraocular muscles
6. Teratogenic
   Thalidomide exposure

dren may be thought to have isolated bilateral sixth nerve paresis if the slow convergence movement and the associated pupillary constriction are not recognized. Another subset exhibits retraction of the globe on attempted adduction.[184] Additional deficits affecting other cranial nerves, particularly V, IX, and XII, may produce feeding and sucking difficulties in the neonatal period and subsequent speech difficulties, with or without atrophy of the tongue.[9]

Möbius syndrome may be associated with a wide variety of associated limb malformations (talipes equinovarus, brachydactyly, syndactyly, congenital amputations) as well as hypoplasia or absence of the branchial musculature, particularly the pectoralis muscle (Poland anomaly).[9] Cardiovascular abnormalities (most commonly dextrocardia, patent ductus arteriosus, and ventricular septal defects), micrognathia, structural abnormalities of the pinna, and mild mental retardation are also occasionally present.[9]

The controversy surrounding the etiology centers around a *peripheral* theory, which proposes that the peripheral muscles or nerves are damaged primarily, resulting in a retrograde degeneration with loss of cranial nerve nuclei, versus a *central* theory, which proposes that the cranial nerve nuclei or supranuclear structures are damaged primarily.[9] The presence of horizontal gaze palsy rather than bilateral sixth nerve palsies in most children would tend to implicate a primary injury involving the caudal brain stem nuclei. Several neuropathologic studies have emphasized the presence of brain stem atrophy and/or necrosis in Möbius syndrome.[71] Recent investigators have suggested that ischemia of the lower cranial nuclei due to an insufficient blood supply in the pontine branches is the cause of Möbius syndrome.[28,71] Intrauterine brain stem infarction could result from premature regression or obstruction of the primitive trigeminal arteries before the establishment of a sufficient blood supply from the vertebral arteries, which may explain the variability in clinical expression.[9] The association of Möbius syndrome with thalidomide embryopathy demonstrates that early embryonic exposure to teratogens may produce a similar malformation complex.[185]

The wide spectrum of systemic malformations complicates the nosology of Möbius syndrome. Miller et al[184] refer to the subgroup with associated limb anomalies as terminal transverse defects with orofacial malformations (TTV-OFM), a term originally used by Temtamy and McKusick.[9] Children with Möbius syndrome have difficulty relating to people in their environment because of inability to convey their reaction of joy or sorrow. They are often incorrectly assumed to be mentally retarded and are predisposed to social and psychiatric problems.[9,184] The successful management of Möbius syndrome entails a multidisciplinary approach, including the medical, speech, education, and mental health disciplines.[9]

Horizons

Current surgical therapies for paralytic strabismus are based primarily upon recession, resection, and transposition of extraocular muscles. Although these techniques improve alignment and motility, they frequently produce an incomplete solution to the complex static and dynamic motility problems that can arise in this setting. Current therapies rarely achieve full rotation in the field of action of the paretic muscle and new limitations of ductions can be created by the surgical attempts to align the eyes in the primary position, resulting in large areas of diplopia. The best rotations following paralytic strabismus are achieved by the various muscle transposition procedures, but a review of the surgical results will illustrate that none achieve normal rotation.

New treatment techniques to provide greater rotation of the eyes in paralytic strabismus are currently being developed. Recent advances in chemodenervation, electrical stimulation, muscle reinnervation, and new muscle growth are promising future additions to the armamentarium of the strabismus surgeon.[20,218]

Substantial research has been undertaken to reanimate or replace paralytic muscle and to extend the length of existing muscle with contractile and noncontractile tissues.[5,16,19,38,53,54,55,62,101,125,217,224,225,248] Synthetic materials have been used to replace the superior oblique tendon and the lateral rectus muscle in selected patients. Research is also under way to reinnervate denervated extraocular muscles and to reestablish the neural supply of damaged extraocular muscles in animals that may be applicable to humans in the near future.

References

1. Abdul-Rahim AS, Savino PJ, Zimmerman RA, et al. Cryptogenic oculomotor nerve palsy: the need for repeated neuroimaging studies. Arch Ophthalmol 1989;107:387-390.
2. Afifi AK, Bell WE, Bale JF, Thompson HS. Recurrent lateral rectus palsy in childhood. Pediatr Neurol 1990;6:315-318.
3. Afifi AK, Bell WE, Menezes AH. Etiology of lateral rectus palsy in infancy and childhood. J Child Neurol 1992;7:295-299.
4. Agostinis C, Caverni L, Moschini L, et al. Paralysis of fourth cranial nerve due to superior cerebellar artery aneurysm. Neurology 1992;42:457-458.
5. Aichmair H. Muscular neurotization in surgery of traumatic abducens paresis. Jpn J Ophthalmol 1977;21:477-487.
6. Alexander JC. Ocular abnormalities among congenitally deaf children. Can J Ophthalmol 1973; 8:428.
7. Altman J, Bayer SA. Development of the brainstem in the rat. IV. Thymidine-radiographic study of the time of origin of neurons in the pontine region. J Comp Neurol 1980;194:905-929.
8. Altman J, Bayer SA. Development of the brainstem in the rat. V. Thymidine-radiographic study of the time of origin of neurons in the midbrain tegmentum. J Comp Neurol 1981;198:677-716.
9. Amaya LG, Walker J, Taylor D. Möbius syndrome. A study and report of 18 cases. Binoc Vis 1990; 5(3):119-132.
10. Anderson L, Baumgartner A. Strabismus in ptosis. Arch Ophthalmol 1980;98:1062-1067.
11. Anderson L, Baumgartner A. Amblyopia in ptosis. Arch Ophthalmol 1980;98:1068-1069.
12. Archer SM, Sondhi N, Helveston EM. Strabismus in infancy. Ophthalmology 1989;96:133-137.
13. Astle WF, Cornock E, Drummond GT. Recession of the superior oblique tendon for inferior oblique palsy and Brown syndrome. Can J Ophthalmol 1993;28:207-212.
14. Bachynski BN, Flynn JT. Direct trauma to the superior oblique tendon following penetrating injuries of the upper eyelid. Arch Ophthalmol 1985;103:1510-1514.
15. Bagolini B, Campos EC, Chiesi C. Plagiocephaly causing superior oblique deficiency and ocular torticollis. A new clinical entity. Arch Ophthalmol 1982;100:1093-1096.
16. Baker RS, Millet AJ, Young AB, Markesbery WR. Effects of chronic denervation of the histology of canine extraocular muscle. Invest Ophthalmol Vis Sci 1982;22:701-705.
17. Baker RS, Buncic JR. Vertical ocular motility disturbance in pseudotumor cerebri. J Clin Neuro-ophthalmol 1985;5:41-44.
18. Baker RS, Conklin JD. Acquired Brown's syndrome from blunt orbital trauma. J Pediatr Ophthalmol Strabismus 1987;24:17-21.
19. Baker R, Noden D. Segmental organization of VIth nerve related motoneurons in the chick hindbrain. Soc Neurosci Abstr 1990;16:318.
20. Baker RS, Steed MM. Restoration of function in paralytic strabismus: alternative methods of therapy. Binoc Vis Q 1990;5(4):203-211.
21. Baker R, Gilland E, Noden D. Rhombomeric organization in the embryonic vertebrate hindbrain. Soc Neurosci Abstr 1991;17:11.
22. Baker RS, Epstein AD. Ocular motor abnormalities from head trauma. Surv Ophthalmol 1991; 35(4):245-267.
23. Baker RS, Stava MW, Nelson KR, et al. Aberrant reinnervation of facial musculature in a subhuman primate: a correlative analysis of eyelid kinematics, muscle synkinesis, and motoneuron localization. Neurology 1994;44:2165-2173.
24. Baldwin L, Baker RS. Acquired Brown's syndrome in a patient with an orbital roof fracture. J Clin Neuro-ophthalmol 1988;8(2):127-130.
25. Balkan R, Hoyt CS. Associated neurological abnormalities in congenital third nerve palsies. Am J Ophthalmol 1984;97:315-319.
26. Barron DL, Galetta SL, Avner JA, Younkin DP. Bilateral ophthalmoparesis associated with bacterial meningitis. Clin Pediatr 1991;30:258-259.
27. Barroso LHL, Abreu SG, Finkel E, Hoyt WF. Cyclic oculomotor paresis in Rio. J Clin Neuro-ophthalmol 1991;11:136.
28. Bavinck JN, Weaver DD. Subclavian artery supply disruption sequence; hypothesis of a vascular etiology for Poland, Klippel-Feil, and Möbius anomalies. Am J Med Genet 1986;23:903-918.
29. Benevento WJ, Tyschen L. Distinguishing compensatory head turn from gaze palsy in children with unilateral oculomotor or abducens nerve paresis. Am J Ophthalmol 1993;115:116-118. Letter.
30. Benson PF. Transient unilateral external rectus muscle palsy in newborn infants. Br Med J 1962; 1:1054-1055.
31. Berkovitz S, Beklin M, Tenenbaum A. Childhood myasthenia gravis. J Pediatr Ophthamol 1977;14: 269-273.
32. Bielschowsky A. Lectures on motor anomalies of the eyes. II: paralysis of individual eye muscles. Arch Ophthalmol 1935;13:33-59.
33. Bixenman WW, von Noorden GK. Benign recurrent sixth nerve palsy in childhood. J Pediatr Ophthalmol Strabismus 1981;18:29-34.
34. Bixenman WW, von Noorden GK. Apparent foveal displacement in normal subjects and in cyclotropia. Ophthalmology 1982;89:58-62.
35. Blinzinger K, Kreutzberg GW. Displacement of synaptic terminals from regenerating motoneurons by microglial cells. Z Zellforsch Mikrosk Anat 1968;85:145-157.
36. Bloom JN, Graviss ER, Mondelli PG. A magnetic resonance imaging study of the up-shoot/downshoot phenomenon of Duane's retraction syndrome. Am J Ophthalmol 1991;111:548-554.

37. Boger WP III, Puliafito CA, Magoon H, et al. Recurrent isolated sixth nerve palsy in childhood. Ann Ophthalmol 1984;16:237-238, 240-244.
38. Bowen SF, Dyer JA. A silicone rubber tendon for extraocular muscle. Invest Ophthalmol Vis Sci 1962;1:579-585.
39. Branley MG, Wright KW, Borchert MS. Third nerve palsy due to cerebral artery aneurysm in a child. Aust N Z J Ophthalmol 1992;20:137-140.
40. Brazis PW. Palsies of the trochlear nerve: diagnosis and localization—recent concepts. Mayo Clin Proc 1993;68:501-509.
41. Brismar G, Brismar J. Spontaneous carotid-cavernous fistulas: clinical symptomatology. Acta Ophthalmol (Copenh) 1976;54:542-552.
42. Brodsky MC, Frenkel REP, Spoor TC. Familial intracranial aneurysm presenting as a subtle stable third nerve palsy. Arch Ophthalmol 1988;106:173.
43. Brodsky MC, Pollock SC, Buckley EG. Neural misdirection in congenital ocular fibrosis syndrome: implications and pathogenesis. J Pediatr Ophthalmol Strabismus 1989;26:159-161.
44. Brushart TM, Mesulam NM. Alteration in connections between muscle and anterior horn motoneurons after peripheral nerve repair. Science 1980;208:603-605.
45. Bryan S, Hamed LM. Levator-sparing nuclear oculomotor palsy: clinical and magnetic resonance image findings. J Clin Neuro-ophthalmol 1992;12:26-30.
46. Buckley EG, Townsend LM. A simple transposition procedure for complicated strabismus. Am J Ophthalmol 1991;111:302-306.
47. Burger LJ, Kalvin NH, Smith JL. Acquired lesions of the fourth cranial nerve. Brain 1970;92:567-574.
48. Burgerman RS, Wolf AL, Kelman SE, et al. Traumatic trochlear nerve palsy diagnosed by magnetic resonance imaging: case report and review of the literature. Neurosurgery 1989;25:978-981.
49. Burian HM, Van Allen MW. Cyclic oculomotor paralysis. Am J Ophthalmol 1963;55:529-537.
50. Cantillo N. A case of superior oblique palsy in an orbital floor fracture. Am Orthop J 1978;28:124-126.
51. Cassin B, Hamed LM. Case corner 1991. Bilateral masked superior oblique palsy. Am Orthop J 1991;41:137-139.
52. Chapman LI, Urist MJ, Folk ER, Miller MT. Acquired bilateral superior oblique muscle palsy. Arch Ophthalmol 1970;84:137-142.
53. Chekhova SP. Surgical treatment of paralytic strabismus using dura mater transplants. Oftalmol Zh 1985;2:80-82.
54. Chen Y, Richards R, Ko W, Finger P. Electrical stimulation of extraocular muscles. In: *Proceedings Ninth Annual Conference IEEE Engineering Medicine Biology Society,* November 13-16, 1987. Boston, MA: IEEE; 1987:649-650.
55. Christiansen S, Madhat M, Baker RS. Histologic consequences of inferior oblique anastomosis to denervated lateral rectus muscle. J Pediatr Ophthalmol Strabismus 1987;24:132-135.
56. Chrousos GA, Dipaolo F, Kattah JC, Laws ER. Paresis of the abducens nerve after trivial head injury. Am J Ophthalmol 1993;116:387-388.
57. Chu MLY, Litman N, Kaufman DM, Shinnar S. Cranial nerve palsies in Streptococcus pneumoniae meningitis. Pediatr Neurol 1990;6:209-210.
58. Cobbs WH, Schatz NJ, Savino TJ. Mid-brain eye signs in hydrocephalus. Trans Am Neurol Assoc 1978;103:130.
59. Cohen RL, Moore S. Primary dissociated vertical deviation. Am Orthop J 1980;30:106-107.
60. Cohen SM, Keltner JL. Thrombosis of the lateral transverse sinus with papilledema. Arch Ophthalmol 1993;111:274-275.
61. Cohn EM. Isolated third nerve palsy caused by an arachnoid cyst. Presented at the Fifth Meeting of the International Neuro-ophthalmology Society. Antwerp, Belgium: May 14-18, 1984.
62. Collins CC, Jampolsky A, Scott AB. Artificial muscles for extraocular implantation. Invest Ophthalmol Vis Sci 1985;26(suppl):80.
63. Collins TE, Mehalic TF, White TK, et al. Trochlear nerve palsy as the sole sign of an aneurysm of the superior cerebellar artery. Neurosurgery 1992;30:258-261.
64. Coppeto JR, Lessel S. Cryptogenic unilateral paralysis of the superior oblique muscle. Arch Ophthalmol 1978;96:275-277.
65. Corbett JJ. Neuro-ophthalmologic manifestations of cluster headaches. Neurol Clin 1983;1:973-995.
66. Corbett JJ. Neuro-ophthalmologic complications of hydrocephalus and shunting procedures. Neurol Clin 1986;6:111-123.
67. Cross HE, Pfaffenbach DD. Duane's retraction syndrome and associated congenital malformations. Am J Ophthalmol 1972;70:442-449.
68. Crouch ER Jr, Urist MJ. Lateral rectus muscle paralysis associated with closed head trauma. Am J Ophthalmol 1975;79:990-996.
69. Cruysberg JRM, Mtanda AT, Duinkerke-Eerola KU, Huygen P. Congenital adduction palsy and synergistic divergence: a clinical and electro-oculographic study. Br J Ophthalmol 1989;73:68-75.
70. Cullen P, Rodgers CS, Callen DF, et al. Association of familial Duane anomaly and urogenital abnormalities with a bisatellited marker derived from chromosome 22. Am J Med Genet 1993;47:925-930.
71. D'Cruz OF, Swisher CM, Jaradeh S, et al. Möbius syndrome: evidence for a vascular etiology. J Child Neurol 1993;8:260-265.
72. de Grauw AJC, Rotteveel JJ, Cruyberg JRM. Transient sixth cranial nerve paralysis in the newborn infant. Neuropediatrics 1983;14:164-165.
73. Dehaene I. Isolated oculomotor palsy. Acta Neurol Belg 1994;94:5-7.

74. De Keizer RJW. Spontaneous carotid-cavernous fistulas. Neuro-ophthalmology 1981;2:35-46.

75. Demer J, Miller J. Magnetic resonance morphometry of the functional anatomy of the superior oblique muscle in normal and pathological states. Invest Ophthalmol Vis Sci 1993;(Suppl):3941-3943.

76. De Respinis P, Caputo A, Wagner R, Suqin G. Duane's retraction syndrome. Surv Ophthalmol 1993; 38:257-288.

77. Dickey CF, Scott WE, Kline RA. Oblique muscle palsies fixating with the paretic eye. Surv Ophthalmol 1988;33:97-107.

78. Dickson JS, Kraft SP, Jay V, Blaser S. A case of unilateral congenitally enlarged extraocular muscles. Ophthalmol 1994;101:1902-1907.

79. Drips RD, Vandam LD. Hazards of lumbar puncture. JAMA 1951;147:1118-1121.

80. Duane A. Congenital deficiency of abduction, associated with impairment of adduction, retraction movements, contraction of the palpebral fissure and oblique movements of the eye. Arch Ophthalmol 1905;34:133-159.

81. Durkan GP, Troost BT, Slamovits TL, et al. Recurrent painless oculomotor palsy in children. A variant of ophthalmoplegic migraine. Headache 1981; 21:58-62.

82. Elliot D, Conningham ET Jr, Miller NR. Fourth nerve paresis and ipsilateral relative afferent pupillary defect without visual sensory disturbance: a sign of contralateral dorsal midbrain disease. J Clin Neuro-ophthalmol 1991;11:169-172.

83. Elston JS, Timms C. Clinical evidence for the onset of the sensitive period in infancy. Br J Ophthalmol 1992;76:327-328.

84. Espinosa JA, Giroux M, Johnston K, et al. Abducens palsy following shunting for hydrocephalus. Can J Neurosci 1993;20:123-125.

85. Fells P, Collin JRO. Cyclic oculomotor palsy. Trans Ophthalmol Soc UK 1979;99:192-196.

86. Fitzsimmons R, Lee JP, Elston JS. Treatment of VIth nerve palsy with combined botulinum toxin chemodenervation in surgery. Ophthalmology 1988;95:1535-1542.

87. Flanders M, Walters G, Draper J, O'Gorman A. Bilateral congenital third nerve palsy. Can J Ophthalmol 1989;24:28-30.

88. Forrester RK, Schatz NJ, Smith JL. A subtle eyelid sign in aberrant regeneration of the third nerve. Am J Ophthalmol 1969;67:696-698.

89. France NK, France TD, Woodburn JD, Burbank DP. Succinylcholine alteration of the forced duction test. Ophthalmology 1980;87:1282-1287.

90. Fredrick DR, Mulliken JB, Robb RM. Ocular manifestations of deformational frontal plagiocephaly. J Pediatr Ophthalmol Strabismus 1993;30:92-95.

91. Friedman AP, Horter DH, Merritt HH. Ophthalmoplegic migraine. Arch Neurol 1962;7:320-327.

92. Friedman DI, Wright KW, Soelan AA. Oculomotor palsy with cyclic spasm. Neurology 1989;39:1263-1264.

93. Frueh BR, Henderson JW. Rectus muscle union in sixth nerve paralysis. Arch Ophthalmol 1971;85:191-196.

94. Gabianelli EB, Klingele TF, Burde RM. Acute oculomotor nerve palsy in childhood. Is arteriography necessary? J Clin Neuro-ophthalmol 1989;9:33-36.

95. Galetta SL, Smith JL. Chronic isolated sixth nerve palsies. Arch Neurol 1989;46(1):79-82.

96. Gilbert PW. The origin and development of the extrinsic ocular muscles in the domestic cat. J Morphol 1947;81:151-193.

97. Gilbert PW. The origin and development of the human extrinsic ocular muscles. Contrib Embryol 1957;36:61-78.

98. Glaser JS. Neuro-ophthalmologic examination: general considerations and special techniques. In: Tasman W, Jaeger EA, eds. Duane's Clinical Ophthalmology, II. Philadelphia, PA: JB Lippincott; 1988:chap 2.

99. Glasier CM, Robbins MB, Davis PC, et al. Clinical, neurodiagnostic, and MR findings in children with spinal and brain stem multiple sclerosis. AJNR 1995;16:87-95.

100. Good WV, Barkovich AJ, Nickel NL, Hoyt CS. Bilateral congenital oculomotor nerve palsy in a child with brain anomalies. Am J Ophthalmol 1991;111:555-558.

101. Gossman MD, Gutman FA, Tucker HM. Extraocular muscle reinnervation by a neuromuscular pedicle. Invest Ophthalmol Vis Sci 1983;24(suppl):23.

102. Gottlob I, Catalano RA, Reinecke RD. Surgical management of oculomotor nerve palsy. Am J Ophthalmol 1991;111(1):71-76.

103. Gradinego G. A special syndrome of endocranial otitic complications (Paralysis of the motor oculi externus of otitic origin). Ann Otol Rhinol Laryngol 1904;13:637.

104. Grafstein B. The nerve cell body response to axotomy. Exp Neurol 1975;48:32-51.

105. Granit R, Leksell L, Skoglund CR. Fibre interaction in injured or compressed region of nerve. Brain 1944;67:125-139.

106. Gross SA, Tien DR, Breinin GM. Aberrant innervational pattern in Duane's type II without globe retraction. Am J Ophthalmol 1994;117:348-351.

107. Gutman I, Levartovski S, Goldhammer Y, et al. Sixth nerve palsy and unilateral Horner's syndrome. Ophthalmology 1986;93:913-916.

108. Guy JR, Savino PJ, Schatz NJ, et al. Superior division paresis of the oculomotor nerve. Ophthalmology 1985;92:777-784.

109. Guy JR, Friedman WF, Mickle JP. Bilateral trochlear nerve paresis in hydrocephalus. J Clin Neuro-ophthalmol 1989;9:105-111.

110. Guyton DL, von Noorden GK. Sensory adaptations to cyclodeviations. In: Reinecke RD, ed. *Strabismus*. New York: Grune & Stratton; 1978:399-403.
111. Hamed LM, Dennehy PJ, Lingua RW. Synergistic divergence and jaw-winking phenomenon. J Pediatr Ophthalmol Strabismus 1990;27:88-90.
112. Hamed LM. Associated neurologic and ophthalmologic findings in congenital oculomotor nerve palsy. Ophthalmology 1991;98:708-714.
113. Hamed LM, Lingua RW, Fanous MM, et al. Synergistic divergence: saccadic velocity analysis and surgical results. J Pediatr Ophthalmol Strabismus 1992;29:30-37.
114. Hamed LM, Maria BL, Quisling RG, Mickle JP. Alternating skew on lateral gaze: Neuroanatomic pathway and relationship to superior oblique overaction. Ophthalmology 1993;100:281-286.
115. Hanna LS, Girgis NI, El Ella A, Farid Z. Ocular complications in meningitis: "Fifteen years study." Metab Pediatr Syst Ophthalmol 1988;11:160-162.
116. Harada M, Ito Y. Surgical correction of cyclotropia. Jpn J Ophthalmol 1964;8:88-96.
117. Hardesty HH. Diagnosis of paretic vertical rotators. Am J Ophthalmol 1963;56:811-816.
118. Harley RD. Paralytic strabismus in children: etiologic incidence and management of the third, fourth, and sixth nerve palsies. Ophthalmology 1980;87:24-43.
119. Harris DJ, Memmen JE, Katz NNK, Parks MM. Familial congenital superior oblique palsy. Ophthalmology 1986;93:88-90.
120. Haymaker W, Kuhlenbeck H. Disorders of the brainstem and its cranial nerves. In: Baker AB, Baker LH, eds. *Clinical Neurology, III*. Philadelphia, PA: JB Lippincott;1988:chap 40.
121. Heath JP, Cull RE, Smith IM, Murray JA. The neurophysiological investigation of Bell's palsy and the predictive value of the blink reflex. Clin Otolaryngol 1988;13:85-92.
122. Heinze J. Cranial nerve avulsion and other neural injuries in road accidents. Med J Aust 1969;2: 1246-1249.
123. Helveston EM. A new 2-step test for diagnosing paresis of a single vertically acting extraocular muscle. Am J Ophthalmol 1967;64:914-915.
124. Helveston EM, Krach D, Plager DA, Ellis FD. A new classification of superior oblique palsy based on congenital variations in the tendon. Ophthalmology 1992;99:1609-1615.
125. Herbison GJ, Teng C, Reyes T, Reyes O. Effect of electrical stimulation on denervated muscle of rat. Arch Phys Med Rehabil 1971;52:516-522.
126. Hermann JS. Masked bilateral superior oblique paresis. J Pediatr Ophthalmol Strabismus 1981;18: 43-48.
127. Hotchkiss N, Miller NR, Clark AW, Green WR. Bilateral Duane's retraction syndrome: a clinical pathologic case report. Arch Ophthalmol 1980;98: 870-874.
128. Hriso E, Masdeu JC, Miller A. Monocular elevation weakness and ptosis: an oculomotor fascicular syndrome? J Clin Neuro-ophthalmol 1991;11(2): 111-113.
129. Huber A. Electrophysiology of the retraction syndromes. Br J Ophthalmol 1974;58:293-300.
130. Hunt WE, Meagher JN, Lefever HE, Zeman W. Painful ophthalmoplegia: its relation to indolent inflammation of the cavernous sinus. Neurology 1961;11:56-62.
131. Hupp SL, Kline LB, Corbett JJ. Visual disturbances of migraine. Surv Ophthalmol 1989;33: 221-236.
132. Ing EB, Sullivan TJ, Clarke MP, Buncic JR. Oculomotor nerve palsies in children. J Pediatr Ophthalmol Strabismus 1992;29:331-336.
133. Jacobson DM. A prospective evaluation of cholinergic supersensitivity of the iris sphincter in patients with oculomotor nerve palsies. Am J Ophthalmol 1994;118:377-383.
134. Jameson NA, Good WV, Hoyt CS. Fat adherence simulating inferior oblique palsy following blepharoplasty. Arch Ophthalmol 1992;110:1369. Letter.
135. Jampolsky A. Surgical leashes and reverse leashes. In: *Strabismus Surgical Management*. Trans New Orleans Acad Ophthalmol. St. Louis: CV Mosby; 1977:244-268.
136. Jampolsky A. A functional classification of the retraction syndromes. Presented as the 19th Jules Stern Lecture, University of California, Los Angeles, April 22, 1988.
136a. Jampolsky A. The superior rectus contracture syndrome. Presented at the combined meeting of the International Strabismological Association and the American Association for Pediatric Ophthalmology and Strabismus, Vancouver, British Columbia, June 18–22, 1994.
137. Jay W, Hoyt CS. Abnormal brainstem auditory evoked potentials in Stilling-Turk-Duane retraction syndrome. Am J Ophthalmol 1980;89:814-818.
138. Jensen CDF. Rectus muscle union: a new operation for paralysis of the rectus muscles. Trans Pacif Coast Ophthalmol Soc 1964;45:359-387.
139. Jones DB, Steinkuller PG. Microbial preseptal and orbital cellulitis. In: Tasman W, Jaeger EA, eds. *Duane's Clinical Ophthalmology, IV*. Philadelphia, PA: JB Lippincott; 1989;25:15.
140. Jones IS, Jakobiec FA, Nolan BT. Patient examination and introduction to orbital disease. In: Tasman W, Jaeger EA, eds. *Duane's Clinical Ophthalmology, II*. Philadelphia, PA: JB Lippincott;1990; 21:23.
141. Katz B, Rimmer S. Ophthalmoplegic migraine with superior ramus oculomotor paresis. J Clin Neuro-ophthalmol 1989;9(3):181-183.
142. Kazarin EL. Congenital third nerve palsy with amblyopia of the contralateral eye. J Pediatr Ophthalmol Strabismus 1972;15:366-370.

143. Keane JR. Fourth nerve palsy opposite a black eye: two patients simulating orbital blowout fractures. J Clin Neuro-ophthalmol 1981;1:209-211.

144. Keane JR. Fourth nerve palsy: historical review and study of 215 patients. Neurology 1993;43:2439-2443.

145. Keith CG. Oculomotor palsy in children. Aust N Z J Ophthalmol 1987;15:181-184.

146. Khawam E, Scott AB, Jampolsky A. Acquired superior oblique palsy: diagnosis and management. Arch Ophthalmol 1967;77:761-768.

147. Killer HE, Matzkin DC, Sternman D, et al. Intracavernous carotid aneurysm as a rare case of isolated sixth nerve palsy in an eight-year-old child. Neuro-ophthalmology 1993;13:147-150.

148. Kirkali P, Topaloglu R, Kansu T, Bakkaloglu A. Third nerve palsy and internuclear ophthalmoplegia in periarteritis nodosa. J Pediatr Ophthalmol & Strabis 1991;28:45-46.

149. Kirkham TH. Duane syndrome and familial perceptive deafness. Br J Ophthalmol 1969;53:335-339.

150. Knapp P. Classification and treatment of superior oblique palsy. Am Orthop J 1974;24:18-22.

151. Knap P. Blow-out fractures. In: Symposium on Strabismus. Trans New Orleans Acad Ophthalmol. St. Louis: CV Mosby; 1978:285-291.

152. Knox DL, Clark DB, Schuster FF. Benign VI nerve palsy in children. Pediatrics 1967;40(4:pt I):560-564.

153. Kodsi SR, Younge BR. Acquired oculomotor, trochlear, and abducent cranial nerve palsies in pediatric patients. Am J Ophthalmol 1992;114:568-574.

154. Kommerell G, Bach M. A new type of Duane's syndrome. Twitch abduction on attempted upgaze and V-incomitance due to misinnervation of the lateral rectus muscle by superior rectus neurons. Neuro-ophthalmology 1986;6:159-164.

155. Kraft SP, Scott WE. Masked bilateral superior oblique palsy: clinical features and diagnosis. J Pediatr Ophthalmol Strabismus 1986;23:264-272.

156. Kraft SP, Clarke MP. Surgical management of Duane's retraction syndrome. Ophthalmol Clin North Am 1992;5:79-92.

157. Kraft SP, O'Donoghue EP, Roarty JD. Improvement of compensatory head postures after strabismus surgery. Ophthalmology 1992;99:1301-1308.

158. Kraft SP, O'Reilly C, Quigly PL, et al. Cyclotorsion in unilateral and bilateral superior oblique paresis. J Pediatr Ophthalmol Strabismus 1993;30:361-367.

159. Ksiazek SM, Slamovits TL, Rosen CE, et al. Fascicular arrangement in partial oculomotor paresis. Am J Ophthalmol 1994;118(1):97-103.

160. Krohel GB, Mansour AM, Petersen WL, Evenchik B. Isolated trochlear nerve palsy secondary to a juvenile pilocytic astrocytoma. J Clin Neuro-ophthalmol 1982a;1:119-123.

161. Kushner BJ. The diagnosis and treatment of bilateral masked superior oblique palsy. Am J Ophthalmol 1988;105:186-194.

162. Kushner BJ. Errors in the three-step test in the diagnosis of vertical strabismus. Ophthalmology 1989;96:127-132.

163. Kushner BJ. 'V' esotropia and excyclotropia after surgery for bilateral fourth nerve palsy. Arch Ophthalmol 1992;110:1419-1422.

164. Lavin PJ, Troost BT. Traumatic fourth nerve palsy: clinicoanatomic correlations with computed tomographic scan. Arch Neurol 1984;41:679-680.

165. Lemoh JN. Traumatic external rectus palsy in a child. Br Med J 1978;1:579-580.

166. Lepore FE, Glaser JS. Misdirection revisited: a critical appraisal of acquired oculomotor nerve synkinesis. Arch Ophthalmol 1980;98:2206-2209.

167. Lesser RL, Kornmehl EW, Pachner AR, et al. Neuro-ophthalmologic manifestations of Lyme disease. Ophthalmology 1990;97:699-706.

168. Lindenberg R. Significance of the tentorium in head injuries from blunt forces. Clin Neurosurg 1966;12:129-142.

169. Loewenfeld IE, Thompson HS. Oculomotor paresis with cyclic spasms. A critical review of the literature in a new case. Surv Ophthalmol 1975;20:81-124.

170. Lumdsen A, Keynes R. Segmental patterns of neuronal development in the chick hindbrain. Nature 1989;337:424-428.

171. Lyle DJ. Experimental oculomotor nerve regeneration. Am J Ophthalmol 1966;61(5):1239-1243.

172. MacDonald JT. Childhood migraine: differential diagnosis and treatment. Postgrad Med 1986;80:301-306.

173. Mandell GL, Bennett JE, Dolin R, eds. Principles and Practice of Infectious Diseases, 4th ed. New York: Churchill Livingstone;1995:84.

174. Maria BL, Rehder K, Eskin TA. Brainstem glioma. I: Pathology, clinical features, and therapy. J Child Neurol 1993;8:112-128.

175. Martonyi EJ. Pediatric sixth nerve palsy: case reviews and management guidelines. Am Orthop J 1990;40:24-31.

176. McKeown CA, Lambert HM, Shore JW. Preservation of the anterior ciliary vessels during extraocular muscle surgery. Ophthalmology 1989;96:498-506.

177. McKinna AJ. Eye signs in 611 cases of posterior fossa aneurysms: their diagnostic and prognostic value. Can J Ophthalmol 1983;18:3-6.

178. McManaway JW III, Buckley EG, Brodsky MC. Vertical rectus muscle transposition with intraoperative botulinum injection for treatment of chronic sixth nerve palsy. Graefe's Arch Clin Exp Ophthalmol 1990;228:401-406.

179. Mein J, Harcourt B. Diagnosis and Management of Ocular Motility Disorders. Oxford: Blackwell Scientific; 1986;288:96-99.

180. Metz HS, Lerner H. The adjustable Harada-Ito procedure. Arch Ophthalmol 1981;99:624-626.
181. Metz HS. Duane's retraction syndrome and severe adduction deficiency. Arch Ophthalmol 1986;104:1586-1587.
182. Metz HS. Muscle transposition surgery. J Pediatr Ophthalmol Strabismus 1993;30:346-353.
183. Miller BA, Pollard ZF. Duane retraction syndrome and arthrogryposis congenita. Surv Ophthalmol 1994;38:395-396.
184. Miller MT, Ray V, Owens P, Cheu F. Möbius and Möbius-like syndromes. J Pediatr Ophthalmol Strabismus 1989;26:176-188.
185. Miller M. Thalidomide embryopathy: a model for the study of congenital incomitant horizontal strabismus. Trans Am Ophthalmol Soc 1991;89:623-674.
186. Miller NR. Solitary oculomotor nerve palsy in childhood. Am J Ophthalmol 1977;83:106-111.
187. Miller NR, Kiel SM, Green WR, Clark AW. Unilateral Duane's retraction syndrome [type I]. Arch Ophthalmol 1982;100:1468-1472.
188. Miller NR. *Walsh and Hoyt's Clinical Neuro-Ophthalmology, II.* 4th ed. Baltimore: Williams and Wilkins; 1985.
189. Miller NR. Superior division paresis of the oculomotor nerve. Ophthalmology 1985;92:783-784. Discussion.
190. Miller NR. *Walsh and Hoyt's Clinical Neuro-Ophthalmology, IV.* 4th ed. Baltimore: Williams and Wilkins; 1991:2533-2538.
191. Mitchell PR, Parks MM. Surgery for bilateral superior oblique palsy. Ophthalmology 1982;89:484-488.
192. Mizen TR, Burde RM, Klingele TG. Cryptogenic oculomotor nerve palsies in children. Am J Ophthalmol 1985;100:65-67.
193. Mottier ME, Mets MB. Vertical fusional vergences in patients with superior oblique palsies. Am Orthrop J 1990;40:88-93.
194. Neetens A. Extraocular muscle palsy from minor head trauma: initial sign of intracranial tumor. Neuro-ophthalmology 1983;3:43-48.
195. Nemet P, Erlich D, Lazar M. Benign abducens palsy in varicella. Am J Ophthalmol 1974;78:859.
196. Nixon RB, Helveston EM, Miller K, et al. Incidence of strabismus in neonates. Am J Ophthalmol 1985;100:798-801.
197. North KN, Antony JH, Johnston IH. Dermoid of cavernous sinus resulting in isolated oculomotor palsy. Pediatr Neurol 1993;9:221-223.
198. O'Hara MA, Anderson RT, Brown D. MR imaging in ophthalmoplegic migraine of children. Presented as a poster at the American Association of Pediatric Ophthalmology and Strabismus, Orlando, FL, April 5-9, 1995.
199. Olivier P, von Noorden GK. Excyclotropia of the nonparetic eye in unilateral superior oblique paralysis. Am J Ophthalmol 1982;93:30-33.
200. Olivier P, von Noorden GK. Results of superior oblique tenectomy and inferior oblique paresis. Arch Ophthalmol 1982;100:581-584.
201. O'Malley ER. Duane syndrome: associated anomalies. Am Orthop J 1993;43:15-17.
202. Osuntokun O, Osuntokun BO. Ophthalmoplegic migraine and hemoglobinopathy in Nigerians. Am J Ophthalmol 1972;74:451-455.
203. Parkinson D, Johnston J, Chaudhuri A. Sympathetic connections to the fifth and sixth cranial nerves. Anat Rec 1978;191:221-226.
204. Parks MM. Isolated cyclovertical muscle palsy. Arch Ophthalmol 1958;60:1027-1035.
205. Patel CK, Taylor DSI, Russel-Eggitt IM, et al. Congenital third nerve palsy associated with mid-trimester amniocentesis. Br J Ophthalmol 1993;77:530-533.
206. Perlman EM, Barry D. Bilateral sixth nerve palsy after water soluble contrast myelography. Arch Ophthalmol 1984;102:968.
207. Plager DA. Tendon laxity in superior oblique palsy. Ophthalmology 1992;99:1032-1038.
208. Pollard ZF. Diagnosis and treatment of inferior oblique palsy. J Pediatr Ophthalmol Strabismus 1993;30:15-18.
209. Porter JD, Baker RS, Ragusa RJ, Brueckner JK. Extraocular muscles: basic and clinical aspects of structure and function. Surv Ophthalmol 1995;39:451-484.
210. Pusateri TJ, Sedwick LA, Margo CE. Isolated inferior rectus muscle palsy from a solitary metastatis to the oculomotor nucleus. Arch Ophthalmol 1987;105:675-677.
211. Raab EL. Clinical features of Duane's syndrome. J Pediatr Ophthalmol Strabismus 1986;23:64-68.
212. Ramsay J, Taylor D. Congenital crocodile tears; a key to the etiology of Duane's syndrome. Br J Ophthalmol 1980;64:518-522.
213. Rasminsky M. Ectopic generation of impulses and cross-talk in spinal nerve roots of "dystrophic" mice. Ann Neurol 1978;3:351-357.
214. Reese PD, Scott WE. Superior oblique tenotomy in the treatment of isolated inferior oblique paresis. J Pediatr Ophthalmol Strabismus 1987;24:4-9.
215. Reinecke RD, Thompson WE. Childhood recurrent idiopathic paralysis of the lateral rectus. Ann Ophthalmol 1981;13:1037-1039.
216. Reisner, SH, Perlman M, Ben-Tovim N, Dubrawski, C. Transient lateral rectus paresis in the newborn infant. J Pediatr 1971;78:461-465.
217. Richards R. Ocular motility disturbances following trauma. Adv Ophthalmic Plast Reconstr Surg 1987;7:133-147.
218. Richards R, Finger PT, Ko WH, Chen Y. Functional electric stimulation of extraocular muscles. Invest Ophthalmol Vis Sci 1988;29(suppl):11.
219. Ro A, Chernoff G, MacRae D, et al. Auditory function in Duane's retraction syndrome. Am J Ophthalmol 1990;109:75-78.

220. Robb RM, Boger WP. Vertical strabismus associated with plagiocephaly. J Pediatr Ophthalmol Strabismus 1983;20:58-62.

221. Robb RM. Idiopathic superior oblique palsies in children. J Pediatr Ophthalmol Strabismus 1990; 27:66-69.

222. Roberts M. Lesions of the ocular motor nerves (III, IV, and VI). In: Vinken PJ, Bruyn GW, eds. *Handbook of Clinical Neurology, XXIV, Part II.* New York: Elsevier; 1976:59-72.

223. Robertson DM, Hines JD, Rucke CW. Acquired sixth nerve paresis in children. Arch Ophthalmol 1970;83:574-579.

224. Robins D. Extraocular intramuscular electrical stimulation in anesthetized cats. Invest Ophthalmol Vis Sci 1988;29(suppl):344.

225. Robins D. Control of contraction length in extraocular muscle using frequency and pulse width modulated electrical stimulation. Invest Ophthalmol Vis Sci 1989;30(suppl):133.

226. Roper-Hall G, Burde RM. Inferior rectus palsies as a manifestation of atypical third cranial nerve disease. Am Orthop J 1975;25:122-130.

227. Rosa L, Carol M, Bellegarrique R, Ducker TB. Multiple cranial nerve palsies due to a hyperextension injury to the cervical spine. J Neurosurg 1984;61:172-173.

228. Rosen E. A post-vaccinal ocular syndrome. Am J. Ophthalmol 1948;31:1443-1453.

229. Rosenbaum AL, Foster RS, Ballard E, et al. Complete superior and inferior rectus transposition with adjustable medial rectus recession for abducens palsy. In: Reinecke RD, ed. *Strabismus II.* Proceedings of the Fourth Meeting of the International Strabismological Association. Orlando: Grune & Stratton; 1982:599-605.

230. Rosenbaum AL, Kushner BJ, Kirschen D. Vertical rectus muscle transposition and botulinum toxin (oculinum) to medial rectus for abducens palsy. Arch Ophthalmol 1989;107:820-823.

231. Rougier J, Girod M, Bongrand M. Considerations sur l'etiologie et sur la recuperation des paralysies du pathetique, en milieu neurologique. A propos de 40 observations. Bull Soc Ophthalmol Fr 1973; 73:739-744.

232. Rucker CW. Paralysis of the third, fourth and sixth cranial nerves. Am J Ophthalmol 1958;6:787-794.

233. Rucker CW. The causes of paralysis of the third, fourth and sixth cranial nerves. Am J Ophthalmol 1966;61:1293-1298.

234. Rush JA, Younge BR. Paralysis of cranial nerves III, IV, and VI: cause and prognosis in 1000 cases. Arch Ophthalmol 1981;99:76-79.

235. Ruttum M, von Noorden GK. The Bagolini striated lens test for cyclotropia. Doc Ophthalmol 1984;58: 131-139.

236. Saad N, Lee J. Medial rectus electromyographic abnormalities in Duane syndrome. J Pediatr Ophthalmol Strabismus 1993;30:88-91.

237. Saunders RA, Sandall GS. Anterior segment ischemia syndrome following rectus muscle transposition. Am J Ophthalmol 1982;93:34-38.

238. Saunders RA. Incomitant vertical strabismus. Treatment with posterior fixation of the inferior rectus muscle. Arch Ophthalmol 1984;102:1174-1177.

239. Saunders RA, Tomlinson E. Quantitated superior oblique tendon tuck in the treatment of superior oblique muscle palsy. Am Ortho J 1985;35:81-89.

240. Saunders RA, Wilson E, Bluestein EC, Sinatra RB. Surgery on the normal eye in Duane retraction syndrome. J Ped Ophthalmol Strabismus 1994;31: 162-169.

241. Saunders RA, Bluestein EC, Wilson ME, Berland JE. Anterior segment ischemia after strabismus surgery. Surv Ophthalmol 1994;38:456-466.

242. Saunders RA, Roberts EL. Abnormal head posture in patients with fourth cranial nerve palsy. Am Orthop J 1995. In press.

243. Schneider RC, Johnson FD. Bilateral traumatic abducens palsy: a mechanism of injury suggested by the study of associated cervical spine fractures. J Neurosurg 1971;34:33-37.

244. Scott AB. Active force tests in lateral rectus paralysis. Arch Ophthalmol 1971;85:397-404.

245. Scott AB, Wong GM. Duane's syndrome: an electromyographic study. Arch Ophthalmol 1972;87: 140-147.

246. Scott AB. Transposition of the superior oblique. Am Ortho J 1977;27:11-14.

247. Scott AB. Botulinum toxin injection of eye muscles to correct strabismus. Trans Am Ophthalmol Soc 1981;79:734-770.

248. Scott AB, Miller JM, Collins CC. Mechanical model applications. Trans Euro Strismol Assn, 14th Meeting. Copenhagen, Denmark: May 18-24, 1984.

249. Scott AB, Kraft SP. Botulinum toxin injection in the management of lateral rectus paresis. Ophthalmology 1985;92:676-683.

250. Scott AB. Change of eye muscle sarcomeres according to eye position. J Pediatr Ophthalmol Strabismus 1994;31:85-88.

251. Scott WE, Kraft SP. Classification and surgical treatment of superior oblique palsies. I: Unilateral superior oblique palsies. In: *Pediatric Ophthalmology and Strabismus: Trans New Orleans Acad Ophthalmol.* New York: Raven Press; 1986;34:15-38.

252. Scott WE, Kraft SP. Classification and treatment of superior oblique palsies. II: bilateral superior oblique palsies. In: *Pediatric Ophthalmology and Strabismus: Trans New Orleans Acad Ophthalmol.* New York: Raven Press; 1986;34:265-291.

253. Seaber JH. Clinical evaluation of superior oblique function. Am Orthop J 1974;24:13-17.

254. Selezinka W, Sandall GS, Henderson JW. Rectus muscle union in sixth nerve paralysis. Arch Ophthalmol 1974;92:382-386.

255. Sevel D. A reappraisal of the origin of human extraocular muscles. Ophthalmology 1981;88:1330-1338.

256. Sevel D. The origins and insertions of the extraocular muscles: development, histologic features, and clinical significance. Trans Am Ophthalmol Soc 1986;84:488-526.

257. Shauly Y, Weissman A, Meyer E. Ocular and systemic characteristics of Duane syndrome. J Pediatr Ophthalmol Strabismus 1993;30:178-183.

258. Sibony PA, Evinger C, Lessell S. Retrograde horseradish peroxidase transport after oculomotor nerve injury. Invest Ophthalmol Vis Sci 1986;27:975-980.

259. Simons K, Arnoldi K, Brown MH. Color dissociation artifacts in Double Maddox Red cyclodeviation testing. Ophthalmol 1994;101:1897-1901.

260. Slee JJ, Smart RD, Viljoen DL. Deletion of chromosome 13 in Möbius syndrome. J Med Genet 1991;28:413-414.

261. Smith JL. The "nuclear third" questions. J Clin Neuro-ophthalmol 1982;2:61-63.

262. Spoor TC, Shippman S. Myasthenia gravis presenting as an isolated inferior rectus paresis. Ophthalmology 1979;86:2158-2160.

263. Sternberg I, Ronen S, Arnon N. Recurrent isolated post-febrile abducens nerve palsy. J Pediatr Ophthalmol Strabismus 1980;17:323-324.

264. Stommel EW, Ward TN, Harris RD. MRI findings in a case of ophthalmoplegic migraine. Headache 1993;33:234-237.

265. Straussberg R, Cohen AH, Amir J, Varsano I. Benign abducens palsy associated with EBV infection. J Pediatr Ophthalmol Strabismus 1993;30:60.

266. Summers CG, Wirtschafter JD. Bilateral trigeminal and abducens neuropathies following low-velocity, crushing head injury: case report. J Neurosurg 1979;50:508-511.

267. Sydnor CF, Seaber JH, Buckley EG. Traumatic superior oblique palsies. Ophthalmology 1982;89:134-138.

268. Thomas R, Mathai A, Gieser SC, Ratnammal J. Bilateral synergistic divergence. J Pediatr Ophthalmol Strabismus 1993;30:122-123.

269. Thorsen G. Neurological complications after spinal anesthesia. Acta Chir Sca 1947;95(suppl 121).

270. Uretsky SH, Kennerdell JS, Gutai JP. Graves ophthalmopathy in childhood and adolescence. Arch Ophthalmol 1980;98:1963-1964.

271. Valls-Sole J, Tolosa ES. Blink reflex excitability in hemifacial spasm. Neurology 1989;39:1061-1066.

272. Van Dalen JTW, Van Mourik-Noodernbos AM. Isolated inferior rectus paresis: a report of six cases. Neuro-ophthalmology 1984;4:89-94.

273. Van Vliet AGM. Post-traumatic ocular imbalance. In: Vinken PJ, Bruyn GW, eds. Handbook of Clinical Neurology, XXIV, Part II. New York: Elsevier; 1976:73-104.

274. Vargus ME, Desrouleaux JR, Kupersmith MJ. Ophthalmoplegia as a presenting manifestation of internal carotid artery dissection. J Clin Neuro-ophthalmol 1992;12:268-271.

275. Verslype LM, Folk ER, Thoms ML. Recurrent sixth nerve palsy. Am Orthop J 1990;40:76-79.

276. Victor DI. The diagnosis of congenital unilateral third-nerve palsy. Brain 1976;99:711-718.

277. Vijayan N. Ophthalmoplegic migraine: Ischemic or compressive neuropathy? Headache 1980;20:300-304.

278. von Noorden GK. Clinical and theoretical aspects of cyclotropia. J Pediatr Ophthalmol Strabismus 1984;21:126-132.

279. von Noorden GK, Murray E, Wong SY. Superior oblique paralysis. A review of 270 cases. Arch Ophthalmol 1986;104:1771-1776.

280. von Noorden GK. Binocular Vision and Ocular Motility: Theory and Management of Strabismus. 3rd ed. St. Louis, MO: Mosby;1990.

281. von Noorden GK. Binocular Vision and Ocular Motility. Theory and Management of Strabismus. 4th ed. St. Louis, MO: CV Mosby; 1990:184-186, 347-349, 387.

282. von Noorden GK, Hansell R. Clinical characteristics and treatment of isolated inferior rectus palsy. Ophthalmology 1991;98:253-257.

283. von Noorden GK. Recession of both horizontal recti muscles in Duane's retraction syndrome with elevation and depression of adducted eye. Am J Ophthalmol 1992;114:311-313.

284. Wagner RS, Caputo AR, Frohman LP. Congenital unilateral adduction deficit with simultaneous abduction. Ophthalmology 1987;94:1049-1053.

285. Wahl CM, Noden DM. Positional specification of extraocular muscles in the chick embryo. Anat Rec 1993;235(suppl):118.

286. Wahl CM, Noden DM. Relation of extraocular muscle precursors to developing hindbrain nuclei of the avian embryo. Invest Ophthalmol Vis Sci 1993;(suppl):2051-2052.

287. Wallace DK, von Noorden GK. Clinical characteristics and surgical management of congenital absence of the superior oblique tendon. Am J Ophthalmol 1994;118:63-69.

288. Walsh JP, O'Doherty DS. A possible explanation of the mechanism of ophthalmoplegic migraine. Neurology 1960;10:1079-1084.

289. Walter KA, Newman NJ, Lessell S. Oculomotor palsy from minor head trauma: initial sign of intracranial aneurysm. Neurology 1991;44:148-150.

290. Warwick R. Representation of the extra-ocular muscles in the oculomotor complex. J Comput Neurol 1953;98:449-503.

291. Werner DB, Savino PJ, Schatz NJ. Benign recurrent sixth nerve palsy in childhood, secondary to immunization or viral illness. Arch Ophthalmol 1983;101:607-608.

292. White WL, Mumma JV, Tomasovic JJ. Congenital oculomotor nerve palsy, cerebellar hypoplasia, and facial capillary hemangioma. Am J Ophthalmol 1992;113:497-500.

293. Wilcox LM, Gittinger JW, Breinin GM. Congenital adduction palsy and synergistic divergence. Am J Ophthalmol 1981;91:1-7.

294. Wilson ME, Hoxie J. Facial asymmetry and superior oblique palsy. J Pediatr Ophthalmol Strabismus 1993;30:315-318.

295. Winterkorn JMS, Baker R. Retraction syndrome: brainstem motoneuron degeneration and aberrant reinnervation of extraocular muscles after peripheral lesions of ocular motor nerves in kittens. Presented at the North American Neuro-ophthalmology Society Meeting. Big Sky, Montana: February, 1993.

296. Wirtschafter J. Verbal communication. February, 1995.

297. Wise J, Gomolin J, Goldberg L. Bilateral superior oblique palsy: diagnosis and treatment. Can J Ophthalmol 1983;18:28-32.

298. Wolf HG. *Headache and Other Head Pain.* 2nd ed. New York: University Press; 1963.

299. Wojno TH. The incidence of extraocular muscle and cranial nerve palsy in orbital blow-out fractures. Ophthalmology 1987;94:682-687.

300. Wolin MJ, Saunders RA. Aneurysmal oculomotor nerve palsy in an 11-year-old boy. J Clin Neuro-ophthalmol 1992;12(3):178-180.

301. Yang MC, Bateman JB, Yee RD, Apt L. Electrooculography and discriminant analysis in Duane's syndrome and sixth-cranial-nerve palsy. Graefe's Arch Clin Exp Ophthalmol 1991;228:52-56.

302. Younge BR, Sutula F. Analysis of trochlear nerve palsies: diagnosis, etiology, and treatment. Mayo Clin Proc 1977;52:11-18.

303. Yoss RE, Rucker CW, Miller RH. Neurosurgical complications affecting the oculomotor, trochlear, and abducent nerves. Neurology 1968;18:594-600.

304. Znajda JP, Krill AE. Congenital medial rectus muscle palsy with simultaneous abduction of the two eyes. Am J Ophthamol 1969;68:1050-1052.

7

Complex Ocular Motor Disorders in Children

Introduction

A number of disparate ocular motility disorders that are not nosologically related will be discussed in this chapter. The diversity of these conditions reflects the need for clinicians to maintain a broad working knowledge of pediatric neurologic disorders along with their ocular motor manifestations. Some clinical features of these conditions (e.g., congenital ocular motor apraxia, congenital fibrosis syndrome) are sufficiently unique that the diagnosis can be established solely on the basis of the clinical appearance. Other disorders either show overlapping manifestations or may effectively masquerade as other entities. Unique features of some conditions, such as conjugate ocular torsion in a subset of patients with skew deviation, have been only recently elucidated and are considered worthy of emphasis since they significantly expand the differential diagnostic paradigms of a number of ocular motility disorders.

The clinical history and physical examinations remain the "gold standard" for establishing the diagnosis, even in this era of high resolution neuroimaging and other sophisticated ancillary testing, but it is doubtful that an adequate history can be elicited by someone unfamiliar with the disorders considered in the differential diagnosis. Therefore, detailed knowledge of the clinical findings that characterize each condition is necessary to perform the diagnostic work-up in an efficient, timely, and less costly manner. A knowledgeable clinician is less likely to embark on "fishing expeditions."

The emphasis of this chapter is on ocular motility disorders of neurologic origin and their differential diagnosis. The most current pathophysiologic concepts of the disorders are summarized. A section at the end of the chapter is devoted to a few common eyelid and pupillary abnormalities encountered in children. Some of these disorders, such as excessive blinking in children, commonly represent benign transient tics that receive very little attention in the ophthalmologic literature but are not rare in clinical practice. These bear only superficial resemblance to the more chronic benign essential blepharospasm of adults, although rarely childhood tics and adult blepharospasm may show clustering in the same family, suggesting a possible link. Occasionally, underlying ocular surface abnormalities and seizure disorders may be uncovered in children with excessive blinking. Other disorders like hemifacial spasm, which is more common in adults, may be the harbingers of more serious central nervous system (CNS) disorders if encountered in very early childhood. Childhood Horner syndrome is treated in some detail at the end of the chapter, because of its potentially ominous association with certain neoplasms, especially neuroblastoma.

The human immunodeficiency virus (HIV) infection has joined the ranks of other great mimickers (e.g., myasthenia gravis, syphilis), with an ever-expanding list of neuro-ophthalmologic manifestations. No part of the nervous system is spared. Even though it is not specifically covered in this chapter, HIV-related neurological disease should now be included in the differential diagnosis of childhood ocular motor disorders of cortical, brain stem,[109] cerebellar, or peripheral nervous system origin.

The common childhood esotropias and exotropias will not be discussed, but that is not to say that these disorders are not neurologically mediated. In fact, recent research has focused on the putative neurophysiological defects that may underly the development of congenital esotropia (e.g., defects in the motion processing pathway) or the hypothetical defects in synaptogenesis in such patients, i.e., insult to the subplate layers that direct neuronal generation and subsequent apostosis (dying back or programmed destruction of cells) during the development of the CNS, as proposed by Flynn.[81] These studies are certain to enhance our understanding of the nature of common strabismic conditions like infantile esotropia and intermittent exotropia.

Skew Deviation

Skew deviation of the eyes is a supranuclear vertical strabismus that is associated with posterior fossa lesions, particularly those affecting the brain stem tegmentum or the cerebellum.[140] While causative lesions are usually structural, skew deviation can rarely result from elevated intracranial pressure due to pseudotumor cerebri.[86] The misalignment may be comitant or incomitant, may simulate a paresis of an extraocular muscle, and may alternate with time (slowly alternating skew deviation) or on lateral gaze (alternating skew on lateral gaze). Skew deviation may occasionally be associated with ocular torsion and torticollis—the so-called ocular tilt reaction (discussed later).

The neurophysiology of skew deviation is still poorly understood, but unilateral damage of tonic otolith-ocular pathways or vestibulo-ocular reflex pathway in the frontal (roll) plane is a popular hypothetical mechanism. Skew deviation has been generally considered to be a nonlocalizing sign, simply indicating involvement of the posterior fossa, without further reference to a specific region. However, recent reports describe at least three distinct types of skew deviation within the context of the ocular tilt reaction, each pointing to involvement of a specific region (i.e., utricle, dorsolateral medulla, midbrain tegmentum).[33]

Much has been learned recently about the interrelationship between skew deviation and ocular torsion.[32,256a] Trobe[256a] had proposed that patients with skew deviation do not show ocular torsion, a feature that may help distinguish them from patients with superior oblique palsy. In his study, the criteria defining skew deviation included a negative Bielschowsky's head tilt test that may have biased the results since patients with skew deviation may show a positive head tilt test.[152] The presence or absence of torsion in his study was measured using a Double Maddox Rod test, which may not detect cyclotorsion of both eyes by the same amount and in the same direction as may be found in the ocular tilt reaction and, possibly, other forms of skew deviation. Evidence has since been presented that some degree of ocular torsion is uniformly found in patients with skew deviation.[31,33] Because the ocular torsion is often, if not always, conjugate, it cannot be effectively evaluated with the Double Maddox Rod test. Indirect ophthalmoscopy and fundus photography are useful in confirming the presence or absence of torsion.

The *ocular tilt reaction* is an oculo-cephalic synkinesis consisting of vertical divergence of the eyes (skew deviation), head tilt in the direction of the lower eye, and ocular torsion in the direction of head tilt[31] (see Figure 9.4). The degree of ocular torsion may or may not be equal in both eyes. The ocular tilt reaction may be associated with pendular nystagmus, lid retraction, symptoms of diplopia, or perception of environmental tilt. Affected patients are often initially thought to have a superior oblique muscle palsy. Both disorders may show a positive head tilt test. The diagnosis of ocular tilt reaction should be considered in patients with suspected superior oblique muscle palsy who show excyclodeviation of the hypotropic eye.[87] The ocular tilt reaction is probably a "righting reflex" that results from alteration in the otolithic and/or vertical semicircular canal pathways that occurs in patients with lesions of either peripheral or central vestibular system. It has been reported in patients with intra-axial brain stem lesions (midbrain tegmentum, dorso-lateral medulla oblongata), unilateral vestibular neurectomy, and labyrinthectomy (performed in patients with severe Meniere's disease or accoustic neuroma).[271] The skew deviation that accompanies the ocular tilt reaction may be subdivided into at least three distinct types, each with distinct clinical features, ocular torsion, and localizing significance:[33]

Type I. There is upward deviation of both eyes associated with some degree of vertical divergence. Both eyes show cyclorotation in the same direction. This type localizes to lesions of the utricle, as may be encountered in the Tullio phenomenon.

Type II. There is hypertropia of one eye while the other eye remains in the primary position. The eyes show disconjugate ocular torsion with predominant excyclotropia of the eye ipsilateral to the lesion. This type localizes to lesions of the dorsolateral medulla oblongata, as may be found in Wallenberg syndrome.

Type III. There is simultaneous hypertropia of one eye and hypotropia of the other eye. The eyes show conjugate ocular rotation toward the hypotropic eye. This type localizes to midbrain tegmentum, as may be encountered in paroxysmal ocular tilt reaction.

In a study of 56 adults with unilateral brain stem infarctions and skew deviations, clinical and neuroimaging analysis revealed the following: (1) The ipsilateral eye was hypotropic with caudal pontomedullary lesions and higher with rostral pontomesencephalic lesions. (2) All patients with skew deviation showed simultaneous conjugate bilateral ocular torsion toward the hypotropic eye. Ocular torsion was evaluated from fundus photographs. In light of these recent studies,[32,33] it has been proposed that skew deviation is a sensitive brain stem sign of localizing and lateralizing value.

Some forms of incomitant skew deviation may mimic a primary overaction of an oblique extraocular muscle. One type of skew deviation, termed alternating skew on lateral gaze or bilateral abducting hypertropia, closely resembles bilateral superior oblique overaction (Figure 7.1).[104,107, 110,187] Affected patients typically display a right hypotropia on downgaze and to the left and left hypotropia on downgaze and to the right. One study of children with brain stem tumors showed

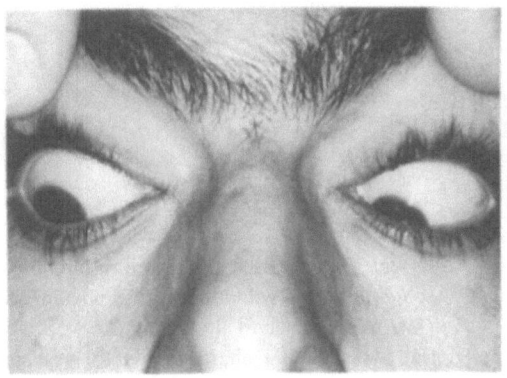
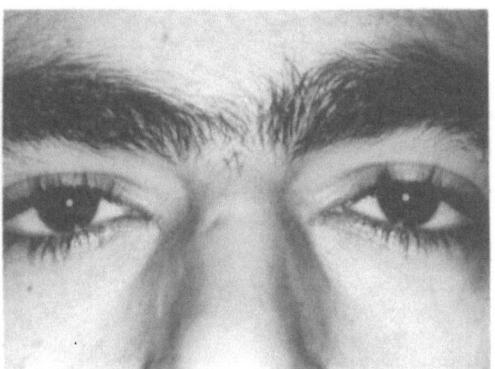
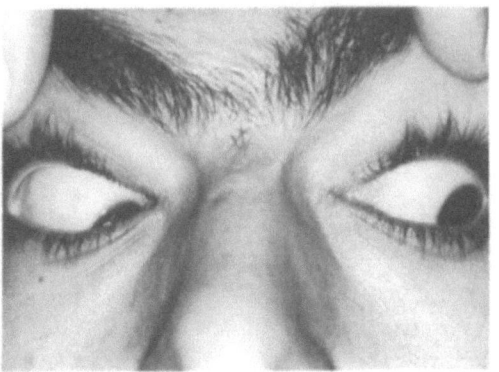

FIGURE 7.1. (A through C) Alternating skew on lateral gaze: This patient presented with new onset of downbeat nystagmus and oscillopsia. He was diagnosed with spinocerebellar degeneration. He was orthotropic in the primary position (B) but displayed left hypotropia on gaze down and to the right (A) and right hypotropia on gaze down and to the left (C). Note similarity to bilateral overaction of the superior oblique muscles.

that alternating skew deviation on lateral gaze localizes to the lower brain stem or cerebellum.[107] Given the similar localization of neuroanatomic lesions in patients with myelomeningocele (the majority of whom have Chiari II malformation) and the observation that these patients show a predilection for superior oblique overaction (Figure 7.2), it has been speculated that, at least in a subset of patients, superior oblique overaction may represent a form of skew deviation.[104,107,113]

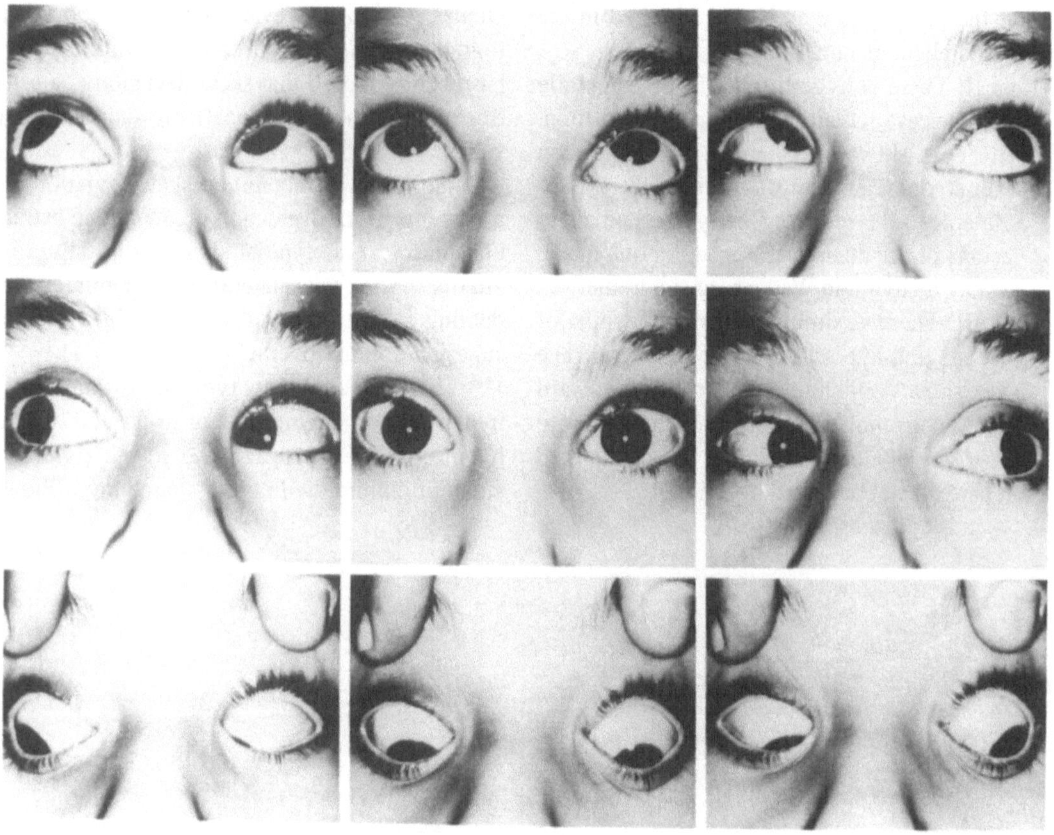

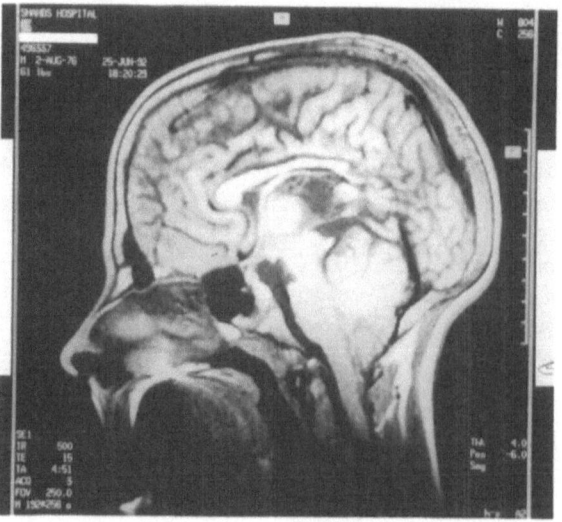

A

B

FIGURE 7.2. (A) Bilateral superior oblique overaction in a child with lumbar myelomeningocele. Note resemblance to alternating skew deviation. (B) MR imaging characteristically associated Chiari II malformation with pronounced peaking of the tectum and herniation of the cerebellar vermis into the cervical spinal canal.

This hypothesis is further supported by the observation that strabismic children who have superior oblique overaction show a higher frequency of associated neurologic disorders when compared with a control population consisting of strabismic children without superior oblique overaction.[104] Superior oblique overaction is commonly seen in conjunction with more generalized neurological disease such as cerebral palsy, myelomeningocele, and hydrocephalus.

Guyton and Weingarten[97] have recently argued that primary oblique muscle overaction and underaction and A- and V-pattern strabismus are a result of sensory torsion that arises when fusion is absent. This "sensory torsion" theory may indeed explain the majority of cases of oblique muscle overaction. Other conditions causing overdepression of the adducting eye (mimicking primary superior oblique muscle overaction) include inferior rectus muscle palsy, apparent overaction of the oblique muscles in exotropia, downshoot of the eye in Duane syndrome, physiologic "overaction" of the oblique muscles in eccentric gaze, and other restrictive or paretic conditions.[113] It is apparent that oblique muscle "overaction" is an ocular sign that may reflect a variety of conditions. It is now possible to conceptualize oblique muscle overaction as comprising a sensory type (congenital esotropia, sensory exotropia), a skew type (meningomyelocele), a leash-effect type (Duane syndrome), a physiologic type, etc.

Strabismus in Children with Neurological Dysfunction

Common neurologic disorders of children are frequently associated with strabismus. These include cerebral palsy, Down syndrome, myelomeningocele, and hydrocephalus. The features of the associated strabismus are often indistinguishable from the varieties found in otherwise normal children, but sufficient differences exist in a distinct minority of neurologically affected children to warrant separate consideration. Children with neurologic disorders who have horizontal strabismus have a higher prevalence of superior oblique overaction than otherwise healthy strabismic children.[106,113]

Cerebral palsy is perhaps one of the most common conditions seen in a pediatric neuro-ophthal-

mology practice. The term cerebral palsy defines a group of chronic neurologic disorders resulting from damage to the immature brain. Most cases nowadays are due to prematurity. Care should be taken to distinguish the static nature of cerebral palsy from the inexorably progressive neurodegenerative disorders such as Pelizaeus–Merzbacher disease.

Cerebral palsy is characterized by onset of neurologic deficits in the neonatal period and absence of progression. In addition to motor disorders such as paralysis, weakness, and incoordination, children with cerebral palsy may display sensory deficits, as exemplified by the frequent finding of optic atrophy, deafness, and cortical visual impairment. Patients with cerebral palsy show ophthalmologic abnormalities with a frequency ranging from 50% to 90%. These include optic atrophy, amblyopia, refractive errors, visual field defects, congenital cataracts, corneal leukomas, retinal dysplasia, choroiditis, macular or iris colobomas, retinopathy of prematurity, ptosis, spastic eyelids, abnormal head postures, and ocular motility disorders.[131,251] The latter include concomitant strabismus, ocular motor nerve palsy, nystagmus, gaze palsy, and other supranuclear disturbances of ocular movements.[165]

Children with cerebral palsy have a markedly increased incidence of strabismus.[165] The strabismic deviations are usually horizontal and nonparalytic, with esotropia exceeding exotropia. Associated vertical incomitance is often seen, with A-pattern strabismus being particularly common. In one series, 54% of strabismic children with cerebral palsy showed A pattern, and 46% showed V pattern.[230] Variability of the magnitude and direction of the strabismus is commonly noted in cerebral palsy. In one series, 22.5% of strabismic children with cerebral palsy showed variable strabismus. Momentary fluctuation from esotropia to exotropia may occur, which has been termed *dyskinetic strabismus* and is considered unique to cerebral palsy.[41] Dyskinetic strabismus is unrelated to accommodative effort or attention. Variable hypertropias may also occur.

In addition to the dyskinetic strabismus of cerebral palsy, the differential diagnosis of a variable strabismus shifting from exotropia to esotropia includes exotropia with a high AC/A ratio, as well as surgically overcorrected accommodative esotropia with high AC/A ratio, and esotropia with dissociated horizontal deviation. The variability in the latter entities is linked to accommodative effort, unlike the dyskinetic strabismus of cerebral palsy. Patients with oculomotor palsy with cyclic spasm may also appear to switch from exotropia to esotropia during a spasm phase, but the associated features are unique enough to obviate diagnostic confusion.

Generally, the subset of children with cerebral palsy who exhibit dyskinetic strabismus are poor candidates for surgical correction. Children with stable deviations respond favorably to strabismus surgery, although their overall outcome is not as good as strabismic children without cerebral palsy.[62,119] Children with cerebral palsy seem to have a strong predilection for surgical overcorrection.[120]

In addition to strabismus, children with cerebral palsy may have abnormalities of gaze affecting pursuit and saccadic movements and vestibulo-ocular reflex suppression by fixation.[137,201]

Gaze Palsies, Gaze Deviations, and Ophthalmoplegia

This section will discuss those conditions causing ophthalmoplegia (i.e., mixed vertical and horizontal ocular paresis) or gaze palsies (either horizontal or vertical). Gaze palsy may reflect abnormalities of saccadic eye movements, as may result from frontal lobe or frontomesencephalic saccadic pathway damage, pursuit eye movements, as may result from occipito-parieto-mesencephalic damage, or both, as may result from damage to the brain stem gaze center. It is sometimes difficult to distinguish a horizontal gaze palsy from a unilateral oculomotor or abducens nerve paresis with a compensatory head turn.[22] An infant or toddler with an abducens nerve palsy may appear to have a gaze palsy when he or she adopts a compensatory head position to achieve binocularity and resists any gaze shift out of the zone of binocularity. In such cases, one must place a patch on the suspected paretic eye, which leads to resolution of the head turn in ocular motor nerve paresis but not in gaze palsy. Complete resolution of such a head turn may occasionally require several days of patching.[22]

Horizontal Gaze Palsy in Children

The causes for horizontal gaze palsy in children are shown in Table 7.1. Generally speaking, inability to conjugately move the eyes horizontally to one side is caused by a lesion in the contralateral frontal eye field or the ipsilateral paramedian pontine reticular formation (PPRF) or abducens nucleus. Such a lesion may be distinguishable with reflex maneuvers (e.g., caloric stimulation, Doll's head maneuver) that would drive the eyes into the paretic gaze if the PPRF and abducens nucleus are intact.

Congenital bilateral paralysis of horizontal gaze has been reported in association with facial paralysis, most likely representing a form of Möbius syndrome (facial diplegia and sixth nerve palsy). It has also been described without facial paralysis. In the latter cases, the most typical findings are total absence of conjugate horizontal gaze, both volitionally and after stimulation of optokinetic and vestibular systems; preserved convergence with substitution of convergence movements for conjugate eye movements upon attempting horizontal lateral gaze; cross fixation; and apparently normal vertical eye movements. These cases have occurred either as an isolated abnormality or in association with other findings that included kyphoscoliosis, facial contracture and myokymia, and the Klippel–Feil syndrome (fusion of cervical and upper thoracic vertebrae) in one patient.[94] The precise cause of these cases is unknown, but the underlying defect has been speculated to represent selective maldevelopment affecting either the horizontal gaze center within the PPRF or the motor neurons and interneurons in the abducens nuclei. Yee et al reviewed current evidence and concluded that a developmental anomaly affecting the abducens nucleus, but not the horizontal gaze center

TABLE 7.1. Causes of horizontal gaze palsy in children.

Leigh syndrome
Pontineglioma
Bilateral Duane syndrome type III
Syndrome of progressive scoliosis and lateral gaze palsy
    (autosomal recessive)
Möbius syndrome
Congenital horizontal gaze paralysis and ear dysplasia
Familial, congenital paralysis of horizontal gaze
Brain stem arteriovenous malformation

in the PPRF, is most consistent with the clinical findings in this syndrome.[278] They further speculated that the involvement of the facial musculature associated with some cases may result from a similar developmental anomaly of the facial nucleus. Some cases of bilateral horizontal gaze paralysis are familial.[278]

Given the propensity of children to develop pontine gliomas, involvement of the abducens nuclei and/or the PPRF may lead to horizontal gaze palsy (Figure 7.3).

Congenital Ocular Motor Apraxia

Apraxia (Greek: inaction) literally denotes inability to perform volitional, purposeful motor activity despite the absence of paralysis. In the context of eye movements, the term apraxia should be limited to describe conditions in which volitional saccades are defective, but reflex and random movements are preserved (i.e., the quick phases of vestibular or optokinetic nystagmus), underscoring the presence of intact lower motor neuron pathways. This apraxic defect becomes more readily understandable by noting the presence of at least two major classes of cerebrally triggered saccades, namely, intrinsically triggered (volitional) saccades and extrinsically triggered (reflexive) saccades. Children with true saccadic apraxia show a defect in the first class of saccades but not in the second.[233]

Ocular motor apraxia is divided into congenital and acquired varieties. The acquired varieties are usually encountered in adults, following bilateral basal ganglia or cerebral hemispheric lesions.[202] Some acquired cases have been reported in children. For example, two children developed isolated ocular motor apraxia following cardiac surgery.[280] In children, the idiopathic form of congenital ocular motor apraxia has to be differentiated from the forms seen in Gaucher disease, ataxia telangiectasia, and Morbus Leigh disease (discussed later).

Congenital ocular motor apraxia is characterized by the selective absence of volitional horizontal saccades with preservation of vertical saccades.[53] Congenital ocular motor apraxia fulfills the strict definition of apraxia outlined above, namely, the reflex and random eye movements as well as the fast phases of optokinetic nystagmus

are preserved. In contrast, acquired ocular motor apraxia seldom fulfills the strict definition of an apraxic disorder.[233] Most acquired cases more closely reflect a global saccadic dysfunction rather than an apraxic disorder and may be better designated as horizontal saccadic palsies or gaze palsies, depending on whether or not smooth pursuit is also affected.

The prominent feature of this syndrome is large horizontal head thrusting to achieve visual fixation. The classical explanation of the head thrusts is that they are compensatory. This explanation states that the head is thrust in the direction of an eccentric target, and the eyes rotate conjugately in the opposite direction under the influence of the resulting vestibulo-ocular reflex. The head excursion must then overshoot the intended target to allow the controversively rotated eyes to fixate the desired target. Once fixation is achieved, the head slowly reassumes its neutral position to allow a direct, straight gaze. The child is usually noted to blink at the onset of head thrusts. The concept that head thrusts are always compensatory has been challenged by evidence suggesting that a thrust-saccade synkinesis is the explanation for head thrusts in that the thrusts may actually facilitate the initiation of saccades in a subgroup of patients.[285]

The head thrusts so characteristic of congenital ocular motor apraxia appear when the baby acquires head and neck control (usually at 6 months). Therefore, although congenital, the disorder is rarely diagnosed until late infancy. At an earlier age, blindness may be suspected due to failure to follow objects. This failure to visually pursue objects is understandable given the defective saccadic system since infants "follow" with a series of hypometric saccades. In this context, failure to pursue may be misconstrued as a visual deficit. Evaluation of the vestibulo-ocular response in such infants by spinning them elicits a slow but not a fast component, which helps establish the diagnosis.

The location and mechanism of the underlying lesion in congenital ocular motor apraxia are not fully known, but a defect of the supranuclear pathway to the PPRF is thought to exist. Some cases are familial.[90] While affected children are often judged to be otherwise healthy, some have associated deficits in other motor spheres resulting in

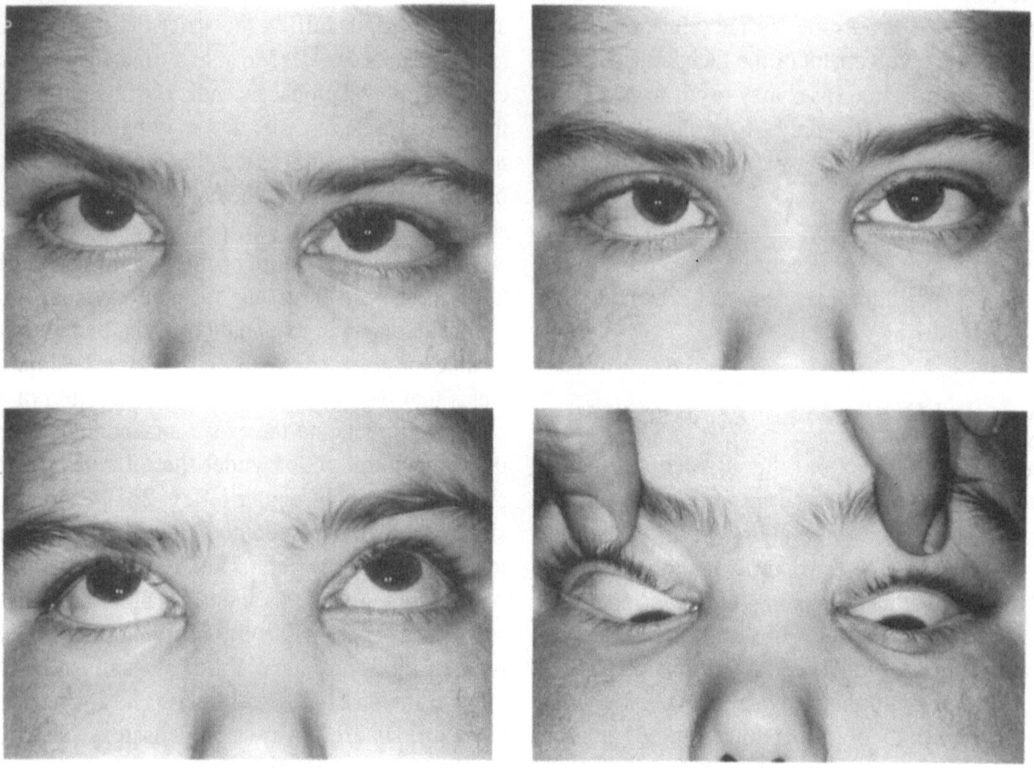

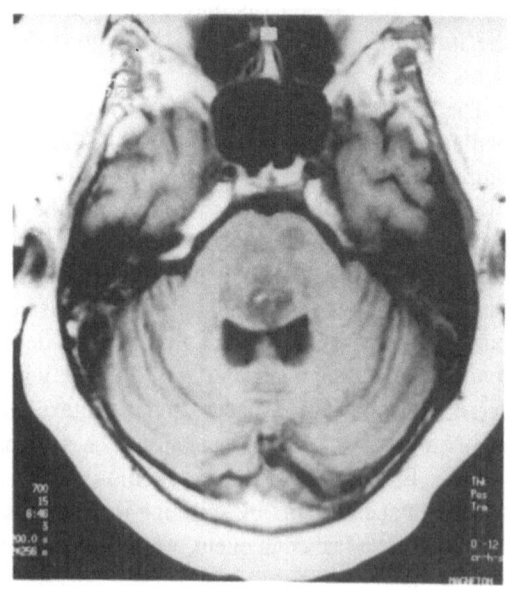

FIGURE 7.3. Horizontal gaze palsy. This child with pontine glioma shows paralysis of (A) right gaze and (B) left gaze but intact (C) upgaze and (D) downgaze. (E) MR imaging shows diffuse enlargement of the pons from a glioma.

problems in oral-motor planning affecting speech output, as well as ataxia, hypotonia, developmental delay, or clumsiness. These findings may indicate that some patients with congenital ocular motor apraxia may have a more general disorder of motor organization.[204,242,243]

The pathogenesis of congenital ocular motor apraxia remains unknown. The results of neuroimaging in patients with congenital ocular motor apraxia are usually normal but occasionally an associated structural lesion has been found. These include porencephalic cyst, agenesis or hypoplasia of the corpus callosum,[30] posterior fossa tumors such as medulloblastoma or lipoma, gray matter heterotopias, and abnormality of the brain stem or hypoplasia of the cerebellar vermis. This broad spectrum of neuroimaging abnormalities precludes meaningful neuroanatomic correlation.[242]

Ocular motor apraxia can also be a clinical manifestation of some well-known neurologic or systemic diseases. The association of congenital ocular motor apraxia and cerebellar vermis hypoplasia should suggest the diagnosis of *Joubert syndrome*. Joubert syndrome, first described in 1969, is characterized by the variable combination of episodic neonatal tachpnea and apnea, rhythmic protrusion of the tongue, ataxia, hypotonia, and a variable degree of psychomotor retardation.[134,223] The episodic tachpnea presents in the neonatal period and alternates with periods of apnea, resembling the panting of a dog, and usually resolves or improves over time. Ocular motor disorders described in Joubert syndrome include slow, hypometric saccades, ocular motor apraxia, strabismus, periodic alternating gaze deviation, pendular torsional nystagmus, seesaw nystagmus, skew deviation, and defective smooth pursuit as well as optokinetic and vestibular responses.[155] Other ophthalmologic findings include retinal dystrophy, ptosis, congenital ocular fibrosis, and colobomas.[155] The associated congenital retinal dystrophy was at first labeled as a variant of Leber congenital amaurosis but subsequently considered different since the visual loss is not as profound (20/60 to 20/200 in Joubert syndrome as compared with counting fingers or worse in Leber congenital amaurosis). In addition, the visual evoked potentials are relatively spared (mild to moderate reduction in amplitudes as compared with absent or highly attenuated signals). Both conditions show flat or highly attenuated electroretinograms (ERGs).

Dysgenesis or hypoplasia of the cerebellar vermis is a typical and a highly characteristic morphological feature of Joubert syndrome. Complete agenesis of the cerebellar vermis may also occur, but this is readily distinguishable from the vermian agenesis that occurs with the Dandy–Walker variant by the associated findings. For instance, hydrocephalus does not occur with Joubert syndrome. Additional sporadic structural defects reported in association with Joubert syndrome include other cerebellar midline defects, a dilated fourth ventricle, short neck, occipital meningoencephalocele, microcephaly, unsegmented midbrain tectum, absence of the corpus callosum, polycystic kidneys, congenital ocular fibrosis, and bilateral retinal colobomas. The condition may be sporadic; familial cases are inherited in an autosomal recessive pattern.

Joubert syndrome has some overlapping features with Arima syndrome (cerebro-oculo-hepato-renal syndrome). The Arima syndrome exhibits pigmentary degeneration, suggestive of Leber congenital amaurosis, severe psychomotor retardation, hypotonia, characteristic facies, polycystic kidneys, and absent cerebellar vermis. Joubert and Arima syndromes may be distinguished by such clinical features as neonatal tachypnea, which is one of the cardinal features of Joubert syndrome.

Occasionally, congenital ocular motor apraxia may be one of the manifestations of a degenerative disorder such as ataxia telangiectasia.[18,244] Some children with ataxia telangiectasia may pose a diagnostic quandary by showing no overt immune dysfunction, inconspicuous oculocutaneous telangiectasia, and an atypical neurological presentation with dystonia predominating over cerebellar ataxia.[46] Vertical saccades are usually involved to some degree when congenital ocular motor apraxia is associated with systemic disease. A syndrome mimicking ataxia telangiectasia with slowly progressive ataxia, choreoathetosis, and ocular motor apraxia in the horizontal and vertical plane has been described.[7] Although the neurological findings were indistinguishable from those of ataxia telangiectasia, the authors noted that the onset tended to be later and that none of the patients showed evidence of multisystem involvement. Ocular motor apraxia is often found in patients with *Gaucher disease*,[76] a lysosomal storage disorder, and may even be the presenting feature of the disease.[95] Other children with Gaucher disease may show a supranuclear horizontal gaze palsy.[200]

In most patients with congenital ocular motor apraxia, the ability to generate saccades improves over the first decade, with better eye movements and less noticeable head thrusts.[49] This spontaneous improvement led Cogan to favor a delayed maturation of the ocular motor pathways rather than congenitally absent initiation pathway for horizontal saccades as the underlying cause. While the ocular motor abnormalities tend to improve with age, most affected children show some degree of delayed motor, speech, or cognitive development.[243] Notwithstanding the benign course in most cases, it is advisable to obtain magnetic resonance (MR) imaging to rule out intracranial pathology (tumor, congenital structural malformations), the occurrence of which has been well documented in a minority of children. Treatment of underlying pathology may ameliorate or cure the apraxia in some cases[282] but not in all.[248] For instance, Zaret et al[282] described a case of congenital ocular motor apraxia that showed rapid improvement after surgical evacuation of a large cystic tumor in the rostral brain stem, while complete resection of a posterior fossa lipoma in a 10-month-old girl had no effect on the apraxia.

Although typical congenital ocular motor apraxia involves a bilateral palsy of volitional horizontal saccades, unilateral cases,[44,145] and cases involving only vertical saccades have been described.[128,211]

Vertical Gaze Palsies in Children

Vertical gaze disturbances are generally less common than horizontal ones and, among vertical disorders, upgaze palsy and combined up- and downgaze paralysis are more common than downgaze palsy (Figure 7.4). The majority of vertical gaze palsies are supranuclear and conjugate (i.e., upgaze palsy, downgaze palsy, vertical gaze palsy). Supranuclear disconjugate vertical gaze syndromes are rare, and their topographic correlation is less precisely determined. They include skew deviation and variants (such as slowly alternating skew deviation), seesaw nystagmus, monocular upgaze palsy, ocular tilt reaction, vertical one-and-a-half syndrome, and V-pattern pseudobobbing. Some of these disorders are not only location-specific but also point to a specific mechanism of injury. (for instance, acute downgaze palsy suggests bilateral infarction of the posterior thalamo-subthalamic paramedian territory). Occasionally, cases involving complete vertical ophthalmoplegia are described that remain unexplained despite thorough evaluation. Nightingale

and Barton[192] described a 6-year-old girl who had episodes of severe ataxia and vertical supranuclear ophthalmoplegia. Horizontal eye movements were not affected, and the patient was normal in between attacks.

Congenital vertical ocular motor apraxia may occur as a benign nonprogressive condition similar to the horizontal variety or may signal the presence of intracranial tumors, especially if other neurological signs are present.[73] Ebner reported a case of purely vertical ocular motor apraxia in a 4-year-old boy whose MR imaging demonstrated bilateral subthalamic lesions.

Downgaze Palsy in Children

Isolated downgaze palsy usually results from a bilateral lesion (usually infarction) involving the midbrain reticular formation and affecting the lateral parts of the rostral interstitial nucleus of the medial longitudinal fasciculus (riMLF) bilaterally. Generally speaking, an acquired isolated downgaze paralysis requires bilateral lesions at the level of the upper midbrain tegmentum, while a unilateral lesion may be sufficient to produce an upgaze palsy or a combined up- and downgaze palsy.[27] Green et al[94] reported a 9-year-old girl with selective downgaze paralysis following pneumococcal meningitis. Magnetic resonance imaging showed bilateral lesions in the riMLF. In adults, downgaze paresis is most commonly an early sign of progressive supranuclear palsy. Kumagai et al[150] described a patient with selective downgaze paresis who had a pineal germinoma with bilateral involvement of the thalamomesencephalic junction. Rhythmic vergence eye movements (alternating convergence and divergence) were observed at a rate of 3 Hz during eyelid closure.

Downgaze palsy in children is a well-known feature of the DAF syndrome, a neurovisceral storage disease considered to be a variant of Niemann-Pick disease (type C). It is characterized by supranuclear gaze palsy in the vertical plane (typically downgaze palsy), hepatosplenomegaly, slowly progressive ataxia, mental deterioration, and other CNS disorders. Foamy cells or sea-blue histiocytes in the bone marrow as well as accumulation of sphingomyelin, cholesterol and other glycosphingolipids are characteristic histopatho-

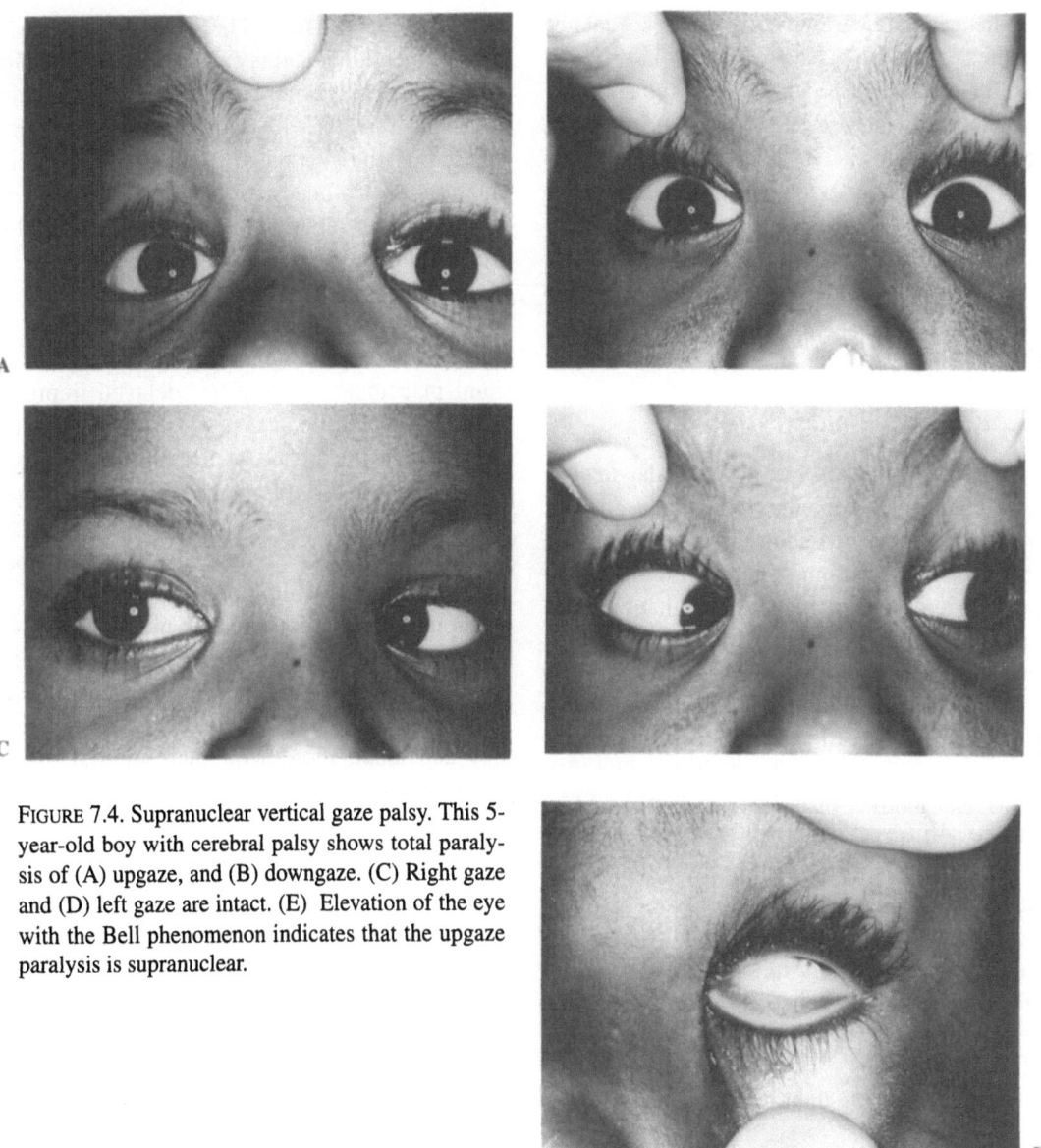

FIGURE 7.4. Supranuclear vertical gaze palsy. This 5-year-old boy with cerebral palsy shows total paralysis of (A) upgaze, and (B) downgaze. (C) Right gaze and (D) left gaze are intact. (E) Elevation of the eye with the Bell phenomenon indicates that the upgaze paralysis is supranuclear.

logic findings. The acronym "DAF" was coined by Cogan to denote the triad of downgaze palsy, ataxia or athetosis, and foam cells in the bone marrow.[48] There has since been one case showing predominantly horizontal supranuclear gaze palsy.[121] An autosomal recessive inheritance pattern is suspected.[16] The age of onset of neurologic symptoms is between 5 and 15 years. In addition to abnormalities indicated by the acronym, affected patients have hepatosplenomegaly, dementia, and widespread CNS dysfunction. Other neurological symptoms and signs include poor

coordination, slurred speech, dysphagia, seizures, cerebellar dysfunction, hyperreflexia, and involuntary movements (dystonia, chorea, or athetosis).[35] The DAF variant of Niemann–Pick disease should be suspected when evaluating school-aged children who have suffered a recent decline in intelligence or school performance and who show progressive neurologic disease and vertical supranuclear ophthalmoplegia.

An acquired condition of bilateral downgaze palsy with monocular elevation palsy, termed the vertical one-and-one-half syndrome, has been reported in a patient with bilateral infarction in the mesodiencephalic region. The authors speculated that the lesions may have affected the efferent fibers of the riMLF bilaterally and the supranuclear fibers to the contralateral superior rectus subnucleus and ipsilateral inferior oblique subnucleus.[60] This disorder should be distinguished from a different condition, also termed a one-and-one-half syndrome, consisting of bilateral upgaze palsy and monocular depression deficit due to thalamo-mesencephalic infarction ipsilateral to the downgaze paresis.[28]

Upgaze Palsy in Children

The most common causes of upgaze palsy in children include hydrocephalus (congenital and acquired) and various conditions associated with the dorsal midbrain syndrome, such as a tumor in the pineal region, arteriovenous malformations, encephalitis, and third ventricular tumors.[142] Midbrain infarction, multiple sclerosis, and syphilis are rare causes in children. The eye signs of hydrocephalus will be detailed in the chapter on neuro-ophthalmologic signs of intracranial disease. Ocular motility disorders reported in hydrocephalus are listed in Table 7.2.

Upgaze paresis is the hallmark of the dorsal midbrain syndrome. Mild cases only involve upward saccades, but severe cases show paralysis of all upward movements. Attempts to produce upward saccades, best elicited by fixating a downward rotating OKN drum, evoke convergence-retraction nystagmus. The pupils are usually mid-dilated and show light-near dissociation. The

TABLE 7.2. Ocular motility disorders in hydrocephalus.[56,160]

Upgaze paralysis (affecting saccades more than pursuit)
Lid retraction
Mydriasis with light-near dissociation
Convergence-retraction nystagmus
Convergence spasm
Pseudo-abducens palsy
Convergence insufficiency
Setting sun sign (in infants)
V-pattern pseudobobbing (with shunt failure)
A pattern esotropia with superior oblique muscle overaction
Superior oblique palsy (unilateral or bilateral)
Skew deviation
Fixation instability

upper eyelid shows pathologic lid retraction (Collier sign) and lid lag. The setting sun sign is unique to children and is suggestive of congenital hydrocephalus. It is not clear why a similar sign is not seen in adults with acquired hydrocephalus. The setting sun sign may be thought of as a combination of Collier sign and tonic downgaze, which has been reported in some children with hydrocephalus, with or without associated intraventricular hemorrhage.[250]

The upgaze palsy of congenital hydrocephalus usually improves dramatically and quickly after shunt placement. Incomplete, delayed improvement over months to years suggests damage to the upgaze pathway either as a result of thalamic hemorrhage and infarction or by the hydrocephalus itself.[250]

Children with severe, congenital visual loss may have difficulty moving their eyes volitionally. In this context, upward gaze is the most severely affected.[129] Jan et al[129] theorized that a selective upgaze deficit exists because children with marked visual impairment rarely look up, since they see much more with their limited vision when viewing closer objects sideways or downward.

Isolated paralysis of upgaze may be the presenting sign of the Miller Fisher syndrome.[139] It may also result from vitamin B_1 or B_{12} deficiency.[221] An occasional case of isolated bilateral elevation deficiency may be due to congenital restriction of the inferior rectus muscles, as occurs in the congenital fibrosis syndrome.[257a] These restrictive phenomena may be readily differentiated from the dorsal midbrain syndrome by demonstration of positive forced ductions or, in sufficiently cooperative patients, differential intraocular pressure measurements, intact upward saccades, intact Bell's phenomenon, and absence of other findings of the dorsal midbrain syndrome.

In adult patients, upgaze palsy is usually less disabling than downgaze palsy, since the superior visual space is comparatively less important. This is in contrast to downgaze palsies that cause significant visual deficits due to the importance of downgaze for such tasks as reading, walking, and eating. However, the visual significance of upgaze palsy is much more profound in children who, by virtue of their short stature, spend a considerable amount of their time looking up.

Diffuse Ophthalmoplegia in Children

There are numerous causes of diffuse ophthalmoplegia in children (Table 7.3). Each has a characteristic clinical profile, making it possible for the diagnosis to be established on clinical grounds in the majority of cases.

Chronic Progressive External Ophthalmoplegia

Chronic progressive external ophthalmoplegia (CPEO) is an umbrella term that includes a number of diverse conditions having in common insidious onset of slowly progressive, typically symmetric, multidirectional external ophthalmoplegia. Although chromosomal alterations are not detected in many patients, CPEO is thought to result from mitochondrial DNA alterations. The various conditions encompassing CPEO range from disorders limited to the eyelids and extraocular muscles to ones that include systemic and encephalopathic features. Mitochondrial encephalopathy is divided into three traditionally distinct clinical phenotypes, namely, the Kearns–Sayre syndrome; the syndrome of mitochondrial encephalopathy, lactic acidosis, and stroke (MELAS); and the syndrome of myoclonus, epilepsy, and ragged red fibers (MERRF). *Kearns–Sayre syndrome* is characterized by the triad of progressive external ophthalmoplegia, pigmentary degeneration of the retina, and heart block. All reported cases are sporadic.

TABLE 7.3. Diffuse ophthalmoplegia in children.

Chronic progressive external ophthalmoplegia
Kearns–Sayre syndrome
Myasthenia gravis
Botulism
Fisher syndrome
Whipple disease
Mitochondrial encephalopathy (e.g., MELAS, MERRF)
Intrinsic brain stem tumors
Toxicity of chemotherapeutic agents (e.g., vincristine)
Olivopontocerebellar degeneration
Medications (e.g., toxic doses of phenytoin, amitriptylene)
Tick fever
Maple syrup urine disease

Other findings may include hearing loss, cerebellar signs, mental retardation, delayed puberty, vestibular abnormalities, and "ragged red fibers" on muscle biopsy. The onset of the disorder occurs before age 20. Affected patients have short stature, other neurologic disorders, and show elevated protein concentration (>100 mg/dL) in the cerebrospinal fluid. In addition to complete heart block, cardiac conduction abnormalities include bundle branch block, bifascicular disease, and intraventricular conduction defects and are thought to result from an associated cardiomyopathy. The heart block generally occurs years after onset of the ocular signs and may cause sudden death. The retinal pigmentary degeneration progresses slowly and may be too subtle early on to detect ophthalmoscopically. The associated ptosis may become visually significant, but surgical correction should be approached with caution since the limited eye movements and the absence of the Bell's phenomenon render patients prone to develop exposure keratopathy.

Myasthenia Gravis in Children

Myasthenia gravis is a disorder of neuromuscular transmission characterized by fatiguability and fluctuating muscular weakness, with a predilection for the extraocular muscles. In severe cases, acute respiratory failure and death may occur. About half of all patients with myasthenia present with ophthalmologic symptoms. These include ptosis, strabismus, and limited ocular ductions, all with a tendency to be highly variable. No pupillary involvement is clinically discerned in myasthenia, and the presence of pupillary signs effectively excludes the diagnosis. Nearly 90% of patients with myasthenia develop ocular involvement at some point during their illness. The majority of patients with ocular myasthenia who develop systemic symptoms and signs do so within 2 years of onset.

Myasthenia gravis assumes more varied clinical and pathogenetic features in the pediatric population as compared with adults. These varied manifestations combined with the rarity of these disorders contribute to the diagnostic difficulty encountered by the clinician. Three distinct myasthenic syndromes may be encountered in the pediatric age group: transient neonatal, congenital, and juvenile. This classification is not based on age at presentation but on pathophysiology. Both congenital myasthenia and juvenile myasthenia may present any time between infancy and adulthood but are distinguished primarily by the fact that congenital myasthenia is not immune-mediated. However, this distinguishing feature is not absolute because juvenile- and adult-onset myasthenia may also be antibody-negative. Also, the defect in acquired myasthenia is postsynaptic, while the defect in congenital myasthenia may be either presynaptic or postsynaptic (subsequently discussed).

Transient Neonatal Myasthenia

Approximately 12% of newborn infants of myasthenic mothers develop transient myasthenic symptoms, presumably due to passive transplacental transfer of anti-AChR IgGs. Serum AChR antibody titers of affected neonates follow the same pattern as their mothers. Neonatal disease does not appear to correlate with the severity of maternal symptoms; affected mothers commonly have active myasthenia, but they may be in remission or may even rarely have undiagnosed subclinical disease. The onset of transient neonatal myasthenia occurs within a few hours after birth in two-thirds of patients, and within the first three days in all of them. Affected infants present with temporary skeletal muscle weakness producing hypotonia, a feeble cry, difficulty sucking and swallowing, facial diparesis, and mild respiratory distress. Occasionally, they may suffer respiratory depression that requires mechanical ventilation. Ocular involvement including ptosis, limited eye movements, and orbicularis weakness affect 15% of infants.

An atypical, more severe form of transient neonatal myasthenia includes the above-mentioned manifestations in addition to multiple joint contractures and occasional prenatal difficulties such as polyhydramnios or decreased fetal movement. Unlike the typical variety, response to oral or parenteral anticholinesterase agents is poor. Severe cases may rarely require assisted mechanical ventilation for up to 1 year.

The pathogenesis of the disorder is incompletely understood. It is not fully explained by passive transplacental IgG transfer since these antibodies are found in the majority of such newborns, but less than half of them are symptomatic. Other infants are symptomatic without detectable antibodies in their mothers. Also, high IgG levels have been found in a few asymptomatic infants. Other factors such as HLA type may play a role.

These difficulties usually last 2 to 3 weeks[186] but may resolve in 1 week or linger on for 2 months before complete recovery. Response to oral (e.g., pyridostigmine bromide) or parenteral anticholinesterase agents is very good, and these agents should be administered until spontaneous resolution occurs. No permanent neuromuscular sequelae are detectable after resolution. If this condition is not recognized and promptly treated, some affected infants may deteriorate from respiratory depression to respiratory arrest and death.

The characteristic clinical features and the history of maternal myasthenia should be enough to confirm the diagnosis, although the diagnosis may be delayed if the mother's disease has not been previously known. Further verification of the diagnosis may be derived from a favorable response to neostigmine methylsulfate with improvement of symptoms 10 to 15 minutes after intramuscular injection of 0.15 mg/kg of body weight. Alternatively, intramuscular edrophonium chloride (Tensilon) may be administered intramuscularly or subcutaneously (0.15mg/kg) or intravenously (0.10 mg/kg).

Sufficient differences exist between transient neonatal myasthenia and the congenital myasthenic syndromes (see below) to render diagnostic confusion rare. Congenital myasthenia does not occur in infants born to mothers with acquired myasthenia. The other condition affecting neuromuscular transmission in this age group, infant botulism, is readily ruled out since it occurs after the second week of life, 5 days after the infant ingests food contaminated with Clostridium botulinum, whereas the onset of transient neonatal myasthenia is within the first three days of life only.

Congenital Myasthenia

Congenital myasthenia is a rare condition that affects individuals born to nonmyasthenic mothers.[235] It results from structural or functional alterations at the myoneural junction.[75,183] Most cases present in the neonatal period or shortly thereafter with poor feeding, failure to thrive, and weakness. In some patients, however, symptoms may not appear until later childhood or even adulthood. Forty-two percent of the cases present before the age of 2 years, and over 60% before the age of 20.[191] A distinction between congenital and acquired myasthenia cannot be made with certainty on the basis of the age of onset since both types may manifest during the neonatal period, infancy, or childhood, and acquired myasthenia may also be antibody-negative. There is usually prominent involvement of the ocular musculature with ophthalmoparesis, orbicularis weakness, and ptosis.

Some cases may be familial with other siblings affected, supporting a genetic basis for the disorder.[249] Congenital myasthenia is not immune-mediated, in contradistinction to juvenile- and adult-onset acquired myasthenia which have an autoimmune basis and are attributed to antibodies that bind to the acetylcholine receptor and cause increased turnover and destruction of the receptor.[11] Serum antiacetylcholine receptor antibodies and other autoantibodies are absent. Congenital myasthenia is not associated with any autoimmune disease or any particular HLA genotype, and cytohistochemical studies fail to reveal immune complexes at the myoneural junction. The condition is generally nonremitting. Once thought to be a single disorder, it is now known to represent a group of diverse disorders distinguishable by the specific site of dysfunction at the myoneural junction (Table 7.4). Multiple inherited defects of neuromuscular transmission at presynaptic or postsynaptic levels are known, but some defects have not yet been characterized. The putative inheritance of most of these defects is autosomal recessive with the exception of the slow channel syndrome, which is autosomal dominant.

The precise characterization of these defects requires the combined use of clinical, electromyographic, in vitro electrophysiological, and morphological data. It is probably impractical to perform all tests needed for accurate characterization of the myoneural defect on each infant suspected with the diagnosis, especially when the infant is ill. However, determination of the specific subtype of congenital myasthenia would be help-

TABLE 7.4. Classification of congenital myasthenia.

I. Presynaptic defects
  A. Abnormal ACh resynthesis or mobilization
  B. Paucity of synaptic vesicles and reduced quantal ACh release
  C. Other putative presynaptic disorders
II. Postsynaptic defects
  A. End-plate congenital acetyl cholinesterase deficiency
  B. AChR abnormalities
    1. Congenital AChR deficiency and short channel open time
    2. Abnormal ACh-AChR interaction
    3. Paucity of synaptic folds
    4. Primary disorder of ACh receptors
    5. Slow channel syndrome (prolonged open time of the ACh-induced channel)
    6. High conductance fast channel syndrome

ful for therapeutic purposes, and would enhance our understanding of the heretofore incompletely understood disorders that constitute congenital myasthenia. Certainly, a detailed history should be obtained on each child regarding the onset and severity of feeding difficulty, breathing dysfunction, choking episodes, drooling, facial weakness, ophthalmoparesis, ptosis, hypotonia, and muscular fatiguability. This would start the process of differentiation between the different syndromes involved. For example, a syndrome characterized by defective AChR shows neonatal respiratory difficulty, feeding difficulty, and ophthalmoparesis, while a syndrome characterized by impaired ACh release shows few if any of these features. The developmental milestones, progression or regression of symptoms and signs during infancy and childhood, response to any therapeutic modalities, and a complete family pedigree should be recorded.

Because the congenital myasthenic syndromes are not immune-mediated, neither plasmapheresis nor immunosuppression have any beneficial effect. Thymectomy usually produces negligible benefits, although a transient improvement has been reported in two patients, one of whom had an abnormal thymus.[47,266] Because of the diversity of the underlying abnormalities, no specific conclusion can be drawn regarding the efficacy of the anticholinesterase preparations. Some types of congenital myasthenia (e.g., congenital acetylcholine receptor deficiency) respond favorably to anticholinesterase preparations while other types (e.g., acetylcholinesterase deficiency, slow channel syndrome) are refractory to such treatment and may even be made worse by it. Therefore, an effort to differentiate juvenile myasthenia from congenital myasthenia and to specifically identify the type of congenital myasthenic syndrome has important therapeutic implications.

Juvenile Myasthenia

Juvenile myasthenia is similar to the adult variety in presentation, pathogenesis, clinical course, and response to therapy. However, some studies reveal the juvenile variety to be more frequently familial, to show more severe ophthalmoplegia, and to have slower progression and a higher rate of spontaneous remissions. An acute fulminating form of myasthenia gravis has been described, with onset between 2 and 10 years of age, with respiratory crisis as the presenting feature of the disorder.[78] The treatment of juvenile myasthenia is similar to that of the adult variety. Although thymectomy is often avoided in myasthenic children for fear of compromising the developing immune system, reports of thymectomy in children have shown favorable results without evidence of immune compromise. Furthermore, thymomas are rare in myasthenic children.[5] Since the disease is immune mediated, unlike congenital myasthenia, immunosuppression and plasmapheresis have a therapeutic role. However, systemic corticosteroids are often avoided because they stunt growth and are generally contraindicated in cases of purely ocular pediatric myasthenia, to avoid treating a non-life-threatening condition with potentially life-threatening medication.

Myasthenia can often be diagnosed on clinical grounds when ptosis or ophthalmoplegia is accompanied by certain neuro-ophthalmologic signs. These include fatiguable ptosis, orbicularis weakness, variable strabismus, quiver-like eye movements, and a Cogan lid twitch sign. A Cogan lid twitch is elicited by having a patient rapidly refixate the eyes from a depressed position to the primary position, with a positive lid twitch sign indicated by the lids overshooting briefly upward before settling to their usual ptotic position. If the lid is first fatigued by sustained upward gaze, the lid twitch sign becomes more exaggerated. Apparently, the short relaxation of the upper lid allowed

by fixating an object in downgaze allows for transient recovery of strength by the myasthenic levator muscle. Although ptosis is the most common sign, lid retraction may occasionally be encountered especially unilaterally in patients with contralateral ptosis. This seemingly paradoxical finding is explained by Hering's law of equal innervation as the patient attempts to elevate the contralateral ptotic lid. Bilateral lid retraction, which is also rarely reported in myasthenia, is not readily explained by Hering's law. In such cases, the possibility of concurrent thyroid eye disease must be excluded.[135]

Rarely, children with diffuse myasthenic ophthalmoplegia can present with *myopia*. This occurs when medial rectus weakness leads to exotropia, which necessitates excessive accommodative convergence to maintain single binocular vision. These children are caught in the unpleasant situation of having to sacrifice clear vision to avoid diplopia.

The diagnosis of myasthenia may be confirmed with certain ancillary tests. The Tensilon test (edrophonium hydrochloride) is the most commonly utilized. Ten milligrams of the drug are placed in a 1 cc tuberculin syringe, and the test is administered by first injecting a 0.2-cc test bolus while observing the patient for side effects. If no side effects occur within 1 to 2 minutes, the remaining Tensilon is injected in 2 to 4 bolus increments separated by 1 minute each while the patient is observed for amelioration of the ocular symptoms (Figure 7.5). A 1 cc tuberculin syringe containing 1 ml (0.4 mg) of atropine should be at hand in case of excessive parasympathetic response to Tensilon administration with significant cardiovascular side effects. Results of the Tensilon test may be equivocal, falsely negative, or falsely positive. False-negative results are more common than false-positive ones. Therefore, if the clinical findings are suggestive of myasthenia, repeating an initially negative Tensilon test is recommended. False-positive results have been reported in patients with compressive lesions (brain tumors, intracranial aneurysm), botulism, the Eaton–Lambert syndrome, amyotrophic lateral sclerosis, poliomyelitis, transverse myelitis, Guillain–Barre syndrome, and myositis.[67,185]

In children, Prostigmine (neostigmine) is administered intramuscularly, which produces a more

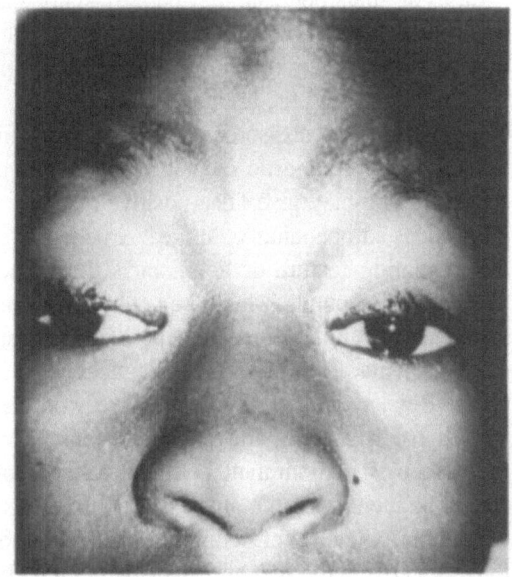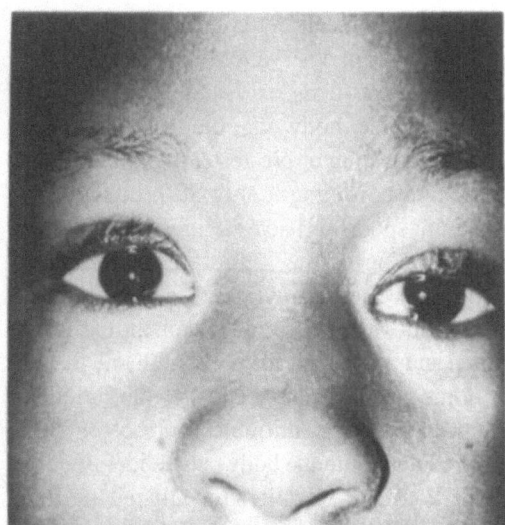

FIGURE 7.5. Positive Tensilon test in juvenile myasthenia gravis. This child presented with variable ptosis and exotropia (A) that showed resolution upon administration of intravenous Tensilon (B).

prolonged response in myasthenic patients than does edrophonium chloride. The patient is examined 30 to 45 minutes after injection. To avoid the complications of pharmacological testing, a sleep test has been suggested wherein the patient is evaluated for improvement of ocular signs immediately after a 30-minute period of sleep, and for worsening of these signs shortly thereafter.[197]

Brain tumors may rarely produce clinical findings that are indistinguishable from myasthenia.[203,247] Ragge and Hoyt[203] described an adolescent girl with neurofibromatosis type I and a dorsal midbrain astrocytoma who had fatiguable ptosis, upgaze paresis, and a positive "lid twitch" sign. These findings improved significantly following radiotherapy of the astrocytoma, confirming that the muscular fatiguability was central in origin. Straube and Witt[247] described four patients with posterior fossa tumors who presented only with fluctuating weakness of the external ocular muscles and/or the pharyngeal muscles, leading to an incorrect diagnosis of ocular myasthenia. Moreover, as noted earlier, false-positive results of Tensilon testing may occur in some instances involving tumors or even aneurysms. Branley et al[34] reported a 7-year-old girl who developed an oculomotor nerve palsy of subacute onset due to a cerebral artery aneurysm. The condition was initially confused with myasthenia gravis because the ptosis improved after Tensilon administration (false-positive result), but the key clinical distinguishing findings were the presence of aberrant innervation and pupillary involvement, which are not features of myasthenia. It should be noted that chemotherapeutic agents like vincristine may cause neurological findings (ptosis, ophthalmoplegia, jaw pain) that may confound the diagnostic picture in children with intracranial tumors.[8]

Systemic therapy of myasthenia helps control ocular symptoms in most patients.[69,70] In selected patients with chronic disability due to strabismus and associated diplopia despite adequate medical therapy, there is a place for strabismus surgery, provided the strabismic angle is sufficiently stable.[3,59,102]

Nonmyasthenic Ophthalmoplegia in Children

Botulism

Clostridium botulinum produces seven distinct protein toxins, of which A, B, and E are the most commonly responsible for human botulism.[273]

The botulism toxin causes neural paralysis of skeletal muscle by disruption of both spontaneous and stimulus-induced release of acetylcholine from the presynaptic nerve terminal, and by interfering with exocytosis of vesicle contents. The toxin enters the body via the following four routes: (1) ingestion of pre-formed toxin, as in the case of food poisoning; (2) toxin production by Clostridium spores or bacteria infecting a wound; (3) colonization of the gastrointestinal tract by Clostridium botulinum with subsequent production of toxin—it is by this mechanism that infant botulism and the "infant form of botulism" that affects some adults occurs; and (4) the "hidden" form in which no identifiable route of entry of toxin or bacteria into the body can be identified.

Infant botulism was first recognized in 1976 and has since become the most frequently reported form of botulism.[226,228,267] The majority of reported cases have been from North America. It results from colonization of the gastrointestinal tract by ingested spores of Clostridium botulinum, which then produce toxin that is absorbed into the circulation. A history of honey ingestion or soil eating is frequently obtained. Because Clostridium botulinum is ubiquitous and is commonly ingested without adverse effects, a number of host factors may render a particular individual predisposed. Constipation, immune dysfunction, gastric pH, and unusual gut flora among others may permit the colonization and germination of Clostridium spores and subsequent local production of toxin. The typical case involves a previously healthy infant who becomes ill at 1 to 5 months of age. The presenting symptoms and signs include hypotonia, hyporeflexia, constipation, and decreased respiratory function. Bulbar signs predominate and include impaired sucking with poor feeding, a feeble cry and external as well as internal ophthalmoplegia. Constipation and feeding difficulties precede the onset of progressive bulbar and skeletal muscle weakness. The muscular weakness progresses in a descending fashion from the cranial nerves to the limbs. Signs of cranial nerve palsy include limited eye movements, ptosis, dilated poorly reactive pupils, drooling, diminished gag reflex, and facial weakness. Respiratory arrest and death may follow, but the majority of infants recover completely in 1 to 5 months.

Cases of infant botulism may be mistakenly diagnosed as crib death, failure to thrive, sepsis, dehydration, viral infection, idiopathic hypotonia, poliomyelitis, meningitis, brain stem encephalitis, or other neuromuscular disorders such as myasthenia. To add to the diagnostic quandary, some patients with botulism may give false-positive response to intravenous edrophonium chloride.[57] One important differentiating feature of botulism is the dilated, poorly reactive pupils, which are not seen in ocular myasthenia. Pupillary involvement is not a feature of myasthenia. The differential diagnosis also includes Reye syndrome, Guillain–Barre syndrome, hypothyroidism, tick paralysis, and toxins. While the diagnosis of noninfant botulism can be confirmed by identifying the organism and toxin in fecal samples, the level of botulinum toxin is too low to be detected in the sera of patients with infant botulism. Electromyographic studies are highly useful in the diagnosis of botulism, with a characteristic electromyogram (EMG) pattern that has been given the acronym BSAP, for "brief duration, small-amplitude, overly abundant, motor-unit action potentials." Fibrillation potentials suggesting functional denervation are observed in about half the cases. Repetitive fast rates of stimulation (20 to 50 Hz) result in marked incremental response, a finding not present in older children and adults with botulism, probably due to the large amount of toxin present. Other conditions showing an incremental EMG response, such as Eaton–Lambert (not seen in infants), hypermagnesemia, and aminoglycoside toxicity, can be readily excluded on clinical and laboratory grounds. Logistical problems in terms of application of EMG to the investigation of infant botulism include the need to transport the cumbersome equipment to the intensive care unit and electrical interference there with the EMG recording.

Signs of total (internal and external) ophthalmoplegia, dry mouth, descending paralysis, obstipation, absence of fever, and lucid sensorium as cardinal symptoms should always raise suspicion of botulism. Spontaneous recovery occurs by sprouting of new nerve endings with formation of new myoneural junctions. Treatment of affected patients includes insertion of a nasogastric tube with suction, enemas, antitoxin administration (benefit controversial), and mechanical ventilation if indicated. The recently introduced botulinum immune globulin (BIG) appears to show promising results.

The Fisher Syndrome—A Variant of Guillain–Barre Syndrome

The Guillain–Barre syndrome (acute infectious polyneuropathy) consists of progressive, usually symmetric muscular weakness that appears several days after a nonspecific infectious prodrome. Mild sensory disturbances such as pain and parasthesias are commonly present. The paralysis usually affects the lower extremities and then ascends. Cranial nerve palsy may appear at any time during the clinical course. Results of electromyographic studies are usually consistent with involvement of the lower motor neurons or peripheral nerves.

The Fisher syndrome is a variant of the Guillain–Barre syndrome with the distinct triad of ataxia, areflexia, and ophthalmoplegia without concurrent peripheral neuropathy. The Fisher syndrome constitutes about 5% of all reported cases of Guillain–Barre syndrome. There appears to be a gender predilection, with the male/female ratio being 2:1. Of the 223 cases reported before 1993, the average age was 43.6 years (range 14 months to 80 years), with 14.3% of these being children.[23]

The majority of patients with the Fisher syndrome suffer a preceding viral prodrome, usually respiratory, 1 to 3 weeks prior to onset of the syndrome.[23] Most patients reach maximum neurologic deficit within 1 week of onset. Diplopia and ataxia are the most common presenting symptoms. Associated ophthalmoplegia is complete (including the parasympathetic fibers to the pupillary sphincter muscle) in about one-half of patients with the Fisher syndrome,[23] but pure external ophthalmoplegia or internal ophthalmoplegia may occur. Isolated ocular motor nerve palsy, and combinations of horizontal and vertical gaze palsies may be noted. Internuclear ophthalmoplegia, one-and-a-half syndrome, gaze-evoked lid nystagmus, convergence spasm, and a dorsal midbrain syndrome with upward gaze paralysis but intact Bell's phenomenon have also been reported.[9,23,174] The presence of these latter disorders and similar findings pointing to brain stem involvement fuels the controversy about the nature of the disease as a peripheral (infranuclear, due to involvement of sensory fibers in the peripheral nerves and dorsal roots) or CNS (supranuclear) disorder or as a combination of both.[174] Some authors consider the Fisher variant to be due to pathologic changes exclusively within the peripheral nervous system. This concept is supported by reports of normal MR imaging scans in affected patients.[214] While pure cases of the Fisher syndrome are apparently attributable to peripheral neuropathy and are not uncommon, overlapping cases occur that bridge the spectrum from the benign Fisher variant to the more virulent Guillain–Barre syndrome. For instance, cases that include limb paralysis do not, strictly speaking, fall within the original definition of the Fisher syndrome and are transitional forms to the Guillain–Barre syndrome. On the basis of current evidence, some authors believe that the Fisher syndrome represents an encephalomyeloneuritis.[23]

Other cranial nerves may be affected, the most common being the facial nerve. Dysphasia and dysarthria may result when the lower cranial nerves are involved. Monoparesis, hemiparesis, or quadraparesis have been described. Patients may have sensory symptoms, including parasthesias, dysesthesia, and headaches. Other symptoms and signs include disturbance of consciousness, seizures, myoclonus, tremors, fever, vomiting, irritability, positive Babinski's sign, and respiratory insufficiency. The cerebrospinal fluid, if examined 2 to 3 weeks or later after onset, usually shows mild elevation in protein, with about 10% of cases in the literature showing pleocytosis.

The triad of severe external ophthalmoplegia, ataxia, and areflexia in an otherwise alert child is fairly unique. The characteristic history and physical findings are usually sufficient to establish the presumptive diagnosis, but differentiation from posterior fossa tumors may be difficult without neuroimaging. Wernicke syndrome and phenytoin intoxication can show a similar syndrome complex, but these entities can be excluded by the clinical history. Both the Fisher syndrome and botulism may show a similar early presentation consisting of extraocular muscle weakness and mydriasis. Other conditions included in the differential diagnosis of the Fisher syndrome are brain stem stroke, pituitary apoplexy, cerebral sinus thrombosis, tick fever, and diphtheria.

While some cases may follow a more virulent course, most cases of the Fisher syndrome resolve spontaneously within 1 to 3 months. Corticosteroids as well as plasmapheresis have been used, but there is little evidence to support their efficacy in the limited form of the condition without brain stem signs. Intravenous immunoglobulin may be helpful in severe cases.[14]

Transient Ocular Motor Disturbances of Infancy

Healthy neonates may exhibit a variety of benign, transient supranuclear eye movement disturbances. These include horizontal heterophorias, tonic downgaze and upgaze, opsoclonus, and skew deviations. As each of these disorders may forebode serious neurological disease, especially in older children, their benign nature in healthy neonates must be recognized to avoid unnecessary diagnostic testing.

Transient Neonatal Strabismus

Several nursery studies have shown that the eyes of otherwise healthy, full-term neonates are commonly misaligned. In one study of 1219 neonates, 48.6% had orthotropia, 32.7% had exotropia, 3.2% had esotropia, and 15.4% were not sufficiently alert to allow determination of ocular alignment.[194] No cases of congenital esotropia were found in any neonate, supporting the concept that congenital esotropia does not manifest at birth. Follow-up studies of these patients have shown that the vast majority of children with transient heterophorias become orthotropic between 2 and 3 months of age, a stage coincident with development of stereoscopic vision.[15,239] Unlike exotropia, which may be found transiently in the neonatal period, the finding of large esotropia within the first several weeks of life should not be classified as congenital esotropia (which usually first appears after 6 weeks of age) until other conditions such as sixth nerve palsy and Moebius syndrome are ruled out (Figure 7.6).

It should also be recognized that the eyes of premature infants may transiently display exotropia with limited adduction. These findings have been speculated to result from immaturity of the medial longitudinal fasciculus in the premature infant.

Tonic Downgaze

Tonic downward deviation of the eyes may occur as a transient phenomenon in neonates and does not necessarily indicate underlying neurologic dysfunction.[124] Both eyes are tonically deviated downward while the infant is awake but can be maneuvered upward with oculocephalic or vestibulo-ocular stimulation; the condition resolves during sleep with both eyes returning to the midline. It usually resolves within the first six months of life. Two infants who displayed this transient tonic downgaze also showed associated upbeat nystagmus, with complete resolution of both findings within the first few months of life.[91] The authors proposed that immaturity of the vestibular system was the cause.

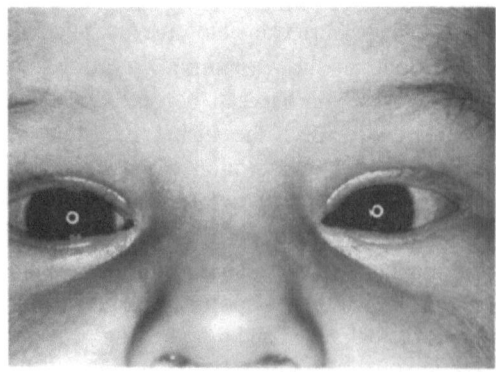
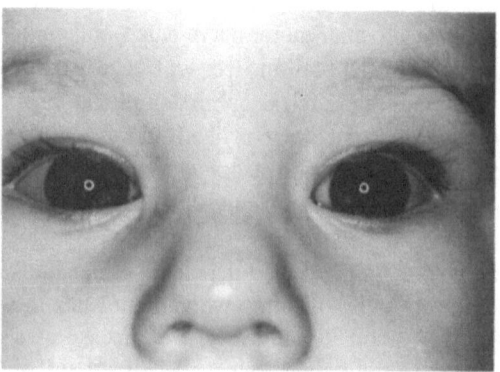

FIGURE 7.6. Transient esotropia in a neonate. This infant showed 30 prism diopters of left esotropia (A) with mild limitation of abduction of the left eye that totally resolved by 5 months of age (B). Perinatal trauma to the abducens nerve was the cause.

The benign, transient form of tonic downgaze differs from the "setting sun sign" associated with hydrocephalus by the absence of eyelid retraction. Yokochi[279] described downward deviations of the eyes of neurologically affected infants that were paroxysmal rather than constant, as in the foregoing benign variety. The paroxysms were not associated with seizure activity. He considered this to be a sign found in brain-damaged infants with cortical visual impairment. The paroxysms spontaneously resolved with time in many patients. We have examined a blind infant with profound bilateral optic nerve hypoplasia, absent septum pellucidum, and developmental delay who showed sudden episodic downward deviations of the eyes occurring every 1 to 2 minutes and lasting 5 to 10 seconds (Figure 7.7). The downward deviation was associated with lid lag. The patient also showed intermittent side-to-side head shaking. Episodic downgaze may be one of the presenting signs of Leigh subacute necrotizing encephalomyelopathy.[171] Mak et al[171] reported a previously healthy infant who, at 6 months of age, showed episodic downgaze with limited horizontal movements that resolved after 5 days then recurred several times along with other abnormalities before a diagnosis of Leigh disease was made.

It is not clear whether congenital hydrocephalus alone results in tonic downgaze. The setting sun sign, a feature of congenital hydrocephalus (Figure 7.8), may be considered a combination of lid retraction (Collier's sign) and tonic downgaze. Acquired hydrocephalus in older patients does not produce tonic downgaze, suggesting a specific susceptibility of the neonatal brain to the mass effect of hydrocephalus on midbrain structures responsible for downgaze or suggesting a higher sensitivity of the pretectal area in infants to hydrocephalus, leading to more severe upgaze palsy (causing the eyes to deviate downward) than is seen in older patients. Tamura and Hoyt[250] reported 11 premature infants with intraventricular hemorrhages who showed acute tonic downward deviation of the eyes, esotropia, and upgaze palsy. All patients showed associated hydrocephalus, shunting of which resulted in gradual improvement in upgaze with persistence of the large-angle esotropia. The authors suggested that the gradual recovery of upgaze indicates that the upgaze palsy may not be simply due to the acute effects of the hydrocephalus. Rather, they suggested that the associated intraventricular hemorrhages act as a mass lesion, compressing (and hence paralyzing) the upgaze centers or irritating (and hence stimulating) the

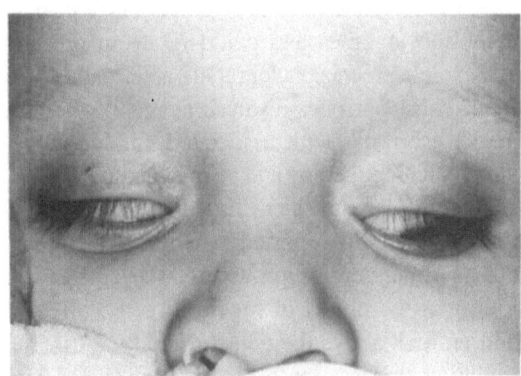

FIGURE 7.7. Episodic tonic downgaze. This blind infant with profound bilateral optic nerve hypoplasia, absent septum pellucidum, and developmental delay showed sudden episodic downward deviations of the eyes occurring every 1 to 2 minutes and lasting 5 to 10 seconds. These have occurred since birth. The downward deviation was associated with lid lag. The infant also showed intermittent side-to-side head shaking.

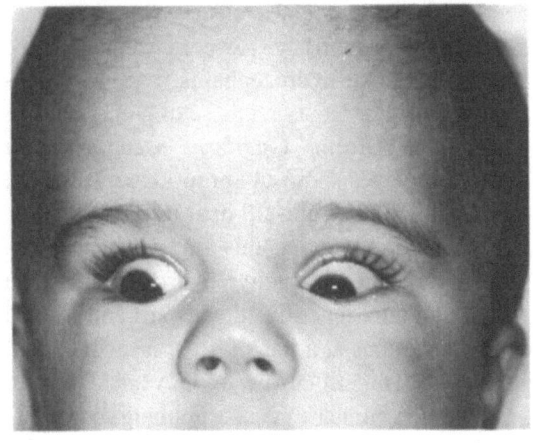

FIGURE 7.8. Setting sun sign in hydrocephalus. This child presented with pronounced lid retraction and mild to moderate tonic downward deviation of the eyes. A disproportionately large head and dilated ventricles on neuroimaging confirmed the diagnosis of hydrocephalus.

downgaze centers within the mesencephalon. They speculated that injury to these mesencephalic structures may contribute to the delay in recovery of upgaze after shunting. In congenital hydrocephalus that is not caused by intraventricular hemorrhage, however, the upgaze palsy and/or the setting sun sign responds quickly to reduction of intracranial pressure. For instance, Hoyt and Daroff[126] described a 3-month-old infant with intermittent hydrocephalus secondary to a tumor of the thalamus and septum pellucidum. The infant displayed tonic downgaze and esotropia whenever the ventricular pressure increased, and eye movements normalized when the ventricular pressure became normal. Such cases demonstrate that a mass effect, independent of the effect of the hydrocephalus itself, need not be present for tonic downgaze to develop in infants with hydrocephalus.

Children with hydrocephalus are predisposed to develop esotropia through several different mechanisms: (1) early-onset childhood esotropia, which is more common in neurologically impaired children; (2) unilateral or bilateral sixth nerve palsy; and (3) intraventricular hemorrhage in premature infants, which may involve the thalamus and mesencephalon and produce neuro-ophthalmologic signs of a thalamic infarction (tonic downward deviation of the eyes, upgaze palsy, and esotropia). The esotropia in these patients usually persists even after the vertical gaze deficits resolve.

Tonic downgaze may be observed in very ill patients with impaired consciousness who have medial thalamic hemorrhage, severe encephalopathy, acute obstructive hydrocephalus, or severe subarachnoid hemorrhage. In this setting, it should be distinguished from *V-pattern pseudobobbing* wherein the eyes show an abrupt downward jerk followed by a slow upward drift to primary position. Keane[141] reported this finding in five patients with acute obstructive hydrocephalus who had arrhythmic, repetitive downward and inward ocular deviations at a rate of 1 per 3 seconds to 2 per second. The fast downward movements render the condition similar to ocular bobbing, but it differs by the presence of a V pattern, a generally faster rate, and associated pretectal, rather than pontine, signs. Keane speculated that V-pattern pseudobobbing represents a variant of convergence-retraction nystagmus that signals the need for prompt shunt placement or revision.

Tonic Upgaze

Tonic upgaze is rarer than tonic downgaze. It also tends to be episodic. In 1988, Ouvrier and Billson[199] described four patients with a new condition they termed "benign paroxysmal tonic upgaze of childhood." This condition was characterized by onset during infancy of episodic tonic conjugate upward deviation of the eyes that was relieved by sleep. The children had impaired downgaze below the primary position with downbeating nystagmus on attempted downgaze and apparently normal horizontal movements. The patients were otherwise neurologically intact with the exception of mild ataxia. Results of metabolic, electroencephalographic, and neuroradiologic investigations were unremarkable. All eventually improved, with one child showing a favorable therapeutic response to levodopa.

The following year, Ahn et al[6] described three infants who had tonic upgaze with no associated seizure activity or neurologic disease. The vestibulo-ocular reflexes were intact, revealing a full range of vertical movements. These episodes were initially noted within the first month or two of life and were most conspicuous when the infant was ill or fatigued. These episodes diminished with time.[6] Mets[175] described a 9-month-old otherwise healthy infant with large-angle esotropia who displayed extreme sustained spasms of upgaze. This infant was noted to have full vertical range of ocular motion at times and could fixate in primary gaze. No electroencephalographic abnormality was found. These episodes resolved at age 3½ months, but the esotropia with associated amblyopia required patching therapy and strabismus surgery.

Tonic upgaze must be distinguished from "overlooking" that was reported by Taylor in patients with neuronal ceroid lipofuscinosis.[252] Instead of looking at the object of regard directly, affected children look above the object. Initially attributed to relative preservation of the inferior visual field associated with certain retinal disorders, it was later reported not to be disease specific but rather to represent a sign of bilateral central scotomas (and vision of 20/200 or worse) in children from a variety of causes.[92] Overlooking may initially be mistaken for either lack of cooperation or comprehension on the part of the patient or may be misinterpreted as a primary ocular motor disorder.

Intermittent episodes of upward ocular deviation may represent an oculogyric crisis or may be a manifestation of a seizure disorder, typically petit mal. Oculogyric crisis denotes an extreme, episodic upward rotation of the eyes, often obliquely either to the right or to the left. The deviation is usually sustained and is often associated with rhythmical jerking or twitching of the eyelid. Each oculogyric movement lasts several seconds, after which the eyes return to the horizontal position, before deviating again a few seconds later until the "crisis" passes, typically in 1 to 2 hours. Patients may have associated thought disorders. Dopamine blocking agents (neuroleptics) are the most common cause of drug-induced acute dystonic reactions such as oculogyric crisis, but other drugs have been incriminated, including carbamazepine, lithium carbonate, metoclopramide, and sulpiride, among others. Oculogyric crisis has also been reported after Tensilon administration.[196] Similar eye movements have been observed in patients with various CNS disorders, such as herpetic encephalitis, Hallervorden–Spatz, and Rett syndrome,[79] and in one patient with cystic glioma in whom the onset of crisis was positional.[241] Oculogyric crisis can be aborted by anticholinergics (e.g., Cogentin) and subsequently controlled by reducing the dosage of the offending medication or changing it altogether. Patients with petit mal seizures may show eye movements similar to oculogyric crisis, usually with concurrent eyelid flutter.[11] Eye movement tics (see later in this chapter) may also superficially resemble intermittent episodic tonic upgaze.

Barontini[19] described two patients who developed upward ocular deviation in association with other neurologic dysfunction that lasted about 1 month. Their review of the literature led them to conclude that either dystonia or downgaze palsy can underlie the phenomenon of tonic upgaze. Acquired tonic upward deviation is also seen in comatose patients, where it indicates a very poor prognosis, or in patients with brain stem disease causing downgaze paralysis.

Opsoclonus

Opsoclonus denotes chaotic repetitive back-to-back saccades in different directions (see Chapter 8). Although usually indicative of an underlying viral encephalitis or neuroblastoma, opsoclonus has been reported as a benign transient finding in healthy neonates. It usually resolves in 1 to 3 months, passing through a phase of ocular flutter. Given the apparent rarity of this observation, it is probably prudent to consider this benign transient variant a diagnosis of exclusion, especially in light of the serious nature of other potentially causative lesions such as neuroblastoma. Interestingly, when opsoclonus accompanies neuroblastoma, it imparts a highly favorable prognosis for survival.[190]

Neonatal Vertical Deviation of the Eyes

A transient vertical deviation of the eyes with or without a horizontal component has been reported in the neonatal period without associated evidence of posterior fossa dysfunction and referred to as skew deviation.[124] Some infants exhibiting this sign may subsequently develop large-angle esotropia typical for congenital esotropia or nystagmus compensation syndrome.[124] Whether this transient vertical deviation of the eyes is a reliable premonitory sign for the subsequent development of congenital esotropia is not known.

Marcus Gunn Jaw Winking (Trigemino-Oculomotor Synkinesis)

A normal synkinesis denotes simultaneous contraction of muscles normally innervated by different peripheral nerves or different branches of the same nerve. A pathologic synkinesis occurs when muscles are reinnervated by nerves other than their own following a nerve injury. Pathologic synkinesis may be congenital (Duane's syndrome, synergistic divergence, Marcus Gunn jaw winking) or acquired (facial synkinesis or oculomotor synkinesis after trauma).

The Marcus Gunn jaw winking (MGJW) synkinesis usually presents as variable unilateral ptosis noted at birth or shortly thereafter. Unlike ordinary congenital ptosis, when the infant nurses, the ptotic lid jerks upward with each suckling movement. In a series of nearly 1500 cases of congenital ptosis,[24] the Marcus Gunn phenomenon accounted for 80 patients (5%). Of these 80 patients, 42 showed right eye involvement, 35 showed left eye involvement, and 3 had bilateral synkinesis. No gender preponderance was identified, and only two cases were familial. Fifty-four percent of patients showed amblyopia, 26% anisometropia. Some form of strabismus was found in 56%, including 19 cases of superior rectus palsy, 19 cases of double elevator palsy, and 2 cases of Duane's retraction syndrome. The natural history of the disorder remains unsettled, with some authors noting that the synkinetic movement becomes less conspicuous with age, although patients may learn to camouflage the lid excursions.

The pathogenesis of the MGJW synkinesis is controversial. The prevalent concept is that the disorder results from aberrant innervation of the levator palpebrae muscle by a branch of the motor division of the trigeminal nerve that supplies the muscles of mastication, hence the designation *trigemino-oculomotor synkinesis.* However, Sano[222] has presented electromyographic evidence that the jaw winking phenomenon is a release phenomenon representing an exaggeration of a normally found but clinically undetectable physiologic cocontraction. Utilizing electromyographic studies of normal subjects, he demonstrated cofiring of the oculomotor-innervated extraocular muscles and the muscles of mastication innervated by the motor branch of the trigeminal nerve. He argues that congenital brain stem lesions may "release" phylogenetically older neural mechanisms such as synkinetic movements from higher central control, which are similar to other synkinetic movements such as the palmo-mental and primitive grasp-feeding reflexes.

Sano[222] has classified the trigemino-ocular motor synkinesis into two major groups: (1) external pterygoid-levator synkinesis (the most common type) with lid elevation upon thrusting the jaw to the opposite side (ipsilateral external pterygoid firing), upon projecting the jaw forward (both external pterygoids firing), or upon opening the mouth widely; and (2) internal pterygoid-levator synkinesis (relatively rare) with lid elevation upon teeth clinching.

In the typical case of MGJW, firing of the motor branch of the trigeminal nerve is associated with firing of the oculomotor branch to the levator. A rare variant of this phenomenon, termed the inverse Marcus Gunn phenomenon,[170] shows firing of the motor branch of the trigeminal nerve synkinetically with inhibition of the oculomotor branch to the levator. Here, the affected eyelid *falls* as the mouth opens or as the jaw moves to the opposite side, without associated activity of the orbicularis oculi.

A frontalis suspension operation is usually recommended for cases severe enough to come to surgery. Some controversy exists regarding whether to disinsert the ipsilateral levator or not and whether to also disinsert the contralateral levator and perform a frontalis suspension on the opposite side for the stated purpose of achieving a greater degree of symmetry.

Pathologic synkineses may cluster together. For instance, the MGJW synkinesis (congenital trigemino-oculomotor synkinesis) has been reported in association with Duane syndrome (congenital oculomotor-abducens synkinesis) and with synergistic divergence.[38,103]

A trigemino-abducens synkinesis may occur after trauma and facial synkinesis is a common finding after facial nerve palsy. It should be noted that various forms of aberrant innervation have been reported in the thalidomide embryopathy, especially Duane retraction syndrome and aberrant lacrimation[180] (crocodile tears). Platysma-levator synkinesis has been documented in a child with congenital third nerve palsy, demonstrating the potential for aberrant regeneration from a portion of the facial nerve.[37]

Rarely, deglutition-trochlear synkinesis may be noted[173] with the affected patient showing torsional diplopia associated with swallowing. This phenomenon suggests a synkinetic movement coupling the trochlear nerve with the bulbar musculature that is innervated by the trigeminal, facial, and hypoglossal nerves.

Some phenomena resemble synkinetic movements but are difficult to explain on the basis of aberrant reinnervation. In some patients, voluntary gaze may evoke such phenomena as vertigo, tinnitus, blepharoclonus, eyelid nystagmus, eyelid closure, facial twitching, arm movements, or seizures.[71,232,260] The pathogenesis of these "synkinetic" movements is unclear but has been speculated to involve ephaptic transmission.[232] Gaze-evoked upper lid jerks (lid nystagmus) may also be seen in patients with the Fisher syndrome and in patients with midbrain pseudomyasthenia (e.g., due to mesencephalic astrocytoma).

Monocular Elevation Deficiency or "Double Elevator Palsy"

"Double elevator palsy" is a descriptive term denoting a congenital deficiency of monocular elevation that is equal in abduction and adduction. Generally speaking, an inability to elevate one eye may occur on a restrictive or paretic basis and may be congenital or acquired. The patient or his family frequently reports that one eye shoots up and disappears under the upper eyelid while in fact the contralateral eye is the one with abnormal motility. The patient frequently has associated hypotropia and ptosis or pseudoptosis. The term "double elevator palsy" was originally coined to reflect what was then thought to be the basis for the disorder, namely, congenital palsy of the ipsilateral inferior oblique and superior rectus muscles,[265] a concept that has since been abandoned. It has since become apparent that the concomitant limited elevation so characteristic of double elevator palsy may result from at least three disparate pathophysiologic disorders, namely, inferior rectus restriction, superior rectus paresis, and a supranuclear disturbance of monocular elevation.[77] In truly paretic cases, dual palsy of the inferior oblique and superior rectus muscles does not occur; paresis of the superior rectus muscle alone (the dominant elevator of the globe) is sufficient to produce the clinical picture. The term *monocular elevation deficiency* is a more accurate descriptive term.

Several large series have shown that the majority of patients with monocular elevation deficiency have a restrictive abnormality to elevation.[177,178,229] Some of these cases represent isolated inferior rectus muscle fibrosis, which generally occurs as part of the autosomal dominantly-inherited congenital fibrosis syndrome.[64,115] Congenital inferior rectus fibrosis and neurogenic double elevator palsy may closely mimic each other since both may exhibit defective elevation associated with ptosis or pseudoptosis. To further confound the picture, it is now apparent that long-standing hypotropia associated with neurogenic

double elevator palsy may result in secondary contracture of the inferior rectus muscle and cause a positive forced duction test. Similar cases of inferior rectus tightness may result from perinatal orbital trauma.[105] The diagnosis of contralateral superior oblique palsy should be considered in any child who appears to have a double elevator palsy since fixation with the "paretic eye" can produce a contralateral inferior rectus contracture. Other conditions to be considered include orbital blowout fractures and orbital fat adherence syndrome. Patients with inferior rectus restriction due to orbital blowout fracture may also show a component of inferior rectus paresis.[153]

Based on studies utilizing scleral search coil techniques, Ziffer et al[286] suggested the existence of at least three distinct pathoetiologic categories: primary inferior rectus restriction, primary superior rectus palsy, and congenital supranuclear elevation defects. The inferior rectus restriction may be present primarily or may secondarily result from longstanding superior rectus weakness. Examination for the status of the Bell's phenomenon and other reflex upward movements is very useful. An intact Bell's phenomenon, or the ability to produce an upward movement of the eye with the oculocephalic maneuver, suggests a supranuclear disturbance. An absent Bell's phenomenon would be indicative of either inferior rectus restriction or superior rectus palsy. The two can be distinguished by saccadic velocity analysis, forced ductions, and active force generation. If restriction is absent and the eyes are orthotropic in the primary position, a superior rectus paresis is most unlikely, and a supranuclear disturbance is inferred.[178] Scott and Jackson have noted that the appearance of an accentuated lower lid fold on attempted upgaze predicts the presence of an inferior rectus contracture.[229]

While the location of the "lesion" in the restrictive variety of the "double elevator palsy" is readily apparent, generally pointing to tightness in the inferior rectus muscle complex, the location of a lesion in the other two classes of the "double elevator palsy" is not as well determined.[179] Cases of superior rectus weakness may result from disorders affecting the muscle or its nerve supply anywhere from the orbit to the superior rectus subnucleus. Mather and Saunders[172] reported a case of bilaterally absent superior rectus muscles. This patient showed paradoxical ocular movements on attempted upgaze. Hoyt[125] described a patient who developed sudden monocular elevation deficit and features of superior rectus paresis, which he attributed to superior rectus subnucleus infarction precipitated by coexisting polycythemia vera. In cases of double elevator palsy with superior rectus weakness and true ptosis, congenital injury to the superior division of the oculomotor nerve may theoretically be responsible. Since oculomotor fascicular fibers destined to the elevators of the eye and eyelid are believed to course laterally in the fascicle as it traverses the midbrain, a midbrain infarction involving a lateral portion of the oculomotor fascicle can cause an acquired unilateral ptosis and elevation deficit.[127] Congenital lesions at this location could also theoretically explain the paretic, infranuclear class of congenital double elevator palsy.

Supranuclear disturbances of monocular eye movements are rare. The neuroanatomic substrate of unilateral supranuclear upgaze deficiency is controversial. It has been attributed to either lesions of the contralateral pretectum, or lesions involving the upgaze efferents from the ipsilateral rostral interstitial nucleus of the medial longitudinal fasciculus. Most reports have been in adults in association with metastatic tumors. Lessell[164] reported a man with bronchogenic carcinoma who developed left monocular elevation deficit but with orthotropia in primary position and an intact Bell's phenomenon. A metastatic tumor was found in the right pretectum at autopsy, which was speculated to have caused the double elevator palsy by interrupting axons destined for the ipsilateral superior rectus subnucleus and the contralateral inferior oblique subnucleus. Ford et al[82] described a 52-year-old woman who developed right monocular elevation paresis who was demonstrated to have a focal, right-sided tumor of the mesodiencephalic junction in the region of the riMLF. Acquired unilateral double elevator palsy has been described in a child with a pineocytoma.[189] The most recent evidence incriminates a lesion of the vertical saccadic burst or pause neurons of the riMLF. A genetic factor is suggested by the finding of identical twins concordant for supranuclear double elevator palsy on the same side with preservation of Bell's phenomenon.[21]

The association of an isolated monocular elevation deficiency with congenital ptosis in general,

and MGJW in particular, implies that aberrant misdirection may play a role in the pathogenesis of some cases of double elevator palsy.[276] This view is supported by the association of the MGJW phenomenon with other misdirection syndromes including various Duane retraction syndrome, (e.g., synergistic divergence) and crocodile tears. It is also supported by reports showing that the superior rectus muscle itself may be involved in the aberrant phenomenon. Oesterle et al[190] described a 9-month-old infant with congenital ptosis without jaw winking who showed an up-and-down movement of the left eye synchronous with nursing movements of the jaw. A second 5-year-old girl with left ptosis, jaw winking, and left double elevator palsy showed up-and-down movements of the left upper lid and the left eye synchronous with chewing. The eye movements persisted after levator excision and fascia lata sling procedures. The authors speculated that the up-and-down eye movements probably represented aberrant innervation of the superior rectus muscle in a manner analogous to the abnormal innervation of the levator muscle in MGJW.

The possible neuroanatomic origins of monocular elevation deficit are summarized in Table 7.5. Patients with superior oblique palsy who habitually fixate with the paretic eye may present with limited monocular elevation of the contralateral (hypotropic) eye due to inhibitional palsy of the contralateral antagonist.[63] This so-called "fallen eye syndrome" may lead to a contralateral inferior rectus contracture and thereby cause a monocular elevation deficiency. The correct diagnosis may be inferred by the three-step test and the comparison of ductions to versions. Cases of vertical retraction syndrome, wherein congenital unilateral restriction of elevation is associated with retraction of the globe and narrowing of the palpebral fis-

TABLE 7.5. Neuroanatomic differential diagnosis of monocular elevation deficiency.

Inferior rectus contracture (e.g., congenital fibrosis syndrome, "fallen eye syndrome")

Superior rectus myoneural junction disease (e.g., myasthenia gravis)

Absence or hypoplasia of the superior rectus (e.g., Crouzon disease)

Superior division oculomotor paresis

Lateral oculomotor fascicular lesion

Superior rectus subnucleus lesion

Supranuclear lesion

sure,[227] have been speculated to arise from a vertical innervational misdirection similar to that observed in Duane syndrome and in some cases of congenital fibrosis syndrome.[89]

Brown syndrome can be distinguished from double elevator palsy by its increasing limitation of elevation in the adducted position. Brown syndrome must also be distinguished from the much less common inferior oblique palsy by the presence of little or no associated superior oblique overaction, a Y-pattern producing exotropia in extreme upgaze, and a positive forced duction test. Brown syndrome results from a congenital or, less commonly, an acquired dysfunction involving the trochlear-superior oblique tendon complex. Either form may be constant or intermittent (Figure 7.9). Intraoperative forced duction testing can help distinguish an inferior rectus restriction from a severe Brown syndrome. Retropulsion of the globe into the orbit while performing forced supraductions reduces or eliminates an inferior rectus restriction but exacerbates tightness due to Brown syndrome. Pulling on the globe does the opposite. Many acquired and some congenital cases of Brown syndrome improve spontaneously so that a conservative approach is reasonable. Treatment is undertaken for persistent cases with significant strabismus in the primary position and/or a significant compensatory anomalous head position. Superior oblique weakening (tenotomy or placement of a silicone spacer to lengthen the tendon)[277] with or without inferior oblique weakening is the treatment of choice in persistent congenital or idiopathic acquired cases with symptomatic diplopia or marked compensatory chin elevation. Local corticosteroid injections around the trochlea may be helpful in acquired inflammatory cases. The occurrence of Brown syndrome in multiple siblings[111] and in monozygotic twins[275] supports a genetic basis in some cases. Causes of acquired Brown syndrome include trauma, a rheumatoid nodule in the vicinity of the trochlea, peribulbar anesthesia, blepharoplasty, pansinusitis, frontal sinus osteoma, metastatic lesions, localized inflammation (orbital pseudotumor), surgical manipulation in the area of the trochlea, and surgical tucking of the superior oblique tendon.

Inferior rectus recession alone or in combination with other procedures ameliorates the restrictive variety of double elevator palsy. Treatment of neurogenic double elevator palsy includes conventional vertical rectus muscle surgery (recess and/or resect), and vertical transposition of the tendons of the medial rectus-lateral rectus superiorly (Knapp procedure).[42] The pseudoptosis disappears upon correction of the vertical deviation, and any residual true ptosis can be addressed after ocular alignment is optimized.[43]

Congenital Fibrosis Syndrome

The congenital ocular fibrosis syndrome is a relatively rare condition that is usually characterized by the presence of congenital restrictive ophthalmoplegia, fixed downgaze, horizontal strabismus,

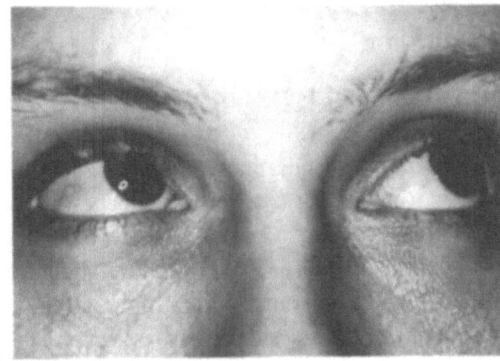 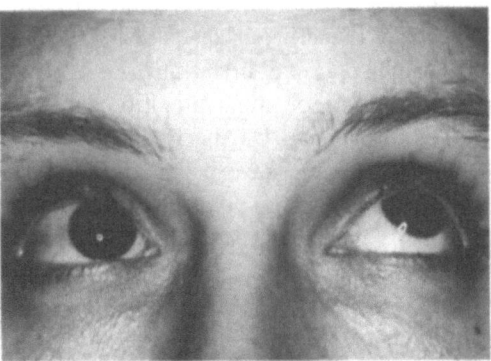

FIGURE 7.9. Intermittent Brown syndrome: This teenager complained of intermittent diplopia. On attempted gaze up and to his left, full ocular ductions and versions were noted on some trials (A), but intermittently, the right eye failed to elevate in adduction (B).

ptosis, and a compensatory backward tilting of the head.[256] In this disorder, the extraocular muscles and the levator muscles are replaced by fibrous tissue to a variable extent.[115] The disorder may be unilateral or bilateral and may be clinically limited to specific muscles in a given individual. The resultant ocular motility deficits are dependent upon which of the extraocular muscles are involved. The inferior rectus muscle is most commonly involved followed by the levator muscle and the lateral rectus muscle. In the presence of ptosis, inferior and lateral rectus muscle involvement may mimic unilateral or bilateral congenital oculomotor palsy. Rarely, all of the extraocular muscles including the levator are affected (generalized fibrosis syndrome). Some investigators prefer to subdivide congenital ocular fibrosis into different subtypes that include congenital fibrosis of the inferior rectus with ptosis, strabismus fixus, congenital unilateral enophthalmos with ocular muscle fibrosis and ptosis,[117] and the vertical retraction syndrome.

The syndrome may be sporadic or familial.[256] In familial cases, the predominant mode of inheritance is autosomal dominant, or rarely X-linked. A gene for the disorder has been recently mapped in several large families to chromosome 12. Affected members of the same family may exhibit widely different clinical manifestations of the syndrome.[1] Refractive errors may be associated and internal ophthalmoplegia may rarely coexist. The condition is usually isolated, and affected patients are otherwise healthy. Sporadic cases have been reported with associated nonocular abnormalities such as ventricular septal defect, facial palsy, and talipes equinovarus. Associated ocular abnormalities include poor vision and hyperopic astigmatism (which are found in half the patients), ocular coloboma, amblyopia, and strabismus.

The pathogenesis of congenital fibrosis syndrome is controversial. On the basis of biopsy studies of affected muscles, it has traditionally been regarded as a primary myopathy localized to the extraocular muscles. Both light and electron microscopy studies show replacement of extraocular muscles by dense fibrous connective tissue and collagen.[115] Histology of an affected levator showed reduction or absence of striations and Z bands and vacuolation of muscle cells. Müller muscle fibers appeared intact. Anomalous insertions of affected muscles may occur, presumably

resulting from a maturational defect at or before the 7th week of gestation.[13] Affected muscles often appear small and atrophic with orbital imaging studies.[268] A primary inflammatory process is unlikely in light of absence of inflammation in cases studied histopathologically. However, an inflammatory process (as occurs within the sternocleidomastoid muscle in congenital muscular torticollis) during fetal development with subsequent fibrosis cannot be excluded.

We have described three patients with congenital ocular fibrosis who displayed both synergistic divergence and MGJW.[38,103] Based upon the existence of such cases, we believe that some forms of congenital fibrosis of the extraocular muscles can result from the absence of normal innervation to orbital striated muscles early in development. (Extraocular muscle fibrosis is also commonly seen in uninnervated portions of the involved lateral rectus muscle in patients with Duane syndrome). A primary failure to establish normal neuronal connections with the extraocular muscles and levator muscle would predispose to neuronal misdirection, which allows for limited preservation of innervated muscle fibers and replacement of the remaining muscle by fibrous tissue.[38,237] Clinically, this would result in the superimposition of synkinetic eye movements upon a diffuse congenital ophthalmoplegia as has been increasingly recognized.[89] Since most patients with congenital ocular fibrosis syndrome do not display signs of neuronal misdirection, we believe that the underlying pathophysiology of congenital fibrosis syndrome can involve a spectrum of localized orbital dysgenesis ranging from a primary myopathy to a primary absence of normal innervation.

Internuclear Ophthalmoplegia

The hallmark of internuclear ophthalmoplegia (INO) is weakness or absence of adduction in one or both eyes on lateral gaze, with nystagmus in the abducting eye.[160,283] Despite this adduction limitation, the eyes remain orthotropic in the primary position. The adduction weakness may be profound and quite noticeable on testing of ocular ductions and versions or may be so subtle as to be discernible only by noting slow adducting saccades in the affected eye. The slow, floating nature of the adducting saccades can be effectively elicited by having the patient fixate an optokinetic nystagmus (OKN) target moving temporally with respect to the eye with limited adduction, which elicits a dysconjugate horizontal nystagmus of greater intensity in the abducting eye. Convergence is usually preserved except in rostral cases that simultaneously affect the medial rectus subnucleus. However, decreased convergence in the setting of bilateral INO with multiple sclerosis may be due to central scotomas caused by optic atrophy as opposed to a primary convergence disorder. Older children may complain of diplopia. A skew deviation often accompanies unilateral INO while vertical upbeating nystagmus in upgaze often accompanies bilateral INO. Unlike most forms of skew deviation in which the lower eye is ipsilateral to the lesion, the higher eye is usually on the same side of the lesion in patients with INO. As INO resolves, the clinical picture evolves from absent or decreased adduction to slow adduction to normal appearing adduction with retention of the abducting nystagmus (i.e., abducting nystagmus is the last to resolve).

Internuclear ophthalmoplegia signifies intrinsic brain stem disease involving the pons or midbrain. It results from injury to axons that originate from interneurons in the abducens nucleus and project via the medial longitudinal fasciculus to the contralateral medial rectus subnucleus of the oculomotor nuclear complex. A number of mechanisms have been suggested to explain the dissociated nystagmus in the abducting eye.[284] One popular explanation suggests that increased innervation to the medial rectus to overcome the adduction weakness is accompanied, under the influence of Hering's law of equal innervation, by a commensurate increase in the innervation to the normal lateral rectus muscle of the contralateral eye. While increased innervation to the paretic medial rectus muscle would improve adduction, the increased innervation to the normal lateral rectus of the other eye would result in abducting saccadic overshoot followed by backward postsaccadic drift. This mechanism is supported by the observation that abducting nystagmus may also be noted in patients with adduction weakness resulting from medial rectus muscle recession.[259] Other mechanisms invoke the possibility that the abducting nystagmus may result from 1) increased convergence tone to improve adduction of the weak eye; 2) interruption of descending internuclear neurons that run in the medial longitudinal fasciculus (MLF) from the oculomotor internuclear neurons to the abducens nucleus; 3) associated injury to fibers other than those of the MLF; and 4) an associated gaze-evoked nystagmus with the component of the nystagmus expected in the adducted eye being dampened by the coexisting adduction paresis.[283,160]

Causes of INO in infants and children include demyelinating disease, stroke, brain stem tumors, particularly pontine glioma, vasculitis,[148] inborn errors of metabolism, parainfectious encephalitis, structural malformations (Arnold-Chiari),[193,274] drug intoxication,[68,210] and trauma. Internuclear ophthalmoplegia in children may rarely be a presenting sign of a brain stem glioma.[52] Another increasingly important cause of INO is HIV encephalitis.

Most cases remit spontaneously. In unilateral cases, diplopia in primary position is often *vertical* rather than horizontal and is attributable to a concurrent skew deviation. It can be eliminated with 2 to 3 prism diopters of vertical prism incorporated into glasses. Nystagmus and oscillopsia may complicate bilateral cases. The oscillopsia is a result of deficient vertical VOR and pursuit movements or the abduction nystagmus. The role of strabismus surgery in selected patients has been recently analyzed.[151] Selected patients with stable ocular alignment despite maximal tolerable medical therapy can benefit from strabismus surgery.[106]

A lesion encompassing both the MLF and the ipsilateral PPRF or the abducens nucleus results in an ipsilateral horizontal gaze palsy and an INO. The only preserved horizontal movement is abduction of the contralateral eye. This constellation of findings is called the "one-and-one-half syndrome." Bilateral INO with unilateral abducens paresis gives a similar motility deficit. The one-and-one-half syndrome has a similar spectrum of causes as INO.

In premature infants, one may occasionally note large-angle exotropia with decreased or no response of the medial recti to vestibular manipulations with rotation or calorics. This has been interpreted as possible bilateral INO, suggesting a maturational delay in the development of the medial longitudinal fasciculus. Such exotropia has a good prognosis for spontaneous ocular alignment as the MLF matures, as compared to the constant large-angle exotropia of infancy that shows no evidence of adduction weakness.[124] This latter variety is usually observed in the setting of neurologic disease, but a subset is seen in otherwise healthy infants in a manner analogous to congenital esotropia. Duane's type 2 syndrome, medial rectus entrapment in a nasal orbital wall fracture with associated paresis, myasthenia gravis, and the Fisher syndrome may produce a similar motility pattern and must be excluded.

Cyclic, Periodic, or Aperiodic Disorders Affecting Ocular Structures

A number of heterogeneous ocular disorders have in common a cyclic, periodic, or aperiodic pattern, that is, an involuntary process that repeats over time (Table 7.6). A major lesson to be learned from these cyclic phenomena is the importance of observing certain ocular disorders over time. The nature of the cyclic phenomenon and the duration of a complete cycle define each disorder.

Cyclic esotropia is a relatively rare condition that is also referred to as alternate day, circadian, or clock-mechanism esotropia.[112] The designation "circadian," which denotes a 24-hour cycle, is a misnomer because the usual cycle duration is 48

TABLE 7.6. Cyclic, periodic, or aperiodic disorders affecting ocular structures.

Cyclic esotropia
Cyclic superior oblique palsy
Cyclic vertical deviation
Periodic alternating nystagmus
Periodic alternating gaze deviation
Periodic alternating skew deviation
Periodic alternating esotropia
Periodic mydriasis
Periodic head turns in congenital nystagmus
Periodic alternating lid retraction
Oculomotor palsy with cyclic spasm
Ping-pong gaze
Rhythmic pupillary oscillations (periodic pupillary phenomenon)
Alternating anisocoria
Migrating pupil

hours. The typical case shows a 24-hour period of manifest esotropia measuring 40 to 50 prism diopters, alternating with a 24-hour period of normal ocular alignment (Figure 7.10). Less common are cycles of 24, 72, or 96 hours in duration. The esotropia is nonaccommodative and nonparalytic, with normal eye movements in both eyes when straight and also when esotropic. On days when the eyes are crossed, diplopia is rare, fusional amplitudes are defective or absent, and sensory anomalies are frequent. Whether other cyclic phenomena occur in association with this condition is debatable. Friendly et al[85] monitored numerous psychological and physiologic functions and found no associated cyclical phenomenon. In contrast, Roper-Hall and Yapp[213] described cyclical changes in behavior, frequency of micturition, and electroencephalographic activity.

Cyclic esotropia may first appear in infancy, but the diagnosis may be delayed months to years, with the average age at diagnosis ranging from 2 to 4 years, although some cases may occur abruptly in adult life. Generally, the condition occurs spontaneously without apparent cause but may be precipitated by strabismus surgery, retinal reattachment surgery, ocular trauma, optic atrophy, or CNS disease.[112] The natural history of this condition is not definitively known, but the cyclicity is thought to diminish with time, leading to a constant esotropia after several months to years. The mechanism of cyclic esotropia remains unknown. One case of cyclic esotropia, developing after unilateral traumatic aphakia, resolved after secondary intraocular lens implantation. This abolition of cyclic esotropia after visual improvement appears analogous to previously reported cases of periodic alternating nystagmus that resolved after visual rehabilitation by removing a cataract or clearing a vitreous hemorrhage. It is therefore advisable to provide maximal optical/refractive correction prior to considering extraocular muscle surgery.

The treatment of cyclic esotropia consists of strabismus surgery to correct the maximum deviation that stops the overt cycles. Richter[208] likened the effect of surgery to "removing the hand of the clock without altering its motor."

Cyclic esotropia should not be confused with periodic alternating esotropia.[114] The latter is a rare condition with cycles of similar duration to periodic alternating nystagmus (about 200 sec-

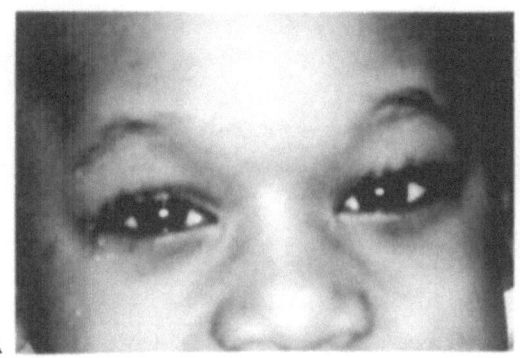
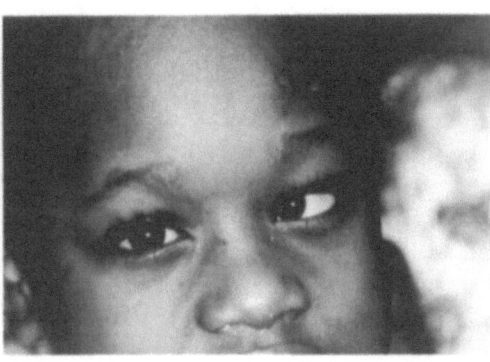
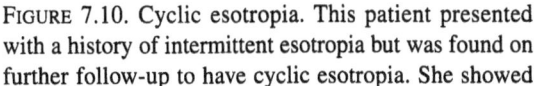

FIGURE 7.10. Cyclic esotropia. This patient presented with a history of intermittent esotropia but was found on further follow-up to have cyclic esotropia. She showed orthotropia (A) and esotropia (B) alternating on a daily basis.

onds). The few reported cases occurred in association with congenital periodic alternating gaze deviation.[108] Such patients probably had the neuroanatomic substrate of periodic alternating nystagmus but with superimposed saccadic palsy leading to absent fast phases of nystagmus.

Periodic alternating gaze deviation (PAGD) is a rare disorder consisting of a slow, conjugate horizontal deviation of the eyes from one side to the other.[114,159,240] It may occur at any age (some cases have been reported in infancy) and is associated with concurrent controversive cyclic face turning to maintain fixation. During a complete cycle, the eyes rotate conjugately toward one side for 1 to 2 minutes, usually with compensatory head turning to the opposite side; return to the midline for a changeover period lasting 10 to 15 seconds; then conjugately deviate to the other side for 1 to 2 minutes, with compensatory head turning to the side opposite the direction of ocular rotation (Figure 7.11). The patient may be orthotropic or esotropic. During eye closure, the alternating turning of the head ceases, even though the eyes continue the rhythmic movement. While the eyes are deviated, they exhibit abnormal voluntary movements, convergence, OKN, and oculocephalic responses, but all of these normalize during the changeover phase. Caloric testing can override the eye and head movements, and the cycling stops during sleep.

Periodic alternating gaze deviation may occur on a congenital basis (Figure 7.11) or may be acquired. Most documented cases reported so far have been due to posterior fossa abnormalities. It has been reported in association with pontine vascular lesions, Arnold–Chiari malformation, Dandy–Walker malformation, congenital hydrocephalus, occipital encephalocele, cerebellar medulloblastoma, spinocerebellar degeneration, and Joubert syndrome with cerebellar vermis hypoplasia.[111, 143,159,240,245] In congenital or early onset PAGD, cerebellar vermis atrophy is the most common neuroradiologic abnormality.

The duration of a complete cycle of PAGD (3 to 4 minutes) is similar to that of periodic alternating nystagmus (PAN), suggesting that the two conditions may have a similar neuroanatomic substrate, the difference being an added saccadic palsy in the case of PAGD. This concept is supported by the findings in a patient with recurrent cerebellar medulloblastoma who sequentially demonstrated PAN, bilateral gaze palsy, PAGD, and then resumption of PAN.[143]

When encountered in a comatose patient, PAGD is usually considered a sign of bilateral cerebral hemispheric dysfunction with a relatively intact brain stem.[245] In this setting, the total duration of the abnormal movements is usually short, a few hours to days, disappearing a few hours before the patient's death.

Ping-pong gaze superficially resembles PAGDs, but the movements are much faster, although some authors have used the two terms interchangeably.[207,231] It consists of conjugate horizontal ocular deviations that alternate rapidly every few seconds. Ping-pong gaze is usually seen in comatose or semicomatose patients and typically denotes cerebellar or bilateral cerebral hemispheric

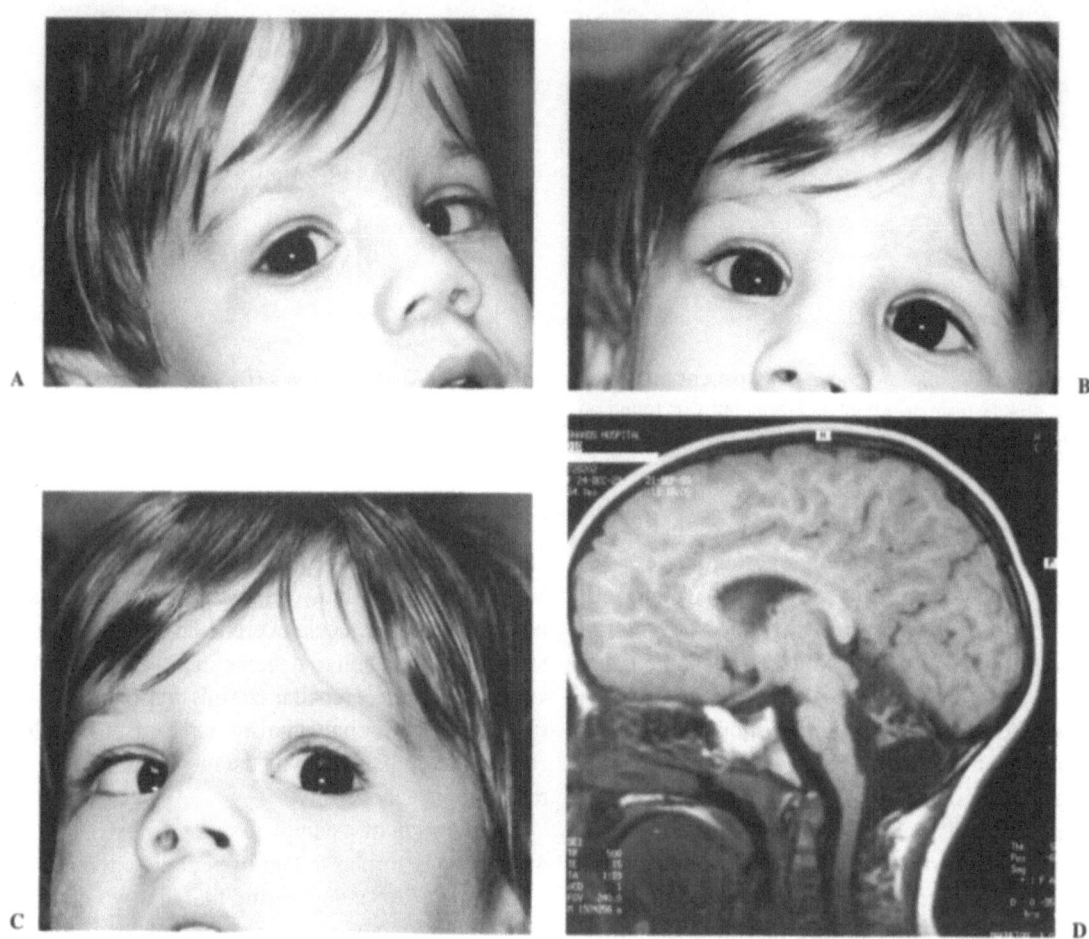

FIGURE 7.11. Congenital PAGD. This 2-year-old girl with Joubert syndrome displayed PAGD with a cycle duration of about 200 seconds. During a complete cycle, (A) the eyes rotated conjugately to the right over 90 seconds, usually with compensatory head turning to the opposite side, (B) returned to the midline for a changeover period lasting seconds, then (C) conjugately deviated to the other side over 90 seconds, with compensatory head turning to the side opposite the direction of ocular rotation. (D) MR imaging showed profound cerebellar vermis hypoplasia.

lesions but a relatively intact brain stem. Ping-pong gaze has been speculatively ascribed to damage of the descending supranuclear inhibitory input on the horizontal gaze centers.

Periodic alternating skew deviation is a rare condition wherein the patient develops right hypertropia lasting one to several minutes alternating with left hypertropia in a cyclic fashion. In some patients, the condition may be aperiodic or intermittent. Downbeat nystagmus may also be present. In one patient, a focal lesion affecting the interstitial nucleus of Cajal was demonstrated with computed tomography. In contrast to seesaw nystagmus, periodic alternating skew deviation has slower movements, larger excursions, and no torsional component. Periodic eye movement disorders with a cycle duration of about 200 seconds, which include PAN, PAGD, and periodic alternating skew deviation, may have similar pathophysiologic mechanisms and have been reported to occur in combinations in the same individual.[143,166]

One case of cyclic superior oblique palsy developed in a 10-year-old patient following trauma to the left trochlear area.[270] Typical left superior oblique palsy alternated daily with orthotropia. A patient with cyclic vertical deviation of an unspecified nature, with a cyclic duration of 48 hours, has been reported following craniofacial surgery.[176] Other cyclic ocular motor disorders include paroxysmal ocular tilt reaction and oculomotor palsy with cyclic spasm. In patients with oculomotor palsy with cyclic spasm, the pupil may reportedly be the only structure to cycle, although more commonly, the extraocular muscles and levator muscle are also involved in the cyclic spasms.

Cyclic or alternating phenomena may affect the pupils. Keane described a patient with traumatic oculomotor palsy in whom the ipsilateral pupil, although unreactive to light, showed continuous rhythmic involuntary oscillations. He speculated that dysfunction of the central parasympathetic nervous system may have been responsible. *Alternating anisocoria* is a rare condition that is characterized by alternating pupillary dilatation, with the dilated pupil showing little or no light reactivity in some cases but normal reactivity in others.[39] This may occur in otherwise neurologically normal children, but a similar phenomenon has been observed in a quadriplegic patient with a posttraumatic syringomyelic cyst.[148] The pathophysiology of this phenomenon is unclear, but it may be due to either episodic oculosympathetic spasm producing alternating Claude Bernard syndrome or episodic oculosympathetic interruption producing Horner's syndrome. Some other pupillary disorders have been intermittent rather than rhythmic and include intermittent mydriasis, cyclic sympathetic spasm with concentric dilatation lasting 40 to 60 seconds, and "tadpole pupils," wherein the sympathetic spasm is sectoral.[254]

Conditions with cycle duration of a few minutes sometimes become apparent when the clinician notices a reversal of a previously noted finding—for example, observation of conjugately turned eyes to the right in a patient whose eyes were previously noted to be conjugately turned to the left brings forth the diagnosis of PAGD. Conditions with a cycle duration of 24 hours or longer cannot be definitively diagnosed from data collected during a single office visit. For instance, a patient with cyclic esotropia may be initially evaluated on a "crossed" day and be labeled as congenital or acquired esotrope. If the subsequent visit occurs on a "crossed" day, it may only consolidate the earlier false diagnosis. If it occurs on a "straight" day, the clinician may suspect spontaneous resolution or an accommodative element with variable angle and either question the observation of esotropia in earlier visits or correctly suspect cyclic esotropia. Conversely, initial evaluation of a patient with cyclic esotropia on a "straight" day may lead to missing the diagnosis, dubbing the condition pseudostrabismus.

Cyclic phenomena in children are not limited to the neuro-ophthalmologic disorders discussed herein but involve other organ systems as well. Other biologic phenomena such as sweating, salivation, and pulse rate also have intrinsic periodicity, as do many manifestations of psychiatric dysfunction. Periodicity appears to be the norm in many biologic phenomena, and a normal person displays a complex array of biorhythms involving the various body systems.[209] Numerous periodic or rhythmic disorders have been described—for example, periodic recurrence of fever, periodic swelling of joints, periodic fluctuations of circulating blood cells (periodic hematopoiesis), and periodic edema. Accumulating evidence points to the existence of a biologic clock mechanism that keeps time with extraordinary accuracy and is independent of internal and external stimuli.

Ocular Neuromyotonia

Myotonia denotes delayed muscle relaxation after sustained contraction as a result of muscle membrane dysfunction. In contrast, *neurotonia* or *pseudomyotonia* represents delayed muscle relaxation as a result of impulse-induced repetitive discharge in a peripheral nerve. *Neuromyotonia* describes neurotonia accompanied by fibrillations, fasciculations, myokymia, or sustained contraction of a muscle group. *Ocular neuromyotonia* describes sustained contraction of one or more extraocular muscles due to involuntary firing of the supplying ocular motor nerve.

Ocular neuromyotonia is a relatively rare ocular motility disorder that manifests with brief paroxysmal monocular deviations with associated diplopia.[236] Episodes generally last 10 to 60 seconds (range of 5 seconds to 3 minutes) and may recur 20 or more times per day. Some episodes occur spontaneously, while others are triggered by gaze in the direction of the involved muscle. Between attacks, affected patients usually show nor-

mal ocular motility, although some may show subtle evidence of aberrant innervation manifesting as
minimal lid retraction in downgaze. The paroxysms result from tonic involuntary contraction of
extraocular muscles innervated by the third (all
muscles supplied by the nerve or any combination
thereof), fourth, or sixth cranial nerves.[20,163]
Spontaneous discharges from axons with unstable
cell membranes are presumed to underlie this condition. Histopathologic studies of peripheral
nerves in nonocular cases of neuromyotonia have
shown segmental demyelination as well as axonal
degeneration, sprouting, and remyelination.[261]
Most patients have a history of brain irradiation,
typically for the treatment of tumors of the skull
base, such as pituitary tumors or craniopharyngiomas.[163,236] Idiopathic cases with no specific
cause have been reported.[236] The interval between
radiotherapy and onset of neuromyotonia may be
months to years.

A favorable response to membrane-stabilizing
medications such as carbamazepine 200 mg bid to
tid) is reported in many patients, supporting
pathoetiology consisting of spontaneous or impulse-induced repetitive discharge of hyperex-
citable trigger zones in ocular motor nerves. In
some instances, the neuromyotonia has not recurred upon cessation of the medication. Some
cases may remit spontaneously.

Ocular Motor Adaptations and Disorders in Patients with Hemispheric Abnormalities

Cerebral hemispheric abnormalities are often associated with ocular motor abnormalities that may
be subtle or profound depending upon the size, location, and other characteristics of the lesion.
These are reviewed in detail elsewhere.

Children with congenital hemianopsia develop a
compensatory saccadic strategy wherein they
overshoot the intended visual target then "find it"
as the eyes drift back.[123] Some patients with congenital homonymous hemianopsia have been
noted to also show concurrent exotropia, usually
also of early onset. Some investigators have suggested that the exotropia in these patients is a
compensatory phenomenon for the hemianopic
field defect, essentially allowing the patient to

have panoramic vision. For this to occur, anomalous retinal correspondence has to coexist, otherwise the patient would be diplopic.[93,118] Some investigators raise the possibility that the exotropia
in such patients is an epiphenomenon, possibly reflecting the type of strabismus one sees in many
children with neurologic disease.[123] It is not clear
whether the concurrent exotropia in these children
truly represents a physiological compensatory
phenomenon, whether it simply represents strabismus precipitated by infantile neurologic disease,
or whether it happens to occur fortuitously in
early life, leading to the development of anomalous retinal correspondence (ARC) and panoramic
vision. Suffice it to say that the latter two mechanisms are probably more likely since most patients with congenital homonymous hemianopia
do not show associated exotropia in our experience. However, in those children who show this
combination of findings, the clinician should understand the possible sensory implications if performing strabismus surgery to straighten the eyes.

Eye Movement Tics

Tics are quick, jerky, sudden, and repetitive movements of circumscribed groups of muscles without
apparent cause or purpose. They occur frequently
in children and most often resolve spontaneously.
Tics most commonly affect facial musculature but
may rarely affect the extraocular muscles causing
eye movement tics.[234] It is important to recognize
eye movement tics as such and not confuse them
with more serious disorders. The few cases of eye
movement tics reported to date have been mostly
associated with facial tics, but isolated ocular tics
may occur and may thus mimic nystagmus.
Frankel and Cummings[83] reported eye rolling tics
in a group of patients with Tourette syndrome. The
tics consisted of eye rolling, gaze abnormalities,
staring, or forced gaze deviations resembling oculogyric crises. Two of the cases described a corneal
sensation preceding their tics. All of these children
also had blepharospasm, and most were taking
neuroleptic or other medications. Neuroleptics
have been implicated in the pathogenesis of a variety of movement disorders including tics and oculogyric crisis. Binyon and Prendergast[25] reported
three cases with conjugate eye movement tics: one

associated with Tourette syndrome, one associated with neurological and behavioral disorders, and one was isolated. The latter resolved spontaneously. Shawkat reported opsoclonus-like ocular tics associated with facial tics in an otherwise healthy child that resolved spontaneously. Affected children are sometimes able to imitate their tics in the clinic upon request, which is a useful indicator that consciousness is not impaired during the tics, allowing the examiner to rule out epilepsy.

Eyelid Abnormalities in Children

Congenital Ptosis

Congenital ptosis can be the presenting sign of several neuro-ophthalmologic disorders (Table 7.7). Specific attention to ocular motility, pupillary examination, and coexisting neurologic signs is imperative. Congenital ptosis must also be differentiated from pseudoptosis due to ipsilateral hypotropia, enophthalmos, or contralateral lid retraction. Motility abnormalities may include congenital oculomotor nerve palsy and double elevator palsy. The latter is associated with congenital ptosis in 20% of cases and is a reason to be conservative with ptosis correction to prevent corneal exposure postoperatively due to absent Bell's phenomenon. Pupillary abnormalities associated with unilateral ptosis may include a large unreactive pupil due to oculomotor palsy or a miotic pupil either due to Horner syndrome or to congenital oculomotor palsy with aberrant regeneration involving the pupil. Causes of pupillary abnormalities

TABLE 7.7. The differential diagnosis of congenital ptosis.

Blepharophimosis syndrome
Myasthenia gravis
Oculomotor nerve palsy
Marcus Gunn jaw winking
Horner syndrome
Cerebral ptosis
Congenital fibrosis syndrome
Hypotropia with pseudoptosis
Microphthalmia, enophthalmos
Myotubular myopathy
Congenital fiber-type disproportion
Congenital myotonia

associated with bilateral early-onset ptosis include the Fisher syndrome and botulism.

Typical cases of congenital ptosis are usually ascribed to levator muscle dystrophy, with variable replacement of muscle fibers with fibrous tissue. As with Duane syndrome and with congenital fibrosis syndrome, some cases of levator fibrosis in children with congenital ptosis could eventuate from absence of normal innervation of the levator muscle with secondary fibrosis. Such cases would be predisposed to developing the MGJW phenomenon.

Rarely, a cerebral hemispheric lesion can cause unilateral or bilateral ptosis (termed *cerebral ptosis*) in the absence of other neurological signs.[149] Lowenstein et al[169] described two children with hemispheric arteriovenous malformations and contralateral ptosis that progressed over several years. In both cases, the ptosis resolved following resection of the AVM. One should consider the rare possibility of cerebral ptosis in the child with progressive nonmyasthenic ptosis, especially when a history of seizures or recurrent unilateral headaches is obtained.

Excessive Blinking in Children

The spontaneous blink rate in infants under 18 months of age is low, ranging from 2 to 5 blinks per minute, while in older children it is about 10, reaching approximately 20 blinks by the age of 20 years and remaining relatively constant throughout adulthood. Benign tics (blinking eyes, twitching mouth, movements of head, jerking shoulders or other body parts) are common in children, with a prevalence as high as 12% between the ages of 6 and 12 years.[158] Benign tics involving the eyes may manifest as excessive intermittent blinking without associated ocular or systemic disorders. Eye winking or blinking tics in children represent exaggerated contractions of the orbicularis muscle. The tics usually increase in frequency when the child is bored, anxious, or tired. The majority of these tics are benign and transient, improving spontaneously with time, without any discernible causation. Unlike essential blepharospasm of adults, there is little if any functional visual impairment. Although tics have been thought to result from an underlying psychological conflict, recent evidence suggests that they may be of organic origin but triggered or exacerbated by stress. Elston et al[74] described a family in which different members in three generations suffered eye-winking tics, excessive blinking, and/or blepharospasm. The proband in that study had eye-winking tics in childhood, then developed excessive blinking evolving to blepharospasm by the age of 21 years. They also described five patients with adult-onset blepharospasm or Meige's syndrome who had a history of excessive blinking dating back to childhood. They speculated that eye-winking tics, excessive blinking, and blepharospasm may represent age-dependent manifestations of a common pathophysiologic disorder.[74]

Frequent eye blinking may be a manifestation of ocular surface, tear film, or eyelid disorders at any age. It may also accompany lacrimal drainage obstruction. Children with congenital glaucoma are classically described as presenting with the triad of epiphora, photophopia, and blepharospasm but may also show frequent blinking as do children with significant intraocular inflammation. Excessive blinking and blepharospasm also occur in conditions with damage to the basal ganglia, such as Wilson's disease and Huntington's chorea.[40]

Seizure activity is associated with a variety of neuro-ophthalmologic signs and symptoms that include nystagmus, gaze deviations, spasm of the near reflex, hemianopsia, cortical blindness, as well as a variety of eyelid signs. Lid signs may consist of eyelid nystagmus or eyelid fluttering resembling tics and spells of eyelid spasms. For instance, Cogan et al[51] described a 7-year-old girl with methylmalonic aciduria and homocystinuria who exhibited spells of fluttering of the eyelids and elevation of the eyes. The EEG showed 2.5-second polyspike and wave discharge during the spells, characteristic of petit mal seizures. Excessive blinking and eyelid myoclonia has been reported in association with typical absence seizures,[12] and this condition has been reported in monozygotic twins.[61] Finger waving and rapid eyelid blinking is a feature of photoconvulsive epilepsy. Eyelid myoclonia may occur upon eye closure in association with electrical status epilepticus without altered consciousness.[258a] Patients with occipital lobe epilepsy may exhibit a variety of neuro-ophthalmologic manifestations including elementary visual hallucinations, ictal or postictal amaurosis, eye movement sensations, eye and/or

head deviation, visual field deficits, and early forced blinking or eyelid flutter.[269] Seizure activity may also be associated with abnormal eye movements such as gaze deviations (usually to the contralateral side) and nystagmus.[136,144,257] Tusa et al[257] described an 11-year-old boy with focal seizures in the right temporo-occipital cortex who showed seizure-associated momentary rightward gaze deviation followed by 10 to 15 seconds of horizontal left-beating jerk nystagmus. They postulated that both the gaze deviation and the slow phases of the nystagmus were caused by seizure activation of a smooth pursuit pathway originating from the temporo-occipital cortex.

The terms "lid nystagmus," "upper lid jerks," and "lid hopping" have all been applied to a neuro-ophthalmologic phenomenon in which a series of rapid, rhythmical, jerky movements of the upper lids occurs alone or in conjunction with specific movements of the eyes or head.[36] Most previously reported cases have been associated with posterior fossa disease and can be subdivided into lid nystagmus evoked by convergence and lid nystagmus evoked by horizontal gaze.[122,218] Howard described a patient with convergence-evoked upbeating eyelid nystagmus, without ocular upbeating nystagmus, who had a large vascular lesion distorting the blood supply to the pontomesencephalic and pontomedullary junctions.[122] Safran et al[218] described two similar patients with convergence-evoked eyelid nystagmus. Patient 1, a 29-year-old man, developed a cerebellar syndrome after sustaining severe head injuries. Patient 2, a 12-year-old girl, had a tumor of the anterior cerebellar vermis. Treatment with corticosteroids (patient 1) and surgery (patient 2) led to gradual resolution of the eyelid nystagmus, which the authors attributed to cerebellar dysfunction. Other rare causes of lid nystagmus include the lateral medullary syndrome, pretectal lesions, and the Fisher syndrome.[220]

Two children have recently been described with signs and symptoms of myasthenic ophthalmoplegia, in whom gaze-evoked lid hopping signaled the presence of intrinsic midbrain tumors.[36,203] While horizontal eye movements in myasthenia gravis may be accompanied by occasional twitching or fluttering movements of the upper lids, lid nystagmus is uncharacteristic of neuromuscular disease and should prompt neuroimaging. Lid nystagmus would appear to necessitate a dissociation between the output of the levator and the superior rectus subnuclei within the oculomotor nuclear complex.

Some children may exhibit lower eyelid pulling as a transient behavior lasting weeks to months.[45] These children are otherwise healthy, and the condition is thought to initially be triggered by ocular irritation but then develops into a "bad habit." This functional disorder is readily distinguishable from eye poking (oculo-digital sign) encountered in children who are blind secondary to congenital retinal disease (i.e., Leber's amaurosis, retinopathy of prematurity, retinal dysplasia)[130] and vigorous eye rubbing seen in patients with Down syndrome.

Eyelid myokymia may occur alone or may be associated with facial myokymia. Facial and eyelid myokymia is characterized by unilateral involuntary fine rippling movements spreading across the surface of affected muscles. Facial myokymia has been reported in association with multiple sclerosis, Guillain–Barre syndrome, Bell's palsy, rattlesnake bites, brain stem tumors, and others. The clinical features of facial myokymia are sufficiently distinctive to avoid confusion with other facial dyskinesias like essential blepharospasm, tardive dyskinesia, facial tics, focal seizures, aberrant regeneration of the facial nerve, hemifacial spasm, and benign facial fasciculations. Some cases of facial myokymia have occurred in association with spastic paretic facial contracture, which is characterized by tonic spasm of the paretic facial muscles, with typical prominence of the nasolabial fold and deviation of the nose toward the affected side. We have examined a patient with diffuse disseminated encephalomyelitis who showed left facial myokymia, spastic paretic facial contracture, and one-and-one-half syndrome and who also showed scattered lesions within the brain stem on MR imaging studies.

Gilles de la Tourette syndrome is a bizarre but relatively common disorder that comprises multiple involuntary motor tics and obscene utterances. There is a predilection for boys (male to female ratio is 3:1 to 5:1) and for whites. The condition is familial in about one-third of cases, appears to be transmitted as an autosomal dominant trait, and has been mapped to the long arm of chromosome 18.

Symptoms usually appear between ages 5 and 10 years, with presenting features consisting of multifocal tics of the face and head. In addition to clonic motor tics (most commonly blinking and facial twitching) and vocal/phonic tics, seen in all patients, many patients exhibit one or more dystonic tics that may include oculogyric deviations, blepharospasm, and dystonic neck movements.[132] The globes may also show dystonic tics. For example, Frankel and Cummings[83] reported eye rolling tics in a group of patients with Tourette syndrome who also had blepharospasm. The motor tics are followed by vocal tics such as grunting, sneezing, coughing, barking, coprolalia (compulsive monosyllabic swearing), and echolalia. Tiqueurs may be able to voluntarily suppress the tics, but a resulting mounting tension eventually leads to further discharge of tics. Patients may show associated obsessive-compulsive traits, self-mutilation, attention deficit disorders, learning disabilities, and serious psychiatric illness. Haloperidol and pimozide are useful in controlling the symptoms.

The workup of tics is conservative, consisting mainly of observation, unless otherwise dictated by the presence of associated clinical findings. Explanation and reassurance of patients and their families is helpful in steering them away from becoming too focused on the tics. Neuroleptics and other drugs should be reserved for severe cases. The long-term prognosis of tics is good, with about two-thirds of cases spontaneously remitting.[55]

Hemifacial Spasm

Hemifacial spasm is primarily a disorder of middle age and older individuals, but a few cases have been reported in childhood. Hemifacial spasm is characterized by involuntary, intermittent unilateral twitching of the muscles innervated by the facial nerve, almost uniformly including the orbicularis oculi. They differ from tics in several ways, including the inability of the patient to suppress the twitches or initiate them, and the absence of compulsion to make them. In approximately half the patients, a particular position of the head (most commonly the contralateral lateral decubitus position) will diminish or halt the spasms. The patient may hear ipsilateral clicking sounds if the stapedius muscle is involved.

It is generally believed that most cases of hemifacial spasm result from microvascular compression of the facial nerve at the root entry zone. "Cross talk" between the sensory and motor branches of the seventh nerve has been suggested as an underlying pathophysiology. Congenital or acquired cholesteatoma is the most common associated tumor. Vascular malformations of the posterior fossa have also been implicated, but the majority of cases are cryptogenic. Rare familial cases suggest a genetic transmission. Friedman et al[84] described a family in which hemifacial spasm occurred in five members through three generations.

The treatment of hemifacial spasm is controversial. Spontaneous resolution may occur in a few cases. A trial of carbamazepine, phenytoin, Baclofen, or tranquilizers can be attempted in mild cases. Local injections of Oculinum provide relief lasting an average of several months. Microvascular decompression of the facial nerve is considered the treatment of choice by some authors. Jho and Jannetta[133] described hemifacial spasm in two children and eight adults who had the onset of hemifacial spasm before the age of 20. Similar to adult cases, all patients showed improvement with microvascular decompression of the facial nerve.

The presence of hemifacial spasm in an infant may be an ominous sign. Langston and Tharp[157] described a case of infantile hemifacial spasm beginning at 6 weeks of age. Surgical exploration at 5 ½ years of age revealed a ganglioneuroma of the fourth ventricle. Flueler et al [80] described three infants who presented with the onset of hemifacial spasm within the first year of life. One patient had occlusion of the straight sinus and large collateral vessels at the base of the brain, supporting the concept of vascular compression of the facial nerve at its exit from the brain stem as a mechanism for the production of hemifacial spasm. Each of the other two patients had an intrinsic mass compressing the fourth ventricle: one was located in the lower pons and extending into the cerebellar vermis and right cerebellar peduncle; the other involved the cerebellar vermis and right middle cerebellar peduncle. Interestingly, hemifacial spasm has been described in some cases of Joubert syndrome, which includes cerebellar vermis aplasia or hypoplasia.[146] Unlike the usually benign nature of the late childhood and adult variety, it appears that early-onset hemifacial spasm should raise suspicion of an underlying CNS malignancy. Neuroimaging is therefore warranted in

cases of hemifacial spasm with onset within the first two years of life. In older children with typical, isolated, hemifacial spasm neuroimaging should be obtained when atypical features (headaches, facial pain, cranial neuropathy, cerebellar dysfunction) are present.[17]

Hemifacial spasm should be differentiated from blepharospasm and facial myokymia. Essential blepharospasm consists of bilateral, localized, repetitive spasms of the orbicularis oculi muscle that, in severe cases, leads to visual impairment. The rare case of bilateral hemifacial spasm can be distinguished from essential blepharospasm because the bilateral contractions do not occur synchronously. Essential blepharospasm is not seen in children, but excessive blinking due to tics, or blepharospasm due to ocular disorders such as congenital glaucoma may bear superficial resemblance to essential blepharospasm. Facial myokymia consists of continuous, fascicular rippling movements of the face that usually begin in the orbicularis muscle. It is not affected by voluntary or reflex activity of the face. The most common causes include multiple sclerosis and brain stem glioma.

Lid Retraction

The margin of the upper eyelid is normally located 1 to 2 mm below the upper corneoscleral limbus. Upper eyelid retraction is more commonly considered in the adult age group where it occurs most commonly in patients with thyroid eye disease, dorsal midbrain syndrome, trauma, proptosis, and seventh nerve palsy, amongst other conditions. The causes of eyelid retraction in children are heterogeneous (Table 7.8).[246] Since Graves ophthalmopathy is rare in children, neurological causes should be primarily considered unless specific clinical or neuroimaging findings suggest the diagnosis.

Lid retraction in children is often intermittent, as in aberrant reinnervation associated with congenital oculomotor palsy or the MGJW phenomenon. Cases of neuromyotonia affecting only the levator muscle would also be expected to show isolated intermittent lid retraction, but such a case has not been reported. Cases of oculomotor palsy with cyclic spasm show intermittent momentary elevation of the eyelid on the affected side, but careful scrutiny of the ocular alignment and the mandatory pupillary involvement in the cyclic

TABLE 7.8. Causes of eyelid retraction in children.

Setting sun sign/hydrocephalus/dorsal midbrain syndrome
   (Collier sign)
Congenital, cryptogenic
Oculomotor palsy with aberrant innervation
Oculomotor palsy with cyclic spasm
Marcus Gunn jaw winking
Eyelid retraction to darkness (normal in first year of life)
Neuromyotonia
Graves disease/hyperthyroidism
Familial periodic paralysis
Orbital hemangioma
Optic nerve anomalies with vertical nystagmus
Contralateral ptosis with compensatory superinnervation of
   both levators (fixation duress)
Myasthenia gravis
Hepatic cirrhosis
Cushing syndrome
Levator muscle fibrosis
Inferior rectus muscle restriction with fixation duress
Iatrogenic after surgical repair of ptosis
Eyelid scarring (e.g., after inflammation from H. Zoster)
Claude Bernard syndrome (sympathetic irritation)
Volitional lid retraction
"Startle" reflex to dimming light in infants

process confirm the diagnosis.[167] A single case of posttraumatic, bilateral, pupillary-involving oculomotor palsy has been reported wherein the patient showed bilateral nonsynchronous episodic eyelid retractions not associated with eye movement or pupillary changes.[154] Patients with unilateral inferior rectus restriction and alternating fixation may show intermittent contralateral eyelid retraction, which occurs as a result of Hering's law when the restricted eye takes up fixation.

Healthy infants also frequently display eyelid retraction to darkness, which resembles the setting sun sign (Figure 7.12). Eyelid retraction to darkness can be elicited by turning off the room lights while observing the palpebral fissures. It can be a clinically useful sign that an apparently blind infant has at least light perception vision. The phenomenon, which appears to be limited to the first year of life, disappears when ambient illumination is restored and is thought to represent a primitive startle reflex.

Apraxia of Eyelid Opening

Apraxia of eyelid opening is a nonparalytic motor disorder of the eyelids. It is characterized by the inability to volitionally initiate eyelid opening despite intact reflex lid elevation, lack of concurrent orbicularis oculi muscle contraction, and intact ocular motor nerves. Affected patients open the eyes manually, or may employ a head thrusting movement to do so.[161] It may be differentiated from blepharospasm by the absence of Charcot's sign (orbicularis contraction forces the eyebrows to a level lower than the superior orbital margin). The condition usually appears in older patients with extrapyramidal disease but may be seen in

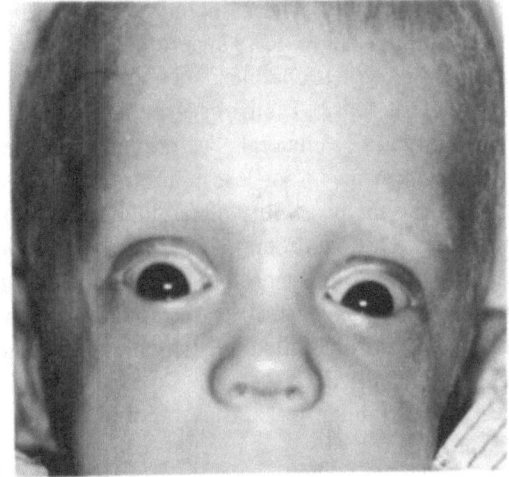
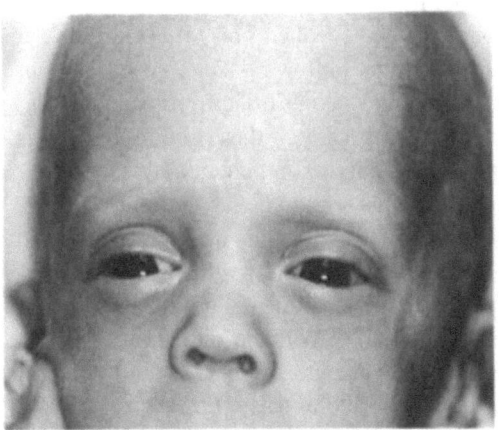

FIGURE 7.12. Pseudo–setting sun sign. This healthy infant showed eyelid retraction immediately after the room light was turned off (A) that resolved when ambient illumination was restored (B).

patients with unilateral or bilateral hemispheric dysfunction. It may favorably respond to local Oculinum injections.[138]

Neurologic Pupillary Abnormalities in Children

Adie Syndrome

Isolated internal ophthalmoplegia either is commonly due to trauma or pharmacological dilatation of the pupil or is a feature of Adie syndrome. Adie syndrome is rare in childhood,[168] having an average age of onset of approximately 32 years and a predilection for females. It is characterized by either unilaterally or bilaterally enlarged, tonic pupils that show markedly slow constriction to either light or near stimulation, followed by a very slow, tonic, redilatation. Patients with Adie syndrome also show regional corneal hypesthesia due to interruption of fibers of the ophthalmic division of the trigeminal nerve as they traverse the ciliary ganglion.

The light-near dissociation found in Adie syndrome differs in pathophysiology from that seen in mesencephalic disease; it may be attributed to either diffusion of acetylcholine from partially innervated or reinnervated ciliary muscle to the supersensitive pupillary sphincter muscle[109] or by aberrant misdirection to the pupillary sphincters of nerve fibers that originally synapsed in the ciliary muscle.[255] An accommodation paresis may also be associated, which is understandable if one considers that the ciliary ganglion has 30 times more neurons destined for the ciliary muscle than for the iris sphincter. Following acute onset, most of the sprouting new axons arise from accommodative neurons, but many of these end up in the iris sphincter (i.e., aberrant regeneration). Hence, although the pupils tend to be large at presentation, they become smaller with the passage of time and may eventually be confused with Argyll Robertson pupils if the examiner is not aware of their earlier dilated status. With the slit lamp, segmental vermiform movements of the iris and sectoral palsy are seen. Sectoral palsy produces shifting of the iris stroma toward the area of active contraction, a phenomenon known as "iris streaming."[253] An associated sectoral palsy of the ciliary muscle

causes lenticular astigmatism that may blur vision during near tasks. The iris vermiform movements noted at the slit lamp represent normal contractile activity of those iris sectors still innervated by light-responsive neurons. Citing two young adults who were found to have long-standing miotic pupils in association with typical features of Adie syndrome, Rosenberg[215] has argued that some cases of Adie syndrome may primarily present with miotic pupils, in a manner analogous to primary aberrant regeneration of the oculomotor nerve. However, the observation of Adie syndrome with dilated pupils in children as young as 4 years[4] (with subsequent development of miosis) argues against this hypothesis.

One case of Adie syndrome involved a 4-year-old boy who developed bilateral consecutive, idiopathic Adie syndrome over a follow-up period of 6 years.[4,72] At the age of 4 years, he was diagnosed with right Adie syndrome and was found to have amblyopia since the associated accommodative difficulty unmasked his latent hyperopia.[4] Examination at age 10 revealed additional myotonic involvement of the left pupil and absent or sluggish deep tendon reflexes.[72]

Thompson[253] has classified patients with tonic pupils into three categories on the basis of their underlying pathophysiologic disorders: (1) Local pathologic disorders within the orbit that involve the ciliary ganglion (e.g., inflammatory processes such as herpes or sarcoid; trauma). These conditions are commonly unilateral. (2) Neuropathic conditions causing diffuse peripheral or autonomic neuropathy. These include syphilis, diabetes, Guillain–Barre, Ross syndrome,[263] and several hereditary neuropathies, such as Shy Drager and Charcot Marie Tooth disease. These conditions are typically bilateral. The presence of Adie-like pupils in an infant less than 1 year of age should raise the possibility of familial dysautonomia (Riley–Day syndrome). (3) Cryptogenic tonic pupils, or true Adie syndrome, begins unilaterally, but eventually at least 20% of patients will develop the syndrome bilaterally. In addition to the ocular signs, the deep tendon reflexes, especially the knee and ankle jerks, may be diminished or absent.

The Adie syndrome bears some resemblance to the Ross syndrome, which is a rare, presumably degenerative peripheral neuropathy characterized by the triad of unilateral or bilateral tonic pupil, hyporeflexia, and segmental anhidrosis.[263] The recent demonstration of subclinical segmental hypohidrosis in patients with Adie syndrome suggests that the two conditions may be related.[99] Tonic pupils have also been described in a child with neuroblastoma and attributed to a paraneoplastic process.[264]

The diagnosis of Adie syndrome can be confirmed by demonstrating constriction of the dilated pupil in response to a dilute solution of pilocarpine (0.125%), which confirms the presence of pupillary supersensitivity due to parasympathetic denervation. This supersensitivity may not be demonstrable acutely, with some acute cases failing to constrict even to strong solutions of pilocarpine, making a differentiation from pharmacologic blockade difficult.

Pharmacological misadventures are a common cause of isolated pupillary dilation, resulting from instillation of mydriatic agents, exposure to certain plants that contain belladonna or atropine-like alkaloids (e.g., jimsonweed), or exposure to certain perfumes or cosmetics. The mydriatic pupils associated with ophthalmoplegic migraine, oculomotor palsy with cyclic spasm, botulism, the Fisher syndrome, and the dilated pupil accompanying the dorsal midbrain syndrome do not usually cause a diagnostic problem due to the other associated features of these disorders. Various infectious diseases have been associated with pupillary mydriasis or tonic pupils including Herpes zoster, measles, diphtheria, syphilis, pertussis, scarlet fever, smallpox, influenza, and hepatitis, but a history of an infectious illness is usually present. Chicken pox may produce a tonic pupil in children, which may present during the incubation period, the active disease stage, or during convalescence.[195,212,217] The mydriasis and decreased accommodation in the setting are presumed to reflect direct infectious or inflammatory involvement of the ciliary ganglion; however, the coexistent iridocyclitis with iris stromal vasculitis and sphincter necrosis could also contribute in some cases. The finding of mutton-fat keratoprecipitates and/or sectoral iris stromal atrophy would favor the latter mechanism.

Traumatic injury, either to the iris sphincter or to the ciliary nerves (e.g., panretinal photocoagulation, orbital surgery), may also produce pupil-

lary mydriasis or tonic pupils.[26] Some children may present with isolated episodic unilateral or bilateral mydriasis accompanied by head pain; [100,281] these may represent a variant of ophthalmoplegic migraine or represent a migraine equivalent and are usually self-limited.[258]

Horner Syndrome

Horner syndrome results from a lesion affecting the sympathetic supply to the eye and may be encountered at any age (Figure 7.13). The clinical features found on the affected side include the following: (1) 1 to 2 mm of miosis with greater anisocoria in dim illumination and a dilation lag. The miosis results from denervation of the sympathetically innervated pupillary dilator muscle. Oculosympathetic denervation of the pupillary dilator muscle can be demonstrated by dimming the ambient light and observing an immediate but transient increase in anisocoria, since the affected pupil does not dilate as rapidly as the normal pupil (dilation lag). (2) Mild upper lid ptosis measuring 1 to 2 mm (due to denervation of the sympathetically supplied superior tarsal muscle), and corresponding elevation of the lower eyelid (upside-down ptosis), due to denervation of the lower eyelid retractors. The upside-down ptosis may be confirmed by matching the lower limbus to the lower lid margin in each eye; more scleral showing would be found on the normal side. The re-

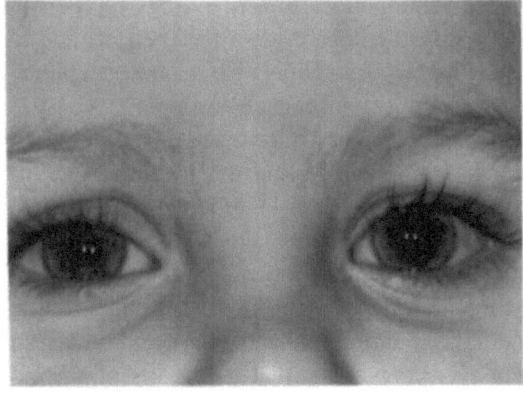

FIGURE 7.13. Congenital Horner syndrome. Note the right upper lid ptosis, right miosis, and mild heterochromia. The right lower lid shows mild reverse ptosis, covering more of the cornea than its left counterpart.

sulting narrowing of the palpebral fissure leads to an apparent enophthalmos. (3) Anhidrosis if the lesion is proximal to the carotid bifurcation. Lesions distal to the carotid bifurcation will not affect sympathetic innervation of facial sweat glands. Congenital or perinatal Horner syndrome results in failure of the iris to become fully pigmented, resulting in heterochromia with the ipsilateral iris appearing lighter in color. Iris heterochromia takes several months to develop and may be difficult to detect in infants who normally have lightly colored irides. Much less commonly, heterochromia may also follow acquired lesions in adults.[65] Subtle iris heterochromia can sometimes be made more visible by examining the child in sunlight. Some congenital cases may present with ipsilateral facial flushing.[219] Patients with acute Horner syndrome may also exhibit decreased Schirmer response, transient myopia, transient hypotony, and transient conjunctival hyperemia. The last three signs are seen only in acquired cases.

The location of the causative lesion along the sympathetic pathway may be inferred clinically and confirmed pharmacologically and/or neuroradiologically.[66] For instance, the combination of Horner syndrome and ipsilateral abducens palsy implicates a lesion in the cavernous sinus. Mesencephalic lesions involving the trochlear nucleus or fascicles, before decussation in the superior medullary velum, and adjacent sympathetic fibers may produce an ipsilateral Horner syndrome and contralateral superior oblique muscle paresis.[96] Pharmacological testing consists of topical instillation of autonomically active drugs to confirm oculosympathetic paralysis (cocaine test) and to distinguish a preganglionic from a postganglionic lesion (hydroxyamphetamine test).

Iris pigmentation, which occurs within the first year of life, requires sympathetic stimulation. Interestingly, Mindel et al [182] reported a 21-year-old woman with neurofibromatosis type I who had a unilateral congenital Horner syndrome with heterochromia. The patient showed symmetric Lisch nodules, which are melanocytic hamartomas, in both eyes, suggesting that unlike iris pigmentation, the formation of Lisch nodules is not influenced by sympathetic innervation of the iris. Other causes of heterochromia such as iris nevus or melanoma, neurofibromatosis, hemosiderosis, hemochromatosis, Waardenburg syndrome, Fuch's

heterochromic iridocyclitis, and essential iris atrophy should be excluded.

Most cases of congenital or early acquired Horner syndrome are of a benign nature. Rarely, congenital Horner syndrome may occur as an autosomal dominant disorder. Hageman et al[98] reported a Dutch family with five cases of congenital Horner syndrome spanning five generations. A history of perinatal trauma, such as brachial plexus injury (Klumpke's paralysis),[10,262] neck or cardiothoracic surgery, peritonsilar lesions, and surgical or nonsurgical intraoral trauma, may be elicited in many cases, but some cases remain cryptogenic despite extensive investigations. Congenital Horner syndrome has also been reported with hemifacial atrophy, synergistic divergence, basilar impression and Arnold–Chiari malformation, cervical vertebral anomaly and an enterogenous cyst, and viral infections such as congenital varicella[156] or cytomegalovirus infections. A case of congenital postganglionic Horner syndrome and fibromuscular dysplasia of the ipsilateral internal carotid artery incited speculation that prenatal or neonatal cervical trauma might have been responsible for both findings.[206] Congenital tumors, including neuroblastoma of the neck, chest, or abdomen have been reported to underlie some cases of congenital Horner syndrome.[224,225,272] Most reported cases of neuroblastoma occurred in the neck,[2] wherein they are frequently mistaken for infectious adenitis, or in the mediastinum,[238] but remote locations have also been described.[88] Lesions acquired in early life may be very difficult to distinguish from congenital cases, but close scrutiny of previous photographs may be helpful.

The rare occurrence of underlying tumors, especially neuroblastoma, in a few congenital cases justifies vigilance in cases with no apparent cause. Gibbs and coworkers[88] reported a 2-year-old child with congenital Horner syndrome who was healthy until the age of 2 when a remote neuroblastoma of the adrenal gland was diagnosed. They argued that both congenital Horner and neuroblastoma may represent widespread dysgenesis of the sympathetic system. Notwithstanding these reports, we have yet to see a patient with isolated congenital Horner syndrome subsequently develop neuroblastoma and do not routinely perform abdominal, thoracic, cervical, and cranial scans on such patients.

Spasm of the Near Reflex

Spasm of the near reflex is characterized by intermittent episodes of miosis, convergence and accommodation. Patients exhibit variable esotropia and varying pupillary size. The designation "spasm of the near reflex" should not be used interchangeably with either accommodation spasm or convergence spasm, each of which may present separately as a distinct entity. Patients may present with diplopia, blurred vision especially for distant objects, fluctuating vision, or nonspecific ocular discomfort. Due to its rarity, affected children may be misdiagnosed as having childhood esotropia, unilateral or bilateral sixth nerve palsy or, less commonly, divergence insufficiency, horizontal gaze palsy, ocular motor apraxia, convergence retraction nystagmus; true myopia, or Tensilon-negative myasthenia gravis.[216] Careful attention to pupillary size, retinoscopy during episodes of spasm to confirm the fluctuating induced myopia, and the variable esotropia should help confirm the diagnosis. The disorder is most commonly considered to be functional in nature, possibly due to underlying emotional conflict, with some patients showing signs of hysteria, malingering, or personality disturbances. However, cases associated with organic disorders are occasionally reported, including head trauma, stroke, pretectal lesions, neurosyphilis, labyrinthine dysfunction, diphenylhydantoin intoxication, Wernicke's encephalopathy, metabolic encephalopathy, the Fisher syndrome (two cases reported so far), and Arnold–Chiari malformation.[29,58,188,205] A few patients with intracranial tumors (two with cerebellar tumors, one with pituitary adenoma) and spasm of the near reflex have been described.[50,58] It should be emphasized that most patients with spasm of the near reflex in association with other neurologic disease manifest other symptoms and signs that can be readily uncovered during a careful neurologic and neuro-ophthalmologic examination.

Spasm of the near reflex in infants and children should be distinguished from nystagmus blockage syndrome and from convergence substitution. The latter is seen in patients with congenital or acquired horizontal gaze paralysis (e.g., Möbius syndrome, multiple sclerosis) wherein the patient substitutes a convergence movement for a lateral version movement when attempting to fixate an eccentric target.

We have examined a 12-year-old boy who had undergone left medial rectus muscle resection (4 mm) for presumed convergence insufficiency, 4 months previously. Shortly postoperatively, he complained of fluctuating vision and varying ocular alignment ranging from orthotropia to 80 prism diopters of esotropia. He was noted to have episodic, pronounced spasm of the near reflex associated with severe spasms involving the eyelids and the facial musculature (Figure 7.14). His neu-

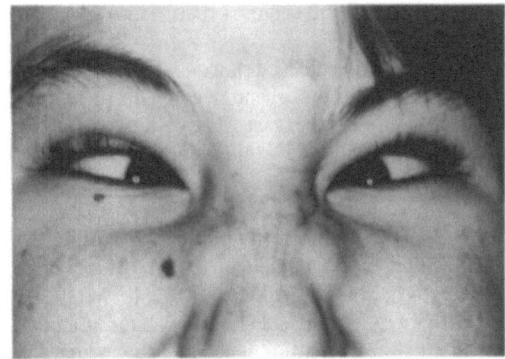 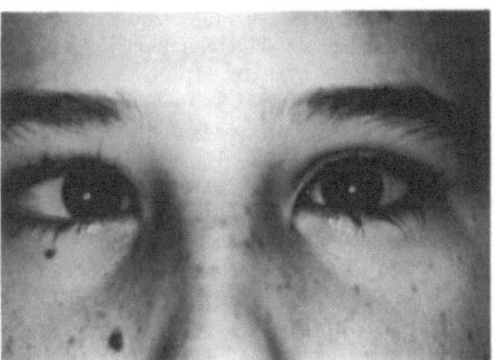

A   B

FIGURE 7.14. Spasm of the near reflex. This 12-year-old boy had undergone a small left medial rectus muscle resection for presumed convergence insufficiency. Four months later he was noted to have episodic, pronounced spasm of the near reflex (large esotropia, miosis, induced myopia with blurred vision) associated with severe spasms involving the eyelids and the facial musculature (A). In between spasms, only a small esotropia was variably present (B).

rological evaluation and MR imaging of the head was totally unremarkable otherwise. His symptoms continued unchanged during a follow-up period of 8 months.

Patients with isolated spasm of the near reflex may improve with reassurance. Some patients require psychiatric counseling. Current ophthalmologic treatment of spasm of the near reflex involves administering cycloplegic eye drops and providing bifocal glasses for reading. Historically, some patients have shown improvement with miotic drops, placebo drops, benzodiazepines, special glasses with occlusion of the inner third of each lens, monocular occlusion, or narcosuggestion during an amobarbital sodium interview. This problem usually resolves spontaneously over months to years except in patients with underlying organic disease.

References

1. Abeloos MC, Cordonnier M, Van-Nechel C, et al. Congenital fibrosis of the ocular muscles: a diagnosis for several clinical pictures. Bull Soc Belge Ophtalmol 1990;239:61-74.

2. Abramson SJ, Berdon WE, Ruzal-Shapiro C, et al. Cervical neuroblastoma in eleven infants—a tumor with favorable prognosis. Clinical and radiologic (US, CT, MRI) findings. Pediatr Radiol 1993; 23(4):253-257.

3. Acheson JF, Elston JS, Lee JP, et al. Extraocular muscle surgery in myasthenia gravis. Br J Ophthalmol 1990;75:232-235.

4. Agbeja AM, Dutton GN. Adie's syndrome as a cause of amblyopia. J Pediatr Ophthalmol Strabismus 1987;24(4):176-177.

5. Aghaji MA, Uzuegbunam C. Invasive thymoma and myasthenia gravis in a three-and-a-half-year-old boy: case report and literature review. Cent Afr J Med 1990;36(10):263-266.

6. Ahn JC, Hoyt WF, Hoyt CS. Tonic upgaze in infancy. A report of three cases. Arch Ophthalmol 1989;107:57-58.

7. Aicardi J, Barbosa C, Andermann E, et al. Ataxia-ocular motor apraxia: a syndrome mimicking ataxia-telangiectasia. Ann Neurol 1988;24:497-502.

8. Albert DM, Wong VG, Henderson ES. Ocular complications of vincristine therapy. Arch Ophthalmol 1967;78:709.

9. al-Din SN, Anderson M, Eeg Olofsson O et al. Neuro-ophthalmic manifestations of the syndrome of ophthalmoplegia, and areflexia: a review. Neurol Scand 1994;89:157-163.

10. al-Rajeh S, Corea JR, al-Sibai MH, et al. Congenital brachial palsy in the eastern province of Saudi Arabia. J Child Neurol 1990;5(1):35-38.

11. Andrews PI, Massey JM, Sanders DB. Acetylcholine receptor antibodies in juvenile myasthenia gravis. Neurology 1993;43(5):977-982.

12. Appleton RE, Panayiotopoulos CP, Acomb BA, et al. Eyelid myoclonia with typical absences: an epilepsy syndrome. J Neurol Neurosurg Psychiatry 1993;56(12):1312-1316.

13. Apt L, Axelrod RN. Generalized fibrosis of the extraocular muscles. Am J Ophthalmol 1978;85:822-829.

14. Arakawa Y, Yoshimura M, Kobayashi S, et al. The use of intravenous immunoglobulin in Miller Fisher syndrome. Brain Dev 1993;15(3):231-233.

15. Archer SM, Helveston EM, Miller KK, et al. Stereopsis in normal infants and infants with congenital esotropia. Am J Ophthalmol 1986;101:591-596.

16. Ashwal S, Thrasher TV, Rice DR, et al. A new form of sea-blue histiocytosis associated with progressive anterior horn cell and axonal degeneration. Ann Neurol 1984;16:184.

17. Auger RG, Piepgaras DG. Hemifacial spasm associated with epidermoid tumors of the cerebellopontine angle. Neurology 1989;39:577-580.

18. Baloh RW, Yee RD, Boder E. Eye movements in ataxia -telangiectasia. Neurology 1978;28:1099-1104.

19. Barontini F, Simonettia C, Ferranini F, Sita D. Persistent upward eye deviation: report of two cases. Neuro-Ophthalmology 1983;3:217-221.

20. Barroso L, Hoyt WF. Episodic exotropia from lateral rectus neuromyotonia—appearance and remission after radiation therapy for a thalamic glioma. J Pediatr Ophthalmol Strabismus 1993;30:56-57.

21. Bell JA, Fielder AR, Viney S. Congenital double elevator palsy in identical twins. J Clin Neuro-Ophthalmol 1990;10:32-34.

22. Benevento WJ, Tychsen L. Distinguishing compensatory head turn from gaze palsy in children with unilateral oculomotor or abducens nerve paresis. Am J Ophthalmol 1993;115:116-118. Letter.

23. Berlit P, Rakicky J. The Miller Fisher syndrome. Review of the literature J Clin Neuro-Ophthalmol 1992;12:57-63.

24. Beyer-Machule CK, Johnson CC, Pratt SG, et al. The Marcus-Gunn phenomenon. Orbit 1985;4:15.

25. Binyon S, Prendergast M. Eye-movement tics in children. Dev Med Child Neurol 1991;33(4):352-355.

26. Bodker FS, Cytryn AS, Putterman AM, et al. Postoperative mydriasis after repair of orbital floor fracture. Am J Ophthalmol 1993;115(3):372-375.

27. Bogousslavsky J, Miklossy J, Regli F, et al. Vertical gaze palsy and selective unilateral infarction of the rostral interstitial nucleus of the medial longitudinal fasciculus (riMLF). J Neurol Neurosurg Psychiatry 1990;53(1):67-71.

28. Bogousslavsky J, Regli F. Upgaze palsy and monocular paresis of downward gaze from ipsilateral thalamo-mesencephalic infarction: a vertical "one-and-a-half" syndrome. J Neurol 1984;231(1): 43-45.

29. Bohlmann BJ, France TD. Persistent accommodative spasm nine years after head trauma. J Clin Neuro-Ophthalmol 1987;7(3):129-134.

30. Borchert MS, Sadun AA, Sommers JD, et al. Congenital oculomotor apraxia: findings with magnetic resonance imaging. J Clin Neuro-Ophthalmol 1987;7:104.

31. Brandt T, Dieterich M. Pathological eye-head coordination in roll: tonic ocular tilt reaction in mesencephalic and medullary lesions. Brain 1987;110: 649.

32. Brandt T, Dieterich M. Skew deviation with ocular torsion: a vestibular brain stem sign of topographic diagnostic value. Ann Neurol 1993;33(5):528-534.

33. Brandt TH, Dieterich M. Different types of skew deviation. J Neurol Neurosurg Psychiatr 1991;54: 549-550.

34. Branley MG, Wright KW, Borchert MS. Third nerve palsy due to cerebral artery aneurysm in a child. Aust N Z J Ophthalmol 1992;20(2):137-140.

35. Breen L, Morris HH, Alperin JB, et al. Juvenile Neimann-Pick disease with vertical supranuclear ophthalmoplegia. Two case reports and review of the literature. Arch Neurol 1981;38:388-390.

36. Brodsky MC, Boop FA. Lid nystagmus in diffuse ophthalmoplegia as a sign of intrinsic midbrain disease. J Neuro-Ophthalmol 1995. In press.

37. Brodsky MC: Platysma-levator synkinesis in congenital third nerve palsy. Arch Ophthalmol 1991;109:620.

38. Brodsky MC, Pollock SC, Buckley EG. Neuronal misdirection in congenital ocular fibrosis syndrome: implications and pathogenesis. J Ped Ophthalmol Strabismus 1989;26:159-161.

39. Brodsky MC, Sharp GB, Fritz KJ, et al. Idiopathic alternating anisocoria. Am J Ophthalmol 1992; 114(4):509-510. Letter.

40. Bruyn GW. Huntington's chorea. In: Vinker PT, Bruyn GW, eds. Handbook of Clinical Neurology. Diseases of the Basal Ganglia. Amsterdam: NVK-Holland Publishing Co; 1968:6;298-378.

41. Buckley E, Seaber JH. Dyskinetic strabismus as a sign of cerebral palsy. Am J Ophthalmol 1981;91: 652-657.

42. Burke JP, Ruben JB, Scott WE. Vertical transposition of the horizontal recti (Knapp procedure) for the treatment of double elevator palsy: effectiveness and long-term stability. Br J Ophthalmol 1992;76(12):734-737.

43. Callahan MA. Surgically mismanaged ptosis associated with double elevator palsy. Arch Ophthalmol 1981;99(1):108-112.

44. Catalano RA, Calhoun JH, Reinecke RD, Cogan DG. Asymmetry in congenital ocular motor apraxia. Can J Ophthalmol 1988;23:318-321.

45. Catalano RA, Trevisani MG, Simon JW. Functional eyelid pulling in children. Am J Ophthalmol 1990;110(3):300-302.

46. Churchyard A, Stell R, Mastaglia FL. Ataxia telangiectasia presenting as an extrapyramidal movement disorder and ocular motor apraxia without overt telangiectasia. Clin Exp Neurol 1991; 28:90-96.

47. Clarke RR, Van der Velde RL. Congenital myasthenia gravis. A case report with thymectomy and electron microscopic study of resected thymus. Am J Dis Child 1971;122:356-361.

48. Cogan DG, Chu FC, Bachman DM, et al. The DAF syndrome. Neuro-Ophthalmology 1981;2:7.

49. Cogan DG, Chu FC, Reingold D, et al. A long term follow-up of congenital ocular motor apraxia: case report. Neuro-Ophthalmology 1980;1:145.

50. Cogan DG, Freese CG. Spasm of the near reflex. Arch Ophthalmol 1955;54:752.

51. Cogan DG, Schulman J, Porter RJ, Mudd SH. Epileptiform ocular movements with methylmalonic aciduria and homocystinuria. Am J Ophthalmol 1980;90:251-253.

52. Cogan DG, Wray SH. Internuclear ophthalmoplegia as an early sign of brain stem tumors. Neurology 1970;20:629-633.

53. Cogan DG. Congenital ocular motor apraxia. Can J Ophthalmol 1966;1:253.

54. Collin JRO, Allen L, Castronuovo S. Congenital eyelid retraction. Br J Ophthalmol 1990;74: 542-544.

55. Corbett JA, Mathews AM, Connell PH, Shapiro DA. Tics and Gilles de la Tourette syndrome: a follow up study and critical review. Br J Psychiatr 1969;115:1229-1241.

56. Corbett J. Neuro-ophthalmic complications of hydrocephalus and shunting procedures. Sem Neurol 1986;6(2):111-123.

57. Critchley EM, Mitchell JD. Human botulism. BR J Hosp Med 1990;43:290-292.

58. Dagi LR, Chrousos GA, Cogan DC. Spasm of the near reflex associated with organic disease. Am J Ophthalmol 1987;103(4):582-585.

59. Davidson JL, Rosenbaum AL, McCall LC. Strabismus surgery in patients with myasthenia. J Pediatr Ophthalmol Strabismus 1993;30:292-295.

60. Deleu D, Buisseret T, Ebinger G. Vertical one-and-a-half syndrome. Supranuclear downgaze paralysis with monocular elevation palsy. Arch Neurol 1989;46:1361-1363.

61. DeMarco P. Eyelid myoclonia with absences (EMA) in two monovular twins. Clin Electroencephalogr 1989;20(3):193-195.

62. de Sa LCF, Good WV, Hoyt CS. Results of initial surgery for comitant strabismus in 25 neurologically impaired children. Binocular Vis Q 1992;7: 165-172.

63. Dickey CF, Scott WE, Cline RA. Oblique muscle palsies fixating with the paretic eye. Surv Ophthalmol 1988;33(2):97-107.

64. Dickey CF. Clinical presentation of congenital fibrosis and double elevator palsy. Am Orthop J 1995;43:40-44.

65. Diesenhouse MC, Palay DA, Newman NJ, et al. Acquired heterochromia with Horner syndrome in two adults. Ophthalmology 1992; 99(12):1815-1817.

66. Digre KB, Smoker WR, Johnston P, et al. Selective MR imaging approach for evaluation of patients with Horner's syndrome. AJNR 1992;13(1): 223-227.

67. Diir LY, Donofrio PD, Patton JF, et al. A false-positive edrophonium test in a patient with a brainstem glioma. Neurology 1989;39:865-867.

68. Donhowe SP. Bilateral internuclear ophthalmoplegia from doxipen overdose. Neurology 1984;34: 259.

69. Drachman DB. Myasthenia gravis. N Engl J Med 1994;330:1797-1810.

70. Drachman DB. Present and future treatment of myasthenia gravis. N Engl J Med 1987;316:743-745.

71. Duncan MB, Jabbari B, Rosenberg ML. Gaze evoked visual seizures in nonketotic hyperglycemia. Epilepsia 1991;32:221-224.

72. Dutton GN, Paul R. Adie syndrome in a child: a case report. J Pediatr Ophthalmol Strabismus 1992;29(2):126.

73. Ebner R, Lopez L, Ochoa S, et al. Vertical ocular motor apraxia. Neurology 1990;40:712-713.

74. Elston JS, Granje FC, Lees AJ. The relationship between eye winking tics, frequent eye blinking, and blepharospasm. J Neurol Neurosurg Psychiatry 1989;52:477-480.

75. Engel AG, Walls TJ, Nagel A, et al. Newly recognized congenital myasthenic syndromes. I: congenital paucity of synaptic vesicles and reduced quantal release. II: high-conductance fast-channel syndrome. III: abnormal acetylcholine receptor (AChR) interaction with acetylcholine. IV: AChR deficiency and short channel-open time. Prog Brain Res 1990;84:125-137.

76. Erikson A, Wahlberg I. Gaucher disease—Norrbottnian type. Ocular abnormalities. Acta Ophthalmol Copenh 1985;63(2):221-225.

77. Fells P, Jampel RS. Supranuclear factors in monocular elevation palsy. Trans Ophthalmol Soc UK 1970;90:471-481.

78. Fenichel GM. Clinical syndromes of myasthenia in infancy and childhood. A review. Arch Neurol 1978;35:97-103.

79. FitzGerald PM, Jankovic J, Glaze DG, et al. Extrapyramidal involvement in Rett's syndrome. Neurology 1990;40:293-295.

80. Flueler U, Taylor D, Hing S, et al. Hemifacial spasm in infancy. Arch Ophthalmol 1990;108(6): 812-815.

81. Flynn JT. Strabismus: A Neurodevelopmental Approach. New York: Springer-Verlag; 1991.

82. Ford CS, Schwartze GM, Weaver RG, et al. Monocular elevation paresis caused by an ipsilateral lesion. Neurology 1984;34(9):1264-1267.

83. Frankel M, Cummings JL. Neuro-ophthalmic abnormalities in Tourette's syndrome: functional and anatomic implications. Neurology 1984;34(3): 359-361.

84. Friedman A, Jamrozik Z, Bojakowski J. Familial hemifacial spasm. Movement Disorder 1989; 4(3):213-218.

85. Friendly DS, Manson RA, Albert DG. Cyclic strabismus—a case study. Doc Ophthalmol 1973; 34:189-202.

86. Frohman LP, Kupersmith MJ. Reversible vertical ocular deviations associated with raised intracranial pressure. J Clin Neuro-Ophthalmol 1985;5: 158-163.

87. Galletta SL, Liu GT, Raps EC, et al. Cyclodeviation in skew deviation. Am J Ophthalmol 1994; 118:509-514.

88. Gibbs J, Appleton RE, Martin J, Findlay G. Congenital Horner syndrome associated with non-cervical neuroblastoma. Dev Med Child Neurol 1992;34(7):642-644.

89. Gillies WE, Harris AJ, Brooks AMV: Congenital fibrosis of the vertically acting extraocular muscles. Ophthalmology 1995;607-612.

90. Godel V, Nemet P, Lazar M. Congenital ocular motor apraxia: familial occurrence. Ophthalmologica 1979;179:90-93.

91. Goldblum TA, Effron LA. Upbeat nystagmus associated with tonic downward deviation in healthy neonates. J Pediatr Ophthalmol Strabismus 1994; 31:334-335.

92. Good WV, Crain LS, Quint RD, Koch TK. Overlooking: a sign of bilateral central scotomata in children. Dev Med Child Neurol 1992;34:61-79.

93. Gote H, Gregersen E, Rindziunski E. Exotropia and panoramic vision compensating for an occult congenital homonymous hemianopia: a case report. Binocular Vision Eye Muscle Surg Q 1993; 8:129-132.

94. Green JP, Newman NJ, Winterkorn JS. Paralysis of downgaze in two patients with clinical-radiologic correlation. Arch Ophthalmol 1993;111(2):219-222.

95. Gross-Tsur V, Har-Even Y, Gutman I, et al. Oculomotor apraxia: the presenting sign of Gaucher disease. Pediatr Neurol 1989;5(2):128-129.

96. Guy J, Day AL, Mickle JP, et al. Contralateral trochlear nerve paresis and ipsilateral Horner's syndrome. Am J Ophthalmol 1989;107(1):73-76.

97. Guyton DL, Weingarten PE. Sensory torsion as the cause of primary oblique muscle overaction/underaction and A- and V-pattern strabismus. Binocular Vision Eye Muscle Surg Q 1994;9:209-236.

98. Hageman G, Ippel PF, te-Nijenhuis FC. Autosomal dominant congenital Horner's syndrome in a Dutch family. J Neurol Neurosurg Psychiatry 1992; 55(1):28-30.

99. Hallermann W. Schweißsekretionsstorungen beim Adie-syndrom. Eine neuropathia multiplex der peripheren autonomen nerven? Aktuel Neurol 1990; 17:179-183.

100. Hallett M, Cogan DG. Episodic unilateral mydriasis in otherwise normal patients. Arch Ophthalmol 1970;84:130-136.

101. Hamanishi C, Tanaka S, Kasahara Y, et al. Progressive scoliosis associated with lateral gaze palsy. Spine 1993;18(16):2545-2548.

102. Hamed LM, Chala P, Fanous M, Guy J. Strabismus surgery in selected patients with stable ocular myasthenia gravis. Binocular Vision Q 1994; 9:283-290.

103. Hamed LM, Dennehy PJ, Lingua RW. Synergistic divergence and jaw-winking phenomenon. J Pediatr Ophthalmol Strabismus 1990;27(2):88-90.

104. Hamed LM, Fang E, Fanous M, et al. The prevalence of neurological dysfunction in children with strabismus who have superior oblique overaction. Ophthalmology 1993;100:1483-1487.

105. Hamed LM, Fang EN. Inferior rectus muscle contracture resulting from perinatal orbital trauma. J Ped Ophthalmol Strabismus 1992;29:387-389.

106. Hamed LM, Lessner A. Fixation duress in the pathogenesis of upper lid retraction in thyroid orbitopathy. Ophthalmology 1994;101:1608-1613.

107. Hamed LM, Maria BL, Quisling RG, Mickle JP. Alternating skew on lateral gaze: Neuroanatomic pathway and relationship to superior oblique overaction. Ophthalmology 1993;100:281-286.

108. Hamed LM, Maria BL, Tusa R, et al. Periodic alternating gaze deviation in Joubert syndrome. Ophthalmology 1995. In press.

109. Hamed LM, Schatz NJ, Galetta SL. Brain stem ocular motility defects and AIDS. Am J Ophthalmol 1988;106:437-442.

110. Hamed LM. Alternating skew on lateral gaze simulating bilateral superior oblique overaction. Binocular Vision Q 1992;7:83-88.

111. Hamed LM. Bilateral Brown's syndrome in three siblings. J Pediatr Ophthalmol Strabismus 1991; 28:306-309.

112. Hamed LM. Cyclic, periodic ophthalmic disorders. In: Margo C, Hamed LM, Mames R, eds. Diagnostic Problems in Clinical Ophthalmology. Philadelphia, PA: W.B. Saunders;1993:711-715.

113. Hamed LM. Superior oblique overaction: some nosologic considerations. Am Orthopt J 1993;43: 82-86.

114. Hamed LM, Silbiger J. Periodic alternating esotropia. J Pediatr Ophthalmol Strabismus 1992; 29(4):240-242.

115. Harley RD, Rodriguez MM, Crawford JS. Congenital fibrosis of the extraocular muscles. Trans Am Ophthalmol Soc 1978;76:197-226.

116. Harriman DGF, Garland H. The pathology of Adie's syndrome. Brain 1968;91:401-418.

117. Hertle RW, Katowitz JA, Young TL, et al. Congenital unilateral fibrosis, blepharoptosis, and enophthalmos syndrome. Ophthalmology 1992;99:347-355.

118. Herzau V, Bleher I, Joos-Kratsch E. Infantile exotropia with homonymous hemianopia: a rare contraindication for strabismus surgery. Graefe's Arch Ophthalmol 1988;226:148-149.

119. Hiles DA, Walla PH, McFarlane F. Current concepts in the management of strabismus in children with cerebral palsy. Ann Ophthalmol 1975;7:789-798.

120. Hollman RE, Merrit JC. Infantile esotropia: results in the neurologic impaired and "normal" child at NCMH (six years). J Pediatr Ophthalmol 1986; 23:41-44.

121. Horikawa H, Juo K, Mano Y, et al. A case of neurovisceral storage disease with sea-blue histiocyte and severe horizontal supranuclear ophthalmoplegia. Rinsho-Shinkeigaku. 1990;30(1):62-67.

122. Howard RS. A case of convergence evoked eyelid nystagmus. J Clin Neuro-Ophthalmol 1986;6(3): 169-171.

123. Hoyt CS, Good WV. Ocular motor adaptations to congenital hemianopia. Binocular Vision Eye Muscle Surg Q 1993;8:125-126.

124. Hoyt CS, Mousel DK, Weber AA. Transient supranuclear disturbances of gaze in healthy neonates. Am J Ophthalmol 1980;89:708-713.

125. Hoyt CS. Acquired "double elevator" palsy and polycythemia vera. J Pediatr Ophthalmol Strabismus 1978;15(6):362-365.

126. Hoyt WF, Daroff RB. Supranuclear disorders of ocular control systems in man: clinical, anatomical, and physiological correlations-1969. In: Bach-Rita P, Collins CC, Hyde JE, eds. The Control of Eye Movements. Orlando, FL: Academic Press Inc; 1971:198-199.

127. Hriso E, Masdeu JC, Miller A. Monocular elevation weakness and ptosis: an oculomotor fascicular syndrome? J Clin Neuro-Ophthalmol 1991;11: 111-113.

128. Hughes JL, O'Conner PS, Larsen PD, et al. Congenital vertical ocular motor apraxia. J Clin Neuro-Ophthalmol 1985;5:153-157.

129. Jan JE, Farrell K, Wong PK, et al. Eye and head movements of visually impaired children. Dev Med Child Neurol 1986;28:285-293.

130. Jan JE, Freeman RD, McCormick AQ, Scott EP, Robertson WD, Newman DE. Eye pressing by visually impaired children. Dev Med Child Neurol 1983;25:755-762.

131. Jan JE, Freeman R, Scott E. Visual impairment in children and adolescents. New York: Grune and Stratton; 1977.

132. Jankovic J, Stone L. Dystonic tics in patients with Tourette's syndrome. Mov Disord 1991;6(3): 248-252.

133. Jho HD, Jannetta PJ. Hemifacial spasm in young people treated with microvascular decompression of the facial nerve. Neurosurgery 1987;20(5): 767-770.

134. Joubert M, Eisenring J, Robb JP, et al. Familial agenesis of the cerebellar vermis. Neurology 1989;19:813-825.

135. Kansu T, Subutay N. Lid retraction in myasthenia gravis. J Clin Neuro-Ophthalmol 1987;7:145-148.

136. Kaplan PW, Lesser RP. Vertical and horizontal epileptic gaze deviation and nystagmus. Neurology 1989;39(10):1391-1393.

137. Katayama M, Tamas LB. Saccadic eye-movements of children with cerebral palsy. Dev Med Child Neurol 1987;29(1):36-39.

138. Katz B, Rosenberg JH. Botulinum therapy for apraxia of eyelid opening. Am J Ophthalmol 1987; 103:718-719.

139. Keane JR, Finstead BA. Upward gaze paralysis as the initial sign of Fisher's syndrome. Arch Neurol 1982;39:781-782.

140. Keane JR. Ocular skew deviation. Analysis of 100 cases. Arch Neurol 1975;32:185-190.

141. Keane JR. Pretectal pseudobobbing. Five patients with 'V'-pattern convergence nystagmus. Arch Neurol 1985;42(6):592-594.

142. Keane JR. The pretectal syndrome: 206 patients. Neurology 1990;40(4):684-690.

143. Kennard C, Barger G, Hoyt WF. The association of periodic alternating nystagmus with periodic alternating gaze. J Clin Neuro-Ophthalmol 1981;1: 191-193.

144. Kernan JC, Devinsky O, Luciano DJ, et al. Lateralizing significance of head and eye deviation in secondary generalized tonic-clonic seizures. Neurology 1993;43(7):1308-1310.

145. Kim WJ, Chang BL. Unilateral congenital ocular motor apraxia: a case report. Korean J Ophthalmol 1992;6(1):50-53.

146. King MD, Dudgeon J, Stephenson JBP. Joubert's syndrome with retinal dysplasia; neonatal tachypnea as the clue to the genetic brain-eye malformation. Arch Dis Child 1984;59:709-718.

147. Kirkali P, Topaloglu R, Kansu T, et al. Third nerve palsy and internuclear ophthalmoplegia in periarteritis nodosa. J Pediatr Ophthalmol Strabismus 1991;28:45-46.

148. Kline KB, McCleur SM, Boniskowski FP. Oculosympathetic spasm with cervical cord injury. Arch Neurol 1984;41:61.

149. Krohel GB, Griffin JF. Cortical blepharoptosis. Am J Ophthalmol 1978;85:632-634.

150. Kumagai N, Yuda K, Ohno S. Abnormal vergence eye movement during eyelid closure caused by a pineal tumor. Nippon Ganka Gakkai Zasshi 1991;95(1):97-102.

151. Kushner BJ, ed. Grand rounds #34. A case of exotropia associated with an internuclear ophthalmoplegia. Binocular Vision Eye Muscle Surg Q 1994;9:112-116.

152. Kushner BJ. Errors in the three-step test in the diagnosis of vertical strabismus. Ophthalmology 1989;96(1):127-132.

153. Kushner BJ. Paresis and restriction of the inferior rectus muscle after orbital floor fracture. Am J Ophthalmol 1982;94(1):81-86.

154. Lam BL, Nerad JA, Thompson HS. Paroxysmal eyelid retractions. Am J Ophthalmol 1992;114(1): 105-107. Letter.

155. Lambert SR, Kriss A, Gresty M, et al. Joubert syndrome. Arch Ophthalmol 1989;197:709-713.

156. Lambert SR, Taylor D, Kriss A, et al. Ocular manifestations of the congenital varicella syndrome. Arch Ophthalmol 1989;107(1):52-56.

157. Langston JW, Tharp BR. Infantile hemifacial spasm. Arch Neurol 1976;33:302-303.

158. Lapouse R, Monk MA. Behaviour deviation in a representative sample of children. Variation by sex, age, race, social class and family size. Am J Orthopsychiatr 1964;34:436-446.

159. Legge RH, Weiss HS, Hedges TR III, Anderson ML. Periodic alternating gaze deviation in infancy. Neurology 1992;42(9):1740-1743.

160. Leigh RJ, Zee DS. The Neurology of Eye Movements (2nd ed.) Philadelphia: F.A. Davis Co; 1991:432-441.

161. Lepore FE, Duvoisin RC. "Apraxia" of eyelid opening: an involuntary levator inhibition. Neurology 1985;53:423-427.

162. Lepore FE. Bilateral cerebral ptosis (Abstract). Neurology 1986(suppl 1);36:251.

163. Lessell S, Lessell IM, Rizzo JF III. Ocular neuromyotonia after radiation therapy. Am J Ophthalmol 1986;102:766-770.

164. Lessell S. Supranuclear paralysis of monocular elevation. Neurology 1975;25(12):1134-1143.

165. Levy NS, Cassin B, Newman M. Strabismus in children with cerebral palsy. J Pediatr Ophthalmol 1976;13:72-74.

166. Lewis JM, Kline LB. Periodic alternating nystagmus associated with periodic alternating skew deviation. J Clin Neuro-Ophthalmol 1983;3:115-117.

167. Loewenfeld IE, Thompson HS. Ocular paresis with cyclic spasms. A critical review of the literature and a new case. Surv Ophthalmol 1975;20:81-124.

168. Loewenfeld IE, Thompson HS. The tonic pupil: a reevaluation. Am J Ophthalmol 1967;63:46-87.

169. Lowenstein DH, Koch TK, Edwards MS. Cerebral ptosis with contralateral arteriovenous malformations: a report of 2 cases. Ann Neurol 1987; 21:404-407.

170. Lubkin V. The inverse Marcus Gunn phenomenon: an electromyographic contribution. Arch Neurol 1978;35:249.

171. Mak SC, Chi CS, Chen CH. Mitochondrial encephalomyopathy presenting with clinical Leigh's disease: report of a case. Chung Hua I Hsueh Tsa Chih Taipei 1991;47(1):54-58.

172. Mather TR, Saunders RA. Congenital absence of the superior rectus muscle: a case report. J Pediatr Ophthalmol Strabismus 1987;24(6):291-295.

173. McLeod AR, Glaser JS. Deglutition-trochlear synkinesis. Arch Ophthalmol 1974;92:171-172.

174. Meienberg O, Ryffel E. Supranuclear eye movement disorders in Fisher's syndrome of ophthalmoplegia,

ataxia, and areflexia. Report of a case and literature review. Arch Neurol 1983;40(7):402-405.

175. Mets M. Tonic upgaze in infancy. Arch Ophthalmol 1990;108:482-483.

176. Metz HS, Searl SS. Cyclic vertical deviation. Trans Am Ophthalmol Soc 1984;82:158-165.

177. Metz HS. Double elevator palsy. Arch Ophthalmol 1979;97(5):901-903.

178. Metz HS. Double elevator palsy. J Pediatr Ophthalmol Strabismus 1981;18(2):31-35.

179. Metz HS. Double elevator palsy: Is there a restriction? Am Orthop J 1993;43:54-58.

180. Miller MT, Stromland K. Ocular motility in thalidomide embryopathy. J Pediatr Ophthalmol Strabismus 1991;28(1):47-54.

181. Miller NR. *Walsh and Hoyt's Clinical Neuro-Ophthalmology*. 4th ed. Baltimore, MD: William & Wilkins; 1985;2:933-938.

182. Mindel JS, Rubenstein AE, Wallace S, et al. Congenital Horner's syndrome does not alter Lisch nodule formation. Ann Neurol 1994;35(1):123-124.

183. Misulis KE, Fenichel GM. Genetic forms of myasthenia gravis. Pediatr Neurol 1989;5(4):205-210.

184. Miyajima Y, Fukuda M, Kojima S, et al. Wernicke's encephalopathy in a child with acute lymphoblastic leukemia. Am J Pediatr Hematol Oncol 1993;15(3):331-334.

185. Moorthy G, Behrens MM, Drachman DB, et al. Ocular pseudomyasthenia orocular myasthenia "plus": A warning to clinicians. Neurology 1989;39:1150-1154.

186. Morel E, Eymard B, Vernet-Der Garabedian B, et al. Neonatal Myasthenia gravis: a new clinical and immunologic appraisal on 30 cases. Neurology 1988;38:138-142.

187. Moster ML, Schatz NJ, Savino PJ, et al. Alternating skew on lateral gaze (bilateral abducting hypertropia). Ann Neurol 1988;23:190-192.

188. Moster ML, Hoenig EM. Spasm of the near reflex associated with metabolic encephalopathy. Neurology 1989;39(1):150.

189. Munoz M, Page LK. Acquired double elevator palsy in a child with a pineocytoma. Am J Ophthalmol 1995;118:810-811.

190. Musarella MA, Ghan HS, DeBoer G, Gallie BL. Ocular involvement in neuroblastoma: prognostic implications. Ophthalmology 1984;91:936-940.

191. Namba T, Brunner NG, Brown SB, et al. Familial myasthenia gravis: report of 27 patients in 12 families and review of 164 patients in 73 families. Arch Neurol 1971;25:49-60.

192. Nightingale S, Barton ME. Intermittent vertical supranuclear ophthalmoplegia and ataxia. Mov Disord 1991;6(1):76-78.

193. Nishzaki T, Tamaki N, Nishida Y, et al. Bilateral internuclear ophthalmoplegia due to hydrocephalus: a case report. Neurosurgery 1985;17:822-825.

194. Nixon RB, Helveston EM, Miller K, et al. Incidence of strabismus in neonates. Am J Ophthalmol 1985;100:798-801.

195. Noel L-P, Watson AG. Internal ophthalmoplegia following chickenpox. Can J Optalmol 1976;11:267-269.

196. Nucci P, Brancato R. Oculogyric crisis after the Tensilon test. Graefe's Arch Clin Exp Ophthalmol 1990;228(4):384-385.

197. Odel JG, Winterkorn JM, Behrens MM. The sleep test for myasthenia gravis. A safe alternative to Tensilon. J Clin Neuro-Ophthalmol 1991;11(4):288-292.

198. Oesterle CS, Faulkner WJ, Clay R, et al. Eye bobbing associated with jaw movement. Ophthalmology 1982;89(1):63-67.

199. Ouvrier RA, Billson F. Benign paroxysmal tonic upgaze of childhood. J Child Neurol 1988;3(3):177-180.

200. Patterson MC, Horowitz M, Abel RB, et al. Isolated horizontal supranuclear gaze palsy as a marker of severe systemic involvement in Gaucher's disease. Neurology 1993;43(10):1993-1997.

201. Picard A, Lacert P. Disorders of horizontal gaze motility in the cerebral palsy patient. J Fr Ophtalmol 1984;7(11):717-720.

202. Pierrot-Deseilligny C, Gautier JC, Loron P. Acquired ocular motor apraxia due to bilateral frontoparietal infarcts. Ann Neurol 1988;23(2):199-202.

203. Ragge NK, Hoyt WF. Midbrain myasthenia: fatigable ptosis, "lid twitch" sign, and ophthalmoparesis from a dorsal midbrain glioma. Neurology 1992;42(4):917-919.

204. Rappaport L, Urion D, Strand K, et al. Concurrence of congenital ocular motor apraxia and other motor problems: an expanded syndrome. Dev Med Child Neurol 1987;29(1):85-90.

205. Raymond GL, Crompton JL. Spasm of the near reflex associated with cerebrovascular accident. Aust N Z J Ophthalmol 1990;18(4):407-410.

206. Reader AL III, Massey EW. Fibromuscular dysplasia of the carotid artery: a cause of congenital Horner's syndrome? Ann Ophthalmol 1980;12:326-330.

207. Reynard M, Wertenbacker C, Behrens M, et al. "Ping pong gaze" amplified. Neurology (NY) 1979;29:757-758. Letter.

208. Richter C. Clock-mechanism esotropia in children. Alternate day squint. Johns Hopkins Med J 1968;122:218-223.

209. Richter CP. *Biological Clocks in Medicine and Psychiatry*. Springfield, IL: Charles C Thomas; 1965.

210. Rizzo M, Corbett J. Bilateral internuclear ophthalmoplegia reversed by naloxone. Arch Neurol 1983;40:242-243.

211. Ro A, Gummeson B, Orton RB, et al. Vertical congenital ocular motor apraxia. Can J Ophthalmol 1989;24(6):283-285.

212. Rogers JW. Internal ophthalmoplegia following chickenpox. Arch Opthalmol 1964;71:617-618.

213. Roper-Hall MJ, Yapp JMS. Alternate day squint. In: *The First International Congress of Orthoptists*, St Louis, MO: CV Mosby; 1968:262.

214. Ropper AH. Three patients with Fisher's syndrome and normal MRI. Neurology 1988;38:1630-1631.

215. Rosenberg ML. Miotic Adie's pupils. J Clin Neuro-Ophthalmol 1989;9(1):43-45.

216. Rosenberg ML. Spasm of the near reflex mimicking myasthenia gravis. J Clin Neuro-Ophthalmol 1986;6(2):106-108.

217. Ross JVM. Ocula varicella with an unusual complication. Am J Ophthalmol 1961;51:1307–1308.

218. Safran AB, Berney J, Safran E. Convergence-evoked eyelid nystagmus. Am J Ophthalmol 1982; 93(1):48-51.

219. Saito H. Congenital Horner's syndrome with unilateral facial flushing. J Neurol Neurosurg Psychiatry 1990;53(1):85-86.

220. Salisachs P, Lapresle J. Upper lid jerks in the Fisher syndrome. Eur Neurol 1977;15:237-240.

221. Sandyk R. Paralysis of upward gaze as a presenting sign of vitamin B_{12} deficiency. Eur Neurol 1984;23:198.

222. Sano K. Trigemino-oculomotor synkinesis. Neuralgia 1959;1:29-51.

223. Saraiva JM, Baraitser M. Joubert syndrome: A review. Am J Genet 1992;43:726–731.

224. Sauer C, Levinsohn MN. Horner's syndrome in childhood. Neurology 1976;26:216-221.

225. Sayed AK, Miller BA, Lack EE, et al. Heterochromia iridis and Horner's syndrome due to paravertebral neurolemmoma. J Surg Oncol 1983;22:15-16.

226. Schmidt RD, Schmidt TW. Infant botulism: a case series and review of the literature. J Emerg Med 1992;10:713-718.

227. Schmidt T, Kreibich S. Vertical retraction syndrome. Klin Monatsbl Augenheilkd 1985;187(2):124-125.

228. Schreiner MS, Field E, Ruddy R. Infant botulism: a review of 12 years' experience at the Childrens' Hospital of Philadelphia. Pediatrics 1991;87:159-165.

229. Scott WE, Jackson OB. Double elevator palsy: the significance of inferior rectus restriction. Opthalmology 1977;27:5-10.

230. Seaber JH, Chandler AC Jr. A five year study of patients with cerebral palsy and strabismus. In: Moore S, Mein J, Stockbridge L, eds. *Orthoptics: Past, Present, and Future.* New York: Grune & Stratton; 1976:271-277.

231. Senelick RC. "Ping pong" gaze: periodic alternating gaze deviation. Neurology (NY) 1976;26:532-535.

232. Sethi KD, Hess DC, Harbour RC, et al. Gaze-evoked involuntary movements. Mov Disord 1990; 5(2):139-142.

233. Sharpe JA, Johnston JL. Ocular motor paresis versus apraxia. Ann Neurol 1989;25:209-210.

234. Shawkat F, Harris CM, Jacobs M, et al. Eye movement tics. Br J Ophthalmol 1992;76(11):697-699.

235. Shillito P, Vincent A, Newsom-Davis J. Congenital myasthenic syndromes. Neuromuscul Disord 1993; 3(3):183-190.

236. Shults WT, Hoyt WF, Behrens M, et al. Ocular neuromyotonia. A clinical description of six patients. Arch Ophthalmol 1986;104:1028-1034.

237. Simonsz HJ. Congenital fibrosis syndrome. J Pediatr Ophthalmol Strabismus 1990;27(6):328-329. Letter.

238. Simpson I, Campbell PE. Mediastinal masses in childhood: a review from a paediatric pathologist's point of view. Prog Pediatr Surg 1991;27:92-126.

239. Sondhi N, Archer SM, Helveston EM. Development of normal ocular alignment. J Pediatr Ophthalmol Strabismus 1988;25:210-211.

240. Staudenmaier C, Buncic JR. Periodic alternating gaze deviation with dissociated secondary face turn. Arch Ophthalmol 1983;101(2):202-205.

241. Stechison MT. Cystic glioma with positional oculogyric crisis. J Neurosurg 1989;71(6):955-957. Letter; comment.

242. Steinlin M, Martin E, Largo R, et al. Congenital ocular motor apraxia: a neurodevelopmental and neuroradiological study. Neuro-Ophthalmology 1990;10:27-32.

243. Steinlin M, Thun-Hohenstein L, Boltshauser E. Congenital oculomotor apraxia. Presentation—developmental problems—differential diagnosis. Klin Monatsbl Augenheilkd 1992;200(5):623-625.

244. Stell R, Bronstein AM, Plant GT, et al. Ataxia telangiectasia: a reappraisal of the ocular motor features and their value in the diagnosis of atypical cases. Mov Disord 1989;4(4):320-329.

245. Stewart JD, Kirkham TH, Mathieson G. Periodic alternating gaze deviation. Neurology 1979;29:222-224.

246. Stout AU, Borchert M. Etiology of eyelid retraction in children: a retrospective study. J Pediatr Ophthalmol Strabismus 1993;30(2):96-99.

247. Straube A, Witt TN. Oculo-bulbar myasthenic symptoms as the sole sign of tumour involving or compressing the brain stem. J Neurol 1990; 237(6):369-371.

248. Summers CG, MacDonald JT, Wirtschafter JD. Ocular motor apraxia associated with intracranial lipoma. J Pediatr Ophthalmol Strabismus 1987; 24(5):267-269.

249. Szobor A. Myasthenia gravis: familial occurrence. A study of 1100 myasthenia gravis patients. Acta Med Hung 1989;46(1):13-21.

250. Tamura EE, Hoyt CS. Oculomotor consequences of intraventricular hemorrhages in premature infants. Arch Ophthalmol 1987;105(4):533-535.

251. Taylor D. The visually handicapped baby and family. In: Taylor D et al (eds). Pediatric Ophthalmology. Boston: Blackwell Scientific Publications; 1990:87.

252. Taylor D, Lake BD, Stephens R. Neurolipidoses. In: Wybar K, Taylor D, eds. *Pediatric Ophthalmology, Current Aspects.* New York: Marcel Dekker; 1983:180-181.

253. Thompson HS. Adie's syndrome: some new observations. Trans Am Ophthalmol Soc 1977;75: 587-626.

254. Thompson HS, Zackon DH, Czarnecki JS. Tadpole-shaped pupils caused by segmental spasm of the iris dilator muscle. Am J Ophthalmol 1983; 96(4):467-477.

255. Thompson HS. Light-near dissociation of the pupil. Ophthalmologica 1984;189(1-2):21-23.

256. Traboulsi ET, Jaagar MD, Kattan HM, Parks MM. Congenital fibrosis of the extraocular muscles: Report of 24 cases illustrating the clinical spectrum and surgical management. Am Orthop J 1993; 43:45–53.

256a. Trobe JD. Cyclodeviation in acquired vertical strabismus. Arch Ophthalmol 1984;102:717-720.

257. Tusa RJ, Kaplan PW, Hain TC, et al. Ipsiversive eye deviation and epileptic nystagmus. Neurology 1990;40(4):662-665.

257a. Tychsen L, Imes RK, Hoyt WF. Bilateral congenital restriction of upward eye movement. Arch Neurol 1986;43:95–96.

258. van-Engelen BG, Renier WO, Gabreels FJ, et al. Bilateral episodic mydriasis as a migraine equivalent in childhood: a case report. Headache 1991; 31(6):375-377.

258a. Veggiotti P, Viri M, Lanzi G. Electrical status epilepticus on eye closure: a case report. Neurophysiol Clin 1992;22(4):281-286.

259. von Noorden GK, Tredici TD, Ruttum M. Pseudointernuclear ophthalmoplegia after surgical paresis of the medial rectus muscle. Am J Ophthalmol 1984;98:602-608.

260. Wall M, Rosenberg M, Richardson D. Gaze-evoked tinnitus. Neurology 1987;37:1034-1036.

261. Warmolts JR, Mendell JR. Neurotonia: impulse-induced repetitive discharges in motor nerves in peripheral neuropathy. Ann Neurol 1980;7:245-250.

262. Weinstein J, Zweifel TJ, Thompson HS. Congenital Horner's syndrome. Arch Ophthalmol 1980;98: 1074-1078.

263. Weller M, Wilhelm H, Sommer N, et al. Tonic pupil, areflexia, and segmental anhidrosis: two additional cases of Ross syndrome and review of the literature. J Neurol 1992;239(4):231-234.

264. West CE, Repka MX. Tonic pupils associated with neuroblastoma. J Pediatr Ophthalmol Strabismus 1992;29:382-383.

265. White JW. Paralysis of the superior rectus and inferior oblique muscles of the same eye. Arch Ophthalmol 1942;27:366-371.

266. Whitely AM, Schwartz MS, Sachs JA, Swash M. Congenital myasthenia gravis: clinical and HLA studies in two brothers. J Neurol Neurosurg Psychiatry 1976;39:1145-1150.

267. Wigginton JM, Thill P. Infant botulism. A review of the literature. Clin Pediatr Phila 1993;32(11): 669-674.

268. Wilder WM, Williams JP, Hupp SL. Computerized tomographic findings in two cases of congenital fibrosis syndrome. Comput Med Imaging Graph 1991;15:361-363.

269. Williamson PD, Thadani VM, Darcey TM, et al. Occipital lobe epilepsy: clinical characteristics, seizure spread patterns, and results of surgery. Ann Neurol 1992;31(1):3-13.

270. Windsor CE, Berg EF. Circadian heterotropia. Am J Ophthalmol 1981;91:8-13.

271. Wolfe GI, Taylor CL, Flamm ES, et al. Ocular tilt reaction resulting from vestibuloacoustic nerve surgery. Neurosurgery 1993;32:417-420, 420-421. Discussion.

272. Woodruf G, Buncic JR, Morin JD. Horner's syndrome in children. J Pediatr Ophthalmol Strabismus 1988;25:40-44.

273. Woodruff BA, Griffin PM, McCroskey, LM, et al. Clinical and laboratory comparison of botulinum from toxin types A, B, and E in the United States, 1975-1988. J Infec Dis 1992; 166:1281-1286.

274. Woody RC, Reynolds JD. Association of bilateral internuclear ophthalmoplegia and myelomeningocele with Arnold-Chiari, type II. J Clin Neuro-Ophthalmol 1985;5:124-126.

275. Wortham EV, Crawford JS. Brown syndrome in twins. Am J Ophthalmol 1988;25:202-204.

276. Wright KW, Liu GY, Murphree AL, et al. Double elevator palsy, ptosis, and jaw winking. Am Orthop J 1989;39:143-150.

277. Wright KW. Superior oblique silicone expander for Brown syndrome and superior oblique overaction. J Pediatr Ophthalmol Strabismus 1991;28(2): 101-107.

278. Yee RD, Duffin RM, Baloh RW, et al. Familial congenital paralysis of horizontal gaze. Arch Ophthalmol 1982;100:1449-1452.

279. Yokochi K. Paroxysmal ocular downward deviation in neurologically impaired infants. Pediatr Neurol 1991;7(6):426-428.

280. Zackon DH, Noel LP. Ocular motor apraxia following cardiac surgery. Can J Ophthalmol 1991; 26(6):316-320.

281. Zak TA. Benign episodic bilateral juvenile internal ophthalmoplegia. J Pediatr Ophthalmol Strabismus 1983;20(1):8-10.

282. Zaret CR, Behrens MM, Eggers HM. Congenital ocular motor apraxia and brain stem tumors. Arch Ophthalmol 1980;98:328-330.

283. Zee DS. Internuclear ophthalmoplegia: pathophysiology and diagnosis. Baillieres Clin Neurol 1992; 1:455-470.

284. Zee DS, Hain TC, Carl JR. Abduction nystagmus in internuclear ophthalmoplegia. Ann Neurol 1987;21:383-388.

285. Zee DS, Yee RD, Singer HS. Congenital ocular motor apraxia. Brain 1977;100:581-599.

286. Ziffer AJ, Rosenbaum AL, Demer JL, et al. Congenital double elevator palsy: vertical saccadic velocity utilizing the scleral search coil technique. J Pediatr Ophthalmol Strabismus 1992;29(3):142-149.

8

Nystagmus in Infancy and Childhood

Introduction

Pediatric nystagmus differs clinically and pathophysiologically from adult-onset nystagmus. Acquired nystagmus in adulthood is usually associated with an acute neurological lesion involving the ocular motor pathways within the brain stem and/or cerebellum. Based upon the clinical characteristics of the nystagmus and the associated neurological signs, a causative lesion can often be inferred clinically and confirmed by neuroimaging.

The initial evaluation of pediatric nystagmus is simplified by the fact that the majority of affected children have congenital nystagmus. The clinical appearance of congenital nystagmus readily distinguishes it from the rarer but more ominous forms of pediatric nystagmus. Unlike adult-onset nystagmus, congenital nystagmus usually reflects a primary visual disturbance at the retinal or optic nerve level. Optic nerve dysfunction is usually recognizable by the presence of optic atrophy or hypoplasia. In contrast, underlying retinal disorders are often clinically occult and may be identifiable only by electrophysiological testing. Because congenital nystagmus is usually an epiphenomenon of bilaterally decreased visual acuity, the identification of congenital nystagmus should be viewed as the initial step in the diagnostic evaluation. Determination of the presence or absence of an underlying sensory visual disturbance should follow.

The most common diagnostic error in the evaluating of congenital nystagmus is the acquisition of neuroimaging studies in the child who is otherwise neurologically normal. Based upon our own experience and a review of the literature, brain tumors do not cause congenital nystagmus in children unless optic atrophy or hypoplasia coexist. Although there are no data to support routine neuroimaging in congenital nystagmus, we continue to be impressed by the fact that parents of the child with congenital nystagmus so often arrive for neuro-ophthalmologic consultation with negative neuroimaging studies in hand.

Congenital Nystagmus

Clinical Features

Congenital nystagmus is an involuntary, conjugate, rhythmical, horizontal oscillation of the eyes. It may appear as a pendular or jerk nystagmus in primary gaze, and it may have a rotary component. The intensity of congenital nystagmus increases on lateral gaze and becomes right-beating in right gaze and left-beating in left gaze. The fact that congenital nystagmus "disobeys" Alexander's law (which states that, in peripheral vestibular nystagmus, the direction of the nystagmus increases in the direction of the fast phase and decreases but never reverses in the direction of the slow phase) is useful in distinguishing it from a horizontal peripheral vestibular nystagmus. Another distinguishing feature of congenital nystagmus is that it remains horizontal in upgaze, in contrast to acquired horizontal vestibular nystagmus, which becomes upbeating in upgaze.

Parents of the child with congenital nystagmus often report that the nystagmus becomes worse with attempted fixation or intense visual effort. This history is useful in further distinguishing the nystagmus from peripheral vestibular nystagmus, which becomes worse with occlusion and is damped by fixation. To confirm this observation, Leigh and Zee have suggested that the examiner observe one optic disc with the direct ophthalmoscope while periodically occluding the other eye. Increased nystagmus intensity with occlusion suggests a peripheral vestibular nystagmus, while either no change or a decrease in nystagmus intensity suggests congenital nystagmus.[175] Anxiety or fatigue will also increase the congenital nystagmus intensity and thereby degrade visual acuity.[5]

Unlike adult-onset nystagmus, it is rare for individuals with congenital nystagmus to experience oscillopsia (an illusory to and fro movement of the environment), although exceptions to this rule are well documented.[9,76,81] The absence of oscillopsia in older children and adults with nystagmus should suggest the diagnosis of congenital nystagmus. Congenital nystagmus usually damps during convergence, which accounts for the observation that near acuity is usually several lines better than distance acuity. Parents will report that children with congenital nystagmus will hold objects close to their faces, which enables them to utilize a combination of axial magnification to see small letters and convergence damping of the nystagmus.

Clinical observation and electro-oculographic recordings have demonstrated that the amplitude, frequency, and waveform of the nystagmus can vary with eye position, giving rise to a region of gaze in which the nystagmus intensity (amplitude × frequency) of the oscillation is minimal (referred to as the null zone).[68] In most individuals with congenital nystagmus, the head position corresponds with the minimal intensity zone of the nystagmus.[7] When the angle of the null zone exceeds 15°, however, the angle of the face turn may fall short of the null zone.[105] In some patients, the anomalous head position appears to be dictated by the velocity distribution of the slow phase (i.e., the percentage of time that the slow phase is less than or equal to 10° per second) and the nystagmus beat direction (which can be influenced both by the prior position of gaze and by the length of time a subject has maintained a fixed gaze position).[7] The multiplicity of factors that influence the null zone in congenital nystagmus might explain why the anomalous head posture in congenital nystagmus might change with time.[7]

Bagolini et al[24] have recognized that some individuals with congenital nystagmus utilize large face turns to place their eyes in extreme sidegaze and actively block their nystagmus. Unlike a null zone, in which electromyographic activity decreases, the mechanism of active blockage utilizes the increased electromyographic activity associated with lateral gaze innervation to damp congenital nystagmus. (The same mechanism of active blockage occurs when congenital nystagmus is damped by convergence.) Individuals with active blockage of nystagmus by sidegaze momentarily move their eyes into extreme lateroversion when they seek good vision, which may cause them to complain of discomfort brought about by the extreme torticollis that is necessary to block their nystagmus.[24] Face turns associated with horizontal null positions are usually less extreme and the nystagmus can be observed to increase if the eyes are carried further into sidegaze.

Congenital nystagmus may be accompanied by head shaking during periods of intense fixation. Head shaking seems to be more common in children (who are presumably less concerned about their cosmetic appearance).[75] Although head oscillations were originally thought to be an adaptive strategy to cancel the effects of the ocular oscillation, such a mechanism has seldom been demonstrated.[175] Furthermore, older children and adults are aware of their head movements and do not feel that these involuntary movements help them to see. With a single exception,[44] simultaneous eye and head movement recordings have demonstrated that head oscillations in individuals with congenital nystagmus represent an associated involuntary movement of pathological origin and not an adaptive strategy to improve vision.[75,175]

Many patients with congenital nystagmus have significant with-the-rule astigmatism that has been attributed to the increased force applied to the corneas by the eyelids when the eyes are oscillating.[214] The clinical characteristics of congenital nystagmus are summarized in Table 8.1.

TABLE 8.1. Clinical findings in congenital nystagmus.

Horizontal pendular or jerk nystagmus
Increased intensity on side gaze
Right-beating in right gaze and left-beating in left gaze
Horizontal in upgaze
Damps during convergence
Null zone, often with associated face turn
Worse with attempted fixation and intense visual effort
No oscillopsia
Appearance of "reversed" horizontal optokinetic responses
With-the-rule astigmatism
Head nodding in approximately 10%

Onset of Congenital Nystagmus

The term *congenital* nystagmus is fundamentally inaccurate since the nystagmus is rarely noted at birth. If carefully questioned, parents and relatives will usually relate an onset of nystagmus between 8 and 12 weeks of age. In hereditary cases, however, congenital nystagmus has been documented at birth by both the obstetrician and the family who are aware of the possibility and carefully observe the infant. Rarely, congenital nystagmus can manifest for the first time in the teens or beyond and can cause blurred vision and oscillopsia by disrupting the long-standing sensory and motor adaptations that the patient has developed to remain asymptomatic.[87,123]

The presence or absence of an underlying visual sensory deficit does not affect the time of onset of congenital nystagmus. Often, the infant is first evaluated in the third month of life when irregular eye movements are noted. The incorrect notion that congenital nystagmus should be present at birth can lead the ophthalmologist or neurologist to conclude that the infant has an acquired form of nystagmus and to suspect an underlying neurological problem. When congenital nystagmus first appears, it is often arrhythmical and intermittent, consisting of a series of irregular horizontal and oblique deviations of the eyes from side to side. At this stage, the erratic eye movements may simulate opsoclonus, leading the infant to be subjected to an unnecessary medical evaluation for neuroblastoma. Although the term *congenital nystagmus* is somewhat misleading, it is deeply entrenched in the literature (much like "congenital esotropia," which is also acquired in early infancy), and we adhere to it for the sake of consistency.

Congenital Nystagmus, Congenital Motor Nystagmus, and Sensory Nystagmus

The term *congenital motor nystagmus* has been applied to individuals with congenital nystagmus in whom the sensory visual system appears intact both clinically and electrophysiologically. This term implies that the oscillation is driven by a primary abnormality within the ocular motor circuitry. The term *sensory* nystagmus has been applied to patients whose congenital nystagmus is attributable to an underlying sensory visual disorder.[50] Cogan proposed that, in sensory nystagmus, the poor visual acuity interrupts sensory afferent input to the oculomotor control system, which causes fixation to become unstable and leads to a pendular oscillation of the eyes. By contrast, *motor nystagmus* was attributed to signal errors intrinsic to the ocular motor control centers, leading to a jerk nystagmus with relatively good visual acuity.[50,216] However, the myth that the presence or absence of a primary sensory deficit can be predicted on the basis of the clinical appearance (i.e., pendular versus jerk nystagmus) has long been dispelled.[68,71,216] A clinical and electro-ocular-graphic study has confirmed that pendular and jerk waveforms often coexist in the same individual with congenital nystagmus so that waveform analysis alone cannot be used to predict the presence or absence of afferent visual pathway dysfunction. The mechanism by which bilateral visual impairment in infancy "unhinges" congenital nystagmus is unknown.

The realization that one cannot predict the presence or absence of an underlying sensory visual disturbance based on the clinical features or electro-oculographic waveform of the nystagmus led some investigators to speculate that all congenital nystagmus may be attributable to a primary sensory disturbance, with occult or subclinical forms simulating what has traditionally been referred to as motor nystagmus. For example, isolated foveal hypoplasia has only recently been recognized as a hereditary cause of congenital nystagmus in individuals with normal ocular pigmentation. Many patients with this condition have undoubtedly been classified as having motor nystagmus. However, there is strong evidence to support the notion that the afferent visual pathways in some individuals with congenital nystagmus are clinically and electrophysiologically normal.[21] We prefer the term *idiopathic congenital nystagmus* to the redundant term *motor nystagmus* in referring to those individuals in whom no clinical or electrophysiological signs of afferent visual pathway dysfunction are found.

Gelbart and Hoyt[108] have emphasized that individuals with idiopathic congenital nystagmus, not surprisingly, have significantly better visual acuities (20/40 to 20/70) than those with primary visual disorders (usually 20/70 or below). Patients with idiopathic congenital nystagmus usually have a positive family history of nystagmus that suggests either an X-linked or autosomal dominant inheritance pattern.[108,282] Any child with idiopathic congenital nystagmus who has no family history should be regarded as being at increased risk of having an underlying neurological disorder.[46,147]

Until recently, it was believed that individuals with primary visual disorders accounted for a minority of congenital nystagmus cases, and electrophysiological testing was not routinely performed. Recent studies utilizing electroretinography and testing of routine and hemispheric visual evoked potentials (VEPs) have demonstrated anterior visual pathway (i.e., bilateral retina or optic nerve) abnormalities in over 90% of patients with congenital nystagmus.[108,275] It is now generally accepted that the great majority of cases of congenital nystagmus are attributable to anterior visual pathway disease. The diagnosis of congenital nystagmus therefore necessitates a directed investigation with the goal of identifying any obvious structural opacity and the deduction of occult retinal dysfunction.[40,41,108,275] Congenital nystagmus associated with bilateral congenital cataracts has been noted to improve or resolve if the cataracts are removed and clear vision is restored within 1 month of the onset of the nystagmus.[286] The decision of whether to perform further electrophysiological studies in an individual patient is predicated on the degree of clinical suspicion that a primary sensory disorder is likely to be present.

History and Physical Examination in Congenital Nystagmus

Although the clinical features and time of onset cannot be used to predict the presence or absence of an underlying visual sensory disorder, other aspects of the history and physical examination are highly suggestive of primary visual impairment as the cause of congenital nystagmus. It is toward the detection of afferent visual pathway disease that the remainder of the parent interview and patient examination is directed.

Relevant History

When evaluating an infant or child with congenital nystagmus for the first time, certain historical points suggest afferent visual pathway dysfunction at the retinal level. A directed history in the child with congenital nystagmus should include the following inquiries:

1. Are the child's eyes unusually light sensitive? Photophobia in a child with congenital nystagmus suggests the presence of a congenital retinal dystrophy (which may be present despite a grossly normal retinal appearance).
2. Does the child see better in daytime or at night? A history of night blindness suggests the possibility of congenital stationary night blindness (CSNB) or a rod-cone dystrophy. Children who are debilitated in daylight but function better in dim illumination may have congenital achromatopsia.
3. Is there a family history of poor vision, nystagmus, hypopigmentation, or easy sunburning? A family history of cutaneous hypopigmentation suggests the diagnosis of oculocutaneous albinism. A family history of nystagmus in the absence of hypopigmentation may be consistent with idiopathic congenital nystagmus, isolated foveal hypoplasia, or a congenital retinal dystrophy but is rare in optic nerve hypoplasia.

Physical Examination

The initial goal of the ocular examination in a child with congenital nystagmus is to rule out ocular structural abnormalities that may reduce vision and lead to congenital nystagmus. Signs of aniridia, congenital cataracts, corneal opacities, iris transillumination defects, and macular hypoplasia are sought. If these features are absent, an examination of the optic discs to look for optic disc anomalies (most notably optic nerve hypoplasia or atrophy) should be undertaken. If the optic nerves are normal in appearance, the possibility of an underlying congenital retinal dystrophy should be considered (Table 8.2). Most congenital retinal dystrophies are characterized by a grossly normal retinal appearance in the early stages (although a sedated examination using direct ophthalmoscopy reveals diffuse narrowing of the retinal arterioles, often accompanied by a subtle wrinkling of the internal limiting membrane over the macula).

If structural ocular abnormalities are absent in congenital nystagmus, the following four clinical signs of congenital retinal dystrophy should be sought (Table 8.3):

1. *Severe photophobia* in a child with congenital nystagmus is strongly suggestive of a congenital retinal dystrophy. (Children with optic nerve hypoplasia, dominant optic atrophy, or cortical visual loss may be mildly photophobic).[148]
2. The finding of bilateral *high myopia* in a child with congenital nystagmus should lead the examiner to suspect a congenital retinal dystrophy.
3. The *paradoxical pupillary reaction* consists of an initial pupillary constriction (rather than dilation) when the room lights are turned off. This phenomenon is best observed by holding a penlight laterally to the globe to dimly illuminate the pupil while turning off the room lights.[29] When a paradoxical pupillary reaction

TABLE 8.3. Clinical signs of congenital retinal dystrophy in congenital nystagmus.

Photophobia
Paradoxical pupils
High myopia
Oculodigital reflex

is observed, there is usually a lag time of approximately 1 second before the initial pupillary constriction is seen. The paradoxical pupillary response were originally described in association with CSNB, and achromatopsia.[28,99] It is now recognized that this phenomenon can rarely be seen in congenital optic nerve disorders and even in normal patients.[40,41,101,221] In the setting of congenital nystagmus, however, the paradoxical pupillary phenomenon remains highly suggestive of a congenital retinal dystrophy. The paradoxical pupillary phenomenon appears to be age-related in that it is difficult to see in adults or in infants younger than 6 months of age.[29]

4. The *oculodigital sign* refers to a repetitive pushing on the eyes with the thumbs or fists. It is speculated that repetitive eye rubbing is a self-stimulatory behavior that elicits phosphenes (entoptic flashes of light) in infants

TABLE 8.2. Congenital nystagmus associated with sensory visual loss.

	Diagnostic modality
Ocular structural abnormalities or media opacities	Ocular examination
Congenital cataracts	
Bilateral vitreous hemorrhage	
Bilateral corneal scarring	
Macular traction (e.g., ROP)	
Inflammatory macular scarring (e.g., toxoplasmosis)	
Isolated foveal hypoplasia	
Nonstructural ocular disease	
Congenital retinal dystrophies	ERG
Leber's congenital amaurosis	
Achromatopsia (complete, blue cone monochromatism)	
Congenital stationary night blindness	
Cone–rod dystrophy, rod–cone dystrophy	
Albinism	
Ocular examination	
Hemispheric VEPs	
Optic nerve dysfunction	Ocular examination,
Optic nerve hypoplasia	MR imaging
Optic atrophy	

with extremely poor vision. The oculodigital sign is commonly described in infants with Leber congenital amaurosis in whom the effects of chronic eye rubbing may contribute to the associated findings of enophthalmos, keratoconus, and cataract.

Electroretinography

If any of the foregoing four signs is present, a congenital retinal dystrophy should be suspected, and electroretinography should be obtained to further characterize it.[108,111,275] When ordering electroretinography in the child with nystagmus, it is important to recognize that the electroretinogram (ERG) can be falsely abnormal in infancy.[103,278] Unless the clinician has access to an electrophysiology laboratory with normative values for infants of different ages, it is best to wait until at least 1 year of age (at which time the amplitude, sensitivity, and latency of the electroretinographic waveform approach adult values) before obtaining this study.[103] If, at that time, the ERG is normal, the diagnosis of a congenital retinal dystrophy can be effectively ruled out. An abnormal ERG obtained after 1 year of age confirms the presence of an underlying congenital retinal dystrophy and, in some cases, establishes a specific diagnosis (discussed later).

Hemispheric Visual Evoked Potentials in the Diagnosis of Albinism

When electroretinography is found to be normal, a careful search for iris transillumination, macular hypoplasia, and chorioretinal hypopigmentation should again be undertaken since these signs may be difficult to detect in infancy. If these signs are equivocal, recording of visual evoked potentials (VEPs) to detect hemispheric asymmetry can be performed. Simonsz and Kommerell[247] studied patients with congenital nystagmus and found a high incidence of subtle oculocutaneous albinism when careful iris transillumination and retinal examinations were performed. Apkarian et al have demonstrated that hemispheric VEPs provide the most sensitive and specific means to establish the diagnosis of albinism.[17] We do not obtain VEPs in children with congenital nystagmus, since we see little prognostic value in distinguishing clinically occult albinism from idiopathic congenital nystagmus.

Overlap of Congenital Nystagmus and Strabismus

Two studies found a 16% incidence of strabismus in congenital nystagmus[100,108] whereas Dell'Osso found a 33% incidence.[73] It has been our clinical impression that strabismus occurs most commonly in congenital nystagmus associated with albinism or bilateral optic nerve hypoplasia. Assessment of the true incidence of strabismus in congenital nystagmus is confounded by the fact that children with Leber congenital amaurosis and other congenital visual disorders lack central fixation, making the assessment of strabismus difficult. The finding of esotropia and nystagmus compels the examiner to rule out manifest latent nystagmus and rotary nystagmus, which are seen in some children with congenital esotropia. These differ from congenital nystagmus in their clinical appearance and in their visual prognosis.

Eye Movement Recordings in Congenital Nystagmus

Immature Congenital Nystagmus Waveforms

Using electro-oculographic recordings, Reinecke et al found a stereotyped waveform evolution in infants with congenital nystagmus.[226] When the nystagmus first appears at 2 to 3 months of age, it takes on a triangular pattern that is occasionally punctuated by small plateaus. At approximately 7 to 12 months of age, the nystagmus transforms into a pendular waveform. Between 10 months and 1½ years of age, the pendular waveform gives way to an increasing-velocity jerk waveform characterized by a saccade to the target of fixation followed by a period of foveation and an increasing-velocity slow phase, which again pulls the fovea away from the object of interest. A few residual triangular and pendular cycles continue to be interspersed within the increasing-velocity waveform.

Mature Congenital Nystagmus Waveforms

Dell'Osso and Daroff have subdivided congenital nystagmus waveforms into 12 distinct categories based upon their electro-oculographic characteristics.[68] Although congenital nystagmus waveforms are often subdivided for classification purposes, it is important to recognize that the majority of congenital nystagmus patients display an average of three to five waveforms. These oscillations exist as a continuum of oscillations characterized by a period of foveation followed by an increasing-velocity slip away from the target and, finally, a corrective saccade back toward the target[68] (Figure

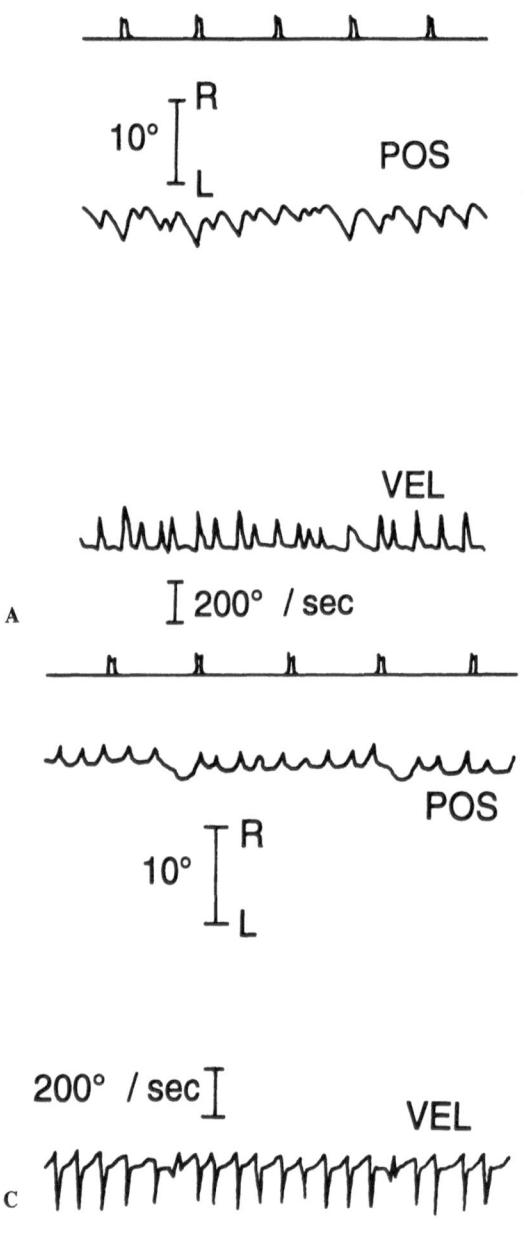

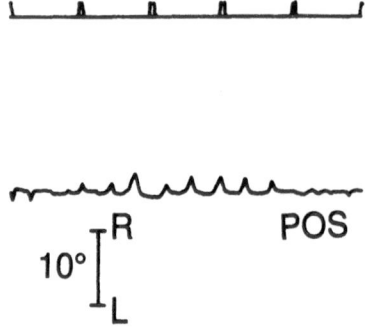

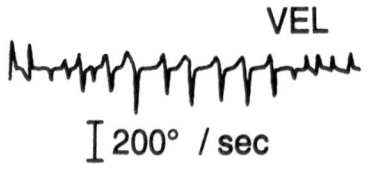

FIGURE 8.1. Eye movement recordings showing three common waveforms in congenital nystagmus. (Upward deflections denote rightward eye movements; downward deflections denote leftward eye movements). (A) Eye position (POS) and velocity (VEL) record of pure jerk nystagmus. Target foveation occurs briefly at the termination of each rightward saccade. Velocity spikes clearly identify the rightward-jerk direction. (B) Eye position (POS) and velocity (VEL) record of jerk nystagmus with extended foveation. Note that the target is foveated for a longer period of time following each saccade compared with pure jerk nystagmus. The velocity waveform readily demonstrates the leftward direction of the saccades, which is difficult to discern from the position tracing alone. (C) Eye position (POS) and velocity (VEL) record of the pseudo-cycloid form of jerk nystagmus. In the waveform, the leftward saccades are corrective in nature but are of insufficient amplitude to fully refoveate the target. Each saccade is followed by a smooth eye movement that refoveates the target. This waveform is often misidentified clinically as pendular nystagmus. The velocity waveform is particularly useful in identifying the saccadic component of each cycle. (Modified from Dell'Osso and Daroff. Congenital nystagmus waveforms and foveation strategies. Doc Ophthalmol 1975;39:155-182. Reprinted by permission of Kluwer Academic Publishers.)

8.1). The visual acuity associated with each waveform is related primarily to the length of the foveation period. It is not clear that any particular waveform is associated with better acuity; in fact, such an assessment would require knowledge of which waveform is predominating at the time acuity is tested. Eye movement recordings raise doubt about the ability to clinically differentiate between pendular and jerk forms of congenital nystagmus, as saccades may be seen in a clinically pendular nystagmus, and a pendular waveform without saccades may be seen in a clinically jerk nystagmus.[68]

Fixation in Congenital Nystagmus

Although congenital nystagmus has often been attributed to a faulty fixation mechanism, Dell'Osso et al have performed detailed examinations of foveation periods (intrabeat dynamics, accuracy of target foveation, effects of gaze angle, convergence, and base-out prisms on foveation period) and found that idiopathic congenital nystagmus is associated with strong fixation reflexes in that individuals are able to accurately achieve and maintain fixation for long periods of time.[79] Bedell et al found greater standard deviations in foveation periods of two albinos than in patients with idiopathic congenital nystagmus and suggested that the effects of macular hypoplasia on the fixation mechanism may have a secondary effect upon vision in albinism.[30] Visual acuity in congenital nystagmus has been found to correlate with fixation parameters, such as the accuracy of target foveation, the duration of target foveation, and the repeatability of foveation from cycle to cycle.[30,79] According to Dell'Osso, the fixation subsystem is only able to prolong foveation and maintain temporary fixation when the target image is on the fovea and moving with a velocity or acceleration that falls below a critical value (estimated at 4° per second).[80,81] This may explain why foveation periods are part of the congenital nystagmus but not the acquired nystagmus waveform, since the initial slow phase velocities in acquired nystagmus are usually too great for the fixation subsystem to extend foveation and improve visual acuity.[84]

While the fixation mechanism appears to be robust in congenital nystagmus, the observation that congenital nystagmus increases during attempted fixation and ceases during nonvisual tasks, such as daydreaming or sleep,[79] suggests that the presence of an abnormal circuitry between the fixation system and the remaining ocular stabilization systems that allows the effort associated with fixation to influence the oscillation.[79]

Smooth Pursuit System in Congenital Nystagmus

The smooth pursuit waveform in the congenital nystagmus patient bears little resemblance to that of the normal individual.[82] This lack of correspondence has, in the past, been misconstrued as a possible smooth pursuit deficit in congenital nystagmus.[162,216,287] Dell'Osso has stressed that the fundamental error of equating the summation of smooth pursuit movements plus the superimposed congenital nystagmus waveform with the pursuit movement alone inevitably leads to the erroneous conclusion that there is an inherent defect in the pursuit system. He has further demonstrated that, during pursuit of a visual target, the slow phases of congenital nystagmus consist of normal pursuit movements plus the nystagmus itself but that the eye position consistently matches the target position during foveation periods.[74,84] If one examines the upper tracing in Figure 8.2 (in which eye position has been superimposed upon target position) and confines this examination to only the foveation periods, it becomes evident that the eye position accurately matches the target position during most of the foveation periods.[74,82] Such findings cast serious doubt upon the hypothesis that defective pursuit is either the cause of, or the necessary result of, congenital nystagmus.[82]

The notion of "inverted pursuit movements" and "inverted optokinetic responses" has created further confusion regarding the role of smooth pursuit in congenital nystagmus. It is widely recognized that patients with congenital nystagmus often show an apparent reversal of their optokinetic responses (i.e., during pursuit of leftward optokinetic stimuli, a left-beating nystagmus rather than a right-beating nystagmus is seen). This clinical observation is consistent with electro-oculographic observation that horizontal optokinetic targets often induce an increasing-velocity slow-phase movement of opposite direction to the target motion in the patient with congenital nystagmus, which has led to the mistaken assumption that congenital nystagmus could be

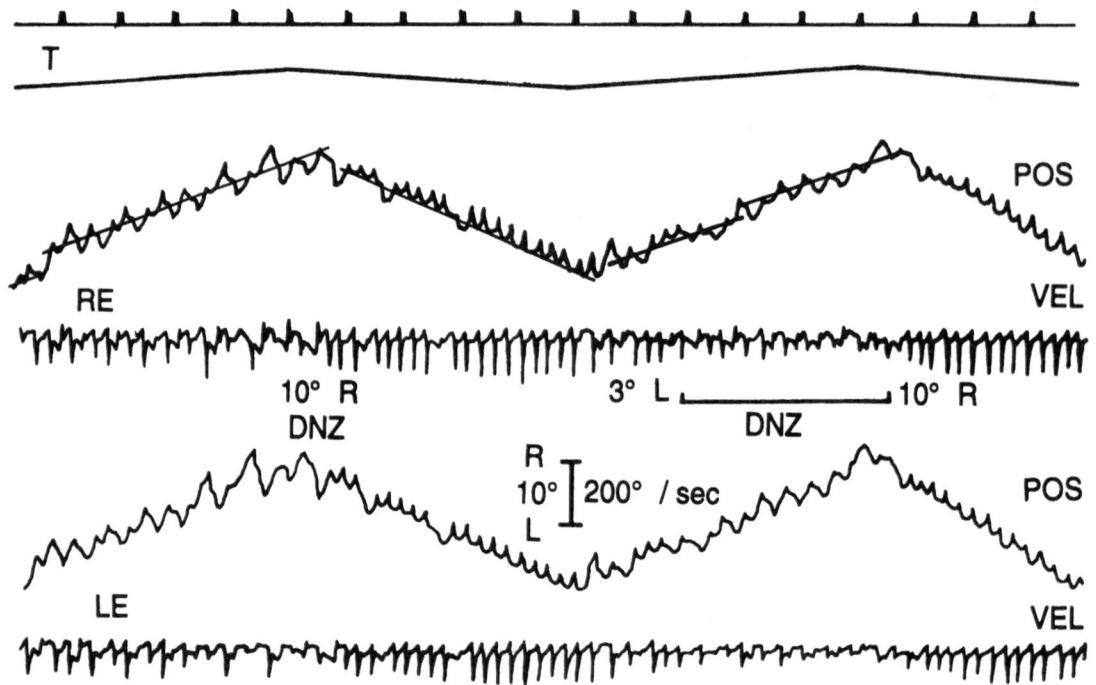

FIGURE 8.2. Eye movement recording from a patient with congenital nystagmus demonstrating smooth pursuit of a moving, constant-velocity target. The upper tracing shows the target position with the right eye (RE) position superimposed. The lower tracing shows the left eye position. (POS = position; VEL = velocity.) Note that the congenital nystagmus waveform is punctuated by brief foveation periods in which the eye position precisely matches the target position. (Modified from Dell'Osso.) Published with permission from the journal Neuro-Ophthalmology. Copyright by Aeolus Press).

caused by an inherent "reversal" in either the smooth pursuit or the optokinetic system.[216] The phenomenon of inverted horizontal pursuit movements in congenital nystagmus is now attributed by most investigators to a dynamic shift in the null zone induced by the moving stimulus.[52,74,82,129,169]

Vestibulo-ocular Reflex in Congenital Nystagmus

Many attempts to evaluate the vestibulo-ocular reflex (VOR) in subjects with congenital nystagmus have failed to successfully separate the slow-phase velocity associated with the underlying nystagmus from that due to the VOR itself.[83] Because of the superimposition of an ever-present and changing congenital nystagmus waveform on the eye movements resulting from the normal VOR, the measured responses do not resemble normal ones. Dell'Osso et al[83] have stressed that calculation of the VOR gain in congenital nystagmus must be limited to foveation periods (Figure 8.3). At any other point in the congenital nystagmus cycle (when there is neither target foveation nor clear vision due to the obligate retinal slip), the calculation of VOR gain is meaningless, both in the mathematical sense and as an indication of the performance of the VOR. Failure to recognize this interrelationship has led some to suggest that the VOR itself is deficient.[44,86,104] Others have recognized that the congenital nystagmus confounds the calculations of VOR gain and have concluded that the VOR was not deficient.[74, 119,122,169,289] Symptomatically, it is noteworthy that patients with congenital nystagmus rarely complain of oscillopsia or exhibit symptoms that normally accompany deficits in the VOR during ambulation.

FIGURE 8.3. Vestibulo-ocular reflex in congenital nystagmus. Note that during head movement, the nystagmus continues to be punctuated by foveation periods (middle tracing) during which the position of gaze remains steady. (From Dell'Osso LF, van der Steen J, Steinman RM, Collewijn H. Foveation dynamics in congenital nystagmus. III. vestibulo-ocular reflex. Doc Ophthalmol 1992;79:51-70.) Reprinted by permission of Kluwer Academic Publishers.

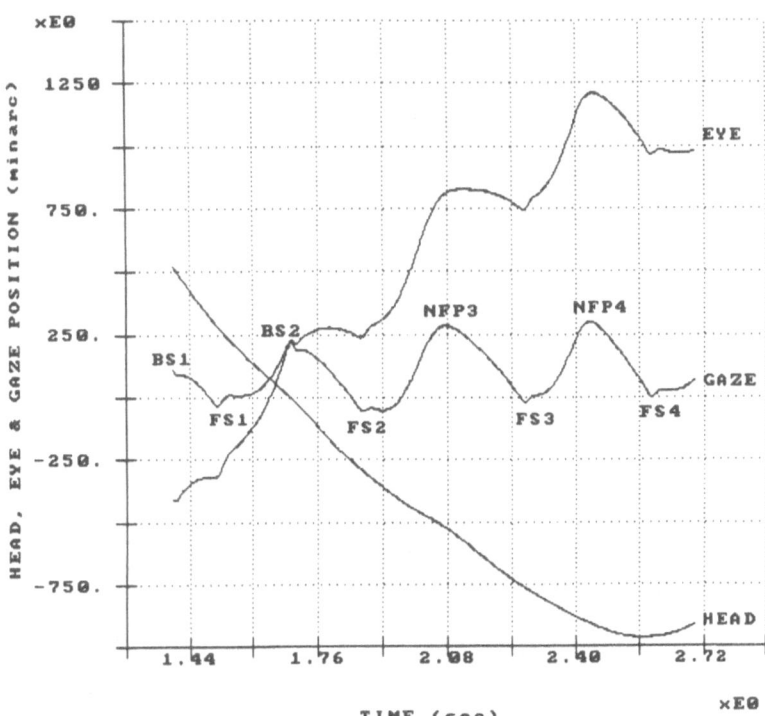

Saccadic System
in Congenital Nystagmus

Although visual feedback provides a means of sampling and assessing the accuracy of foveation periods in congenital nystagmus, a number of observations suggest that fast phases are not produced in response to a retinal displacement error signal between the fovea and the target image.[285] Worfolk and Abadi[285] have offered the following evidence to support this supposition:

1. Jerky congenital nystagmus can continue with the eyes closed.
2. Congenital nystagmus continues and its parameters remain unchanged as individuals track paracentral afterimages, suggesting that the timing and direction of the fast phases are not dependent on retinal feedback.[163]
3. In pendular congenital nystagmus with foveating saccades (Figure 8.1(B)), the retinal displacement error signal is opposite in sign to the forthcoming fast phase until approximately 70 milliseconds before the saccade, allowing insufficient time to program the quick phases using visual information.

The foregoing evidence suggests that the fast phases in congenital nystagmus are likely to be initiated on a predictive basis or in response to efference copy information.[285]

The peak fast-phase velocity in congenital nystagmus is reduced by approximately 10% with respect to normals.[6] This finding is consistent with the slightly reduced saccadic velocity in normals who are making saccades based upon nonvisual information rather than visually guided saccades[6] and further suggests that factors responsible for the fast phase in congenital nystagmus may include nonvisual elements.[6,163] To date, there is no evidence to suggest that congenital nystagmus either results from or involves an abnormality of saccadic velocity.[6]

Suppression of Oscillopsia
in Congenital Nystagmus

Several mechanisms have been proposed to account for the stability of the perceived world in the face of nearly constant motion across the retinas in individuals with congenital nystagmus. These include the notion of visual information sampling only during foveation periods with suppression at other times, use of an extraretinal signal to cancel out the visual effects of eye motion, central elevation of motion detection threshold, and postsaccadic backward masking of motion.[9] The suggestion that individuals with congenital nystagmus periodically sample their visual environment only during foveation periods with total suppression at all other times (i.e. "stroboscopic" vision) was a simplistic inference drawn from the observation that clear and stable vision was possible only during foveation periods and has been dispelled.[10]

Temporal modulation studies demonstrate that individuals with congenital nystagmus process retinal information continuously rather than selectively during foveation periods.[151,274] It is not surprising that congenital nystagmus patients have elevated motion detection thresholds when compared to normal patients with still eyes.[89] The fact that these individuals are unable to see their nystagmus in a mirror presumably results from the simultaneous movement of the mirror images with the eyes (retinal image stabilization) since these same individuals can recognize their nystagmus on a videotape. The observation that the vision is clearest during foveation periods when the eyes are relatively still and degraded during ocular movement is a normal physiological finding that should not be misconstrued as an a priori elevation in motion detection thresholds.

Bedell has found no evidence of decreased sensitivity to oscillatory target motion in patients with congenital nystagmus when comparing them to control patients viewing a target with sinusoidal or ramp motion to simulate the retinal image motion that occurs with retinal eye movements.[31] Based upon his experimental results, an abnormally low sensitivity to oscillatory target motion cannot be invoked to explain the absence of oscillopsia in individuals with congenital nystagmus. The fact that retinal image stabilization produces oscillopsia in individuals with congenital nystagmus suggests that an extraretinal signal (efference copy) may be used by the brain to cancel out the congenital nystagmus waveform.[163,174] Dell'Osso and coworkers[78,82] have demonstrated that individuals with congenital nystagmus also require well-defined, repeatable foveation periods from one cycle to the next to perceive a nonmoving visual world (Figure 8.4).[78,82] Perturbations in the congenital nystagmus cycle related to external or internal factors (e.g., head trauma, medications) can result in oscillopsia.[9] In one case oscillopsia was present only when the waveform failed to enter the foveation window[80]; in another, when the foveation period fell below a minimal duration.[9]

Summary of Ocular Stabilization Systems in Congenital Nystagmus

In examining how the ocular stabilization systems function in the setting of congenital nystagmus, one must confine the analysis to the foveation periods. It is during this portion of the congenital nystagmus waveform that the oscillation has subsided, vision is clear, and some degree of ocular stabilization is possible. Eye movement recordings and phase plane portraits in congenital nystagmus demonstrate the following:[38a]

1. The oscillations of congenital nystagmus supersede the ocular stabilization systems but do not extinguish them.
2. Amidst the ongoing oscillations of congenital nystagmus, these systems exert their primary influence on vision during foveation periods.
3. Defects in ocular stabilization are neither the cause nor the necessary result of congenital nystagmus.

Contrast Sensitivity and Pattern Detection Thresholds in Congenital Nystagmus

A reduction in contrast sensitivity for medium to high spatial frequency vision and increased pattern detection thresholds in congenital nystagmus impairs the detection of vertically oriented stationary and moving grating patterns more so than horizontal ones. The increased contrast sensitivity and pattern detection thresholds are secondary to the oscillation itself and improve when the congenital nystagmus oscillation is reduced.[1,2,3,4,88]

Cause of Congenital Nystagmus

Early theories regarding the cause of congenital nystagmus focused on the notion that the oscillation must result from an inherent abnormality in one of the ocular stabilization systems (i.e., the smooth pursuit system, the optokinetic system, the

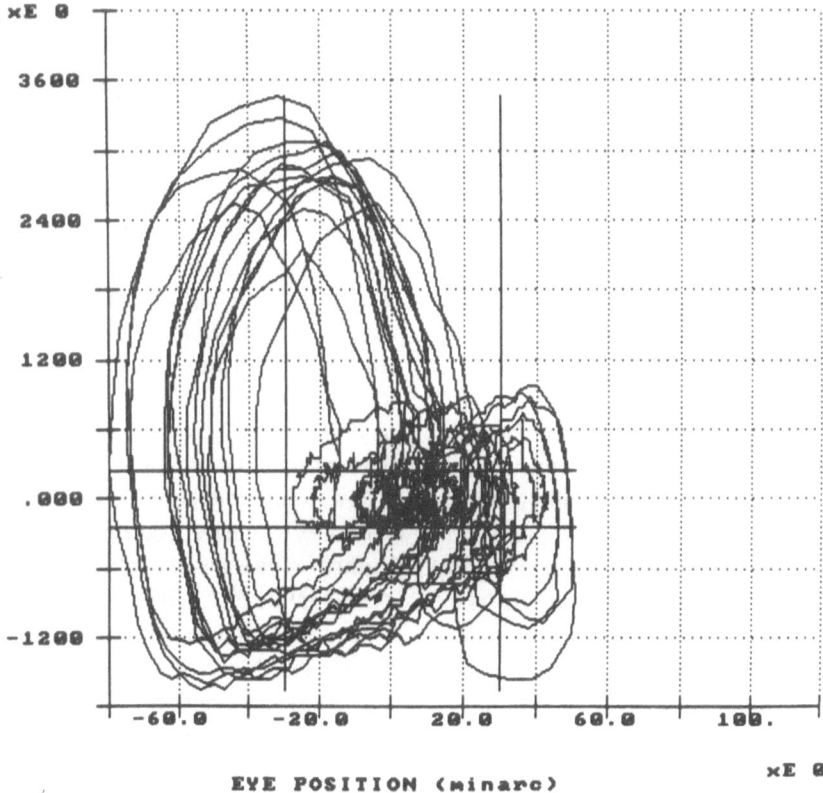

FIGURE 8.4. Phase plane portrait demonstrating multiple consecutive cycles in a patient with congenital nystagmus. This figure does not depict the trajectory of the eyes. Its purpose is to simultaneously display the position of the eye and the velocity of the eye at any point in the nystagmus cycle. By touching a line at any point with a pencil, the examiner can simultaneously assess the position and the velocity of the eyes at that point in time. Phase plane portraits are useful in understanding visual acuity and suppression of oscillopsia in congenital nystagmus. For good visual acuity, the eye position must simultaneously fall within 1/2° of the fovea (bracketed by vertical lines) and have a velocity of less than approximately 4° per second (bracketed by vertical lines). Time function is not linear along each tracing; relatively less time is spent in positions of high velocity, and more time is spent in positions of low velocity. Note the stereotyped appearance of each repetitive cycle, which appears to be a prerequisite for the suppression of oscillopsia. (From Dell'Osso LF, van der Steen J, Steinman RM, Collewijn H. Foveation dynamics in congenital nystagmus. I: fixation. Doc Ophthalmol 1992;79:1-23. Reprinted by permission of Kluwer Academic Publishers.)

VOR, or the fixation system). Over the last decade, however, the accumulated clinical and electro-oculographic evidence has refuted these hypotheses. Attempts to attribute the oscillation to a neuronal misdirection involving the retinogeniculate or subcortical visual pathways seem equally untenable, given the wide variety of visual disorders associated with congenital nystagmus in the absence of chiasmal misdirection and the absence of electrophysiological abnormalities in idiopathic congenital nystagmus. The recent finding of congenital nystagmus in achiasmatic dogs[281] further belies the hypothesis that abnormal contralateral projections of optic axons through the chiasm, as is seen in albinos, could be a neuroanatomical substrate for all congenital nystagmus. As succinctly stated by Kommerell, "The pathogenesis of congenital nystagmus is still an unresolved riddle."[163]

Visual Deficits Precipitating Congenital Nystagmus

Albinism

Albinism is not a single entity; it encompasses a heterogenous group of congenital hypomelanotic disorders.[5,160] These disorders can be divided into three general categories of regional hypopigmentation involving neuroectoderm (ocular albinism), neural crest (albinoidism), or both (oculocutaneous albinism).[139] In ocular albinism, there is hypopigmentation of ocular neuroectoderm (iris and retinal pigment epithelium) that manifests clinically with iris transillumination, macular hypoplasia, chorioretinal hypopigmentation, photophobia, and nystagmus. The term *albinoidism* is applied to a condition in which hypopigmentation is limited to tissues of neural crest origin (skin, hair, and iris stroma). Unlike patients with ocular albinism, those with albinoidism do not manifest macular hypoplasia, nystagmus, photophobia, or decreased vision.[139] In oculocutaneous albinism, there is diffuse hypopigmentation involving tissue of neuroectodermal and neural crest origin. Considerable clinical heterogeneity occurs within human albinos, as evidenced by the existence of at least 10 distinct forms of oculocutaneous albinism and four types of ocular albinism.[5]

The normal process of melanogenesis involves conversion of the amino acid tyrosine into melanin by the action of the enzyme tyrosinase.[5,160] In albinism, there appears to be an intracellular block of this metabolic pathway. Pigmentary dilution in oculocutaneous albinism is due to inadequate melanization of a normal number of melanosomes,[5] while in ocular albinism, it is due to an abnormally low number of mature ocular melanosomes.[213]

Individuals with mild ocular or oculocutaneous albinism are often misdiagnosed as having idiopathic congenital nystagmus.[246] The finding of subtle signs of ocular hypopigmentation in some congenital nystagmus patients with good vision has led to speculation that patients with idiopathic congenital nystagmus may actually be heterozygous for albinism. Simon et al have demonstrated that when patients with congenital nystagmus are carefully examined, many show iris transillumination, blunting of the macular reflex, and chorioretinal hypopigmentation consistent with albinism.[246] In evaluating the congenital nystagmus patient, it is critical to perform a careful slit lamp examination with the room lights turned off, the door closed, and a retro-illumination through a thin, axial light beam to detect basal iris transillumination. Varying degrees of macular hypoplasia (absence of the foveal pit, absence of macula lutea pigment, absence of normal macular pigment epithelial hyperpigmentation, and passage of retinal vessels through the fovea), together with other signs of ocular hypopigmentation, suggest the diagnosis of albinism. However, isolated foveal hypoplasia may also occur as a hereditary condition in children with normal pigmentation.[215] This finding should be sought in all children who seem to have idiopathic congenital nystagmus. Schatz and Pollock[233] have identified a characteristic optic disc appearance in albinos consisting of a small, cupless disc, with temporal entrance and situs inversus of the vessels, an oblique long axis of the disc (see Figure 8.2). It has been our observation that most infants with albinism also have gray optic discs and that the gray cast often disappears over the first few years of life.[37] Although some have contended that optic nerve hypoplasia is a component of albinism, electrophysiological and neuroimaging studies cast doubt on the validity of this purported association.[38]

The visual and auditory pathways in albinos have anomalous neuroanatomical connections that are similar in all types of animals studied.[5] Initially, the loss of a nonpigmentary function of tyrosinase was considered responsible for these neural defects, but work by Silver and Sapiro, and Strongin and Guillery has implicated the presence of melanin and the stage-specific lysis of melanosomes at the distal end of the developing optic stalk close to the optic disc as being vital for normal retinofugal axonal migration.[245,258]

Neuroanatomical and electrophysiological studies of albino visual pathways have demonstrated that retinogeniculate axons arising from ganglion cells in the portion of the temporal retina within 20° of the vertical meridian decussate abnormally in the optic chiasm to synapse in the contralateral lateral geniculate nucleus (Figure 8.5).[56,57,59,124–126,240] Apkarian et al have found that hemispheric VEPs provide the most sensitive and specific means by which to establish the diagnosis of albinism.[17]

FIGURE 8.5. Distribution of optic axons from nasal and temporal retina in the left eye (viewed from above) of an ocularly pigmented and albino human. In ocularly pigmented humans, the nasotemporal border corresponds with the fovea. In the human albino, the nasotemporal border is shifted approximately 20° into the temporal retina, resulting in a majority of retinal ganglion fibers crossing at the optic chiasm. (From Brodsky MC, Glasier CM, and Creel DJ. Magnetic resonance imaging of the human albino visual pathways. J Pediatr Ophthalmol Strabismus 1993;30:382-385, with permission.)

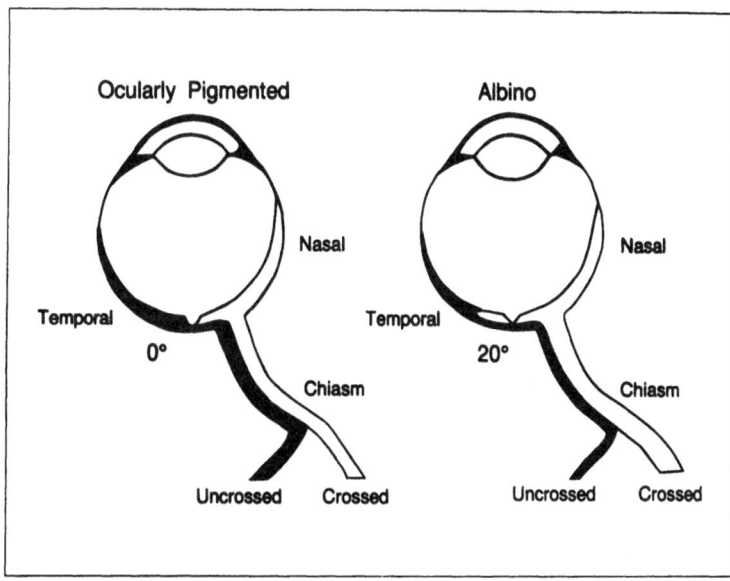

Other ocular and systemic hypopigmentation disorders should be considered in the differential diagnosis of albinism. Creel et al[58] have reported asymmetrical hemispheric VEPs in patients with Prader–Willi syndrome (a condition characterized by hypotonia, hypomentia, hypogonadism, and hyperphagia).[58] Albinism is seen in approximately 1% of patients with Prader–Willi syndrome.[176] In contradistinction, Apkarian et al found no evidence of hemispheric VEP asymmetry in the Prader–Willi syndrome but noted lateralization of the VEP response to the right or left hemisphere regardless of which eye was stimulated in half of their Prader–Willi patients.[19] Since both studies were carried out by highly experienced investigators, the discrepancy in findings may merely reflect the greater degree of albinism in the small group of patients tested by Creel et al.

Patients with oculocutaneous albinism, ocular albinism, Prader–Willi syndrome, and Angelman syndrome have been recently found to have mutations of the P gene, which has been mapped to 15 q11-q13.[176] The P gene codes for a polypeptide that appears to be an integral membrane protein with structural homology to transporters of amino acids, and it has been speculated that this gene might transport tyrosine (the precursor of melanin).[176] Interestingly, Prader–Willi syndrome is associated with deletions of the paternally inherited P gene, whereas Angelman syndrome (the happy puppet syndrome), which has an entirely

different phenotype, is associated with deletions of the maternally inherited P gene.[209] Differential expression of genetic material depending on the gender of the transmitting parent is referred to as *genomic imprinting.*

Aland Island eye disease (Forsius–Eriksson syndrome) is a form of ocular hypopigmentation associated with electroretinographic findings of CSNB.[109] Although it is classified as a form of ocular albinism, patients with this disorder do not manifest hemispheric VEP asymmetry. Waardenburg re-examined the original Finnish family with this disorder and found the multiple areas of focal fundus depigmentation in Aland Island eye disease to differ from the diffuse hypopigmentation of albinism.[109,272] Other ocular and systemic hypopigmentation disorders such as Waardenburg syndrome and phenylketonuria also lack the hemispheric VEP asymmetry seen in albinism.[166]

The consistent finding of asymmetrical hemispheric VEPs in human albinos provides an electrophysiological correlate to the neuroanatomical finding of abnormal decussation in animals. For example, a light or pattern stimulus to the albino's right eye would produce a signal of larger amplitude over the left occipital cortex than the right, due to the preponderance of crossing optic axons in albinos (Figure 8.6). This finding initially led to speculation that patients with idiopathic congenital nystagmus may too have afferent visual pathway miswiring as the neuroanatomical substrate

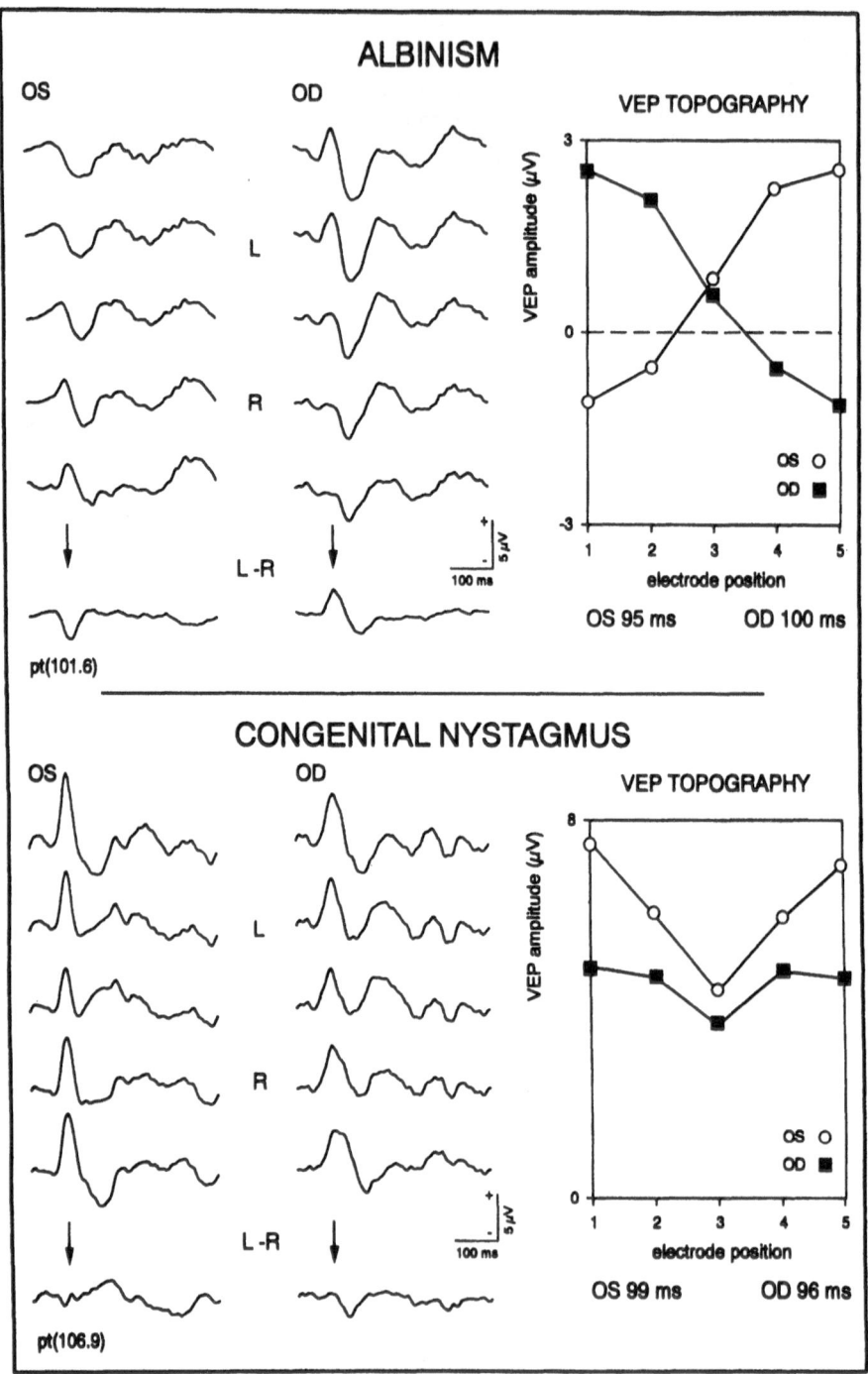

FIGURE 8.6. Hemispheric VEP asymmetry to pattern on-set responses in an adult albino (top), and absence of hemispheric VEP asymmetry in an adult with idiopathic congenital nystagmus (bottom). The five traces for each patient are derived from electrodes positioned from the left (trace 1) to right occiput (trace 5). The bottom trace is obtained by subtracting trace 4 (right) from trace 2 (left). Contralateral asymmetry in the upper figure is shown by the polarity reversal of the difference poten-tials (arrows) and by the crossover of the CI component measured at the time instant indicated and plotted as a function of electrode for OD and OS. VEP topography for the patient with congenital nystagmus shows a slight interocular amplitude difference and midline response attenuation. (From Apkarian and Shallo-Hoffman: VEP projections in congenital nystagmus; VEP asymmetry in albinism: a comparative study. Invest Ophthalmol Vis Sci 1991;32:2653-2661, with permission.)

for their nystagmus.[185] However, most studies have found that no electrophysiological evidence of afferent visual pathway misrouting in idiopathic congenital nystagmus.[21,127] The absence of hemispheric VEP asymmetry in patients with aniridia and macular hypoplasia further suggests that it is the ocular hypopigmentation rather than the associated macular hypoplasia in albinism that alters the trajectory of retinogeniculate axons.[166]

Shatz has performed neuroanatomical studies in albino (Siamese) cats and found an altered visual cortical topography and abnormal interhemispheric connections via the splenium of the corpus callosum.[240] Although albino cats demonstrated different targets for their visual callosal connections, the organization of fibers was similar to that seen in normally pigmented cats. Apkarian and Reits have demonstrated that, despite the paucity of binocularly driven cortical neurons in areas 17, 18, and 19 of the albino visual cortex, many patients with albinism retain global stereopsis.[18] We have examined the afferent visual pathways of human albinos using high-resolution MR imaging and found no structural abnormalities.[30] Although it has been suggested that nystagmus in albinism is the direct result of retinogeniculate and/or subcortical visual pathway misrouting, occasional patients with albinism and asymmetrical hemispheric VEPs show no nystagmus.[21] Furthermore, the nystagmus waveform is identical in idiopathic congenital nystagmus (in which there is no afferent visual pathway rerouting) and albinism, suggesting that it is the decreased vision associated with macular hypoplasia that is primarily responsible for congenital nystagmus in albinism.[21]

Apkarian has suggested a testing paradigm for full field monocular stimulation in the testing of hemispheric VEPs, consisting of a luminance flash stimulus in children younger than 3 years of age, both luminance flash and pattern onset for children between 3 and 6 years of age, and a pattern onset stimulus in older patients.[22] Pattern reversal VEP waveforms are not generally used to test for hemispheric VEPs since it has been shown that pattern reversal stimulation produces small VEPs in albinos compared to pattern-onset stimulation.[166,167] Confirmation of hemispheric VEPs in neonates can be obtained using special testing methods.[20]

Although periodic alternating nystagmus is said to be particularly common in albinism,[5,128,166]

this finding has heretofore eluded us in our albino patients. Abadi and Pascal claim to have found periodic alternating nystagmus in over 30% of their albino population.[5] Albino infants may rarely display seesaw nystagmus, which later reverts to horizontal nystagmus.[143]

In addition to retinogeniculate, cortical, and intracortical neural misrouting, albino animals have also been found to have misrouting of their subcortical visual pathways, which are intimately involved in optokinetic responses. This finding has led some to attribute the ocular instability in the albino rabbit to an abnormality in the opticokinetic pursuit system.[283] In the rabbit, retinal error signals reach the inferior olivary nucleus through the accessory optic tract independent of geniculocortical projections.[259] The nucleus of the optic tract plays an important role in mediating the opticokinetic response in rabbits. In the normal animal, opticokinetic mechanisms act as a negative feedback system using retinal motion as input. If the visual world (e.g., an optokinetic drum) is rotated about the animal, a smooth ocular rotation is reflexly elicited in the direction of drum rotation by the movement of the image of the visual world across the retina.[283] This negative feedback system normally acts to stabilize the eye with respect to the visual surroundings. If the "sign" of the signal flowing through the optokinetic system were to be inverted, there would be a positive feedback system that would then destabilize the eyes with respect to the visual surroundings (once the eye moves, it continues to move).[128,283] Such is the case in the albino rabbit, in which anomalous retinal innervation inverts the directional selectivity of those cells in the nucleus of the optic tract that have receptive fields in the temporal retina.[283]

The notion that misrouting of the accessory optic tract through the inferior olive is the cause of nystagmus in albino rabbits[51,181,182] has led to the inference that it may also cause congenital nystagmus in humans.[216] However, the existence of similar pathways have not been confirmed in humans.[128] More importantly, the frequent finding of congenital nystagmus in nonalbinos with no misrouting (who constitute the great majority of individuals with congenital nystagmus) makes it difficult to invoke a unique mechanism for the identical nystagmus in albinos.[82] Boylan and Harding have argued that congenital nystagmus in albinos is more likely attributable to poor central fixation due to lack of foveal differentiation but that afferent visual pathway miswiring might be related to the high prevalance of strabismus in albinos.[35]

Leber Congenital Amaurosis

Leber congenital amaurosis is an autosomal recessive rod–cone dystrophy characterized by congenital blindness, nystagmus, sluggish pupillary responses to light, and minimal retinal abnormalities in infancy. Affected patients may manifest roving eye movements or a large-amplitude, low-frequency nystagmus (in keeping with the low visual acuity).[147] Less commonly, the nystagmus may be upbeating, in which case it may be asymmetrical.[112] Pupillary responses are absent or sluggish. These infants characteristically demonstrate the "oculodigital" sign in which the thumbs or fists are habitually used to apply pressure to the closed eyes. Facial features of Leber congenital amaurosis may include enophthalmos (possibly from chronic eye rubbing) and maxillary hypoplasia. Unlike other congenital retinal dystrophies that are characterized by myopia, high hyperopia is seen in approximately half of patients with Leber congenital amaurosis. The diagnosis is established by a nonrecordable or highly attenuated ERG. Over time, retinal pigmentary abnormalities become evident and the optic discs become pale. Acquired retinal pigmentary abnormalities can range from a fine pigment granularity to diffuse marbleization of the fundus. Occasional infants with Leber congenital amaurosis will have bilateral staphylomatous macular lesions. Despite the fact that retinal pigmentary changes are acquired, the majority of patients do not experience progressive visual loss.[136]

Early studies noted a high incidence of mental retardation and neurological problems in Leber congenital amaurosis. It is likely that these studies included patients with a variety of primary neurometabolic and neurodegenerative diseases that would be more readily detected with modern diagnostic techniques. Although the great majority of children with Leber congenital amaurosis appear to be intellectually and neurologically normal, mental retardation, developmental delay, hearing loss, epilepsy, hypotonia, and cerebellar abnor-malities are seen in a small subset of patients. Leber congenital amaurosis is an autosomal recessive condition that is genetically heterogenous.

Achromatopsia

Achromatopsia is an autosomal recessive condition characterized by decreased visual acuity, absent color vision, photophobia, and nystagmus. Although histopathological studies have demonstrated conelike structures in the retina,[93,110,132] psychophysical studies have shown that the achromat has no functional cone vision.[239] Parents of a child with this condition typically give a history that the child shuns daylight and "comes to life when the twilight falls." The photophobia in children with achromatopsia may more accurately be designated as a light aversion (photodysphoria), since the children become debilitated when light bleaches their rods. Although children with this condition are unable to distinguish colors, many can identify basic colors based on hue discrimination. Children with achromatopsia frequently demonstrate a paradoxical pupillary phenomenon.[106]

Yee et al studied eye movement recordings in patients with achromatopsia and found a lower amplitude, higher frequency nystagmus than seen in congenital nystagmus.[289] Monocular optokinetic stimulation in achromats demonstrates marked directional asymmetry characterized by a higher gain during rotation of the drum in the temporal-nasal direction of the visual field than during the same rotation in the nasal-temporal direction.[25,289] Similar directional asymmetry is seen in afoveate animals. Additionally, achromats and afoveate animals also demonstrate a slow buildup of slow-phase optokinetic velocity during monocular optokinetic stimulation that is not seen in humans with congenital nystagmus.[25,289]

Gottlob and Reinecke[116] believe that patients with achromatopsia and blue cone monochromatism have a distinct form of nystagmus characterized by an oblique trajectory in younger patients, decreasing-velocity slow phases, oscillations of equal frequency that may be in phase or out of phase but retain equal frequencies, and head nodding. This constellation of findings may mimic spasmus nutans (discussed later).

The diagnosis of achromatopsia is established by electroretinography that shows normal rod function with absent cone function (absent flicker response). The dark adaptation curve is monophasic; achromats have no Purkinje shift, and spectral sensitivity studies show that rods mediate thresholds under both photopic and scotopic conditions.[212,239] In older children, the Sloan Achromatopsia test utilizes the superior ability of achromats over normals to match central hues with surrounding shades of gray on the basis of brightness.[207,212]

Although associated systemic findings are usually absent, a child with congenital achromatopsia with short stature, mild developmental delay, premature puberty, small hands and feet, minimal dysmorphism, and unilateral parental isodisomy of chromosome 14 has recently been described.[218]

Blue Cone Monochromatism

Blue cone monochromatism is a partial form of achromatopsia in which the blue cone mechanism predominates. The diagnosis is suggested by the presence of X-linked inheritance and high myopia in a child with achromatopsia.[276] In 1957, Blackwell and Blackwell first described this disorder in three brothers with congenital achromatopsia who had the residual ability to discriminate blue and yellow colored objects.[34] Lewis et al[177] have defined two classes of mutations localized to the long arm of the X chromosome (Xq28) which are responsible for blue cone monochromatism.[177,203]

These defects involve one or more regions of the contiguous red and green cone pigment genes on the terminal end of the long arm of the X-chromosome, causing affected individuals to have minimal functional red or green cone pigments.[203,204] Blue cone pigments, which are coded on chromosome 7, are unaffected.

Clinically, patients with blue cone monochromatism present with congenital nystagmus, although nystagmus is occasionally absent. Gottlob and Reinecke[116] believe that individuals with blue cone monochromatism and achromatopsia share an electro-oculographically distinct form of nystagmus (see *achromatopsia*). The finding of a fine-amplitude, upbeat, jerk-type nystagmus in carrier females with normal visual acuity raises the possibility that the nystagmus may be caused independently by the mutation in the absence of an underlying visual deficit.[117] Unlike in achromatopsia, in which visual acuity is usually no bet-

ter than 20/200, children with blue cone monochromatism (and other less-common forms of incomplete achromatopsia) often have acuities better than 20/200, indicating residual cone function.[276] Affected patients show a preferential ability to identify blue-yellow color plates. Farnsworth Panel D-15 tests show consistent errors directed along the protan and deutan axis but not the tritan axis, in contrast to the random pattern of errors seen in complete achromatopsia.[276] The long-term visual prognosis of blue cone monochromatism is paradoxically worse than that of complete achromatopsia, as teenagers and adults develop a progressive atrophic maculopathy that secondarily reduces central acuity.[98,204]

Electroretinography is useful in establishing the diagnosis of achromatopsia (minimal photopic response with preservation of scotopic response), but it does not separate out the blue cone response unless special techniques are used. Spectral sensitivity testing shows maximum sensitivity near 440 nm in the blue region, dropping rapidly at longer wavelengths.[276] The basis of the better acuities in children with blue cone monochromatism in comparison to those with complete achromatopsia is difficult to explain since psychophysical data suggests that the center of the normal fovea is tritanopic.[133] It is possible that functioning blue cones in the parafoveal region account for the slightly improved acuity. Some have suggested that the improved acuity results not from residual blue cone function but from retention of a lesser degree of additional residual red and green cone function,[276] since some blue cone monochromats have residual sensitivity to longer wavelengths,[249] as evidenced clinically by their ability to correctly identify some red-green color plates. The observed genetic heterogeneity in blue cone monochromatism could account for this observation.[204]

Congenital Stationary Night Blindness

Congenital stationary night blindness is characterized by night blindness, nystagmus, decreased visual acuity, and a normal retinal examination. Visual acuity can range from 20/20 to 20/200. High myopia is common, and affected children frequently have paradoxical pupillary responses to light.

Congenital stationary night blindness can be inherited in an autosomal dominant, autosomal recessive, or X-linked fashion, with X-linked inheritance being the most common pattern. Decreased visual acuity, myopia, and nystagmus are seen in X-linked CSNB and in some patients with autosomal recessive CSNB, but not in autosomal dominant CSNB.[139,207] In X-linked CSNB, visual acuity generally ranges from 20/30 to 20/100.[207] Congenitally tilted discs and optic disc pallor have been noted in some patients with X-linked CSNB.[135,139]

The diagnosis of CSNB is established by electroretinography. Most patients with the X-linked and autosomal recessive forms of CSNB have a near-normal a wave and a substantially reduced b wave (referred to as an *electronegative* ERG) when tested under dark-adapted bright-flash conditions (Schubert–Bornschein type). When the intensity of the test stimulus is increased, the amplitude of the a wave increases while that of the b wave remains unchanged. The photopic b wave may also be reduced, together with a characteristic loss of the early components of the oscillatory potentials, leading to a "squared-off" appearance to the photopic ERG a wave.[135,279]

Miyake has subdivided patients with CSNB and electronegative ERGs into complete or incomplete types. A particular type is consistently found within a given pedigree.[230] In the complete type, there is no electrophysiological evidence of rod function, while the incomplete type has some residual rod function.[109,195] In pedigrees with the autosomal dominant form of CSNB (Riggs type), the scotopic ERG is electropositive, and there is a reduced but normal-appearing photopic response that does not increase in amplitude under scotopic conditions,[210] although rare autosomal dominant pedigrees with electronegative ERGs have been reported.[134,210] Miyake et al[195] have attributed the Riggs-type response obtained in autosomal dominant pedigrees to the weaker stimulus used in earlier studies and demonstrated that a stronger intensity stimulus converts the Riggs-type response to an electronegative (Schubert–Bornschein) waveform. This finding has raised the possibility that the incomplete type of CSNB and the Riggs type may be the same clinical entity, although this has been disputed.[195,210] There is usually a monophasic dark adaptation curve in the X-linked and autosomal recessive forms, whereas a rod contribution is evident in the autoso-

mal dominant form, but the rod threshold is slowed and elevated. A tight genetic linkage between the complete form of X-linked CSNB and the Xp11.3 DNA marker, DXS7, has been established.[107,198] Recent linkage data support a similar Xp11.3 localization of incomplete CSNB.[199] No clear genetic localization has been defined in the autosomal dominant or recessive forms of CSNB.

No histologic abnormality of the retina in CSNB has been identified, and rhodopsin concentration and regeneration, as determined by retinal densitometry, is also normal.[279] Congenital stationary night blindness is believed to result from a selective defect in scotopic neurotransmission of the visual signal from the photoreceptors to the middle retinal neurons, possibly from the congenital absence or deficiency of a specific neurotransmitter required for the scotopic, rod-mediated vision.[228,279] An acquired form of night blindness with electronegative ERGs that are similar but not identical to those in CSNB can be seen as a paraneoplastic effect in patients with cutaneous malignant melanoma. Immunohistochemistry has demonstrated heavy immunostaining of rod bipolar cells in two patients with this condition.[190]

The combination of ocular hypopigmentation and an electronegative ERG may be seen in Forsius–Erickson syndrome (Aland Island eye disease). Aland Island eye disease is an X-linked disorder characterized by subnormal visual acuity, myopia, astigmatism, dyschromatopsia, night blindness, nystagmus, hypopigmentation of the iris and chorioretinal hypopigmentation, foveal hypoplasia, normal skin melanosomes, and an electronegative ERG.[219] Alitalo et al[14] have localized Aland Island disease to the pericentromeric region of the X chromosome.[14,109] Although this condition has been considered a form of ocular albinism, its nosology is open to question since affected patients do not have the hemispheric VEP asymmetry seen in ocular albinism.[266] Weleber et al have suggested that Aland Island eye disease and the incomplete form of CSNB may be the same disease.[279] Recent linkage data from patients with incomplete CSNB support this hypothesis.[199]

It has recently been recognized that approximately 80% of patients with Duchenne muscular dystrophy have electronegative ERGs that are similar to but distinguishable from those seen in CSNB.[48] Most affected patients have point mutations in the dystrophin gene. Unlike in CNSB, patients with muscular dystrophy are not myopic, photophobic, or nyctalopic, either clinically or by dark adaptation studies.[66] Visual acuity is generally unaffected, although many patients have increased macular pigmentation.[244] Fitzgerald et al were the first to localize the abnormal retinal signal transmission in Duchenne muscular dystrophy to the photoreceptor/depolarizing bipolar cell synapse.[97] Pillers et al have identified an additional subgroup of patients with muscular dystro-

phy, glycerol kinase deficiency, and adrenal hypoplasia that appears to be attributable to a contiguous gene syndrome that includes the muscular dystrophy gene. They have termed this disorder "Oregon Eye disease" and tentatively mapped the deletion to Xp21.[219]

Rarely, the nystagmus associated with CSNB can mimic spasmus nutans.[171] Lambert and Newman have therefore recommended that patients with spasmus nutans who are myopic undergo electroretinography to rule out CSNB.[171]

Figure 8.7 summarizes the electroretinographic features that distinguish the more common congenital retinal dystrophies.

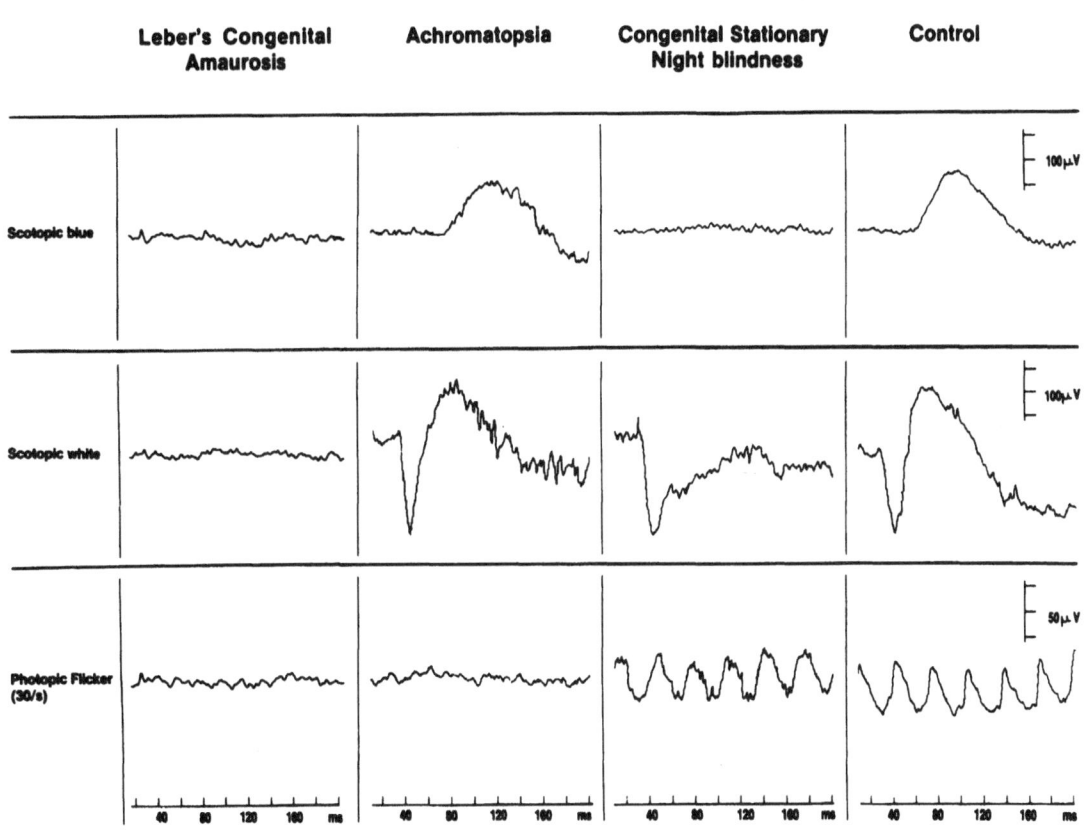

FIGURE 8.7. Comparison of ERG responses to scotopic blue, scotopic white, and photopic flicker (30/second) stimulation of a 3-year-old with Leber congenital amaurosis, a 5-year-old boy with X-linked incomplete achromatopsia, a 5-year-old boy with X-linked CSNB, and a 4- year-old normal control. ERG responses were recorded using corneal electrodes and a ganzfeld stimulator. (From Lambert SR, Taylor D, Kriss A. The infant with nystagmus, normal appearing fundi, but an abnormal ERG. Surv Ophthalmol 1989;34:173-186. With permission.)

Prognostic Value of Optokinetic Nystagmus Testing in Infants with Congenital Nystagmus

In children with relatively good vision, targets on a vertically moving optokinetic drum will elicit a vertical optokinetic nystagmus superimposed upon the child's ongoing horizontal nystagmus. When vision is poor, a vertical optokinetic response cannot be elicited. Long ago, Cogan pointed out the importance of eliciting vertical optokinetic nystagmus in prognosticating vision in the infant with congenital nystagmus.[49] The ability of a child to follow vertical optokinetic targets can be used to identify children who will be "mainstreamed" and educable in regular schools from those with severe visual impairment who will probably require visual aids and special services. Since infants with sensory nystagmus may have a superimposed delayed visual maturation within the first six months of life, it is important to wait until this age before conferring a poor visual prognosis on the child based upon absent vertical optokinetic responses.

When to Obtain Neuroimaging Studies in Children with Nystagmus

We have emphasized that it is a common mistake to obtain neuroimaging studies in a neurologically normal infant or child with congenital nystagmus since brain tumors and other compressive central nervous system (CNS) lesions generally do not cause congenital nystagmus. Nevertheless, there are three clinical situations in which neuroimaging is warranted:

1. In infants with congenital nystagmus and optic nerve hypoplasia, we obtain MR imaging to evaluate the structural status of the pituitary infundibulum, cerebral hemispheres, and midline intracranial structures (septum pellucidum, corpus callosum). Since it is understood that the nystagmus is sensory in nature (resulting from optic nerve hypoplasia), the purpose of neuroimaging is not to delineate the cause of the nystagmus, but rather to search for associated CNS anomalies that commonly coexist with optic nerve hypoplasia. It should be parenthetically noted that congenital suprasellar tumors (e.g., craniopharyngioma, chiasmal glioma)

can rarely disrupt optic axonal migration during embryogenesis and present with optic nerve hypoplasia, tilting of the optic discs, or other disc anomalies.[261] Routine MR imaging of infants with optic nerve hypoplasia insures that this rare association will not be overlooked.

2. We obtain MR imaging in any infant with congenital nystagmus and optic atrophy to rule out a congenital suprasellar tumor (chiasmal glioma, craniopharyngioma) or hydrocephalus. In our experience, there are few noncompressive causes of congenital or early infantile optic atrophy (see Chapter 4).

3. We routinely obtain MR imaging in children in whom the diagnosis of congenital nystagmus is uncertain and the possibility of spasmus nutans exists to rule out chiasmal gliomas or other suprasellar tumors.

Treatment of Congenital Nystagmus

Nonsurgical Treatment

Medical Treatment

Drug therapy for acquired nystagmus has been directed toward augmenting the inhibitory neurotransmitter system (e.g., gamma-amino-butyric acid (GABA)) or inhibiting the excitatory neurotransmitter system (e.g., glutamate).[45] Most notably, downbeat nystagmus has been treated successfully with clonazepam (a GABA-ergic inhibitor), and acquired periodic alternating nystagmus has been successfully treated with Baclofen (an inhibitor of glutamate release).

The pharmacological treatment of congenital nystagmus has met with limited success. One study noted objective improvement in visual acuity by one or two lines together with subjective improvement in four of seven congenital nystagmus patients who were treated with Baclofen.[290] Another study purported improved vision in two congenital nystagmus patients with 5-hydroxytryptophan therapy.[172] Given the well-documented visual improvement obtained by optical and surgical treatment of congenital nystagmus, drug therapy is not usually included in the therapeutic armamentarium for congenital nystagmus.[45]

Optical Treatment

Since congenital nystagmus is damped by physiological convergence, some authors have advocated incorporating base-out prisms into spectacle lenses to increase tonic convergence.[188] It is now widely accepted that base-out prisms can be incorporated into spectacle lenses to increase foveation time and to improve vision in congenital nystagmus.[80] However, glass prisms are thick and cumbersome, which reduces patient acceptance, especially in children. More recently, the value of biofeedback in reducing the intensity of congenital nystagmus and improving vision has been demonstrated in several independent studies.[4,11,61,189] Several forms of cutaneous stimulation (including acupuncture) are said to reduce congenital nystagmus. [77,144] Dell'Osso and coworkers have also demonstrated that congenital nystagmus is markedly reduced simply by placing contact lenses on the eyes,[76,231] as well as by cutaneous stimulation in the dermatome supplied by the ophthalmic division of the trigeminal nerve (e.g., tactile or vibrational stimulus applied to the forehead).[78]

Surgical Treatment of Congenital Nystagmus

Strabismus surgery in the treatment of congenital nystagmus falls into three general categories:

1. Surgery to eliminate torticollis,
2. Recession of the four horizontal rectus muscles to improve acuity, and
3. Artificial divergence surgery to improve visual acuity.

Surgery to Eliminate Torticollis

For the most part, treatment of congenital nystagmus has consisted of transferring the null position into primary gaze and thereby eliminating the prominent face turn in some patients with congenital nystagmus.[165] This is accomplished by performing a horizontal recess-resect procedure on both eyes (Kestenbaum–Andersen procedure), moving all four horizontal rectus muscles. For example, a child who assumes a right face turn to maintain the eyes in left gaze is treated with a left lateral rectus recession, left medial rectus resection, right medial rectus recession, and right lateral rectus resection to surgically rotate the eyes conjugately to the right and effectively transfer the null zone to primary gaze. The frequent recurrence of a face turn following an initally successful Kestenbaum–Andersen procedure has led to utilization of increasingly large recess-resect procedures. Even with "augmented" Kestenbaum–Andersen procedures, late regression continues to be a problem that limits long-term efficacy. Reports touting the efficacy of this procedure should therefore be interpreted with caution in the absence of long-term (several years) follow-up data.

Bagolini et al[24] have emphasized that large face turns should be conceptually distinguished from null positions; such patients utilize active blockage of nystagmus associated with increased innervational effort (similar to that seen with active convergence) to damp their nystagmus. Such patients may require supramaximal (11 to 13 mm) recessions of two yoke muscles that produce a horizontal gaze palsy to eliminate the face turn.

In addition to shifting the null zone, Dell'Osso and Flynn have shown that the Kestenbaum–Anderson procedure expands the null zone and improves visual acuity in some cases.[69] Serial electro-oculographic studies performed by Abadi and Whittle have demonstrated that the final face position following a Kestenbaum procedure does not always correspond precisely to the null zone, suggesting that other unrecognized factors influence the outcome.[7,8]

Rare patients with congenital nystagmus may assume a vertical head posture or a head tilt to achieve their null position. Vertical null positions can be eliminated with a recess-resect procedure of the vertical rectus muscles. (In a patient with a chin-down position, the inferior rectus muscles are resected, and the superior rectus muscles are recessed.) However, children with congenital nystagmus and vertical head positions may have unrecognized A or V patterns that cause them to assume a vertical head position to produce a large exophoria that allows them to converge and damp their nystagmus. It is therefore important to search carefully for an A or V pattern (which is difficult to detect in a child with nystagmus) before attributing a vertical head position to a vertical null position.

Head tilts resulting from torsional null positions are rare but well recognized in congenital nystagmus.[243] Head tilts resulting from a torsional null point can be treated by "torsional Kestenbaum procedures" that involve transposition of the vertical or horizontal rectus muscles or oblique muscle surgery to produce bilateral ocular torsion.[53,65,67, 253,270] In a child with a right head tilt, the goal of surgery would be to surgically induce clockwise torsion in both globes to induce a rightward environmental tilt that can only be compensated for by straightening the head.[271] The surgical aspects of "vertical Kestenbaum" and "torsional Kestenbaum" procedures are detailed in textbooks on strabismus surgery.

Recession of the Four Horizontal Rectus Muscles to Improve Acuity

Numerous authors have advocated simultaneous large recessions of four horizontal rectus muscles in the treatment of congenital nystagmus.[32, 137,267,270] In this procedure, the medial rectus muscles must be recessed less than the lateral rectus muscle to avoid postoperative exotropia. Although this procedure remains controversial,[99] results suggest that it generally improves acuity measurements by an average of one line and produces considerable subjective visual improvement without inducing oscillopsia or diplopia.[137] Because many early investigators recessed all four horizontal rectus muscles equally, which may have resulted in large exophorias, it is difficult to assess the degree to which any postoperative improvement resulted from an unintentional artificial divergence effect, as opposed to the recessions per se.

In evaluating the purported benefits of this procedure electro-oculographically, it should be recalled that increased foveation time (rather than decreased intensity of the nystagmus) is the fundamental correlate with acuity.

Artificial Divergence Surgery

Cüppers has advocated strabismus surgery in congenital nystagmus to diverge the eyes, requiring active convergence for fusion, which dampens the nystagmus.[62] In planning artificial divergence surgery, it is important to first confirm the presence of fusion and quantitate fusional convergence amplitudes by placing base-out prisms before the eyes. The goal of artificial divergence surgery is to produce a large exophoria that allows the patient to utilize fusional convergence and thereby damp the nystagmus. Overcorrection to exotropia negates any surgical benefit and requires reoperation to reduce the deviation in an attempt to convert the exotropia to an exophoria. Spielmann[255] has coined the term "pseudo-latent-congenital nystagmus" to describe the dramatic increase in congenital nystagmus intensity when convergence is blocked by monocular occlusion. This finding provides indirect evidence of active convergence in the binocular state and is therefore indicative of an ideal result following artificial divergence surgery.[254] Medical and surgical treatments of congenital nystagmus are summarized in Table 8.4.

Zubcov et al recently compared the efficacy of the artificial divergence procedure of Cüppers with the Kestenbaum–Andersen procedure in improving visual acuity. They found that a visual improvement of approximately one line is seen in approximately half of patients following either

TABLE 8.4. Treatment of congenital nystagmus.

Treatment to improve visual acuity
  Medical treatment
    1. Base-out prisms to induce convergence and dampen nystagmus
    2. Biofeedback to improve acuity during periods of attention or concentration
    3. Contact lenses
  Surgical treatment
    1. Cüppers divergence procedure to induce convergence and dampen nystagmus
    2. Large recession of four horizontal rectus muscles to reduce the intensity of nystagmus

Procedures to relocate the null zone to primary position
  Horizontal null zone
    1. Kestenbaum–Andersen procedure (recess-resect procedure of horizontal rectus muscles of both eyes)
  Vertical null zone
    1. Recess-resect procedure of four vertical rectus muscles
  Torsional null zone
    1. Horizontal transposition of vertical rectus muscles
    2. Vertical transposition of horizontal muscles (DeDecker procedure)
    3. Spielmann procedure: slanting of the insertion of the rectus muscles
    4. Recess-resect procedure of four oblique muscles

procedure and that combining the two procedures further improves vision.[300]

Spasmus Nutans

The term spasmus nutans (Latin: nodding spasm) refers to the constellation of nystagmus, head nodding, and torticollis. Although the term "acquired nystagmus" has been applied to spasmus nutans as a differentiating feature from congenital nystagmus, it should be remembered that congenital nystagmus is also "acquired," albeit usually earlier in infancy. Unlike congenital nystagmus, which becomes apparent between 8 and 12 weeks of age, the age of onset in spasmus nutans is generally quoted as 6 to 12 months of age,[217] although cases with onset ranging from 2 weeks to 3 years of age have been documented.[211] Spasmus nutans remits spontaneously, usually within 1 to 2 years of onset, but may rarely persist for up to 8 years.[175,211] It resolves with no lasting effect on vision,[191] except in the rare cases in which a markedly asymmetrical nystagmus leads to amblyopia.

Spasmus nutans appears as an extraordinarily fine and rapid nystagmus that has been likened to an ocular quiver.[141,211] It is usually horizontal in direction but may also be vertical or rotary.[140] It is often described as an intermittent nystagmus that is asymmetrical in appearance and occasionally monocular.[115,277] A key clinical electro-oculographic observation is the variable phase difference between the two eyes, which is reflected clinically as an asymmetry in the oscillations between the two eyes.[277] On lateral gaze, the dissociation may increase, with nystagmus of the abducting eye predominating.[211]

Some case series suggest an increased prevalence of esotropia in spasmus nutans,[211] although such children may have actually had manifest latent nystagmus associated with congenital esotropia (discussed later). In contradistinction to congenital nystagmus, visual acuity is minimally affected in spasmus nutans. Spasmus nutans is more common in black children and has been reported in several sets of identical twins.[96,138,140,141,156]

The head nodding associated with spasmus nutans is a combination of true (anteroposterior) head nodding together with a lateral shaking of the head in an unpredictable pattern.[140,257] The head nodding is of lower frequency than the nystagmus[115] and becomes prominent when the child attempts to inspect something of interest. It disappears during sleep but may persist when the child is lying down.[140] Since some children with congenital nystagmus also have head nodding, this finding alone cannot be used to confirm the diagnosis of spasmus nutans in the child with nystagmus. Earlier controversy surrounding the issue of whether associated head nodding in spasmus nutans is compensatory (i.e., performed for the purpose of improving vision) or an involuntary movement of pathologic origin similar to the nystagmus itself is now resolved. Gresty and coworkers examined patients with spasmus nutans in whom head nodding abolished the nystagmus, and a normal VOR stabilized the eyes during head movements.[118–120] These authors were the first to demonstrate electro-oculographically that the head nodding in spasmus nutans is an adaptive behavior that serves to improve visual acuity by suppressing the nystagmus, rather than a separate pathological phenomenon.[118–120] Eye movement recordings from these patients demonstrated that the head nodding in spasmus nutans functions to abolish the nystagmus through some mechanism independent of the vestibulo-ocular response.[121] Gottlob et al recently confirmed and refined these conclusions in a large number of patients with spasmus nutans using electro-oculographic recordings.[115] In their patients, the head nodding changed the spasmus nutans waveform from a fine, pendular, dissociated nystagmus of high frequency to a larger slower waveform that is symmetrical between the two eyes (Figure 8.8). There is now general agreement that head nodding in spasmus nutans is compensatory.

The head tilt in spasmus nutans is a variable finding that is present in less than half of cases. Although the reason for the associated head tilt is unclear, Gottlob et al have suggested that it may serve to directionalize the head nodding to its optimal trajectory.[115] Although early authors stated that the head nodding was the first sign of spasmus nutans to appear and the last to resolve, it is now generally agreed that the nystagmus is the most constant feature of spasmus nutans and that it probably precedes the head nodding, although the

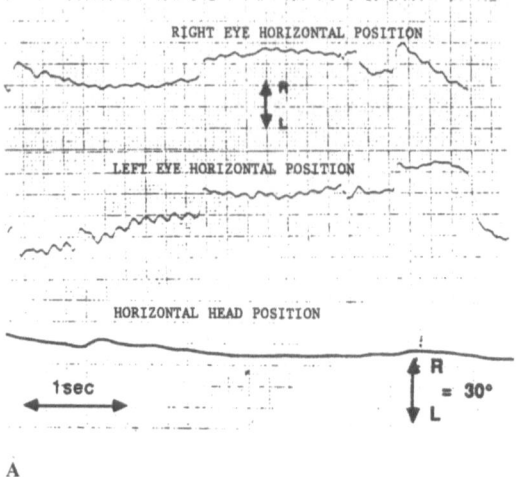

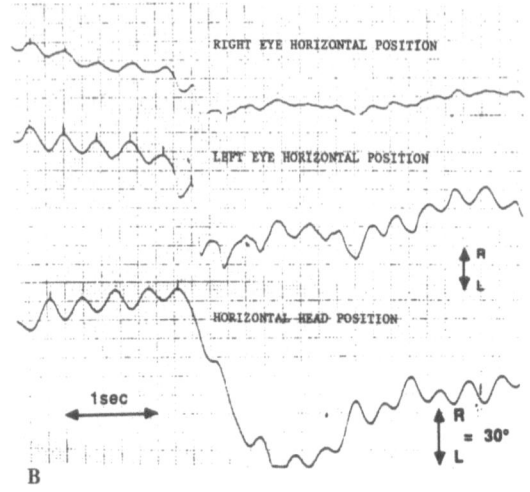

FIGURE 8.8. Eye movement recording from a child with spasmus nutans. (A) When the head is still, the eyes oscillate disconjugately and rapidly. (B) During periods of head nodding, the eyes oscillate conjugately and oppo- sitely to the head, resulting in a steady gaze that is con- jugate in space. (From Gottlob et al. Head nodding is compensatory in spasmus nutans. Published courtesy of Ophthalmology 1992;99:1024-1031.)

head nodding may be the abnormality that first at- tracts attention.[175,191] The clinical characteristics of spasmus nutans are summarized in Table 8.5.

Weissman found persistence of the nystagmus in some of their patients, and Gottlob et al found persistence of nystagmus on electro-oculographic recordings in all patients who had clinical resolu- tion of the condition, suggesting that the nystag- mus diminishes to a subclinical level but does not entirely resolve.[115,277]

Early reports considered spasmus nutans to be pathogenetically related to diverse causes that in- cluded light deprivation, dietary factors, season, rickets, epilepsy, autoarousal, and poor socio-eco- nomic conditions.[60,96,152,217,224,257,277] Hermann noted a strong predisposition for the onset of spas- mus nutans to occur during the winter months, with 70% of cases having their onset during December, January, and February.[138] In 1897, Raudnitz[224] published the classical description of spasmus nu- tans in which he collated previously reported cases with 15 cases of his own. He emphasized the fact that virtually all of his patients belonged to a cer- tain dark quarter of Prague. When this district was later sanitized, no further cases of spasmus nutans developed.[217] Raudnitz viewed darkness as the pri- mary etiologic factor, speculating that the eyes of affected children were somehow damaged by the "irritant effect" of insufficient light during a critical period of fixation development. According to the translation by Osterberg, Raudnitz believed that "efforts at fixing resulted in erratic movements of the eye as certain ganglion cells cannot settle down till the eyes are satisfactorily focused, incidents will still be asserting themselves, they extend into larger areas of innervation, and head-nystagmus etc. are brought about secondarily."[217] Raudnitz noted that pups who were reared in total darkness for several months developed eye nystagmus and head nystag- mus.[224] Still attributed spasmus nutans to "an index of nervous instability" associated with rickets and with "confinement in a closed, ill-ventilated room" and directed therapy toward remediating these problems.[257]

TABLE 8.5. Clinical findings in spasmus nutans.

Rapid, small amplitude, "ocular shiver"
Variable phase in nystagmus of both eyes
Horizontal, vertical, or oblique
Intermittent, asymmetrical, or monocular
Head nodding
Variable head tilt
Onset between 6 months and 1 year of age
Visual acuity normal or nearly so
Spontaneously resolves over months to years

For a century, numerous reports emphasized that spasmus nutans was a visually and systemically benign and self-limited clinical entity.[140,211] Since 1967, however, many infants with spasmus nutans have been found to have congenital suprasellar tumors (most commonly chiasmal gliomas).[90] (In retrospect, it seems likely that some children with spasmus nutans who were felt to have either rickets or malnutrition might have harbored suprasellar tumors and would currently be classified as having the Russell diencephalic syndrome, discussed below.) While there is no longer any question that congenital suprasellar tumors can produce a constellation of neuro-ophthalmologic signs that are clinically and electro-oculographically indistinguishable from spasmus nutans,[13,94,114,157] it is curious that this association went largely unnoticed for over a century of observation.

Based upon these previous reports, we advocate MR imaging in all children in whom the diagnosis of spasmus nutans is being entertained. Although King et al have emphasized that the absence of afferent pupillary defects, optic atrophy, or papilledema in spasmus nutans is reassuring and makes the possibility of chiasmal glioma less likely,[159] children with chiasmal gliomas and paradigmatic findings of spasmus nutans without pupillary or optic nerve abnormalities have been reported, demonstrating that the absence of these abnormalities does not totally preclude an underlying neoplasm.[16,161,208] With MR imaging now readily available at most institutions, it would seem prudent to resist the temptation to "play the odds." The systemic findings of hydrocephalus, café au lait spots, or other physical findings of neurofibromatosis increase the relative likelihood that an infant with spasmus nutans may harbor a chiasmal/hypothalamic glioma.

Neurodegenerative disorders such as Pelizaeus–Merzbacher disease and Leigh disease may produce nystagmus and head nodding that are indistinguishable from spasmus nutans.[23,238] These disorders should be suspected in children with clinical signs of ataxia or developmental delay or with MR evidence of white matter signal abnormalities. Achromatopsia and CSNB can also masquerade as spasmus nutans. However, the findings of photophobia and decreased vision in achromatopsia, and night blindness with myopia in

CSNB, should suggest an underlying congenital retinal dystrophy.[116,171]

The fact that rare infants with spasmus nutans are later found to have congenital retinal dystrophies or neurodegenerative disease, has led some authorities to conclude that spasmus nutans is a diagnosis that can only be made in retrospect once the nystagmus has resolved.[46,150,263] In our experience, the clinical appearance of the nystagmus, together with the absence of decreased vision or other signs or symptoms of a congenital retinal dystrophy, allows us to assign the diagnosis of spasmus nutans and order MR imaging on the initial visit.

After a century of observation and conjecture, the pathogenesis and neuroanatomical substrate of this self-limiting form of transient vertical disconjugate nystagmus are still unknown.[277]

Russell Diencephalic Syndrome

An infant with congenital chiasmal/hypothalamic glioma is often brought to medical attention because of weight loss and failure to thrive after a period of normal growth.[173] Russell diencephalic syndrome refers to the constellation of emaciation, hyperactivity, and euphoria.[54] Radiological examination shows an almost complete absence of subcutaneous fat in the extremities.[54] Affected infants often display a euphoria and affectionate spontaneity that contrasts strikingly with their profound emaciation[54,192] (Figure 8.9(A)). Minor features of the syndrome include skin pallor despite a normal hemoglobin, hypotension, hypoglycemia, and an alert appearance that has been attributed to Collier sign. Neuro-ophthalmologic examination may reveal spasmus nutans or see-saw nystagmus, with a variable degree of optic atrophy.[54]

The great majority of children with Russell diencephalic syndrome have been found to have chiasmal/hypothalamic glioma (Figure 8.9(B)). Children with the diencephalic syndrome usually have elevated growth hormone levels that may be an important factor in causing emaciation despite adequate food intake. Infantile diencephalic gliomas appear to be unusually radiosensitive, with a return to normal weight gain and normal growth hormone levels following treatment in many patients.[202] Burr found an average survival time in tients.[42] The natural history of the Russell diencephalic syndrome following radiation therapy is extremely variable,[54] however, with survival of up to 12 years being documented.[54,202]

Monocular Nystagmus

In 1956, Cogan stated that spasmus nutans is the most common if not the only cause of unilateral horizontal nystagmus in infancy.[49] With the added caveat that chiasmal gliomas can present with paradigmatic spasmus nutans,[90] this generalization still applies to the majority of infants with monocular nystagmus (Table 8.6). Rarely, severe unilateral visual loss can cause a slow, unilateral horizontal peculiar nystagmus in the affected eye.[37,113]

In the second decade of life, a monocular vertical oscillation may develop in an eye with reduced vision (20/200 or less) of long duration (the Heimann–Bielschowsky phenomenon). Yee et al described the vertical drift with monocular visual loss as small-amplitude, low-frequency pendular and accentuated by refixation or eccentric gaze.[288] Smith et al subsequently described this oscillation as large in amplitude and low in frequency.[248] Pritchard et al attempted to reconcile these two views by demonstrating that some patients have small rapid oscillations superimposed upon larger oscillations of lower frequency.[222] There is some suggestion that the amplitude of the larger waveform may correlate with the duration of visual loss.[222] In our experience, most affected patients display a slow-velocity and large-amplitude oscillation that makes it easily distinguishable from other forms of nystagmus.

Episodic monocular nystagmus can also be a rare manifestation of epilepsy.[145]

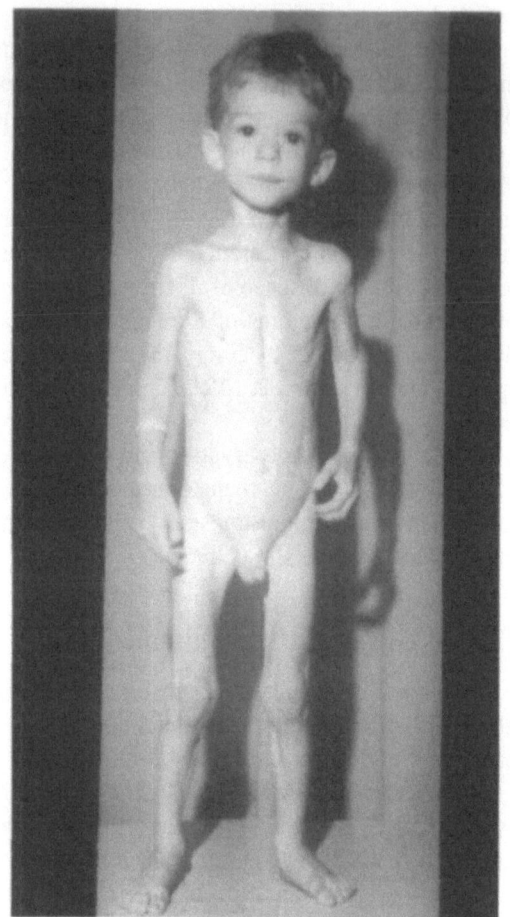
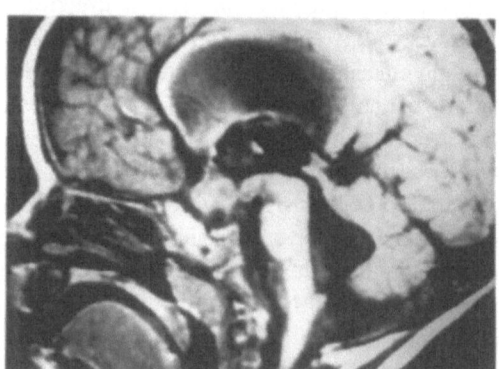

FIGURE 8.9. (A) Two-year-old boy with thalamic glioma and Russell diencephalic syndrome. (Courtesy of William F. Hoyt, M.D.) (B) MR scan demonstrating chiasmal glioma and hydrocephalus in a child with Russell diencephalic syndrome. (Courtesy of Neil R. Miller, M.D.)

TABLE 8.6. Monocular nystagmus in children.

Infants and young children
Spasmus nutans
Chiasmal/hypothalamic glioma
Congenital unilateral visual loss
Teenage years
Heimann–Bielschowsky phenomenon

untreated patients averaging 12.3 months compared to at least 25 months in the treated pa-

Nystagmus Associated with Congenital Esotropia

Rotary Nystagmus

Children with congenital esotropia often display a subtle conjugate rotary nystagmus that lacks a horizontal component and therefore does not resemble congenital nystagmus. These conjugate ocular rotations do not have any recognized clinical or prognostic significance.

Manifest Latent Nystagmus

Latent nystagmus refers to a bilateral conjugate horizontal jerk nystagmus that occurs when either eye is occluded. It is most commonly seen in children with a history of congenital esotropia. In latent nystagmus, the nasally-directed slow phase in the fixating eye is followed by a temporally-directed corrective saccade. The amplitude of latent nystagmus increases when the fixating eye is moved into abduction and decreases in adduction. Unlike congenital nystagmus, latent nystagmus obeys Alexander's law (which states that, in patients with peripheral vestibular nystagmus, the amplitude of the jerk nystagmus increases in the direction of the fast phase and decreases but never reverses in the direction of the slow phase). The fact that manifest latent nystagmus obeys Alexander's law suggests that it may be tied into the same circuitry as peripheral vestibular nystagmus.[229]

The finding of latent nystagmus correlates with the finding of nasotemporal disparity when a monocularly occluded child follows horizontal optokinetic targets. Nasotemporal disparity refers to the clinical finding of normal nasally directed optokinetic responses and impaired temporally directed optokinetic responses under conditions of monocular viewing (clinical optokinetic testing evokes a pursuit response rather than a true optokinetic response). It is thought to reflect the effect of the immature visual motion processing system (which has a nasal pursuit bias) on the smooth pursuit movements.[264,265] The extrastriate motion processing system is localized to the dorsal parieto-occipital pathways that extend from the primary visual area to the extrastriate middle temporal visual area (MT). It receives its major inputs from the magnocellular neurons in the geniculate body.

Nasotemporal pursuit disparity is normal in infants until approximately 22 weeks of age.[200] Absence of binocularity (usually in congenital esotropia) during this critical period leads to retention of nasal pursuit bias that manifests clinically as nasotemporal disparity and latent nystagmus. Since nasotemporal disparity is always present in patients with latent nystagmus, the nasal slow-phase drift of latent nystagmus is the clinical manifestation of a nasal pursuit bias. Although nasotemporal disparity is usually observed in the setting of congenital esotropia, it may occur with other forms of early infantile strabismus as well. In older children with a history of strabismus, the finding of nasotemporal disparity confirms that the eyes were misaligned within the first year of life.

Manifest latent nystagmus can be viewed as a latent nystagmus that is made manifest by amblyopia or strabismus. In manifest latent nystagmus, the brain suppresses one eye, which causes it to be physiologically "occluded." Under such circumstances, both eyes develop a small-amplitude conjugate horizontal jerk nystagmus that increases when the fixating eye moves toward abduction and decreases when the fixating eye is in adduction. Affected children assume a face turn to place the fixating eye in adduction and thereby dampen the nystagmus (Table 8.7). The association between manifest latent nystagmus and congenital esotropia and a face turn has also been given the eponym of *Ciancia syndrome*.

A rotary component is occasionally seen in children with otherwise typical manifest latent nystagmus. It is possible that this may represent a rotary component of dissociated vertical deviation that, like latent nystagmus, often accompanies congenital esotropia.[70] In contradistinction to congenital

TABLE 8.7. Manifest latent nystagmus.

Small-amplitude, horizontal jerk nystagmus
Fast phase to the right when left eye occluded; fast phase to the left when right eye occluded
Increases in abduction, dampens in adduction of the fixating eye
Face turn to fixate in adduction with the preferred eye
May improve or resolve with treatment of amblyopia or strabismus

nystagmus, eye movement recordings in manifest latent nystagmus show a rapid slip off the fovea following refixation saccades (referred to as a decreasing-velocity or decreasing-exponential waveform) (Figure 8.10). Dell'Osso has recently demonstrated that some patients with manifest latent nystagmus will develop a strategy of making a saccade beyond the target, thereby allowing the decreasing-velocity tail of the waveform to provide foveation.[84] This adaptive strategy serves to transfer the slow component of the drift onto the fovea, which probably accounts for the good visual acuity in these children.

Manifest latent nystagmus may be mistaken for acquired nystagmus since it may not become clinically apparent for several years. Affected children may be subjected to an extensive neurological workup if the associated ocular findings are not recognized. The characteristic clinical finding is that manifest latent nystagmus changes direction when the eyes are alternately occluded (i.e. it is right-beating when the left eye is occluded and left-beating when the right eye is occluded). Although this clinical finding is highly suggestive of manifest latent nystagmus, it can also reflect congenital nystagmus with a latent component.

In the child with congenital esotropia, latent nystagmus, and alternating fixation, the manifest latent nystagmus may superficially resemble periodic alternating nystagmus.[131] Some patients with latent nystagmus can induce a manifest latent nystagmus by simply imagining that one eye is occluded. Bright illumination in one eye will often have a similar effect to occlusion and cause a latent nystagmus to become manifest.[247] Rare patients have been reported to release and suppress latent nystagmus at will.[164]

In addition to occurring in patients with congenital esotropia and amblyopia, manifest latent nystagmus is a common manifestation in infants with congenital unilateral visual loss resulting from microphthalmos, congenital cataract, or optic disc anomalies.[47,178] These infants develop a face turn toward the good eye (i.e., an infant with left mi-

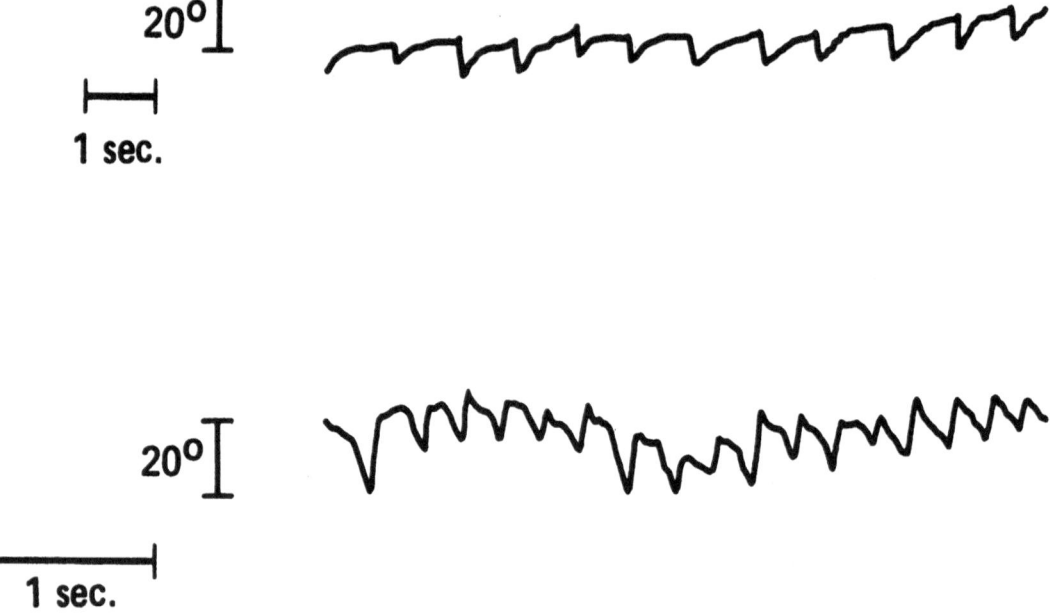

FIGURE 8.10. Comparison of eye movement recordings (position tracings) in manifest latent nystagmus and congenital nystagmus. An upward deflection corresponds to a rightward eye movement. In manifest latent nystagmus (top) each leftward fast phase is followed by a decreasing-velocity drift off the target with no intervening foveation period. In congenital nystagmus (bottom), each rightward fast phase is followed by a foveation period before the eyes drift off the target in an increasing-velocity slow phase. (From von Noorden et al. Compensatory mechanisms in congenital nystagmus. Am J Ophthalmol 1987;103:87-89. Published with permission from The American Journal of Ophthalmology. Copyright by the Ophthalmic Publishing Company.)

crophthalmos will take a right face turn to dampen the nystagmus in the right eye by keeping it positioned in adduction). Parents may misinterpret this phenomenon and believe that the child is turning his face to view objects with his bad eye. Infants with congenital unilateral visual loss also tend to develop a sensory esotropia. Adults who develop manifest latent nystagmus occasionally note oscillopsia.[178]

Treatment of Manifest Latent Nystagmus

Manifest latent nystagmus should be viewed as a treatable form of nystagmus. Zubcov et al have shown that either successful occlusion therapy or surgical realignment of the eyes will diminish the intensity of manifest latent nystagmus.[299] It is a common misconception that occlusion therapy is futile or even contraindicated in patients with amblyopia and latent nystagmus.[268] Some authors have advocated optical or atropine penalization for amblyopia treatment in patients with latent nystagmus. It is now well established, however, that occlusion therapy is effective in patients with latent nystagmus.[268] Simonsz and Kommerell have demonstrated that the slow-phase speed of latent nystagmus in the amblyopic eye diminishes over 2 to 3 days during prolonged occlusion of the better eye and that the slow-phase speed in the better eye increases by a commensurate amount.[247] They caution that early visual improvement during occlusion therapy probably reflects an occlusion-induced short-term change in the nystagmus waveform rather than true sensory visual improvement.

Since manifest latent nystagmus often occurs in the setting of congenital esotropia with superimposed amblyopia, it is not surprising that treatment of the underlying conditions can convert a manifest-latent nystagmus to a latent nystagmus (i.e., eliminate the manifest component).[298] Children who have manifest-latent nystagmus associated with unilateral congenital visual loss (unilateral microphthalmos, congenital cataract, or optic disc anomalies) may require a large recession of the medial rectus muscle of the adducted eye to transfer the null zone into primary position and eliminate the sensory esotropia.[146,252] Jampolsky has cautioned that, in this particular situation, it is often necessary to perform additional recessions of the medial and lateral rectus muscles of the

normal contralateral eye to eliminate horizontal incomitance.[146] Adults with congenital blindness in one eye and large face turns associated with manifest-latent nystagmus may benefit from oculinum injection into the medial rectus muscle of the fixating eye or from a recess-resect procedure of the fixating eye to simultaneously eliminate the face turn and the large esotropia.[178]

Nystagmus Blockage Syndrome

The nystagmus blockage syndrome is a rare variant of congenital nystagmus. It is characterized by an intermittent horizontal nystagmus accompanied by a large-angle, variable esotropia. The following three clinical characteristics typify the nystagmus blockage syndrome:

1. The esotropia increases as the nystagmus dampens and decreases as the intensity of the nystagmus increases.
2. The esotropia disappears or markedly diminishes when one eye is occluded and the fixating eye is moved into abduction.
3. The angle of esotropia increases when prisms are placed before the eyes to neutralize the deviation.

The child with nystagmus blockage syndrome invokes excessive convergence to dampen an underlying congenital nystagmus or convert it to a low-amplitude manifest latent nystagmus by a purposive esotropia and improve acuity.[72] During periods of convergence, pupillary constriction may or may not be observed, suggesting that some children have the ability to partially dissociate accommodation from convergence, which would predispose to nystagmus blockage syndrome by making it a visually beneficial adaptive strategy. When viewing objects of interest, children with nystagmus blockage syndrome display tonic convergence that may simulate a bilateral sixth nerve palsy. Fixation with the adducted eye necessitates a face turn toward the fixating eye to view objects that are in primary position.[75] An alternating face turn may signify alternating fixation during periods of esotropia. Many children with nystagmus blockage syndrome eventually develop a constant esotropia, suggesting that a progressive medial rectus contracture gradually develops.

Treatment of Nystagmus Blockage Syndrome

Nystagmus blockage syndrome can be successfully treated with strabismus surgery that consists of bilateral medial rectus posterior fixation sutures (if the eyes are straight during periods of relaxation) or bimedial recessions with posterior fixation sutures (if a superimposed esodeviation develops).

Vertical Nystagmus

Neuroimaging is warranted to rule out a posterior fossa lesion in children with acquired vertical nystagmus. When the onset of vertical nystagmus is noted within the first three months of life, neuroimaging studies are frequently normal. In this, context, upbeating and downbeating nystagmus in infancy are each associated with a distinct clinical profile and visual prognosis.

Upbeating Nystagmus in Infancy

Unlike upbeating nystagmus in adulthood, which is associated with a structural lesion involving the brain stem or cerebellum, upbeating nystagmus in infancy is usually associated with anterior visual pathway disease.[112,143] Good et al[112] found anterior pathway disease in 11 children who presented with upbeating nystagmus in infancy. The underlying diagnosis included Leber congenital amaurosis (seven cases), optic nerve hypoplasia (two cases), aniridia (one case), and congenital cataracts (one case). Upbeating nystagmus in infancy may be asymmetrical and may convert to a horizontal nystagmus within the first two years of life.[112] In the absence of structural CNS abnormalities on neuroimaging studies and no structural ocular abnormalities, electroretinography should be performed to rule out a congenital retinal dystrophy.

If electroretinography is also negative, the diagnosis of hereditary vertical nystagmus should be considered (discussed later).[155,184,250] The positive family history and good visual acuity in patients with familial upbeating nystagmus readily distinguishes it from infantile upbeating nystagmus associated with anterior visual pathway disease.[112]

Downbeat Nystagmus

In any child with downbeat nystagmus, MR imaging should be obtained to rule out an underlying CNS malformation at the level of the craniocervical junction, such as Arnold–Chiari malformation, basilar impression, platybasia, syringobulbia, and Klippel–Feil anomaly.[235] In many of these conditions, the downbeat nystagmus results from compression of the herniated cerebellum against the caudal brain stem rather than an intrinsic abnormality of the ocular motor pathways, as demonstrated by the clinical improvement that often follows surgical decompression.[26,235]

Downbeat nystagmus in infancy is rare. The infant with downbeat nystagmus and negative neuroimaging is likely to have a benign familial form of downbeat nystagmus characterized by the following constellation of findings: (1) a chin-down position, (2) some degree of ataxia and imbalance when learning to walk, (3) resolution of the nystagmus and head position over the first two years of life, and (4) a first-degree relative with a history of a chin-down position in infancy that resolved.[33] A parent may also show subtle evidence of central vestibular imbalance (gaze-evoked nystagmus, subtle, downbeating nystagmus on oblique gaze downward).[33] Unlike acquired hereditary forms of downbeat nystagmus that may have their onset in childhood and may be harbingers of spinocerebellar degeneration, congenital hereditary downbeating nystagmus seems to impart a benign neurological prognosis. Eye movement recordings have demonstrated a linear slow-wave configuration, unlike the increasing exponential waveform considered classic for congenital nystagmus. In contradistinction to the anterior visual pathway disease that frequently underlies upbeating nystagmus, patients with transient familial downbeating nystagmus of infancy have good vision once the nystagmus resolves.

Benign familial downbeat nystagmus of infancy probably results from an imbalance in central vestibular tone that is gradually compensated. Infants with familial tonic upgaze have a similar constellation of findings, suggesting that it may share a similar pathogenesis.[43]

Hereditary Vertical Nystagmus

Several families have been described with vertical pendular (or occasionally upbeating) nystagmus, cerebellar ataxia, and negative neuroimaging studies.[155,184] In one report, the cerebellar findings were progressive, suggesting that these patients had a hereditary, cerebellar degeneration.[155] Hereditary vertical nystagmus can rarely occur as an intermittent phenomenon.[250]

Periodic Alternating Nystagmus

A subgroup of patients with congenital nystagmus will be found on prolonged observation to have a reversal in the direction of their nystagmus at approximately 2-minute intervals. As the nystagmus finishes one half cycle (e.g., right-beating nystagmus), there is a brief transition period in which upbeating nystagmus, downbeating nystagmus, or square wave jerks may be seen before the next half cycle (e.g., left-beating nystagmus) commences.[175] Careful examination usually shows that the nystagmus is actually *aperiodic* in that one phase generally predominates. It is also common for the duration of each phase of the cycle to vary from one cycle to the next. It is important (and often difficult) to distinguish periodic alternating nystagmus from congenital nystagmus with "double torticollis," in which two separate horizontal null points exist, and the patient randomly utilizes one or the other. Although Kalyanaranman reported three siblings who had periodic alternating nystagmus with associated head nodding as part of a cerebrocerebellar degeneration,[152] structural CNS lesions are rarely seen in congenital periodic alternating nystagmus, and the underlying pathophysiology remains elusive.

Acquired periodic alternating nystagmus is usually seen in older children or adults but may present in early childhood. Causes of acquired periodic alternating nystagmus include multiple sclerosis, posterior fossa lesions, encephalitis, otitis media, syphilis, aqueductal stenosis, and Arnold–Chiari malformation.[131] Unlike congenital periodic alternating nystagmus, acquired periodic alternating nystagmus is usually associated with structural lesions involving the cerebellum or its central connections. Reports of acquired periodic alternating nystagmus following visual loss (e.g., vitreous hemorrhage or cataract) and its disappearance with restoration of vision provide an important clue to the underlying pathophysiology.[149]

Animal experiments combined with additional data in humans suggest that acquired periodic alternating nystagmus probably requires concurrent CNS dysfunction at two separate levels. The nodulus and uvula of the cerebellum are believed to control post-rotational nystagmus, which is prolonged following ablation. Periodic alternating nystagmus can be produced in animals following ablation of these structures if visual deprivation is superimposed. It is believed that normal vestibular repair mechanisms act to reverse the direction of the nystagmus. Under normal circumstances, the oscillations of periodic alternating nystagmus would be blocked by visual fixation, smooth pursuit, and optokinetic mechanisms. When these visual stabilization systems are held in abeyance (as a result of either visual deprivation with concurrent disease of the cerebellar flocculus), the acquired form of periodic alternating nystagmus develops. It has been suggested that patients who acquire periodic alternating nystagmus following loss of vision may be harboring a congenital lesion of the brain stem or cerebellum that is clinically silent until there is a reduction in retinal input.[128]

Pharmacological evidence suggests that the nodulus and uvula maintain inhibitory control on the vestibular rotational responses via the inhibitory neurotransmitter GABA.[45] Halmagyi et al[130] were the first to report the successful treatment of the acquired form of periodic alternating nystagmus with the GABA-ergic drug Baclofen. The finding that acquired periodic alternating nystagmus is abolished by Baclofen, both in humans and in animals following ablation of the nodulus and uvula, further supports this pathogenetic mechanism in acquired period alternating nystagmus. Although congenital periodic alternating nystagmus is reportedly refractory to Baclofen, occasional patients improve with treatment.[45]

Seesaw Nystagmus

Seesaw nystagmus is an uncommon form of pendular nystagmus characterized by simultaneous elevation and intorsion of one eye with depression and extorsion of the other eye, followed by a reversal of the cycle.[63,175] Seesaw nystagmus usually occurs in patients with large suprasellar tumors involving the optic chiasm and extending into the third ventricle. These children usually have a bitemporal hemianopia.[63] Less commonly, focal lesions confined to the rostral mesencephalon may produce seesaw nystagmus in conjunction with other brain stem ocular motility disorders. Mild seesaw nystagmus is easily misinterpreted as rotary nystagmus if the vertical component of the nystagmus is overlooked.

Congenital seesaw nystagmus can rarely be seen in infants with albinism and other sensory visual disorders who later convert to a horizontal nystagmus.[143] It has been noted that congenital forms of seesaw nystagmus may lack the torsional components or even show the opposite pattern (i.e., extorsion with elevation and intorsion with depression).[63,234] Zelt and Biglan have stressed that the direction of cyclodeviation of the globes on vertical excursion cannot be relied upon to clinically differentiate the congenital from the acquired form of seesaw nystagmus.[297]

Seesaw nystagmus characteristically increases in bright light and dampens with accommodation or convergence.[297] Acquired seesaw nystagmus in children is most commonly caused by craniopharyngioma and other parasellar tumors but may also be seen with other neurological conditions (hydrocephalus, acute febrile illness), trauma, and rarely with congenital retinal dystrophies,[297] septo-optic dysplasia,[64] Arnold–Chiari malformation,[297] and syringobulbia.[95] Strabismus, most commonly exotropia, is frequent in children with seesaw nystagmus.[91,297]

Although it is accepted that seesaw nystagmus can be an ominous neuro-ophthalmologic sign and that it often correlates with the presence of a suprasellar mass lesion, the precise neuroanatomical site of injury remains speculative. The two major theories of causation center around abnormal ocular motor output and anomalous visual sensory input. The motor theory states that large parasellar lesions compress the adjacent diencephalon and compress, injure, or disrupt the adjacent interstitial nucleus of Cajal. Discrete lesions involving the interstitial nucleus of Cajal at the junction of the rostral midbrain and diencephalon have been described in two patients with seesaw nystagmus.[154,223] Furthermore, it is known that stimulation of the interstitial nucleus of Cajal in the monkey produces an ocular tilt reaction consisting of extorsion and depression of the eye on the stimulated side and intorsion and elevation of the other eye, which is similar to a half cycle of seesaw nystagmus.[280]

The sensory hypothesis of Nakada and Kwee purports that chiasmal lesions disrupt subcortical pathways that carry signals from the inferior olive and cerebellar flocculus which may normally be used for adaptive control of vestibular responses.[201] According to this hypothesis, associated bitemporal

hemianopia alters retinal error signals that reach the inferior olivary nucleus through two discrete pathways independent of the geniculocortical projections.[259] Retinal error signals in the inferior olivary nucleus and their connections with Purkinje cells in the cerebellum are utilized for vestibulo-ocular reflex adaptation, which renders the visuovestibular control system unstable,[201] while the pursuit system is unaffected. Nakada and Kwee have speculated that integrity of the inferior-olivary nodulus connections in seesaw nystagmus could explain the 180° phase difference that distinguishes it from the midline form of oculopalatal myoclonus, where these connections are disrupted.[201]

Williams et al have recently reported seesaw nystagmus in combination with congenital nystagmus in a strain of achiasmatic dogs.[281] Apkarian et al[22a] recently described two unrelated children with congenital achiasmia who had see-saw nystagmus. These observations suggest that chiasmal anomalies alone can cause seesaw nystagmus.

Alcohol,[102] Baclofen,[45] and Clonazepam[45] have been reported to abolish seesaw nystagmus.

Saccadic Oscillations that Simulate Nystagmus

Convergence-Retraction Nystagmus

Convergence-retraction "nystagmus" is a disorder in which attempted upward saccades evoke repetitive, simultaneous saccadic contractions of all rectus muscles, producing a series of rapid, jerky convergent movements with associated retraction of the globes.[175] It is seen almost exclusively in the setting of dorsal midbrain syndrome, which is characterized by impaired upgaze, upper lid retraction (Collier sign), pupillary dilation with light-near dissociation, and impairment of either convergence or divergence.[175] Infants with dorsal midbrain syndrome from congenital hydrocephalus may display the "setting sun" sign in which upper lid retraction and an upgaze palsy occur together with tonic downward deviation of the eyes. Convergence-retraction nystagmus is best elicited by having a child follow downward-moving optokinetic targets that necessitate repetitive upward saccades. It may be overlooked if only vertical pursuit movements are examined.

The invariable association of convergence-retraction nystagmus with dorsal midbrain syndrome (which results from a lesion of the posterior commissure) gives it strong localizing value to the dorsal mesencephalon. Dorsal midbrain syndrome in infancy suggests the diagnosis of aqueductal stenosis, while its recurrence in children who have had a ventriculoperitoneal shunt placed for hydrocephalus usually signifies shunt failure.[55] The onset of dorsal midbrain syndrome in an older child is suggestive of pineal tumor. Midbrain vascular malformations or traumatic injury may also cause dorsal midbrain syndrome in childhood.[175,263] We have observed convergence-retraction nystagmus as the presenting sign of Leigh disease in a 4-year-old boy, and Plange has documented a similar case.[220]

Opsoclonus

Opsoclonus is a rare but striking ocular motility disorder characterized by involuntary, chaotic bursts of multidirectional, high-amplitude saccades, without an intersaccadic interval.[241] When purely horizontal, such oscillations are termed ocular flutter.[175] Opsoclonus differs from nystagmus in that the oscillations are saccadic and not rhythmical and consist of long silent periods punctuated by intermittent bursts of activity.

Childhood opsoclonus forebodes a different set of diseases than adult opsoclonus. Hoyt et al have reported that opsoclonus may occur as a transient phenomenon in healthy neonates.[142] Acquired opsoclonus in infancy or preschool years necessitates a workup for neuroblastoma. Altman and Baehner have reported that the finding of opsoclonus in a child with neuroblastoma imparts a favorable prognosis for survival.[15] Musarella et al found a 100% 3-year survival rate in children with neuroblastoma who presented with opsoclonus, compared with 78.6% in those who presented with Horner syndrome and 11.2% in those with orbital metastasis.[197] Improved survival in the subgroup with opsoclonus could not be accounted for by earlier diagnosis or a higher percentage of low-staged cases. It has been hypothesized that the opsoclonus myoclonus in these patients may be pathogenetically related either to a peptide produced by the tumor directly causing myoclonus and opsoclonus, or to an immunological cross-reactivity between the tumor and normal cerebellar neurons, with persistent anticerebellar antibodies being produced long after the tumor is removed.[15,194,197]

Opsoclonus may also occur as part of a "benign" encephalitis (Kinsbourne's myoclonic encephalopathy, dancing eyes and dancing feet).[194] In affected patients, vertigo and truncal ataxia follow a prodrome of malaise and fever. Cerebellar and long-tract signs accompany shivering movements of the head and body. Along with the constantly changing, often forceful myoclonic jerking of the extremities and trunk (polymyoclonia), there are shocklike torsions of the head and neck as well as opsoclonus.[206] Spinal fluid protein may be elevated. Although the illness usually resolves over weeks to months, the clinical course may be protracted and recovery incomplete. Recent findings of small neuroblastomas or ganglioneuroblastomas in children with the chronic form of myoclonic encephalopathy have led some investigators to suggest that myoclonic encephalopathy may reflect the presence of an indolent neural crest tumor that was previously impossible to identify without high-resolution CT scanning or MR imaging.[194] This theory is compatible with the finding that several neuroblastic tumors in infancy tend to regress or mature into tissue with benign neural crest cells.[36] Many children fail to improve neurologically following resection of the tumor and develop a chronic ataxic syndrome that worsens with minor febrile illnesses and is associated with chronic symptoms of delayed speech and motor development.[194] The favorable response to steroid treatment suggests possible immunologic mechanisms, although an autoimmune pathogenesis has yet to be proven.[241] Isolated reports suggest that Clonazepam and Propranolol may occasionally be effective in the treatment of this disorder.[45,175]

Opsoclonus has less commonly been attributed to exposure to toxins or drugs, systemic disease, trauma, meningitis, hydrocephalus, and intracranial tumors. Although opsoclonus has a fairly characteristic clinical appearance, Leigh and Zee have alluded to inherent uncertainty in diagnosing opsoclonus without eye movement recordings since it is impossible to ascertain the pattern of back-to-back saccades with no intersaccadic interval by mere clinical observation.[175]

The anatomical localization of the abnormality underlying opsoclonus is unknown.[241] Early findings of abnormal cerebellar Purkinje cells led to the supposition that opsoclonus resulted from cerebellar dysfunction.[92] The clinical observation that opsoclonus regresses through phases of flutter and dysmetria lends credence to this hypothesis.[232] The subsequent discovery of burst neurons (that are active immediately prior to saccades and carry information specifying the parameter of the imminent saccade) and pause neurons (that function to inhibit burst neurons which generate saccades) led Zee and Robinson to hypothesize that disorders that selectively impair pause cell function could lead to opsoclonus.[296] Pause cells lie in the nucleus raphe interpositus, which is located in the midline between rootlets of the abducens nerves. They discharge continuously except immediately prior to and during saccades, when they pause. They pause either before eye movements in a specific direction (directional pause neurons) or before eye movements in all directions (omnipause neurons). Their function is to inhibit saccades. However, an autopsy study of opsoclonus patients showed no abnormalities in the pontine region where pause cells are located.[227] Patients who display MR signal abnormalities in the pontine tegmental raphe (where pause cells are located) demonstrate gaze palsies or internuclear ophthalmoplegia with slowing of saccades rather than opsoclonus.[39] Likewise, experimentally induced lesions of the pause cell region in monkeys have produced slow saccades rather than opsoclonus, although some areas of burst cells may have also been affected.[153] It is possible that pause cell dysfunction could result from metabolic or neurotransmitter abnormalities in the absence of a discrete lesion or visible histopathological changes.[227]

It has also been suggested that any input driving the burst cells could also inhibit the pause cells via inhibitory burst neurons, thereby resulting in opsoclonus.[175,237,241] Shawkat et al have demonstrated overshoot dysmetria on eye movement recordings of patients with opsoclonus who had no concurrent abnormalities of smooth pursuit, optokinetic nystagmus, or VOR. They suggested that these findings are compatible with a lesion of affecting the cerebellar fastigial nuclei that spares the flocculus and paraflocculus.[241]

Voluntary Nystagmus

The diagnosis of voluntary "nystagmus" should be considered in any child who appears to have ocular flutter or opsoclonus. Voluntary nystagmus is usually brought on by a strong convergence effort that causes the patient to display a strained facial expression, mild widening of the palpebral fissures, and occasional fluttering of the eyelids. Voluntary nystagmus appears as an extremely fine-amplitude rapid, conjugate, horizontal oscillation that resembles an ocular shiver. The strong convergence effort necessary to evoke the oscillation usually dissipates after 20 to 30 seconds, after which the facial appearance normalizes. The inability to sustain the oscillation provides a clue to the diagnosis. The ability to generate voluntary ocular tremor appears to be familial in some instances. Rare cases of voluntary vertical nystagmus have also been reported.[168]

Eye movement recordings have shown that, unlike true nystagmus, voluntary "nystagmus" consists of a series of back-to-back horizontal saccades with no intersaccadic interval (Figure 8.11).[242] Electro-oculographically, this oscillation is indistinguishable from opsoclonus.

Neurological Nystagmus

The term *neurological nystagmus,* which has been used to describe pediatric nystagmus associated with neurodegenerative disorders, is somewhat ambiguous since all nystagmus is fundamentally neurological in origin. As is clear from the preceding discussion, some of the rarer forms of nystagmus (spasmus nutans, monocular nystagmus, seesaw nystagmus, convergence-retraction nystagmus) should be recognized as ominous neuro-ophthalmological signs as they often portend intracranial lesions at specific neuroanatomical sites. These forms of nystagmus are readily distinguishable from congenital nystagmus by their clinical appearance.

Neurodegenerative disease may occasionally produce a horizontal nystagmus in infancy prior to the development of other neurological signs.[46, 179,282,291,292] In our experience, it is not uncommon for infants with neurodegenerative disease to be initially diagnosed as having congenital nystagmus, only to have the diagnosis amended as developmental delay, hypotonia, seizures, or other neu-

FIGURE 8.11. Electro-oculographic recording of voluntary "nystagmus" demonstrating that it consists of a series of back-to-back saccades with no intersaccadic intervals. The same electro-oculographic pattern is seen in opsoclonus. (From Shults WT, Stark L, Hoyt WF, et al. Normal saccadic structure of voluntary nystagmus. Arch Ophthalmol 1977;95: 1399-1404. Copyright 1977, American Medical Association.)

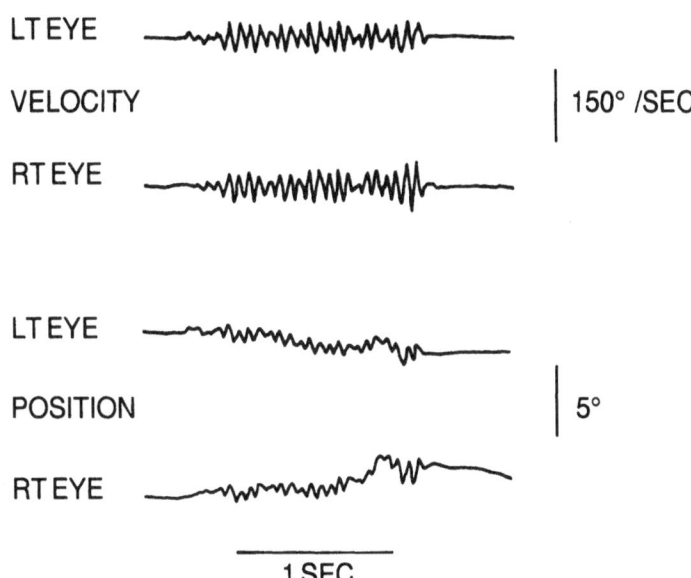

rological problems supervene. The prevalence of children with neurodegenerative congenital nystagmus in our pediatric patient population is less than 5%. By contrast, retrospective neurological reviews that purport a high prevalence of neurodevelopmental delay in "nonhereditary congenital nystagmus"[147,256] probably draw from neurological pediatric populations biased toward these disorders.

The clinical overlap between congenital nystagmus and the horizontal pendular nystagmus associated with neurological disease should not be misconstrued as an indication for neuroimaging in infants with paradigmatic congenital nystagmus, since neuroimaging is rarely helpful early in the course of a neurodegenerative disorder if no other neurological signs are apparent.

The neurodegenerative disorders discussed below are particularly prone to cause nystagmus.

Leigh Subacute Necrotizing Encephalomyelopathy

Leigh disease is an autosomal recessive mitochondrial disorder leading to progressive neurological degeneration in infancy or childhood. Its onset is usually heralded by the insidious development of psychomotor retardation and brain stem and cerebellar dysfunction resulting in ataxia, dystonia, and nystagmus. Limb weakness and optic atrophy are often noted. T2-weighted MR imaging in Leigh disease shows characteristic symmetrical hyperintense lesions involving the basal ganglia and brain stem with predominant involvement of the putamen.[187] Patients with Leigh disease usually have metabolic acidosis with elevated lactate and pyruvate concentrations in the blood and CSF, suggesting that a disorder of pyruvate metabolism may be the primary biochemical defect. Specific mitochondrial enzyme deficiencies associated with Leigh disease have been reported to include pyruvate carboxylase deficiency, pyruvate dehydrogenase complex defects, and cytochrome c oxidase deficiency.[187] Current evidence suggests that a nuclear DNA-encoded factor is responsible for the mitochondrial enzyme deficiencies in Leigh disease.[193]

Nystagmus, ophthalmoplegia and optic atrophy are the predominant neuro-ophthalmologic findings in Leigh disease. In addition to nystagmus of virtually any type, children with Leigh disease can manifest with a variety of brain stem ocular motility deficits including dorsal midbrain syndrome,[220] internuclear ophthalmoplegia, and horizontal gaze palsy. Leigh disease can also produce nystagmus and head nodding and thereby mimic spasmus nutans.[238]

Pelizaeus-Merzbacher Disease

Pelizaeus-Merzbacher disease is an X-linked recessive leukodystrophy with a fairly characteristic clinical picture.[12] It often presents in infancy with abnormal tremulous movements of the eyes and intermittent shaking movements of the head that may simulate spasmus nutans.[12,23,183] Electro-oculography shows a distinctive combination of elliptical pendular and upbeat nystagmus which has not been described in other neurodegenerative diseases.[263a] These early findings are followed by loss of developmental milestones, choreiform and athetoid movements, severe cerebellar signs and difficulty initiating saccades. Seizures, pyramidal signs, and spasticity appear later. Standing and talking are not possible, and some infants do not even develop head control.[12] By contrast, intellectual function is often preserved until the terminal stages of the disease. The MR imaging shows lack of myelination without frank evidence of white matter destruction.[27] The presumptive clinical diagnosis is confirmed on postmortem examination that shows a diffuse, patchy, "tiger-stripe" demyelination throughout the brain.

Joubert Syndrome

Joubert syndrome comprises the triad of congenital retinal dystrophy, episodic panting tachypnea, and variable absence of the cerebellar vermis.[158] Affected infants also exhibit profound developmental delay and hypotonia.[170] The congenital retinal dystrophy in Joubert syndrome was initially classified as Leber congenital amaurosis.[196] Unlike Leber congenital amaurosis, however, Joubert syndrome is associated with good visual acuity (visual acuity may be as high as 20/60) and relatively preserved VEPs.[170]

The nystagmus in Joubert syndrome may consist of a torsional pendular nystagmus or a seesaw nystagmus.[170] Alternating hyperdeviation of the eyes, tonic deviation of the eyes laterally, periodic alternating gaze deviation,[131] and abnormal saccadic movements (decreased velocity, hypometria, increased latency) have also been described.[170,196] Children may have congenital ocular motor apraxia and utilize head thrusts to view objects of interest in the lateral visual field.[170,196] The important role of the cerebellar vermis in stabilizing saccades suggests that the severe vermal hypoplasia must significantly contribute to the complex ocular motility dysfunction seen in this condition.

Haltia-Santivouri Syndrome

This congenital form of ceroid lipofucsinosis differs from acquired forms in that poor vision, nystagmus, and retinal lesions are present early in the course of the disease. Death usually ensues by 2 years of age.

Infantile Neuroaxonal Dystrophy

Infantile neuroaxonal dystrophy is an autosomal recessive neurodegenerative disorder with onset within the first or second year of life.[260] Clinically, affected children show difficulty walking, psychomotor regression, marked hypotonia, muscular atrophy, pyramidal tract signs, and optic atrophy progressing to blindness.[260] The MR imaging demonstrates marked cerebellar atrophy with a striking diffuse hyperintensity of the cerebellar cortex on T2-weighted imaging that is probably secondary to extensive gliosis and shrinkage of the cerebellar cortex.[260] The basic metabolic defect is unknown. The diagnosis can be established by skin, nerve, conjunctiva, or muscle biopsy that shows large dystrophic axons (spheroids).[284] Children with infantile neuroaxonal dystrophy may have a pendular nystagmus that is clinically indistinguishable from congenital nystagmus.[225]

Systemic Disorders Associated with Nystagmus in Children

Down Syndrome

Nystagmus is seen in 30% of patients with Down syndrome. While a visual sensory etiology (e.g., congenital cataract, high myopia) is occasionally present, many children with Down syndrome and nystagmus have no visually significant ocular disease.[273] Patients with Down syndrome may display a fine rapid horizontal nystagmus. Less commonly, a dissociated pendular nystagmus or a manifest latent nystagmus may be seen. Most children with Down syndrome and nystagmus have associated esotropia.[273]

Hypothyroidism

Approximately 10% of children with hypothyroidism are reported to have a high-frequency, low-amplitude nystagmus.[180] Strabismus, most commonly esotropia, is seen in approximately half of hypothyroid

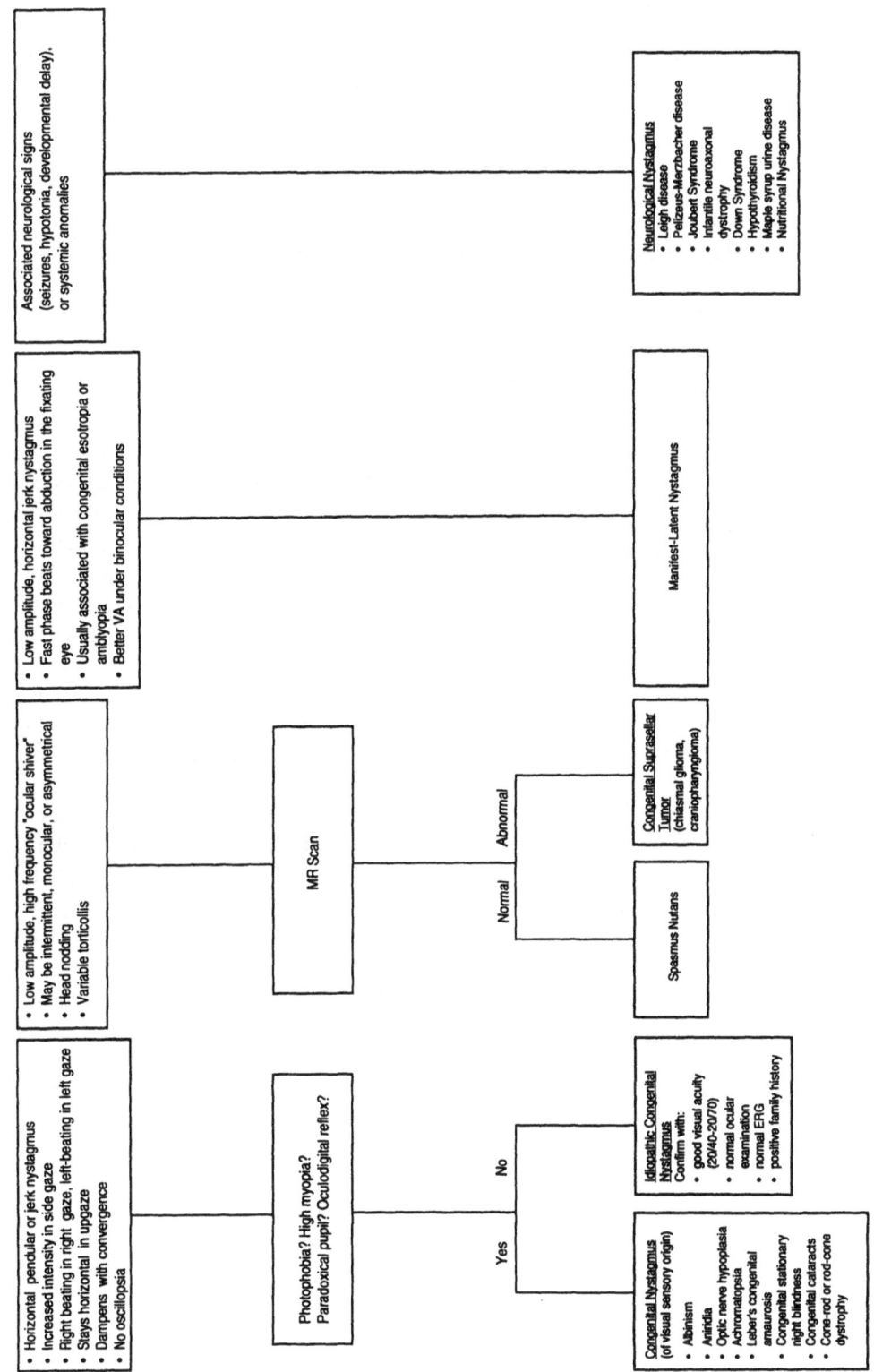

FIGURE 8.12. Differential diagnosis of horizontal nystagmus in children.

children.[180] We suspect that some children reported to have hypothyroidism and nystagmus actually had bilateral optic nerve hypoplasia with anterior pituitary hormone deficiency.[236]

Maple Syrup Urine Disease

Maple syrup urine disease is an autosomal recessive disorder of amino acid catabolism in which affected infants present with intermittent lethargy, poor feeding, irregular respirations, and fluctuating muscle tone.[295] Biochemical studies show severe metabolic acidosis and ketosis. Older children can present with ataxia or dystonia.[263] Various forms of gaze palsies (upgaze paresis, mixed vertical and horizontal paresis, adduction paresis) are frequently seen, as is bilateral ptosis.[262] Nystagmus is usually confined to the recovery phase (after dietary restrictions are instituted) and consists of intermittent, brief bursts of flutterlike movements of the eyes and lids.[175,262,295] Rapid diagnosis is essential as the outcome is worse after the first 24 hours, with progressive and permanent neurological sequelae.[205,263]

Nutritional Nystagmus

Young children with severe malnutrition may develop an acquired, gaze-evoked nystagmus with a Wernicke type of encephalopathy that resolves following administration of B group vitamins.[263,293]

Summary

Congenital nystagmus is the most common form of nystagmus in infants and children. Our understanding of congenital nystagmus has evolved to incorporate two new concepts: (1) the majority of individuals with congenital nystagmus have a primary disturbance of the anterior visual pathways, and (2) the nystagmus waveform in idiopathic cases is indistinguishable from the waveform seen in patients with sensory visual loss. Attempts to adjust the nomenclature to reflect these concepts have generated considerable confusion. Some authorities apply the term *sensory nystagmus* to patients in whom a bilateral visual sensory deficit is identified and *congenital motor nystagmus* when no clinical or electrophysiological evidence of a sensory visual deficit can be found. They discour-

age the rubric congenital nystagmus pointing out that its application is counterproductive in that it tends to discourage further investigation into an underlying cause. Others argue the term sensory nystagmus engenders confusion by suggesting that the nystagmus waveform differs fundamentally from that seen in idiopathic congenital nystagmus. They further contend that the term congenital motor nystagmus is redundant since all congenital nystagmus is motor nystagmus in that the oscillation is identical and therefore tied to the same neurological circuitry whether or not an underlying sensory etiology is present.

The recent recognition that congenital nystagmus usually is precipitated by a primary visual deficit, has unfortunately fueled speculation that the presence of a primary visual disturbance may be a prerequiste for the development of congenital nystagmus. Based in part upon this uncertainty, the clinical pendulum has swung toward obtaining electrophysiological studies in all children with congenital nystagmus. However, it has now been demonstrated that some individuals with congenital nystagmus have no ocular or electrophysiological abnormalities that are detectable using currently available methodology. We believe that routine electrophysiological testing is not mandatory in the diagnostic evaluation of congenital nystagmus. When the ocular examination reveals no structural abnormalities, the four clinical signs of congenital retinal dystrophy (photophobia, paradoxical pupil, myopia, oculodigital reflex) serve to facilitate the identification of those patients who are likely to have a congenital retinal dystrophy and thereby render the routine electrophysiological investigation of every child with congenital nystagmus unnecessary.

A clinical algorithm to assist in the differential diagnosis of horizontal nystagmus in children is provided in Figure 8.12.

References

1. Abadi RV. The effects of early anomalous visual inputs on orientation selectivity. Perception 1974; 3:141-150.
2. Abadi RV, Sandikcioglu M. Visual resolution in congenital pendular nystagmus. Am J Optom Physiol Opt 1975;52:573-581.
3. Abadi RV, King-Smith PE. Congenital nystagmus modifies orientational detection. Vision Res 1979; 19:1409-1411.

4. Abadi RV, Carden D, Simpson J. A new treatment for congenital nystagmus. Br J Ophthalmol 1980; 64:2-6.

5. Abadi R, Pascal E. The recognition and management of albinism. Ophthalmic Physiol Opt 1989;9: 3-15.

6. Abadi RV, Worfolk R. Retinal slip velocities in congenital nystagmus. Vision Res 1989;29:195-205.

7. Abadi RV, Whittle J. The nature of head postures in congenital nystagmus. Arch Ophthalmol 1991; 110:216-220.

8. Abadi RV, Whittle J. Surgery and compensatory head postures in congenital nystagmus: a longitudinal study. Arch Ophthalmol 1992;110:632-635.

9. Abel LA, Williams IM, Levi L. Intermittent oscillopsia in a case of congenital nystagmus. Invest Ophthalmol Vis Sci 1991;32:3104-3108.

10. Abel LA, Dell'Osso LF. Congenital nystagmus mechanism. Invest Ophthalmol Vis Sci 1993; 34:282.

11. Abplanalp P, Bedell H. Visual improvement in an albinotic patient with an alteration of congenital nystagmus. Am J Optom Physiol Opt 1987;64: 944-951.

12. Adams RD, Lyon G. Neurology of Hereditary Metabolic Diseases of Children. New York: McGraw-Hill; 1982:65-68.

13. Albright AL, Sclabassi RJ, Slamovits TL, et al. Spasmus nutans associated with optic gliomas in infants. J Pediatr 1984;105:778-780.

14. Alitalo T, Kruse TA, Forsius H, et al. Localization of the Aland island eye disease locus to the pericentromeric region of the X chromosome by linkage analysis. Am J Hum Genet 1991;48:31-38.

15. Altman AJ, Baehner RL. Favorable prognosis for survival in children with coincident opsomyoclonus and neuroblastoma. Cancer 1976;37: 846-852.

16. Antony JH, Ouvrier RA, Wise G. Spasmus nutans: a mistaken identity. Arch Neurol 1980;37:373-375.

17. Apkarian P, Reits D, Spekreijse H, van Dorp D. A decisive electrophysiological test for human albinism. Electroencephalogr Clin Neurophysiol 1983;55:513-531.

18. Apkarian P, Reits D. Global stereopsis in human albinos. Vision Res 1989;29:1359-1370.

19. Apkarian P, Spekreijse H, van Swaay E, van Schooneveld HM. Visual evoked potentials in Prader-Willi syndrome. Doc Ophthalmol 1989;71: 355-367.

20. Apkarian P, Eckhardt PG, van Schooneveld MJ. Detection of optic pathway misrouting in the human albino neonate. Neuropaediatrics 1991;22: 211-215.

21. Apkarian P, Shallo-Hoffmann J. VEP projections in congenital nystagmus; VEP asymmetry in albinism: a comparison study. Invest Ophthalmol Vis Sci 1991;32:2653-2661.

22. Apkarian P. A practical approach to albino diagnosis: VEP misrouting across the age span. Ophthalmic Paediatr Genet 1992;13:77-82.

22a. Apkarian P, Bour L, Barth PG. A unique achiasmatic anomaly detected in non-albinos with misrouted retino-fugal projections. European J Neuroscience 1994;6:501-507.

23. Arnoldi KA, Poulos M, Tychsen L. Prevalence of intracranial lesions in children presenting with disconjugate nystagmus (spasmus nutans). Presented to the Joint Meeting of the International Strabismological Association & the American Academy of Pediatric Ophthalmology and Strabismus. Vancouver, BC: June 1994.

24. Bagolini B, Campos E, Fonda S, et al. Active blockage and rest position nystagmus electromyographic demonstration of two types of ocular induced head turn. Doc Ophthalmol 1986;62:149-159.

25. Baloh RW, Yee RD, Honrubia V. Optokinetic asymmetry in patients with maldeveloped foveas. Brain Res 1980;186:211-216.

26. Baloh RW, Spooner JE. Downbeat nystagmus: a type of central vestibular nystagmus. Neurology 1981;31:304-310.

27. Barkovich AJ. Pediatric Neuroimaging, I. New York: Raven Press; 1990:38-39.

28. Barricks ME, Flynn JT, Kushner BJ. Paradoxical pupillary responses in congenital stationary night blindness. Arch Ophthalmol 1977;95:1800-1804.

29. Barricks ME, Flynn JT, Kushner BJ. Paradoxical pupillary responses in congenital stationary night blindness. Neuro-ophthalmology Update. New York: Masson; 1986:31-38.

30. Bedell HE, White JM, Abplanalp PL. Variability of foveation in congenital nystagmus. Clin Vis Sci 1989;4:247-252.

31. Bedell HE. Sensitivity to oscillatory target motion in congenital nystagmus. Invest Ophthalmol Vis Sci 1992;33:1811-1821.

32. Bietti GB, Bagolini B. Traitement medicochirurgical du nystagmus. Anneé Ther Clin Ophtalmol 1960;11:269-296.

33. Bixenman WW. Congenital hereditary downbeat nystagmus. Can J Ophthalmol 1983;18:344-348.

34. Blackwell HR, Blackwell OM. Blue mono-cone monochromacy: a new color vision defect. J Opt Soc 1957;47:338-344.

35. Boylan C, Harding GFA. Investigation of visual pathway abnormalities in human albinos. Ophthalmic Physiol Opt 1983;3:273-85.

36. Brandt S, Carlsen N, Glenting P, Helweg-Larsen J. Encephalopathia myoclonica infantilis (Kinsbourne) and neuroblastoma in children. A report of three cases. Dev Med Child Neurol 1974;16:286-294.

37. Brodsky MC, Buckley EG, McConkie-Rosell A. The case of the gray optic disc! Surv Ophthalmol 1989;33:367-372.

38. Brodsky MC, Glasier CM, Creel DJ. Magnetic resonance of the visual pathways in human albinos. J Pediatr Ophthalmol Strabismus 1993;30:382-385.

38a. Brodsky MC. Ocular stabilization systems in congenital nystagmus. Am Orthop J 1995, in Press.

39. Bronstein AM, Rudge P, Gresty MA, et al. Abnormalities of horizontal gaze. Clinical oculographic and magnetic resonance imaging findings. II. gaze palsy and internuclear ophthalmoplegia. J Neurol Neurosurg Psychiatry 1990;53:200-207.

40. Buckley EG. Evaluation of the child with nystagmus. Semin Ophthalmol 1990;5:131-137.

41. Buckley EG. The clinical approach to the pediatric patient with nystagmus. Int Pediatr 1990;5:225-231.

42. Burr IM, Slonim AE, Danish RK, et al. Diencephalic syndrome revisited. J Pediatr 1976;88:439-444.

43. Campistol J, Prats JM, Garaizar C. Benign paroxysmal tonic upgaze of childhood with ataxia: a neuro-ophthalmological syndrome of familial origin? Dev Med Child Neurol 1993;35:431-448.

44. Carl JR, Optican LM, Chu FC, Zee DS. Head shaking and the vestibuloocular reflex in congenital nystagmus. Invest Ophthalmol Vis Sci 1985;26:1043-1050.

45. Carlow TJ. Medical treatment of nystagmus and ocular motor disorders. In: Beck RW, Smith CH, eds. Neuro-ophthalmology. Boston, MA: Little-Brown; 1986:251-264.

46. Casteels I, Harris CM, Shawkat F, Taylor D. Nystagmus in infancy. Br J Ophthalmol 1992;76:434-437.

47. Ciancia AO. Infantile esotropia with abduction nystagmus. Int Ophthalmol Clin 1989;29:24-29.

48. Cibis GW, Fitzgerald KM, Harris DJ, et al. The effects of dystrophin gene mutations on the ERG in mice and humans. Invest Ophthalmol Vis Sci 1993;34:3646-3652.

49. Cogan DG. Neurology of the Ocular Muscles. 2nd ed. Springfield, IL: Charles C. Thomas; 1956.

50. Cogan DG. Congenital nystagmus. Can J Ophthalmol 1967;2:4-10.

51. Collewijn H, Winterson BJ, Dubois MFW. Optokinetic eye movements in albino rabbits: inversion in anterior visual field. Science 1978;199:1351-1353.

52. Collewijn H, van der Steen J, Ferman L, Jansen TC. Human ocular counter-roll: assessment of static and dynamic properties from electromagnetic scleral coil recordings. Exp Brain Res 1985;59:185-196.

53. Conrad HG, de Decker W. Torsional Kestenbaum procedure: evolution of a surgical concept. Proceedings of 4th Meeting of the International Strabismological Association. 1982;301-305.

54. Cooper TD, Jun CL. Diencephalic syndrome of emaciation in infancy and childhood. In: Smith JL, ed. Neuro-ophthalmology Update. New York: Masson; 1977:253-260.

55. Corbett J. Neuro-ophthalmic complications of hydrocephalus and shunting procedures. Semin Neurol 1986;6(2):111-123.

56. Creel DJ, Witkop CJ, King RA. Asymmetric visual evoked potentials in human albinos: evidence for visual system anomalies. Invest Ophthalmol 1974;13:430.

57. Creel D, Spekreijse H, Reits D. Evoked potentials in albinos: efficacy of pattern stimuli in detecting misrouted optic fibers. Electroencephalogr Clin Neurophysiol 1981;52:595-603.

58. Creel DJ, Bendel CM, Wiesner GL, et al. Abnormalities of the central visual pathways in Prader-Willi syndrome associated with hypopigmentation. N Engl J Med 1986;314:1606-1609.

59. Creel DJ, Summers CG, King RA. Visual anomalies associated with albinism. Ophthalmic Paediatr Genet 1990;11:193-200.

60. Cox R. Congenital head nodding and nystagmus: report of a case. Arch Ophthalmol 1936;15:1032-1036.

61. Cuiffreda KJ, Goldrich SG, Neary C. Use of eye movement auditory biofeedback in the control of nystagmus. Am J Optom Physiol Opt 1982;59:396-409.

62. C,ppers C. Probleme der operativen Therapie des okularen Nystagmus. Klin Monatsbl Augenheilkd 1971;159:145-157.

63. Daroff RB. Seesaw nystagmus. Neurology 1965;15:874-877.

64. Davis GV, Shock JP. Septo-optic dysplasia associated with seesaw nystagmus. Arch Ophthalmol 1975;93:137-139.

65. de Brown EL, Bernadeli J, Corvera-Bernardelli J. Metodo debiltante para el tratamiento del Nistagmus. Rev Mex Oftalm 1989;63:65-67.

66. de Becker I, Dooley J, Tremblay F. Pathognomonic negative electroretinogram but not congenital stationary night blindness in Duchenne muscular dystrophy. Invest Ophthalmol Vis Sci 1993;34:1076. Abstract.

67. de Decker W. Rotatischer Kestenbaum an geraden Augenmuskeln. Z Prakt Augenheilkd 1990;11:111-114.

68. Dell'Osso LF, Daroff RB. Congenital nystagmus waveforms and foveation strategy. Doc Ophthalmol 1975;39:155-182.

69. Dell'Osso LF, Flynn JT. Congenital nystagmus surgery: a quantitative evaluation of the effects. Arch Ophthalmol 1979;97:462-469.

70. Dell'Osso LF, Schmidt D, Daroff RB. Latent, manifest latent, and congenital nystagmus. Arch Ophthalmol 1979;97:1877-1885.

71. Dell'Osso LF, Daroff RB. Achromatopsia and congenital nystagmus. J Clin Neuro-ophthalmol 1983;3:152.

72. Dell'Osso LF, Ellenberger C, Abel LA, Flynn JT. The nystagmus blockage syndrome: congenital nystagmus, manifest latent nystagmus or both? Invest Ophtahlmol Vis Sci 1983;24:1580-1587.

73. Dell'Osso LF. Congenital, latent and manifest-latent nystagmus-similarities and differences and relation to strabismus. Jpn J Ophthalmol 1985;29:351-368.

74. Dell'Osso LF. Evaluation of smooth pursuit in the presence of congenital nystagmus. Neuro-ophthalmology 1986;6:381-406.

75. Dell'Osso LF, Daroff RB. Abnormal head position and head motion associated with nystagmus. In: Keller EL, Zee DS, eds. *Adaptive Processes in Visual and Oculomotor Systems.* Oxford: Pergamon Press; 1986:473-478.

76. Dell'Osso LF, Taccis S, Abel LA, Erzurum SI. Contact lenses and congenital nystagmus. Clin Vision Sci 1988;3:229-232.

77. Dell'Osso LF, Leigh RJ, Daroff RB. Suppression of congenital nystagmus by cutaneous stimulation Neuro-ophthalmology 1991;11:173-175.

78. Dell'Osso LF. Eye movements, visual acuity and spatial constancy. Acta Neurol Belg 1991;91:105-113.

79. Dell'Osso LF, van der Steen J, Steinman RM, Collewijn H. Foveation dynamics in congenital nystagmus. I: fixation. Doc Ophthalmol 1992;79: 1-23.

80. Dell'Osso LF, Leigh RJ. Foveation period stability and oscillopsia suppression in congenital nystagmus: an hypothesis. Neuro-ophthalmology 1992; 12:169-183

81. Dell'Osso LF, Leigh RJ. Ocular motor stability of foveation periods. Required conditions for suppression of oscillopsia. Neuro-ophthalmology 1992;12:303-326.

82. Dell'Osso LF, van der Steen J, Steinman RM, Collewijn H. Foveation dynamics in congenital nystagmus. II: smooth pursuit. Doc Ophthalmol 1992;79:25-49.

83. Dell'Osso LF, van der Steen J, Steinman RM, Collewijn H. Foveation dynamics in congenital nystagmus. III: vestibulo-ocular reflex. Doc Ophthalmol 1992;79:51-70.

84. Dell'Osso LF. Foveation dynamics and oscillopsia in latent/manifest latent nystagmus. Invest Ophthalmol Vis Sci 1993;34(suppl):1125. Abstract.

85. Dell'Osso et al. Seesaw nystagmus in achiasmatic dogs. Vision Res, 1995; In press.

86. Demer JL, Zee DS. Vestibulo-ocular and optokinetic defects in albinos with congenital nystagmus. Invest Ophthalmol Vis Sci 1984;25:739-745.

87. de Sa LC. Congenital-type nystagmus emerging in later life. Surv Ophthalmol 1992;36:389. Comment.

88. Dickinson CM, Abadi RV. The influence of nystagmoid oscillation on contrast sensitivity in normal observers. Vision Res 1985;25:1089-1096.

89. Dieterich M, Brandt TH. Impaired motion perception in congenital nystagmus and acquired ocular motor palsy. Clin Vis Sci 1987;1:337-347.

90. Donin JF. Acquired monocular nystagmus in children. Can J Ophthalmol 1967;2:212-215.

91. Druckman R, Ellis P, Kleinfeld J, et al. Seesaw nystagmus. Arch Ophthalmol 1966;76:668.

92. Ellenberger C, Campa JF, Netsky MG. Opsoclonus and parenchymatous degeneration of the cerebellum. The cerebellar origin of an abnormal ocular movement. Neurology 1968;18:1041-1046.

93. Falls HF, Wolter JR, Alpern M. Typical total monochromacy. Arch Ophthalmol 1965;74:610-616.

94. Farmer J, Hoyt CS. Monocular nystagmus in infancy and early childhood. Am J Ophthalmol 1984;98:504-509.

95. Fein JM, Williams RDB. Seesaw nystagmus. J Neurol Neurosurg Psychiatry 1969;32:202-207.

96. Fineman JAB, Kuniholm P, Seridan S. Spasmus nutans: a syndrome of auto-arousal. J Am Acad Child Psychiatr 1971;10:136.

97. Fitzgerald KM, Cibis GW, Giambrone SA, Harris DJ. Retinal signal transmission in Duchenne Muscular Dystrophy: evidence for dysfunction in the photoreceptor/depolarizing bipolar cell pathway. J Clin Invest 1994;93:2425-2430.

98. Fleischman JA, O'Donnell FE. Congenital X-linked incomplete achromatopsia: evidence for slow progression, carrier fundus findings, and possible genetic linkage with glucose-6-phosphate dehydrogenase locus. Arch Ophthalmol 1981;99:468-472.

99. Flynn JT, Scott WE, Kushner BJ. Large rectus muscle recessions for the treatment of congenital nystagmus. Arch Ophthalmol 1991;109:L1636-1637.

100. Forssman B. A study of congenital nystagmus. Acta Otolaryngol 1964;57:427-449.

101. Frank JW, Kushner BJ, France TD. Paradoxical pupillary phenomena. a review of patients with pupillary constriction to darkness. Arch Ophthalmol 1988;106:1564-1566.

102. Frisén L, Wikkelsø C. Posttraumatic seesaw nystagmus abolished by ethanol ingestion. Neurology 1986;36:841-844.

103. Fulton AB, Hansen RM. Electroretinography: application to clinical studies of infants. J Pediatr Ophthalmol Strabismus 1985;22:251-255.

104. Furman JM, Stoyanoff S, Barber HO. Head and eye movements in congenital nystagmus. Otolaryngol Head Neck Surg 1984;92:656-661.

105. Fujiyama Y, Ozawa H, Ishikawa S. Study on abnormal head position in patients with congenital nystagmus. Agressolog 1983;24:231-232.

106. Flynn JT, Kazarian E, Barricks M. Paradoxical pupil in congenital achromatopsia. Int Ophthalmol 1981;3:91-96.

107. Gal A, Schinzel A, Orth U, et al. Gene of x-chromosomal congenital stationary night blindness is closely linked to DXS7 on Xp. Hum Genet 1989;81:315-318.

108. Gelbart SS, Hoyt CS. Congenital nystagmus: a clinical perspective in infancy. Graefeís Arch Clin Exp Ophthalmol 1988;226:178-180.

109. Glass IA, Good P, Coleman MP, et al. Genetic mapping of a cone and rod dysfunction (Aland Island eye disease) to the proximal short arm of the human X chromosome. J Med Genet 1993;30: 1044-1050.

110. Glickstein M, Heath GG. Receptors in the monochromat eye. Vision Res 1975;15:633-636.

111. Good PA, Searle AET, Campbell S, Crews SJ. Value of the ERG in congenital nystagmus. Br J Ophthalmol 1989;73:512-515.

112. Good WV, Brodsky MC, Hoyt CS, Ahn JC. Upbeating nystagmus in Infants: a sign of anterior visual pathway disease. Binoc Vis Q 1990;5:13-18.

113. Good WV, Koch TS, Jan JE. Monocular nystagmus caused by unilateral anterior visual pathway disease. Dev Med Child Neurol 1993;35: 1106-1110.

114. Gottlob I, Zubcov A, Catalano RA. Signs distinguishing spasmus nutans (with and without central nervous system lesions) from infantile nystagmus. Ophthalmology 1990;97:1166-1175.

115. Gottlob I, Zubcov AA, Wizov SS, et al. Head nodding is compensatory in spasmus nutans. Ophthalmology 1992;99:1024-1031.

116. Gottlob I, Reinecke RD. Eye and head movements in patients with achromatopsia. Graefe's Arch Clin Exp Ophthalmol 1994;232:392-401.

117. Gottlob I. Eye movement abnormalities in carriers of blue cone monochromatism. Invest Ophthalmol Vis Sci 1994;35:3556-3560.

118. Gresty M, Leech J, Sanders H, Eggars H. A study of head and eye movement in spasmus nutans. Br J Ophthalmol 1976;60:652-654.

119. Gresty M, Halmagyi GM, Leech J. The relationship between head and eye movement in congenital nystagmus with head shaking: objective recordings of a single case. Br J Ophthalmol 1978;62: 533-656.

120. Gresty MA, Ell JJ. Spasmus nutans or congenital nystagmus? Classification according to objective criteria. Br J Ophthalmol 1981;65:510-511. Correspondence.

121. Gresty MA, Halmagyi GM. Head nodding associated with childhood nystagmus. Ann NY Acad Sci 1981;374:614-618.

122. Gresty MA, Barratt HJ, Page NG, Ell JJ. Assessment of vestibulo-ocular reflexes in congenital nystagmus. Ann Neurol 1985;17:129-136.

123. Gresty MA, Bronstein AM, Page NG, et al. Congenital-type nystagmus emerging in later life. Neurology 1991;41:653-656.

124. Guillery RW, Okoro AN, Witkop CJ. Abnormal visual pathways in the brain of a human albino. Brain Res 1975;96:373-377.

125. Guillery RW. Neural abnormalities of albinos. TINS 1986;364-367.

126. Guillery RW. Normal and abnormal visual field maps in albinos: central effects of non-matching maps. Ophthalmic Paediatr Genet 1990;3:177-183.

127. Guo S, Reinecke RD, Fendick M, Calhoun JH. Visual pathway abnormalities in albinism and infantile nystagmus: VEPs and stereoacuity measurements. J Pediatr Ophthalmol Strabismus 1989;26: 97-104.

128. Guyer DR, Lessell S. Periodic alternating nystagmus associated with albinism. J Clin Neuro-ophthalmology 1986;6(2):82-85.

129. Halmagyi GM, Gresty MA, Leech J. Reversed optokinetic nystagmus (OKN): mechanism and clinical significance. Ann Neurol 1980;7:429-435.

130. Halmagyi GM, Rudge P, Gresty MA, et al. Treatment of periodic alternating nystagmus. Ann Neurol 1980;8:609-611.

131. Hamed LF, Silbiger J. Periodic alternating esotropia. J Pediatr Ophthalmol Strabismus 1992;29: 240-242.

132. Harrison R, Hoefnagel D, Hayward JN. Congenital total color blindness, a clinicopathological report. Arch Ophthalmol 1960;4:685-692.

133. Hart WM. Acquired dyschromatopsias. Surv Ophthalmol 1987;32:10-31.

134. Hayakawa M, Imai Y, Wakita M, et al. A Japanese pedigree of autosomal dominant congenital stationary night blindness with variable expressivity. Ophthalmic Paediatr Genet 1992;13:211-217.

135. Heckenlively JR, Martin DA, Rosenbaum AL. Loss of electroretinographic oscillatory potentials, optic atrophy, and dysplasia in congenital stationary night blindness. Am J Ophthalmol 1983; 96:526-534.

136. Heher KL, Traboulsi EI, Maumenee IH. The natural history of Leber's congenital amaurosis: age-related findings in 35 patients. Ophthalmology 1992;99:241-245.

137. Helveston EM, Ellis FD, Plager DA. Large recession of the horizontal recti for treatment of nystagmus. Ophthalmology 1991;98:1302-1305.

138. Hermann C. Head shaking with nystagmus in infants. AJDC 1918;16:180-194.

139. Hittner HM, King RA, Riccardi VM, et al. Oculocutaneous albinoidism as a manifestation of reduced neural crest derivatives in the Prader-Willi syndrome. Am J Ophthalmol 1982;94:328-337.

140. Hoefnagel D, Biery B. Spasmus nutans. Dev Med Child Neurol 1968;10:32-35.

141. Hoyt CS, Aicardi E. Acquired monocular nystagmus in monozygous twins. J Pediatr Ophthalmol Strabismus 1979;16:115-118.

142. Hoyt CS, Mousel DK, Weber AA. Transient supranuclear disorders of gaze in healthy neonates. Am J Ophthalmol 1980;89:708-711.

143. Hoyt CS, Gelbart SS. Vertical nystagmus in infants with congenital ocular abnormalities. Ophthalmic Pediatr Genet 1984;4:155-162.

144. Ishikawa S, Ozawa H, Fujiyama Y. Treatment of nystagmus by acupuncture. In: *Highlights in Neuro-ophthalmology.* Proceedings of 6th Meeting of the International Neuro-Ophthalmology Society (INOS), Amsterdam: Æolus Press; 1987:227-232.

145. Jacome DE, Fitzgerald R. Monocular ictal nystagmus. Arch Neurol 1982;39:653-656.

146. Jampolsky A. When is supermaximal surgery safe? Am Orthop J 1987;37:33-44.

147. Jan JE, Carruthers JDA, Tillson G. Neurodevelopmental criteria in the classification of congenital motor nystagmus. Can J Neurol Sci 1992;19: 76-79.

148. Jan JE, Groenveld M, Anderson DP. Photophobia and cortical visual impairment. Dev Med Child Neurol 1993;35:473-477.

149. Jay WM, Marcus RW, Jay MS. Periodic alternating nystagmus clearing after cataract surgery. J Clin Neuro-ophthalmology 1985;5:149-152.

150. Jayalakshmi P, Scott TF, Tucker SH, Schaffer DB. Infantile nystagmus: a prospective study of spasmus nutans, congenital nystagmus, and unclassified nystagmus of infancy. J Pediatr 1970;77: 177-187.

151. Jin YH, Goldstein HP, Reinecke RD. Absence of visual sampling in infantile nystagmus. Invest Ophthalmol Vis Sci 1989;30(suppl):50.

152. Kalyanaranman K, Jagannathan K, Ramanujam RA, et al. Congenital head nodding and nystagmus with cerebrocerebellar degeneration. J Pediatr 1973;83:1023-1026.

153. Kaneko CRS, Fuchs AF. The effect of ibotenic acid lesions of the omnipause neurons on saccadic eye movements in the monkey. Neuroscience 1987; 13:392. Abstract.

154. Kanter DS, Ruff RL, Leigh RJ, Modic M. Seesaw nystagmus and brain stem infarction. MRI findings. Neuro-ophthalmology 1987;7:279-283.

155. Kattah JC, Kolsky MP, Guy J, O'Doherty D. Primary position vertical nystagmus and cerebellar ataxia. Arch Neurol 1983;40:310-314.

156. Katzman B, Lu LW, Tiwari RP. Spasmus nutans in identical twins. Ann Ophthalmol 1981;13: 1193-1195.

157. Kelly TW. Optic glioma presenting as spasmus nutans. Pediatrics 1970;45:295-296.

158. King MD, Dudgeon J, Stephenson JBP. Joubert's syndrome with retinal dysplasia: neonatal tachypnea as the clue to a genetic brain-eye malformation. Arch Dis Child 1984;59:709-718.

159. King RA, Nelson LB, Wagner RS. Spasmus nutans. A benign clinical entity. Arch Ophthalmol 1986;104:1501-1504.

160. Kinnear PE, Jay B, Witkop CJ. Albinism. Surv Ophthalmol 1985;30:75-101.

161. Koenig SB, Naidich TP, Zaparackas Z. Optic glioma masquerading as spasmus nutans. J Pediatr Ophthalmol Strabismus 1982;19:20-24.

162. Kommerell G, Mehdorn E. Is an optokinetic defect the cause of congenital or latent nystagmus? In: Lennerstrand G, Zee DS, Keller EL, eds. Functional Basis of Ocular Motility Disorders. Elmsford: Pergamon Press; 1982:159-167.

163. Kommerell G. Congenital nystagmus control of slow tracking movements by target offset from the fovea. Graefe's Arch Clin Exp Ophthalmol 1986; 224:295.

164. Kommerell G, Zee DS. Latent nystagmus: release and suppression at will. Invest Ophthalmol Vis Sci 1993;34:1785-1792.

165. Kraft SP, O'Donoghue EP, Roarty JD. Improvement of compensatory head postures after strabismus surgery. Ophthalmology 1992;99:1301-1308.

166. Kriss A, Russell-Eggitt I, Harris CM, et al. Aspects of albinism. Ophthalmol Pediatr Genet 1992;13: 89-100.

167. Kriss T, Harris C, Lambert SR. Ocular motility anomalies in developmental misdirection of the optic chiasm. Am J Ophthalmol 1992;113: 601-602.

168. Krohel G, Griffen JF. Voluntary vertical nystagmus. Neurology 1979;29:1153-1154.

169. Kurzan R, Büttner U. Smooth pursuit mechanisms in congenital nystagmus. Neuro-ophthalmology 1989:313-325.

170. Lambert SR, Taylor D, Kriss A. The infant with nystagmus, normal appearing fundi, but an abnormal ERG. Surv Ophthalmol 1989;34:173-186.

171. Lambert SR, Newman NJ. Congenital stationary night blindness masquerading as spasmus nutans. Neurology 1993;43:1607-1608.

172. Larmande P, Pautrizel B. Tritement du nystagmus congenital par le 5-hydroxytryptophance. Presse Med 1981;10:3166.

173. Lavery MA, O'Neill JF, Chu FC, et al. Acquired nystagmus in early childhood: a presenting sign of intracranial tumor. Ophthalmology 1984;91: 425-435.

174. Leigh RJ, Dell'Osso LF, Yaniglos SS. Oscillopsia, retinal image stabilization, and congenital nystagmus. Invest Ophthalmol Vis Sci 1988;29:279-282.

175. Leigh RJ, Zee DS, eds. The Neurology of Eye Movements, 2nd ed. Philadelphia, PA: F.A. Davis; 1991.

176. Lee S-T, Nicholls RD, Bundey S, et al. Mutations of the P gene in oculocutaneous albinism, ocular albinism, and Prader-Willi syndrome plus albinism. N Engl J Med 1994;330:529-534.

177. Lewis RA, Holcom JD, Bromley WC, et al. Mapping X-linked ophthalmic diseases. III: provisional assignment of the locus for blue cone monochromacy to Xq28. Arch Ophthalmol 1987;105: 1055-1059.

178. Liu C, Gresty M, Lee J. Management of symptomatic latent nystagmus. Eye 1993;7:550-553.

179. Lo CY. Brain lesions in congenital nystagmus as detected by computed tomography. Jpn J Clin Ophthalmol 1982;36:871.

180. MacFaul R, Dorner S, Brett EM, Grant DG. Neurological abnormalities in patients treated for hypothyroidism from early life. Arch Dis Child 1978;53:611-619.

181. Maekawa K, Simpson JI. Climbing fiber activation of Purkinje cells in the flocculus by impulses transferred through the visual pathway. Brain Res 1972;39:245-250.

182. Maekawa K, Simpson JI. Climbing fiber responses evoked in vestibulocerebellum of rabbit from visual system. J Neurophysiol 1973;36:649-665.

183. Mallinson AI, Longridge NS, Dunn HG, et al. Vestibular studies in Pelizaeus-Merzbacher disease. J Otolarayngol 1986;12:361-364.

184. Marmor MF. Hereditary vertical nystagmus. Arch Ophthalmol 1973;90:107-111.

185. McCarty JW, Demer JL, Hovis LA, et al. Ocular motility anomalies in developmental misdirection of the optic chiasm. Am J Ophthalmol 1992;113: 86-95.

186. McFaul R, Dorner S, Brett EM, et al. Neurological abnormalities in patients treated for hypo-thy-

roidism from early life. Arch Dis Child 1978; 53:611-619.

187. Medina L, Chi TL, DeVivo DC, Hilal SK. MR findings in patients with subacute necrotizing encephalomyelopathy (Leigh's syndrome). AJNR 1990;11:379-384.

188. Metzger EL. Correction of congenital nystagmus. Am J Ophthalmol 1950;33:1796-1797.

189. Mezawa M, Ishikawa S, Ukse K. Changes in waveform of congenital nystagmus associated with biofeedback treatment. Br J Ophthalmol 1990; 74:472-476.

190. Milam AH, Saari JC, Jacobson SG, et al. Autoantibodies against retinal bipolar cells in cutaneous melanoma-associated retinopathy. Invest Ophthalmol Vis Sci 1993;34:91-100.

191. Miller NR. *Walsh and Hoyt's Clinical Neuro-ophthalmology, II.* 4th ed. Baltimore, MD: Williams and Wilkins; 1985:898.

192. Miller NR. *Walsh and Hoyt's Clinical Neuro-ophthalmology, III.* 4th ed. Baltimore, MD: Williams and Wilkins; 1988;1157-1158.

193. Miranda AF, Ishii S, DiMauro S, et al. Cytochrome c oxidase deficiency in Leigh's syndrome: genetic evidence for a nuclear DNA-encoded mutation. Neurology 1989;39:697-702.

194. Mitchell WG, Snodgrass SR. Opsoclonus-Ataxia due to childhood neural crest tumors: a chronic neurologic syndrome. J Child Neurol 1990;5: 153-158.

195. Miyake Y, Yagasaki K, Horiguchi M, et al. Congenital stationary night blindness with negative electroretinogram: a new classification. Arch Ophthalmol 1986;104:1013-1020.

196. Moore AT, Taylor DSI. A syndrome of congenital retinal dystrophy and saccade palsy—a subset of Leber's congenital amaurosis. Br J Ophthalmol 1984;68:421-431.

197. Musarella MA, Chan HS, DeBoer G, Gallie BL. Ocular involvement in neuroblastoma: prognostic implications. Ophthalmology 1984;91:936-940.

198. Musarella MA, Weleber RG, Murphey WH, et al. Assignment of the gene for complete x-linked congenital stationary night blindness (CSNB1) to human chromosome Xp11.3. Genomics 1989;5: 727-737.

199. Musarella MA, Kirshgessner C, Trofatter J, et al. Assignment of the gene for incomplete congenital stationary night blindness (CSNB2) to proximal Xp. Invest Ophthalmol Vis Sci 1992;33:792. Abstract.

200. Naegele JR, Held R. The postnatal development of monocular optokinetic nystagmus in infants. Vision Res 1982;22:341-346.

201. Nakada T, Kwee IL. Seesaw nystagmus: role of visuovestibular interaction in its pathogenesis. J Clin Neuro-ophthalmology 1988;8(3):171-177.

202. Namba S, Nishimoro A, Yagyu Y. Diencephalic syndrome of emaciation (Russell's syndrome). Long-term survival. Surg Neurol 1985;23: 581-588.

203. Nathans J, Davenport CM, Maumenee IH, et al. Molecular genetics of human blue cone monochromacy. Science 1989;245:831-838.

204. Nathans J, Maumenee IH, Zrenner E, et al. Genetic heterogeneity in blue cone monochromatism. Am J Hum Genet 1993;53:987-1000.

205. Naughten ER, Jenkins J, Francis DEM, et al. Outcome of maple syrup urine disease. Arch Dis Child 1982;57:918-921.

206. Nellhaus G. Abnormal head movements of young children. Dev Med Child Neurol 1983;25: 384-389.

207. Nelson LB, Calhoun JH, Harley RD. *Pediatric Ophthalmology.* 3rd ed. Philadelphia, PA: WB Saunders; 1991:497.

208. Newman SA. Spasmus nutans—Or is it? Surv Ophthalmol 1990;34:453-456.

209. Nicholls RD. Genomic imprinting and uniparental disomy in Angelman and Prader-Willi syndromes: a review. Am J Med Genet 1993;46:16-25.

210. Noble KG, Carr RE, Siegel IM. Autosomal dominant congenital stationary night blindness with an electronegative electroretinogram. Am J Ophthalmol 1990;109:44-48.

211. Norton EWD, Cogan DG. Spasmus nutans: a clinical study of twenty cases followed two or more years since onset. Arch Ophthalmol 1954;52: 442-446.

212. O'Connor PS, Tredici TJ, Ivan DI, et al. Achromatopsia: clinical diagnosis and treatment. J Clin Neuro-ophthalmology 1986; 2:219-226.

213. O'Donnell FE, Hambrick GW, Green WR, et al. X-linked ocular albinism: an oculocutaneous macromelanosomal disorder. Arch Ophthalmol 1976;94:1883-1892.

214. Ohmi G, Reinecke RD. Astigmatism of nystagmus subjects. Invest Ophthalmol Vis Sci 1993;34: 1125-1143.

215. Oliver MD, Dotan SA, Chemke J, Abraham FA. Isolated foveal hypoplasia. Br J Ophthalmol 1987; 71:926-930.

216. Optican LM, Zee DS. A hypothetical explanation of congenital nystagmus. Biol Cybernet 1984;50: 119-134.

217. Osterberg G. On spasmus nutans. Acta Ophthalmol 1937;15:457-467.

218. Pentao L, Lewis RA, Ledbetter DH, et al. Maternal uniparental isodisomy of chromosome 14: association of with autosomal recessive rod monochromacy. Am J Hum Genet 1992;50: 690-699.

219. Pillers DM, Seltzer WK, Powell BR, et al. Negative-configuration electroretinogram in Oregon eye disease: consistent phenotype in Xp21 deletion syndrome. Arch Ophthalmol 1993;111:1558-1563.

220. Plange H. Augensymptome bei der subakuten nekrotisierenden enzephalomyelopathie. Klin Monatsbl Augenheikd 1976;168:146-149.

221. Price MJ, Thompson HS, Judisen GF, Corbett JT. Pupillary constriction to darkness. Br J Ophthalmol 1985;69:205-211.

222. Pritchard C, Flynn JT, Smith JL. Waveform characteristics of vertical oscillations in long-standing visual loss. J Pediatr Ophthalmol Strabismus 1988;25:233-239.

223. Ranalli PJ, Sharpe JA, Fletcher WA. Palsy of upward and downward saccadic, pursuit, and vestibular movements with a unilateral midbrain lesion: pathophysiologic correlations. Neurology 1988; 38:114-122.

224. Raudnitz R. Zer Lehre vom Spasmus Nutans. Jahrb Kinderh 1897;45:146.

225. Ray C, Skarf B. New onset pendular nystagmus in a 12-month old. Presented at 25th Annual Frank B. Walsh Society Meeting. New York: 1993.

226. Reinecke RD, Guo S, Goldstein HP. Waveform evolution in infantile nystagmus: an electro-oculographic study of 35 cases. Binoc Vis Q 1988; 31:191-202.

227. Ridley A, Kennard C, Scholtze CL, et al. Omnipause neurons in two cases of opsoclonus associated with oat cell carcinoma of the lung. Brain 1987;110:1699-1709.

228. Ripps H. Night blindness revisited: from man to molecules. Proctor Lecture. Invest Ophthalmol Vis Sci 1982;23:588-609.

229. Robinson DA, Zee DS, Hain TC, et al. Alexander's law: its behavior and origin in the human vestibulo-ocular reflex. Ann Neurol 1984;16:714-722.

230. Ruether K, Apfelstedt-Sylla E, Zrenner E. Clinical findings in patients with congenital stationary night blindness of the Schubert-Bornschein type. Ger J Ophthalmol 1993;2:429-435.

231. Safran AB, Gambazzi Y. Congenital nystagmus: rebound phenomenon following removal of contact lenses. Br J Ophthalmol 1992;76:497-498.

232. Savino PJ, Glaser JS. Opsoclonus: pattern of regression in a child with neuroblastoma. Br J Ophthalmol 1975;59:696-698.

233. Schatz MP, Pollock SC. Optic disc morphology in albinism. Presented at the North American Neuro-ophthalmology Society Meeting. Durango, CO: February 27-March 3, 1994.

234. Schmidt D, Kommerell G. Congenitaler Schaukelnystagmus (seesaw nystagmus). Graefeís Arch Clin Exp Ophthalmol 1976;191:265-272.

235. Schmidt D. Downbeat nystagmus: a clinical review. Neuro-ophthalmology 1991;11:247-262.

236. Schulman JD, Crawford JD. Congenital nystagmus and hypothyroidism. N Engl J Med 1969;280: 708-710.

237. Scudder CA, Fuch AF, Langer TP. Characteristics and functional identification of saccadic inhibitory burst neurons in the alert monkey. J Neurophysiol 1988;59:1430-1454.

238. Sedwick LA, Burde RM, Hodges FJ. Leigh's subacute necrotizing encephalomyelopathy manifesting as spasmus nutans. Arch Ophthalmol 1984; 102:1046-1048.

239. Sharpe LT, van Norrend D, Nordby K. Pigment regeneration, visual adaptation, and spectral sensitivity in the achromat. Clin Vis Sci 1988;3:9-17.

240. Shatz C. A comparison of visual pathways in Boston and Midwestern Siamese cats. J Comp Neurol 1977;171:205-208.

241. Shawkat FS, Harris CM, Wilson J, Taylor DSI. Eye movements in children with opsoclonus. Neuropaediatrics 1993;24:218-223.

242. Shults WT, Stark L, Hoyt WF, et al. Normal saccadic structure of voluntary nystagmus. Arch Ophthalmol 1977;1399-1404.

243. Sigal MB, Diamond GR. Survey of management strategies for nystagmus patients with vertical or torsional head posture. Ann Ophthalmol 1990; 22:134-138.

244. Sigesmund DA, Weleber RG, Pillers DM, et al. Characterization of the ocular phenotype of Duchenne and Becker muscular dystrophy. Ophthalmology 1994;101:856-865.

245. Silver J, Sapiro J. Axonal guidance during development of the optic nerve. The role of pigmented epithelia and other extrinsic factors. J Comp Neurol 1981;202:521-538.

246. Simon JW, Kandel GL, Krohel CB, Nelsen PT. Albinotic characteristics in congenital nystagmus. Am J Ophthalmol 1984;97:320-327.

247. Simonsz HJ, Kommerell G. Effect of prolonged occlusion on latent nystagmus. Neuro-ophthalmology 1992;12:185-192.

248. Smith JL, Flynn JT, Spiro HJ. Monocular vertical oscillations of amblyopia. The Heimann-Bielschowsky phenomenon. J Clin Neuro-ophthalmology 1982;2:85-91.

249. Smith VC, Pokorney J, Delleman JW, et al. X-linked incomplete achromatopsia with more than one class of functional coneness. Invest Ophthalmol Vis Sci 1983;23:451-457.

250. Sogg RL, Hoyt WF. Intermittent vertical nystagmus in a father and son. Arch Ophthalmol 1962;68:515-517.

251. Spicer WTH. Head shaking with nystagmus in infancy. Lancet 1906;2:207-209.

252. Spielmann A. Sensorial strabismus in infants: the congenital functional monophtalme syndrome. J Fr Orthoptie 1989;21:23-33.

253. Spielmann A. Pediatric nystagmus and strabismus. Curr Opin Ophthalmol 1990;1:621-626.

254. Spielmann A, Spielmann AC. The surgical treatment of exodeviations with congenital nystagmus: Problems related to exodeviations with blocking convergence. Presented to the Joint Meeting of the International Strabismological Association and the American Academy of Pediatric Ophthalmology and Strabismus. Vancouver, BC: June 1994.

255. Spielmann A. Nystagmus. Curr Opin Ophthalmol 1994;5:20-24.

256. Stang HJ. Developmental disabilities associated with congenital nystagmus. Dev Behav Pediatr 1991;12:322-323.

257. Still GF. Head nodding with nystagmus in infants. Lancet 1906;2:207-209.

258. Strongin AC, Guillery RW. The distribution of melanin in the developing optic cup and stalk and its relation to cellular degeneration. J Neuroscience 1981;1:1193-1204.

259. Takeda T, Maekawa K. Bilateral visual inputs to the dorsal cap of inferior olive: differential localization and inhibitory interactions. Exp Brain Res 1980;39:461-471.

260. Tanabe Y, Iai M, Ishii M, et al. The use of magnetic resonance imaging in diagnosing infantile neuroaxonal dystrophy. Neurology 1993;43: 110-113.

261. Taylor D. Congenital tumours of the anterior visual system with dysplasia of the optic discs. Br J Ophthalmol 1982;66:455-463.

262. Taylor D. Ophthalmological features of some human hereditary disorders with demyelination. Bull Soc Belge Ophtalmol 1983;1:405-413.

263. Taylor D. *Pediatric Ophthalmology*. Boston, MA: Blackwell; 1990:38.

263a Trobe JD, Sharpe JA, Hirsh DK, Gebarski, SS. Nystagmus of Pelizeus Merzbacher disease: A magnetic search coil study. Arch Neurol 1991;48: 87-91.

264. Tychsen L, Hurtig RR, Scott WE. Pursuit is impaired but the vestibulo-ocular reflex is normal in infantile strabismus. Arch Ophthalmol 1985;103: 536.

265. Tychsen L, Lisberger SG. Visual motion processing for the initiation of smooth-pursuit eye movements in humans. Neurophysiology 1986;56: 953-967.

266. van Dorp DB, Eriksson AW, Dellman JW, et al. Aland eye disease: no albino misrouting. Clin Genet 1985;28:526-531.

267. von Noorden GK, La Roche R. Visual acuity and motor characteristics in congenital nystagmus. Am J Ophthalmol 1983;95:748-751.

268. von Noorden GK, Avilla C, Sidkaro Y, et al. Latent nystagmus and strabismic amblyopia. Am J Ophthalmol 1987;103:87-89.

269. von Noorden GK, Munoz M, Wong SY. Compensatory mechanisms in congenital nystagmus. Am J Ophthalmol 1987;104:387-397.

270. von Noorden GK, Sprunger DT. Large rectus muscle recessions for the treatment of congenital nystagmus. Arch Ophthalmol 1991;109:221-224.

271. von Noorden GK, Jenkins RH, Rosenbaum AL. Horizontal transposition of the vertical rectus muscles for treatment of ocular torticollis. J Ped Ophthalmol Strabismus 1993;30:8-14.

272. Waardenberg PJ. Some notes on publications of Professor Arnold Sorsby and on Aland eye disease (Forsius-Erickson syndrome). J Med Genet 1970;7:194-199.

273. Wagner RS, Caputo AR, Reynolds RD. Nystagmus in Down syndrome. Ophthalmology 1990;97: 1439-1444.

274. Waugh SJ, Bedell HE. Sensitivity to temporal luminance modulation in congenital nystagmus. Invest Ophthalmol Vis Sci 1992;33:2316-2324.

275. Weiss AH, Biersdorf WR. Visual sensory disorders in congenital nystagmus. Ophthalmology 1989;96: 517-523.

276. Weiss AH, Biersdorf WR. Blue cone monochromatism. J Pediatr Ophthalmol Strabismus 1989;26: 218-223.

277. Weissman BM, Dell'Osso LF, Abella, Leigh RJ. Spasmus nutans. A quantitative prospective study. Arch Ophthalmol 1987;105:525-528.

278. Weleber RG, Tongue AC. Congenital stationary night blindness presenting as Leber's congenital amaurosis. Arch Ophthalmol 1987;105:360-365.

279. Weleber RG, Pillers DM, Powell BR, et al. Aland Island Eye Disease (Forsius-Eriksson Syndrome) associated with contiguous gene deletion syndrome at Xp21: similarity to incomplete congenital stationary night blindness. Arch Ophthalmol 1989;107:1170-1179.

280. Westheimer G, Blair SM. The ocular tilt reaction— a brain stem oculomotor routine. Invest Ophthalmol 1975;14:833-839.

281. Williams RW, Garraghty PE, Goldowitz D. A new visual system mutation. Achiasmatic dogs with congenital nystagmus. Soc Neuroscience 1991;17: 187.

282. Willshaw HE. Assessment of nystagmus. Arch Dis Child 1993;69:102-103.

283. Winterson BJ, Collewijn H. Inversion of direction-selectivity to anterior fields in neurons of nucleus of the optic tract in rabbits with ocular albinism. Brain Res 1981;220:31-49.

284. Wisniewski K, Wisniewski HM. Diagnosis of infantile neuroaxonal dystrophy by skin biopsy. Ann Neurol 1980;7:377-379.

285. Worfolk R, Abadi RV. Quick phase programming and saccadic re-orientation in congenital nystagmus. Vision Res 1991;31:1819-1830.

286. Yagasaki T, Sato M, Awaya S, Nakamura N. Changes in nystagmus after simultaneous surgery for bilateral congenital cataracts. Jpn J Ophthalmol 1993;37:330-338.

287. Yamazaki A. Abnormalities of smooth pursuit and vestibular eye movements in congenital jerk nystagmus. In: Shimaya K, ed. *Ophthalmology*. Amsterdam: Exerpta Medica; 1979:1162-1165.

288. Yee RD, Jelks GW, Baloh RW, et al. Uniocular nystagmus in monocular visual loss. Ophthalmology 1979;86:511-518.

289. Yee RD, Baloh RW, Honrubia V. Eye movement abnormalities in rod monochromacy. Ophthalmology 1981;88:1010-1018.

290. Yee RD, Baloh RW, Honrubia V. Effect of Baclofen on congenital nystagmus. In: Lennerstrand G, Zee DS, Keller EL, eds. *Functional Basis of Ocular Motility Disorders*. Oxford: Pergamon Press; 1982:151-158.

291. Yee RD. Evaluating nystagmus in young children. Arch Ophthalmol 1990;108:793.

292. Yee RD. In Reply: Choice of initial tests for nystagmus in infants. Arch Ophthalmol 1991;109:64.

293. Zak TA, Ambrosio A. Nutritional nystagmus in infants. J Pediatr Ophthalmol Strabismus 1985;22: 141-142.

294. Zauberman H, Magora A. Congenital "seesaw" movement. Br J Ophthalmol 1969;53:418-421.

295. Zee DS, Freeman JM, Holtznan NA. Ophthalmoplegia in maple syrup urine disease. J Pediatr 1974;84:113-115.

296. Zee DS, Robinson DA. A hypothetical explanation of saccadic oscillations. Ann Neurol 1981;5: 405-414.

297. Zelt RP, Biglan AW. Congenital seesaw nystagmus. J Pediatr Ophthalmol Strabismus 1985;22: 13-16.

298. Zimmerman CF, Roach ES, Troost BR. Seesaw nystagmus associated with Chiari malformation. Arch Neurol 1986;43:299-300.

299. Zubcov AA, Reinecke RD, Gottlob I, et al. Treatment of manifest latent nystagmus. Am J Ophthalmol 1990;110:160-167.

300. Zubcov AA, Stark N, Weber A, et al. Improvement of visual acuity after surgery for nystagmus. Ophthalmology 1993;100: 1488-1497.

9

Torticollis and Head Nodding

Introduction

Children with neuro-ophthalmologic disorders often develop anomalous head postures (torticollis) or rhythmical movements of the head. The neuro-ophthalmologic evaluation of *torticollis* is greatly simplified by the probable association of a head tilt with superior oblique palsy and a horizontal or vertical head posture with incomitant strabismus or nystagmus. When strabismus and nystagmus are absent, the differential diagnosis includes a long list of ocular and systemic conditions. *Head nodding* in children usually signifies spasmus nutans or congenital nystagmus; however, an awareness of other rare causes is necessary to provide a complete evaluation. Abnormal head movements are less likely to be overlooked by parents than are abnormal head positions.

In this chapter, we use the term head nodding generically to describe an abnormal oscillation of the head in any direction. Many sources limit use of the term head nodding to describe anteroposterior oscillations of the head and apply the term *head shaking* to side-to-side oscillations. However, some children display a combination of horizontal and vertical oscillations, and it is convenient to apply a single descriptive term in such cases. The term *head tremor* has the advantage of being directionally nonspecific, but it connotes a rapid, small-amplitude head movement (as seen in benign essential tremor) that differs from the slower, larger-amplitude oscillations seen in children with neurological disease.

This chapter will focus on the clinical manifestations of those neuro-ophthalmologic and sys-temic conditions that lead to torticollis, head nodding, or both. It includes extensive discussion of common conditions and brief mention of rare disorders that warrant consideration once common conditions are excluded. Other forms of abnormal head movement (head thrusting, myoclonus, tics, and habit spasms) are covered in Chapter 7 in the context of their associated neuro-ophthalmologic findings.

Torticollis

Torticollis, derived from the Latin tortus (twisted) and collum (neck) is defined as "a contracted state of the cervical muscles, producing twisting of the neck and an unnatural position of the head."[34] In clinical practice, torticollis refers to any abnormal head tilt, face turn, or vertical position of the head. Also known as "wryneck" or "caput obstipum," torticollis was first alluded to by Hippocrates (c. 500 BC) and later detailed by Plutarch (356 to 232 BC).[66] Throughout history, treatments for torticollis have ranged from elaborate splints and traction techniques to tenotomy of the neck muscles. In 1873, Cuignet described torticollis as a manifestation of misalignment of the eyes.[35]

Head posture is maintained anatomically by the vertebral column supporting the head and the muscles of the neck and shoulders (the sternocleidomastoid, thoracic, and cervical semispinalis muscles).[120] An erect head posture will not be maintained by these muscles unless the brain has the ability to recognize the position of the head in relation to the body and to the pull of gravity. This

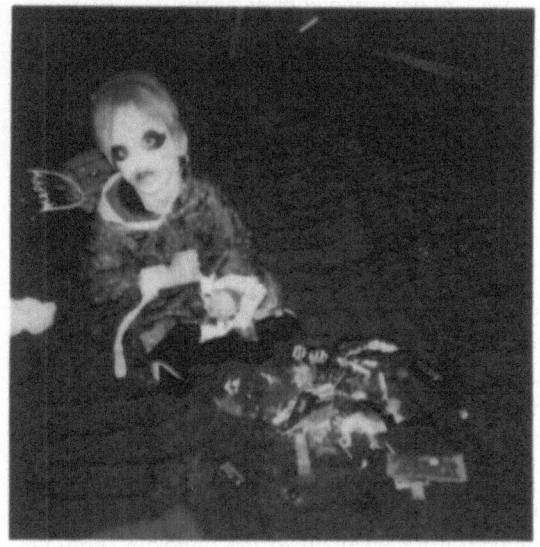

FIGURE 9.1. Child with ocular torticollis in costume for Halloween. Note simultaneous head tilt and face turn.

information is supplied by the proprioceptive impulses from the cervical muscles, by the labyrinthine and vestibular reflexes, and by the centers for balance in the brain. Further adjustments in head position are made following ocular muscle activity as a result of retinal stimulation.[120]

Abnormal head positions involve rotation of the head around one of the three primary axes: the vertical axis for head rotation, the horizontal axis for chin elevation and depression, and the anterior-posterior axis for head tilting toward the shoulder.[120] Some patients utilize a head position that involves simultaneous rotation around two or more axes (Figure 9.1). Rarely, the entire head can be retracted or pushed forward with respect to the median axis of the body.

Ocular Torticollis

Since the eyes receive stimuli for finer adjustments of head posture, visual or motor abnormalities often produce compensatory activity.[120] An abnormal head posture related to vision only develops if it offers some visual reward. In children with noncomitant strabismus, the anomalous head position is a good prognostic sign since it usually signifies the preservation of fusion. When the abnormal head position becomes too uncomfortable to sustain, then other compensations such as suppression or amblyopia develop, and the head resumes its normal position.[120]

Most ocular disorders that result in torticollis reflect a disturbance of neural input from the ocular motor nerves, the vestibular apparatus, or the afferent visual pathways. The abnormal head position may serve to restore single binocular vision, improve visual acuity, or centralize a partial visual field with respect to the body.[120] Rarely, central innervational anomalies may simultaneously produce ocular misalignment, torsion, and torticollis which is not visually compensatory, as in the ocular tilt reaction (discussed later). Most forms of ocular torticollis (Table 9.1) are associated with a distinct constellation of clinical and neuroimaging abnormalities that allow definitive diagnosis of the underlying condition. Once the specific cause of the ocular torticollis is established, appropriately planned strabismus surgery has a high rate of success in eliminating the abnormal head position.[71]

TABLE 9.1. Ocular torticollis.

Head tilt	Face turn	Vertical head position
Superior oblique palsy	Incomitant strabismus	A or V pattern
Plagiocephaly (synostotic)	Congenital nystagmus	Congenital nystagmus with null point
Spasmus nutans	Congenital homonymous hemianopia	Congenital nystagmus with A or V pattern
Congenital nystagmus	Horizontal gaze palsies or gaze deviation	Congenital ptosis (unilateral or bilateral)
Dissociated vertical deviation	Macular heterotopia	Noncomitant strabismus (e.g., Brown
Photophobia, epiphora, torticollis		syndrome)
Paroxysmal torticollis of infancy		Vertical gaze palsies or gaze deviation
Ocular tilt reaction		
Oblique astigmatism		
Lens subluxation		

Head Tilts

Noncomitant Strabismus

Any vertical extraocular muscle paresis may necessitate a compensatory head tilt to achieve binocular vision. Head tilting may be the salient clinical feature of an isolated oblique muscle palsy. An isolated vertical rectus muscle palsy may produce a head tilt that occurs in conjunction with an abnormal vertical head position. Isolated vertical muscle weakness resulting from disease involving the neuromuscular junction or the muscle itself can lead to similar findings.

Superior oblique palsy is the most common cause of a head tilt.[73,93,112,121] The long intracranial course of the fourth cranial nerve, which innervates the superior oblique muscle, renders it particularly susceptible to injury from head trauma. Unilateral superior oblique paresis produces excyclodeviation and a hyperdeviation of the involved eye. Patients with uncomplicated unilateral superior oblique palsy tilt their head contralaterally to the side of the injured nerve to restore single binocular vision. This compensatory head posture causes the otolith apparatus to increase innervation to the extorters (inferior oblique muscle and inferior rectus muscle) of the involved eye and decrease innervation to the intorters (superior rectus muscle and superior oblique muscle), thus minimizing the mechanical advantage of the superior rectus muscle (an elevator) over the paretic superior oblique muscle (a depressor). Tilting the head ipsilaterally to the side of the injured nerve causes the otolith apparatus to stimulate the intorters (the superior rectus muscle and superior oblique muscle) and inhibit the extorters (the inferior rectus muscle and inferior oblique muscle) of the involved eye, which provides a mechanical advantage to the superior rectus muscle over the paretic superior oblique muscle, resulting in worsening of the hyperdeviation.

The patient with superior oblique palsy tilts his or her head to eliminate the *vertical* deviation rather than the torsional deviation, which can be overcome by adaptive mechanisms including sensory cyclofusion, as well as other psychological-experiential and physiological-sensory adaptations.[51,115] (Placing a prism in front of either eye of a patient with superior oblique palsy to match the vertical deviation eliminates the vertical deviation and causes the head tilt to resolve, despite persistence of the torsion.)[115]

Occasionally, children with superior oblique palsy are unable to adapt to a cyclotropia, in which case the cyclotropia (without an accompanying vertical deviation) can be the exclusive source of the torticollis.[115] Children whose head tilt disappears on covering the paretic eye and persists when the nonparetic eye is covered probably fall into this group. Since binocular vision is disrupted when either eye is covered and symptoms of hypertropia are thus eliminated, only cyclotropia could explain the persistence of the head tilt when the sound eye is covered.[115] Under binocular conditions, such a child would assume a compensatory head tilt to the opposite shoulder when the involved eye fixates and would have no compensatory head posture when the uninvolved eye fixates.[71,114,115] Some children with superior oblique palsy maintain a contralateral head tilt even though a manifest vertical strabismus exists and fusion is absent in the preferred head position.[115] In such children, a long-standing head tilt may persist on a habitual basis, it may be secondary to unilateral contracture of the neck muscles, or it may serve to provide anomalous fusion on the basis of anomalous retinal correspondence.[115] A child with superior oblique palsy may rarely tilt the head toward the side of the hypertropic eye to maximize separation of diplopic images.[71,115] The finding of a paradoxical head tilt should also lead one to consider the possibility of dissociated vertical deviation, which can be associated with a head tilt toward or away from the side of the hypertropic eye.[21]

Congenital and acquired superior oblique palsies differ with respect to their clinical manifestations and their underlying etiologies. In acquired palsies, the head position is marked, a noncomitant deviation is present, intermittent diplopia is common, and there is no facial asymmetry, except in long-standing deviations.[116] By contrast, congenital superior oblique palsy is often associated with milder torticollis that has persisted since infancy (evident in old photographs)[89] together with facial asymmetry (see Chapter 6).[121] Large vertical fusional vergence amplitudes are also highly characteristic of congenital or longstanding superior oblique palsy.[116] Recognition of these features is crucial in establishing the diagnosis of congenital fourth nerve palsy, since spread of comitance may develop over many years, obscuring the characteristic ocular motility pattern. Many patients with congenital superior oblique palsy and torticollis deny diplopia, but some present with acute vertical diplopia when they lose control of their deviation. Unlike patients who acquire superior oblique palsy from an injury to the trochlear nerve, many patients with congenital superior oblique palsy are found at surgery to have a lax, misdirected, or absent superior oblique tendon.[94] Such cases of congenital superior oblique palsy actually represent a primary myopathy and could arguably be classified as a unique form of congenital muscular torticollis.

Synostotic Plagiocephaly

Patients with synostotic plagiocephaly have premature fusion of the coronal suture on one side of the skull.[5,32] This cranial abnormality leads to ipsilateral forehead and orbital retrusion, contralateral forehead protrusion, orbital and lateral canthal dystopia, and contralateral zygomatic and occipital flattening[32] (Figure 9.2). Affected infants manifest unilateral superior oblique dysfunction and tilt their head contralateral to the side of the retruded orbit.[5,32,40] Weakness of the superior oblique muscle results from a desagittalization and laxity of the superior oblique tendon within the retruded orbit (Figure 9.3). As will be discussed, a separate form of plagiocephaly (deformational) results from the asymmetrical effects of congenital muscular torticollis on craniofacial growth. Unlike synostotic plagiocephaly, deformational plagiocephaly is not associated with strabismus.[40]

We have grown attuned to the notion that a dichotomy exists in which head tilting in infancy can be assigned to a purely neurogenic or myogenic category. This nosologic distinction has become nebulous in congenital fourth nerve palsy and is even more so in synostotic plagiocephaly, wherein malpositioning of the trochlea associated with an osseous (i.e., musculoskeletal) abnormality leads to superior oblique tendon laxity and signs and symptoms of superior oblique palsy.

Spasmus Nutans

Nystagmus accompanied by head nodding and torticollis in an infant or young child is highly suggestive of spasmus nutans. In 1906, Still[107] rhapsodically summarized the sensation of observing a child with spasmus nutans:

Hardly less striking than this rhythmic unsteadiness of the head is the curious way the child has of looking at objects out of the corner of his eyes with the head slightly averted and the face turned slightly downwards, reminding one of the behavior of the Beaver in *The Hunting of the Snark,* for as you may remember,

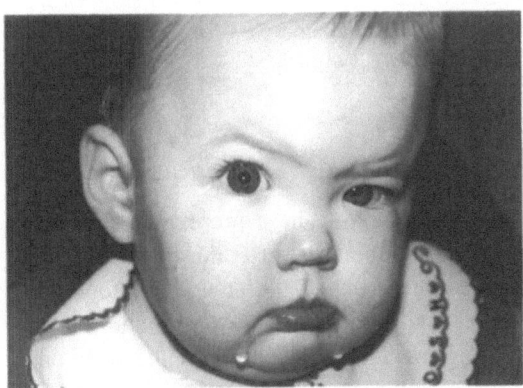

FIGURE 9.2. Infant with right synostotic plagiocephaly. Note retrusion of the right forehead and orbit, elevated right superior orbital rim, widened right palpebral fissure, left forehead protrusion, and head tilt to the left.

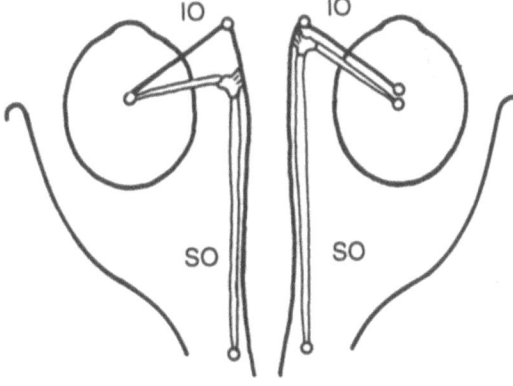

FIGURE 9.3. Relationship between the inferior oblique muscle and the superior oblique tendon in synostotic plagiocephaly. Desagittalization of the superior oblique tendon occurs due to the retruded right orbit and right trochlea relative to the inferior orbital rim.

'Whenever the butcher was by,
The Beaver kept looking the opposite way
And appeared unaccountably shy.'

The other feature which attracts attention is the exceedingly fine rapid nystagmus which is peculiar in being so much more marked in one eye than the other, that it may appear to be actually limited to one eye, a point which the mother herself has usually noticed.

The appearance of the nystagmus alone in spasmus nutans is fairly distinct in that it resembles an ocular shiver that may be so fine and rapid as to be barely visible.[45] It may be horizontal, vertical, or rotary in direction.[55] The clinical appearance of spasmus nutans differs from that of congenital nystagmus in that spasmus nutans is often asymmetrical and may actually be monocular. It also differs in its usual time of onset (4 months to a year in spasmus nutans versus 2 to 3 months of age in congenital nystagmus). Although usually a benign, self-limited entity, MR imaging is warranted in children with spasmus nutans since children with congenital suprasellar tumors may present with an identical constellation of findings.[44,87] Neurodegenerative disorders[104] and congenital retinal dystrophies[46,74] may also rarely masquerade as spasmus nutans.

The compensatory nature of the head nodding in spasmus nutans is discussed below. While the cause of the associated head tilt and face turn remains speculative, Gottlob et al[45] have recently suggested that it may serve to directionalize the visually compensatory head nodding to its optimal trajectory.

Congenital Nystagmus

Children with congenital nystagmus may infrequently utilize a head tilt to dampen their nystagmus. In this setting, a careful search for an underlying cyclovertical muscle palsy should be undertaken before attributing the head tilt to a torsional null position. Congenital nystagmus with a torsional null position should also become visibly worse when straightening the head or tilting it to the opposite side. Several "torsional Kestenbaum" procedures are effective in eliminating the null-point–associated head tilt in congenital nystagmus.[26,106] These procedures involve transposing the horizontal, vertical, or oblique muscles to rotate the eyes in the direction of the head tilt. Tor-

sional Kestenbaum procedures induce an adverse stimulus (tilting of the visual world) that can only be compensated for by straightening the head. Unlike Kestenbaum procedures, which effectively transfer the null position to primary gaze, torsional Kestenbaum procedures impede utilization of the compensatory head tilt, thereby eliminating access to the null position.[117] Notwithstanding the efficacy of these procedures, it is important to realize that they effectively eliminate access to the torsional null zone.

Paroxysmal Torticollis of Infancy

In 1969, Snyder[105] described 12 infants with paroxysmal head tilts that lasted from 10 minutes to 2 days. In some infants, the torticollis was accompanied with vomiting, pallor, and agitation. When the torticollis resolved, the infants appeared normal until the next attack. After a period of months to years, the attacks subsided. Subsequent reports have shown a female predominance and a tendency for the attacks to occur upon awakening.

Paroxysmal torticollis of infancy is now considered to be a migraine equivalent that primarily affects the vestibular system.[92] Older children may complain of headache or vertigo during the attack. Later in life, some children develop benign paroxysmal vertigo, which may be a migraine variant. Affected children often have a strong family history of migraine headache. An infant with an episodic torticollis, complete interval recovery, a suggestive past history, and a family history of migraines need not be subjected to invasive and expensive diagnostic studies.[92]

Photophobia, Epiphora, and Torticollis

Torticollis can rarely be a presenting sign of a posterior fossa tumor.[7,68] Marmor et al[78] recently described three young children with photophobia, epiphora, and torticollis who were found to have posterior fossa tumors. In one child, the symptoms improved following surgical resection. Posterior fossa tumors could theoretically cause torticollis by irritation of the vestibular nuclear complex, dural stretch, tonsillar herniation, cyclovertical muscle paresis, or any combination thereof.[78] Torticollis in the absence of photophobia or epiphora has also been reported in association with infratentorial tumors.

Ocular Tilt Reaction

The ocular tilt reaction consists of vertical divergence of the eyes, bilateral ocular torsion, and tilting of the head.[53] The ocular tilt reaction appears to be a compensatory postural reflex of otolithic origin.[52] The physiological basis of this reaction is best understood when one considers its phylogenetic origin. Part of the role of the otolithic (static) vestibular system is to maintain verticality. Tilting a fish about its long axis produces a hypotropia of the uppermost eye.[52] A chicken or an owl will keep its head gravitationally vertical during lateral tilting of its trunk.[52] Tilting a frontal-eyed animal about its sagittal axis evokes a graviceptive response, leading to bilateral ocular torsion, vertical divergence, and a head tilt.

A pathological ocular tilt reaction results from a central nervous system (CNS) lesion that affects either the vestibular nucleus or its central connections to the contralateral interstitial nucleus of Cajal (a paramedian structure located near the junction of the thalamus and the midbrain). The imbalance in central vestibular tone created by such a lesion presumably simulates the situation in which the entire body is tilted to one side, resulting in a "righting response" to reestablish verticality (Figure 9.4). For example, an irritative lesion that stimulates the ipsilateral interstitial nucleus of Cajal at the junction of the thalamus and the midbrain can produce an "ipsiversive" tilt reaction, characterized by a head tilt toward the side of the lesion, hypotropia on the side of the lesion, and torsion of both eyes toward the side of the lesion. A destructive or inhibitory lesion does the opposite. The ocular tilt reaction is a rare but recognizable cause of torticollis. Magnetic resonance imaging with special attention to the brain stem and thalamomesencephalic junction should be obtained in suspected cases.

Face Turns

Neurovisual disturbances may produce compensatory face turns in three ways. (Table 9.1):

1. A face turn is often adopted to restore binocular single vision in patients with incomitant paralytic or restrictive strabismus. Almost any patient who assumes an abnormal head posture for visually related reasons does so at

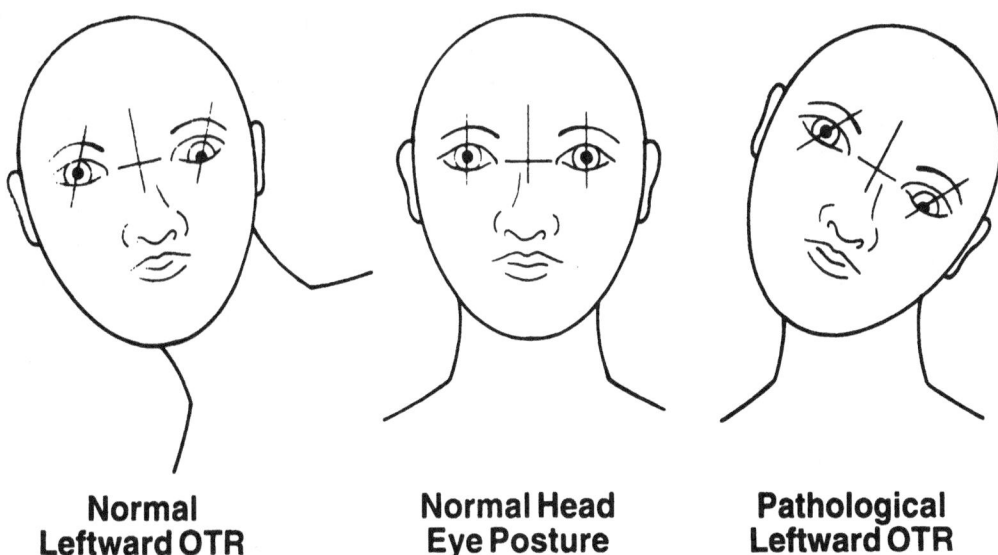

**Normal
Leftward OTR**   **Normal Head
Eye Posture**   **Pathological
Leftward OTR**

FIGURE 9.4. The normal ocular tilt reaction in a subject tilted to the right about his sagittal axis (left), showing the normal compensatory leftward head tilt, vertical divergence of the eyes, and bilateral ocular torsion in the absence of any rotation of the trunk. (Modified from Halmagyi et al. Neurology 1990;40:1508.)

least partly to frontalize their field of vision relative to their body.[120] For example, a child with a sixth nerve palsy will prefer to turn his or her face toward the affected side to realign the eyes, despite the fact that ocular alignment could also be obtained without a face turn by shifting the head and trunk laterally together while maintaining fixation in the direction opposite to that of the paresis.

2. Face turns are utilized by patients with congenital or manifest-latent nystagmus to move the eyes into a null zone where the nystagmus is reduced and optimal visual acuity is achieved. At times, a subtle nystagmus may not be visible unless the optic disk is viewed with a direct ophthalmoscope. Children with unilateral microphthalmos, unilateral aphakia, or other conditions associated with congenital visual loss often develop manifest latent nystagmus with a large face turn toward the better-seeing eye. Similarly, children with congenital esotropia and manifest latent nystagmus often turn their face to dampen the nystagmus by placing the better-seeing eye in adduction. Face turns in spasmus nutans are probably not associated with a null position but are utilized to directionalize the head nodding to the specific trajectory necessary to effectively dampen the nystagmus.

3. Children with congenital homonymous hemianopia often turn their face toward the hemianopic field while maintaining fixation on objects of interest.[59,120] Since this maneuver does not change the position of the intact visual field in space, centralization of the intact visual field with respect to the body seems to be the only function subserved by a face turn in this particular setting. Because these children are often exotropic, it has been suggested that the development of exotropia may be an adaptive mechanism to expand their limited visual field.[43] However, Hoyt and Good[59] have argued that the exotropia seen in children with congenital homonymous hemianopia could well be an epiphenomenon rather than a visual adaptation.

Other disorders have also been documented to produce face turns in children. The combination of a large convergent or divergent ocular deviation and limited ocular movements will cause a child to turn the face to direct the preferred eye toward the object of fixation.[120] Face turns may also be seen in children with horizontal gaze palsy or gaze deviations without strabismus. Children with retinopathy of prematurity and macular heterotopia may take a face turn to fixate eccentrically with the better-seeing eye.[73] Children with nystagmus blockage syndrome must take a large face turn to foveate objects of interest while utilizing excessive convergence.[73]

Vertical Head Postures

Most abnormal vertical head postures occur in children with congenital ptosis, A- or V-pattern horizontal strabismus, restrictive vertical strabismus, or incomitant vertical strabismus (Table 9.1). Children with unilateral congenital ptosis will raise the chin to obtain binocular vision; those with bilateral congenital ptosis will raise the chin to increase their field of vision. Children with congenital fibrosis syndrome may have a combination of bilateral ptosis and fixed downgaze, each necessitating a chin-up position.[73] In the setting of either A- or V-pattern strabismus or vertical restrictive strabismus, the chin-up or chin-down position places the eyes in a position of minimal deviation to establish some degree of binocularity.[120]

Some children with congenital nystagmus have a vertical null zone, necessitating a chin-up or chin-down position. Congenital nystagmus patients with even small A or V patterns may utilize a vertical head position to create a large exophoria, which enables them to increase convergence tone and improve visual acuity. It is therefore critical in the child with congenital nystagmus to search for an associated exophoria in the preferred field of gaze before concluding that the vertical head position results from a vertical null position, since the appropriate surgical management varies according to the underlying condition.

Rarely, the two problems can coexist, as exemplified by the following case:

A 5-year-old girl had been followed since infancy with congenital nystagmus and a marked chin-down position. Numerous examinations showed that the intensity of the nystagmus dampened in upgaze and increased in downgaze. Additionally, she had a V pattern with orthophoria in upgaze and esotropia in downgaze. The child was treated with bilateral superior rectus recessions and inferior rectus resections with lateral transpositions of the inferior rectus muscles. This procedure transferred the null zone to primary gaze and eliminated the V pattern.

Vertical head positions are also seen in children with vertical gaze palsy or vertical gaze deviations who must assume an abnormal head position to fixate. Rarely, children with retinal or optic nerve disease associated with altitudinal visual field defects may assume chin-up or chin-down positions, presumably to centralize the remaining visual field relative to the body.[25]

Refractive Causes of Torticollis

Rarely, ocular refractive errors can lead to anomalous head positions that serve to improve vision (Table 9.1). Patients with bilateral oblique astigmatism may tilt their head to directionalize the astigmatic blur with respect to the vertical meridian.[14,73,100,120] Undercorrected myopia may cause a patient to elevate the chin or turns the face to gain increased strength from the spectacle lenses.[35,120] An 8-year-old girl with homocystinuria and bilateral ectopia lentis was reported to utilize a head tilt to recenter one of the crystalline lenses and obtain phakic vision.[72] Although rare, these conditions should be included in the differential diagnosis of enigmatic torticollis.

Neurological Causes of Torticollis

Central nervous system pathology unrelated to the visual system should also be considered in patients with enigmatic torticollis (Table 9.2). Acquired torticollis may be the presenting sign of syringomyelia and spinal cord tumors,[68,109] as well as cervical epidural abscess with osteomyelitis.[80] Torticollis associated with hyperactive tendon reflexes, ankle clonus, or extensor plantar responses suggests a cervical spinal cord disturbance and is an indication for MR imaging of the cervical spine.[37]

If evidence of dystonia in the face or limbs is present, the diagnosis of *spasmodic torticollis* should be considered. Spasmodic torticollis refers to a dystonia of the facial and cervical muscles resulting from neurological disease or medications affecting the basal ganglia.[10,22] Spasmodic torticollis associated with neurological disease has been successfully treated with botulinum toxin therapy and with selective surgical peripheral denervation of the sternocleidomastoid and splenius capitus muscle.[9] Spasmodic torticollis in children may occur as an idiosyncratic reaction following a first dose of phenothiazine or haloperidol.[37] In this setting, it may be accompanied by other dystonic reactions including trismus, opisthotonos, and oculogyric crises.[69] Drug-induced spasmodic torticollis resolves promptly when the child is treated with anticholinesterase medications (e.g., Cogentin). Spasmodic torticollis is uncommon in children except when drug induced.[37] The highest frequency of drug-induced dystonia and oculogyric crises occurs in children under 15 years of age.[69] Spasmodic torticollis may rarely occur as a familial condition.[41]

Head tilting has recently been described in the infectious disease literature as a rare manifestation of nuchal rigidity in three patients with acute bacterial meningitis,[79] however, no neuro-ophthalmologic examinations were performed to rule out the possibility of a fourth nerve palsy. Given the strong association between acute bacterial meningitis and cranial nerve palsies, an inflammatory fourth nerve palsy must be the primary diagnostic consideration in the child with acute bacterial meningitis and an unexplained head tilt.

Paroxysmal dystonia in infancy is a condition that usually has its onset in the first months of life. Motor symptoms are characterized by torsion of the neck or trunk, opisthotonos, hypertonus of the

TABLE 9.2. Nonocular torticollis.

Musculoskeletal	Systemic	Neurologic
Congenital muscular torticollis	Unilateral deafness	Spasmodic torticollis
Congenital deformities	Compensation for pain	Syringomyelia
of the cervical spine	arthritis	Spinal cord tumor
Klippel–Feil anomaly	mastoiditis	Meningitis
Occipitocervical synostosis	Gastroesophageal reflux (Sandifer syndrome)	
	Psychiatric	

upper limbs with flexion or extension of the arms and hyperpronation of the wrist, and no disturbance of consciousness.[3] The attacks usually last several minutes and occur with a frequency ranging from several times a day to once a month. This entity differs from paroxysmal torticollis in infancy in that the trunk and arms are also involved and no autonomic symptoms are detected.[3] The attacks spontaneously remit in most cases.

Paroxysmal choreoathetosis is a rare disorder with onset between 1 and 2 years of age. It consists of paroxysmal episodes of abnormal posturing and choreoathetoid movements that may include torticollis and facial grimacing. The child is conscious and often uncomfortable during the episode.[96] These children are otherwise in good health and neurologically normal between attacks.[98] The disorder can be familial or sporadic. The episodes occur several times a month, but may vary in frequency from several times a day to several times a year. They last for 5 minutes to an hour and often appear to be related to excitement or fatigue.[98] These transient episodes do not appear to be epileptiform or migrainous in nature.

Congenital Muscular Torticollis

Congenital muscular torticollis is diagnosed in an infant or young child with a unilateral head tilt associated with limited rotation of the head to the opposite side (Figure 9.5).[56] It is differentiated from the more common head tilt associated with superior oblique palsy by its restriction to passive motion and its failure to normalize when one eye is patched. The presence of facial asymmetry, which was once considered to be a distinguishing feature of congenital muscular torticollis, is now also well recognized in children with congenital superior oblique palsy.[121]

Soon after birth, a mass appears in the belly of the sternocleidomastoid muscle, and the patient develops a head tilt to the side of the involved muscle.[24,66] After several months, the mass or tumor disappears as signs of facial asymmetry become more evident (Figure 9.5). In the majority of cases, the head tilt subsequently resolves, and the facial asymmetry normalizes over the first year of life, with or without physical therapy.[24] When the head tilt persists, the affected sternocleidomastoid muscle is found to be hard and tight to palpation.[61]

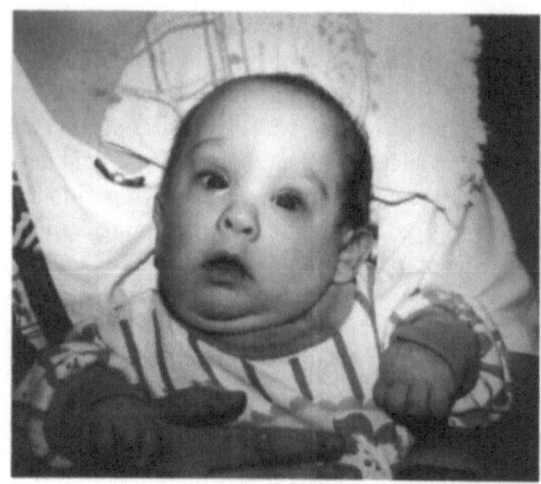

FIGURE 9.5. Five-month old girl with congenital muscular torticollis. Note facial asymmetry (deformational plagiocephaly).

The pathogenesis of congenital muscular torticollis is obscure. It is frequently, although not necessarily, associated with a history of some obstetrical difficulty.[58] Clinically, congenital muscular torticollis consists of a contracture of the sternocleidomastoid muscle, without osseous deformity, local inflammation, or primary neural abnormality.[12] Excisional biopsies of the tumor have shown a hard, white, fibrous lesion that resembles a fibroma with no evidence of hematoma or injury.[76] The sternal head of the muscle is almost completely replaced by fibrous tissue. Sarnet and Morrissy[102] suggested that the separate arterial supply of the sternal head predisposes to ischemia, focal myopathy, and fibrosis, while the grouped atrophy in the clavicular head was consistent with the combination of secondary entrapment neuropathy of the spinal accessory nerve resulting from its passage through a myopathic sternal head on its way to the clavicular head.

Facial asymmetry (termed "facial scoliosis" in the older literature) is generally regarded as a ubiquitous finding in children whose congenital muscular torticollis fails to resolve spontaneously. It is therefore considered to be an inevitable consequence of a permanent oblique head posture of long duration.[58] As the neck and facial bones assume larger proportions, the fibrotic sternocleidomastoid muscle fails to elongate normally, producing pathological changes of the face and skull.

The eyebrow on the side of the shortened muscle tends to slope downward, and the portion of the face below the level of the eye becomes shorter and wider on the affected side than the corresponding normal side (Figure 9.5). The frontal eminence is flattened on the affected side, and there is a well-marked bulge in the occipital region, while on the other side, the eminence is unduly prominent and the occipital region is rather flat. The vault of the skull is "thrown back" on the affected side and "pushed forward" on the opposite side, resulting in "deformational plagiocephaly." Facial asymmetry progressively increases as growth continues and the cervical curve continues. It often resolves following early surgical intervention and, in some older children, shows a gradual reversal following surgical repair.[11,61,77]

An association of congenital muscular torticollis with congenital hip dysplasia is now well established. Hummer and MacEwen[62] retrospectively reviewed records from 70 children with congenital muscular torticollis and found congenital dislocation of the hip in 5% and congenital subluxation of the hip in 15%. The authors noted that only patients with some physical abnormality had radiographic studies, so that silent or subclinical cases were probably overlooked. There was no statistically significant relationship between the side of the torticollis and the side of the hip dysplasia. Interestingly, Busch and Westin[12] found congenital hip dislocation or dysplasia in 9 of 36 patients, which always involved the hip ipsilateral to the tight cervical muscles. Clinical and neuroradiographic examination of the hip joints is now considered a part of the routine evaluation of congenital muscular torticollis.

Conservative treatment of congenital muscular torticollis consists of passive tilting of the head in the direction opposite the deformity, rearrangement of the crib to encourage the infant to lie on the affected side, and special neck braces in some cases.[12] Approximately 80% of infants respond to conservative measures and do not require surgical release.[12,15] Canale et al[15] found that an exercise program is more likely to be successful when the restriction of motion is less than 30° and there is little or no facial asymmetry.

Beyond 1 year of age, congenital muscular torticollis does not generally respond to conservative measures. Early or previous surgical treatment of congenital muscular torticollis consisted of surgical transection of the contracted sternocleidomastoid muscle. It is now evident that this procedure is often associated with unsightly clavicular prominence and neck asymmetry.[12,58] Bipolar release (i.e., complete release of the mastoid and clavicular attachments) combined with Z plasty of the sternal head has been recommended to avoid this complication.[12,15]

Other Musculoskeletal Causes of Torticollis

Musculoskeletal torticollis can also be a secondary manifestation of cervical skeletal abnormalities, such as occipitocervical synostosis, Klippel–Feil syndrome, scoliosis, basilar impression, atlanto-axial displacement, Sprengel's deformity, and congenital subluxations of cervical disks (Table 9.2).[54,95,100]

Systemic Causes of Torticollis

Torticollis can rarely be auditory, gastrointestinal, rheumatologic, or psychiatric in origin (Table 9.2). An intermittent unilateral face turn in infancy may be the presenting sign of unilateral deafness.[118] An extremely large, intermittent head tilt can be a sign of gastrointestinal disease.[90] *Sandifer syndrome* is a rare disorder in which a child with hiatal hernia and gastroesophageal reflux takes a large head tilt to prevent regurgitation.[119] Children with Sandifer syndrome typically have a history of vomiting and are thin. Compensation for pain may necessitate an abnormal head position in a variety of other conditions such as cervical arthritis or mastoiditis.[118] Psychiatric patients with no neurologic or systemic disease may occasionally assume large head tilts for no apparent reason.[54]

Head Nodding

Early in this century, rhythmical oscillations of the head were termed *head nystagmus*. In current usage, a nonsaccadic oscillation of the eyes is designated as *nystagmus*, while a similar oscillation of the head is often referred to as a *tremor*.[28] Head nodding can still be conceptually viewed as a form of "head nystagmus," since it represents a central disorder of the cephalomotor control system.[16] Its neuro-ophthalmologic intrigue lies primarily in its association with pediatric nystagmus, where it may be compensatory (i.e., serving to reduce the intensity of nystagmus and improve vision) or noncompensatory (i.e., a centrally driven oscillation similar to the nystagmus itself).

Several distinct forms of head nodding can be observed in children (Table 9.3).[30] Some are benign, while others provide a decisive clinical clue to a potentially life-threatening neurological or systemic disorder that may be treatable.[30] Our rudimentary understanding of the phenomenology of head nodding is exceeded by our ability to identify the underlying neurological or systemic disorders that produce it in the majority of cases.

Head Nodding with Nystagmus

In children with head nodding and nystagmus, the pathogenetic interrelationship between the ocular and cervical oscillations depends upon the underlying condition. In order to understand how these oscillations interrelate under pathological circumstances, one must first understand the role of the vestibulo-ocular reflex (VOR) under normal conditions. In normal individuals, the VOR causes any movement of the head to be accompanied by eye movements that are equal in velocity and opposite in direction to that of the head.[82] This reflex serves to stabilize the position of the eyes in space so that the direction of gaze remains constant during head movements. Thus, in children

with nystagmus, head nodding would not be expected to change the waveform of nystagmus since the head movements will be countered by the VOR, leaving the nystagmus to determine the position of the eyes.[49] It is now clear, however, that this rule cannot be applied to individuals with congenital nystagmus, because head or total body movements effect a dynamic shift in the null position (see Chapter 9) which secondarily modifies the congenital nystagmus waveform.[29] The change in the overall congenital nystagmus waveform induced by vestibular stimulation is often misconstrued as evidence of an underlying deficit in the VOR in individuals with congenital nystagmus.

In the child with nystagmus, head oscillations could function to improve vision only if (1) the VOR gain was inherently abnormal, (2) a normal VOR gain was somehow actively suppressed by the head movements, or (3) activation of a normal VOR could somehow "override" the nystagmus. Regardless of any clinically apparent effect of head oscillations upon the overall intensity of congenital nystagmus, compensatory head movements would have to prolong foveation time to improve vision.[16,28]

Spasmus Nutans

Spasmus nutans is the most common condition associated with head nodding in children.[18] The head nodding of spasmus nutans consists of a combination of true (anteroposterior) head nodding together with lateral shaking of the head in an unpredictable pattern.[55,107] It becomes prominent when the child inspects an object of interest

TABLE 9.3. Head nodding in children: Differential diagnosis.

I. Neurological disorders	II. Visual disorders	III. Systemic disorders
Spasmus nutans	Blindness	Aortic regurgitation
Congenital nystagmus	Intermittent esotropia	Acute metabolic abnormalities
Bobble-headed doll syndrome		(hypomagnesemia, hypocalcemia,
Neurodegenerative, metabolic,		uremia, thyrotoxicosis)
or multisystem genetic diseases		
Cerebellar disease		
Infantile spasms		
Congenital ocular motor apraxia		
Opsoclonus/Myoclonus		
Autism		
Benign essential tremor		

and it seems to increase with the complexity of the fixation target.[45,47]

Gresty and coworkers[47,48] were the first to describe simultaneous eye and head movement recordings in three children with spasmus nutans in whom head nodding abolished the nystagmus and activated normal VORs and suppressed the nystagmus. These children had better vision when they nodded their heads. Gresty and coworkers concluded that the head nodding was an operant-conditioned phenomenon, which served to suppress the nystagmus and improve visual acuity, and not a separate pathological phenomenon.

More recently, Gottlob et al[45] analyzed simultaneous head and eye movement recordings in 35 children with spasmus nutans. In 21 of these patients, the fine, fast dissociated nystagmus changed during head nodding to larger and slower symmetrical eye movements with both eyes oscillating in phase at the same amplitude and 180° out of phase to the head movements (see Figure 8.8). The ocular oscillations during head nodding corresponded to a normal VOR. These investigators concurred with Gresty and coworkers in concluding that head nodding in spasmus nutans is an adaptive strategy to improve vision rather than an involuntary movement of pathological origin. Head nodding in spasmus nutans could reduce or abolish the nystagmus through an unclear mechanism that functioned independently of the VOR or by stimulating the powerful VOR to override the nystagmus.[110]

Gottlob et al[45] also found that passive horizontal shaking of the patient's head by the examiner suppressed mainly the horizontal nystagmus, whereas passive vertical shaking suppressed mainly the vertical nystagmus. This finding would suggest that the principle direction of the head nodding in spasmus nutans may be dictated by the trajectory of the nystagmus. The associated head tilt in spasmus nutans may help to directionalize the head nodding to most effectively suppress the nystagmus.[45]

Gresty and Halmagyi[49] questioned whether a child's ability to cancel nystagmus and improve vision by shaking the head (as seen almost exclusively in spasmus nutans) could be construed as a predictive neurodevelopmental sign that the nystagmus would eventually resolve. The initial neurodevelopmental adaptation to the nystagmus (head oscillation) is achieved through an overt behavioral maneuver whereas the final adaptation (suppression of the nystagmus without head nodding) is internalized. This sequence of events recapitulates the developmental scheme proposed by Piaget in which, at the earliest developmental stage, the child is trying to solve problems by overt behavioral acts of experimentation, but as he develops into a stage of formal reasoning, he gains the ability to construct an internal model of control processes that enables him to suppress the involuntary movements without resorting to overt maneuvers.[49] Whether the eventual disappearance of spasmus nutans requires active suppression or whether it represents recovery of normal ocular stabilization systems is unclear.

Congenital Nystagmus

Approximately 10% of individuals with congenital nystagmus display a rapid, horizontal pendular shaking of the head.[39,88] According to Jan et al[63] this head shaking occurs in bursts lasting from 5 to 30 seconds and only during intense visual fixation. It occurs only with visual activity and does not involve any other part of the body. Head nodding in congenital nystagmus is a subconscious act that ceases when it is called to the individual's attention and cannot be willfully reactivated.[63]

Head nodding can be associated with a fine-amplitude nystagmus in several congenital retinal dystrophies (achromatopsia, blue-cone monochromatism, congenital stationary night blindness), producing a clinical appearance that may mimic spasmus nutans.[46,74] Unlike the head nodding in spasmus nutans, however, electro-oculographic recordings in congenital nystagmus have shown that the associated head oscillations do not contribute to an improvement in vision. On the contrary, it is now believed to be an involuntary cephalomotor tremor that presumably shares a common pathogenic origin with the nystagmus.[28]

Many of the conclusions drawn from studies pertaining to the interrelationship of congenital nystagmus and head shaking were based on clinical observations regarding the overall waveform of the nystagmus without objective documentation of the effect of head shaking on foveation periods. Thus, for many years, head shaking in congenital nystagmus has been thought to be compensatory in nature (i.e., synchronous with but opposite in direction to the ocular nystagmus, thereby serving to stabilize the eyes on the object of attention).[19] This idea was attractive because it seemed consistent with the clinical observation that the head nodding increased noticeably during periods of fatigue, anxiety, and intense curiosity, when the intensity of the nystagmus also increased.[63] Numerous electro-oculographic studies claiming to show that the VOR was defective in congenital nystagmus (see Chapter 8) seemed to provide a pathophysiological basis for the notion that head oscillations could stabilize the position of the eyes in space without being neutralized by a normal VOR.

These early studies were inherently flawed either in premise or implementation. Some investigators provided only verbal descriptions of congenital nystagmus in which the head oscillations appeared to be equal and opposite to the ongoing eye movements (with a VOR gain somehow reduced to zero) or in which the head oscillations seemed to cancel the ocular oscillations by a central mechanism as in spasmus nutans without providing simultaneous eye and head movement recordings to support these claims.[48,49] One report contained simultaneous head and eye movement recordings but showed jerky head movements of approximately 30° that were supposedly compensating for a nystagmus of approximately 7°.[81] In another case, eye movement recordings showed convergent nystagmus (which is consistent with spasmus nutans but not with congenital nystagmus) and head movements that canceled the nystagmus.[110] As with smooth pursuit, the sustained vestibular input from head nodding produces a dynamic shift in the null zone, which changes the overall waveform of the nystagmus. As mentioned earlier, the failure to recognize the significance of this observation has contributed to the conclusion that the VOR is inherently defective in congenital nystagmus.

As discussed in Chapter 8, this myth has now been largely dispelled.[16,29,50] Electro-oculographic recordings of congenital nystagmus have shown that, during foveation periods, the position of gaze remains stable during head rotation despite the superimposed oscillations of congenital nystagmus. With rare exceptions, the VOR is preserved, and electro-oculographic recordings show no flattening of foveation periods.[16,28,75] These findings are consistent with the fact that older children and adults are often aware of their intermittent head shaking and state that they do not believe it helps them to see.[28]

Carl et al[16] documented an exception to this rule in a patient who showed true compensation of congenital nystagmus by the head movements. This patient suppressed his VOR gain and improvement occurred only during foveation periods. Simultaneous eye and head movement recordings showed that the foveation periods were not flat when the head was still, but they became flat when the head movements occurred. Four other individuals who were studied showed no improvement in foveation periods during head shaking. Dell'Osso and Daroff[28] have stressed that most individuals with congenital nystagmus have flat foveation periods and can therefore achieve no visual benefit from shaking their head.[28] From both a theoretical and an evidentiary standpoint, head nodding in congenital nystagmus is almost never visually adaptive.

Neurodegenerative Disorders, Metabolic Defects, and Genetic Syndromes

Pelizaeus Merzbacher disease may be associated with intermittent shaking movements of the head and a rapid, irregular, often asymmetric pendular nystagmus.[1] Children with 3-methyl-glutaconic aciduria and neurological signs of Behr syndrome may display head nodding, nystagmus, and optic atrophy.[103] Dhir et al[31] described two siblings with reduced visual acuity, nystagmus, hypopigmentation of the maculae, head nodding, dysarthria, and other neuromuscular coordination resulting from histidinemia. Reports from the Japanese literature have described a newly recognized condition in boys characterized by ataxic diplegia, mental retardation, horizontal pendular nystagmus, head nodding, and abnormal auditory brain stem responses.[2] Head nodding and nystagmus can occasionally be seen in multisystem genetic disorders.[33,85]

Head Nodding without Nystagmus

Bobble-Headed Doll Syndrome

Children with large third ventricular cysts or tumors that are associated with obstructive hydrocephalus occasionally develop a to-and-fro bobbing or nodding of the head and trunk. This 1- to 3-Hz anterior-posterior movement is named for its resemblance to the movement of a doll whose weighted head is mounted on a coiled spring.[6] This disorder can be distinguished from benign familial tremor by its slower rate, its invariable association with hydrocephalus, and by the child's ability to volitionally inhibit it.[30] With rare exceptions, it is unique to children, with an average age of 7 years at diagnosis.[65]

The head nodding of the bobble-headed doll syndrome is a slow (1 to 3 Hz) anteroposterior movement that disappears with sleep and in the lying position and can be suppressed or decreased at will or decreases during voluntary head motion or activity.[30,111] The head nodding may be accompanied by a synchronous gentle rocking of the trunk or movement of the hands.[86]

The cause of the head and trunk movements is unclear. Rapidly progressive hydrocephalus is not associated with this disorder. Similarly, the classic setting sun sign of infantile hydrocephalus has not been reported in conjunction with the bobble-headed doll syndrome, although it too is related to third ventricular dilatation or periaqueductal dysfunction. The bobble-headed doll syndrome seems to signify a slowly progressive hydrocephalus, while the setting sun sign is a sensitive sign of rapidly progressive hydrocephalus or shunt blockage in shunt-dependent hydrocephalus.[30]

Most children with bobble-headed doll syndrome have been found to have a cyst or mass in or near the anterior part of the third ventricle.[65] Most of the remaining cases have been found to have hydrocephalus secondary to aqueductal stenosis or, rarely, ventricular shunt obstruction,[27] suggesting a slow dilation of the third ventricle as the possible common denominator. It may be that head nodding in the bobble-headed doll syndrome shares a common pathogenesis with the head nodding in spasmus nutans associated with large suprasellar tumors, namely, compression of the floor of the third ventricle[42] (i.e., some children with bobble-headed doll syndrome may harbor a subclinical nystagmus, and the head nodding may actually contribute to an improvement in vision).

In some children, the head bobbing precedes other signs or symptoms of intracranial pressure by as much as 6 months.[111] Associated neurological and endocrinological abnormalities are common. Apart from a large head size, neurological findings may include abnormal pyramidal-tract findings, ataxia or intention tremor of the trunk, and optic disc pallor—which may reflect compression of the optic nerves, chiasm, or tract, depending on the underlying cause. Endocrinological abnormalities may also be present, including diabetes insipidus, precocious puberty, and advanced bone age.[111] Resolution or improvement of the tremor following surgical removal of the cyst or tumor is noted in some patients.[65]

Cerebellar Disease

Midline cerebellar lesions may give rise to a slow (3 to 4 cps) predominantly anteroposterior oscillation of the head (titubation) which may simulate the bobble-headed doll syndrome.[17,111] However, cerebellar head tremors are accompanied by other cerebellar signs such as truncal ataxia and motor incoordination, as well as cerebellar eye signs (ocular dysmetria, impaired pursuits, gaze-evoked nystagmus, impaired VOR suppression).[20] Kalyanaraman et al[66a] described three related children with head nodding and nystagmus associated with a cerebrocerebellar degeneration of unclear etiology.

Benign Essential Tremor

Benign essential tremor is a hereditary, monosymptomatic condition in which an intermittent, involuntary, high-frequency tremor affects the head and hands. It may appear as early as 2 years of age, although it more commonly develops during later childhood or adolescence. The head movements may precede the hand movements by several years. Benign essential tremor may initially manifest as shuddering or shivering attacks in which the head flexes and turns along with other body movements.[113] Because these brief shuddering attacks can occur several times a day then cease spontaneously for a week or two, affected children may be misdiagnosed as having epilepsy, psychogenic disturbances, tics, or paroxysmal choreoathetosis.[86]

The high frequency of benign essential tremor (5 to 15 cps) distinguishes it from the bobble-headed doll syndrome. Unlike the bobble-headed doll syndrome in which the head movements are inhibited by activity, benign essential tremor persists or worsens with activity.[111] Ingestion of small amounts of alcohol (one drink) abates the tremor, whereas ingestion of larger volumes exacerbates it. Treatment with propanolol effectively abolishes the tremor. Autopsy studies of the basal ganglia and other structures have failed to detect any pathological abnormality.[97]

Paroxysmal Dystonic Head Tremor

Paroxysmal dystonic head tremor is a rare, nonfamilial disorder characterized by attacks of horizontal head tremor (frequency 5 to 8 Hz).[37,99] The attacks last from 1 to 30 minutes and cannot be suppressed. They begin in adolescence, but some children may have an associated head tilt that predates the onset of the tremor by 5 to 10 years.[37] Neuroimaging studies are negative. The condition is nonprogressive and its cause is unknown.[60] Daily clonazepam reduces the frequency and severity of attacks.[37]

Autism

Autistic children may display rocking of the head and trunk along with other motor stereotypes (hand flapping and spinning), sensory stereotypes, and impaired communication and socialization. Recent necropsy studies implicate severe Purkinje cell loss in the posterior cerebellar vermis and cerebellar hemispheres as a neuroanatomical correlate of autism.[23] This abnormality is reflected on MR imaging as either hypoplasia or hyperplasia of the cerebellar vermis, causing previous quantitative MR estimates of the mean posterior cerebellar size to fall within the normal range. Autism is one developmental neuropsychiatric deficit for which substantial concordance exists among several independent microscopic and macroscopic studies as to the location and type of neuroanatomic maldevelopment.[23]

Infantile Spasms

Infantile spasms may manifest with nodding attacks that occur in isolation or together with mental retardation, myoclonic jerks, or various neurological deficits.[36,83] Morimoto et al[83] described such nodding attacks in a 2-year-old boy whose nodding disappeared immediately following surgical resection of a right temporal astrocytoma.

Congenital Ocular Motor Apraxia

We have observed infants with congenital ocular motor apraxia who, in addition to head thrusting, show intermittent head nodding during fixation of a nonmoving object. This nodding may persist at an age when the head thrusting has resolved. We assume it somehow serves to fine-tune or recalibrate the fixation mechanism in this disorder.

Opsoclonus/Myoclonus

Severe myoclonus associated with opsoclonus can cause incessant, rapid, irregular head movements. Kinsbourne[67] described wobbling, titubation, or rapid irregular jerking movements of the head in three of six young children with acute postviral myoclonic encephalopathy associated with opsoclonus. The associated myoclonus distinguishes this disorder from other causes of head nodding. In the absence of an underlying neuroblastoma, the illness may resolve over weeks to months, although the course may be protracted and recovery incomplete in some children.[75]

Visual Disorders

Blindness

Jan[64] has extensively reviewed the numerous abnormal head movements in visually impaired children. Head oscillations are among the sophisticated adaptations that blind children develop to interact more effectively with their physical surroundings. Head oscillations in the visually impaired child may appear as stereotyped purposeless movements to the examiner if their numerous adaptive functions go unrecognized. Children with tunnel vision may make side-to-side oscillating head movements when walking in order to scan the environment. Many blind children use their hearing to avoid obstacles with surprising efficiency. Jan[64] has noted that, in the corridors of schools for the blind, it is not uncommon to see children walking with their heads slowly turning from side to side while making clicking or chirping noises, in order to use their "radar systems." The rhythmical front-to-back or side-to-side rocking movements of the head or trunk seen in blind children may start as a response to understimulation or overstimulation and later become a habit. These self-stimulating movements tend to be slow and rhythmical with boredom and fatigue and become faster and irregular with stress or excitement.[63,64]

Intermittent Esotropia

Rubin and Slavin[101] reported a neurologically normal infant without nystagmus but with intermittent esotropia and intermittent head nodding whose head movements manifested only when his eyes were straight. The head movements ceased with the spontaneous onset of esotropia or with the occlusion of either eye. When his head was forcibly stabilized, he immediately developed esotropia. The authors concluded that the head nodding somehow facilitated ocular alignment.

Otological Abnormalities

Labyrinthine Fistula

"Head nystagmus" was alluded to in the older literature as a sign of labyrinthine fistula.[28,91] Despite the recent flurry of interest in this controversial condition, its association with head shaking seems to have disappeared.[8,13,57,70]

Systemic Disorders

Aortic Regurgitation

Patients with severe aortic regurgitation may display a bobbing motion of the head together with a jarring motion of the body with each systole due to a widened arterial pulse pressure (de Musset sign).[108] The head bobbing of aortic regurgitation is accompanied by a high-pitched, decrescendo, diastolic murmur along the left sternal border. Originally considered a sign of syphilitic aortitis, de Musset sign may rarely develop in children with Marfan syndrome.

Endocrine and Metabolic Disturbances

A gross tremor of the head and hands may occur in endocrine and metabolic disturbances such as hypomagnesemia,[38] hypocalcemia (including hypoparathyroidism), uremia, and thyrotoxicosis.[86] These findings may also be seen in untreated phenylketonuria and in citrullinemia.[86]

References

1. Adams RD, Lyon G. *Neurology of Hereditary Metabolic Diseases of Children.* New York: McGraw-Hill;1982:65.
2. Aiba K, Yokochi K, Ishikawa T. A case of ataxic diplegia, mental retardation, congenital nystagmus, and abnormal auditory brainstem responses showing only waves I and II. Brain Dev 1986;8:630-632.
3. Angelini L, Rumi V, Lamperi E, et al. Transient paroxysmal dystonia in infancy. Neuropediatric 1988;19:171.
4. Angelini L, Nardocci N, Rumi V, et al. Idiopathic dystonia with onset in childhood. J Neurol 1989;236:319.
5. Bagolini B, Campos EC, Chiesi C. Plagiocephaly causing superior oblique deficiency and ocular torticollis. Arch Ophthalmol 1982;100:1093-1096.
6. Benton JW, Nellhaus G, Huttenlocher PR, Ojemann RG, Dodge PR. The bobble-headed doll syndrome. Neurology 1966;16:725-729.
7. Boisen E. Torticollis caused by infratentorial tumor: three cases. Br J Psychiatry 1979;134:306-307.
8. Bower CM, Martin PF. Diagnosis, treatment, and rehabilitation of pediatric sensorineural hearing loss. Curr Opin Otolaryngol Head Neck Surg 1993;1:161-166.

9. Braun V, Richter HP. Selective peripheral denervation for the treatment of spasmodic torticollis. Neurosurgery 1994;35:58-63.

10. Bronstein AM, Rudge P. The vestibular system in abnormal head postures and in spasmodic torticollis. Adv Neurol 1988;50:493-500.

11. Brown JB, McDowell F. Wryneck facial distortion prevented by resection of fibrosed sternomastoid muscle in infancy and childhood. Ann Surg 1950;131:721.

12. Busch MT, Westin GW. Muscular torticollis. Orthop Consult 1988:8-12.

13. Calhoun KH. Perilymph fistula. Arch Otolaryng Head Neck Surg 1992;118:693-694.

14. Campos EC. Ocular torticollis. Int Ophthalmol 1983;6:49-53.

15. Canale ST, Griffen DW, Hubbard CN. Congenital muscular torticollis. J Bone Joint Surg 1982;64: 810-816.

16. Carl JR, Optican LM, Chu FC, Zee DS. Head shaking and vestibulo-ocular reflex in congenital nystagmus. Invest Ophthalmol Vis Sci 1985;26: 1043-1050.

17. Cleeves L, Findley LJ, Marsden CD. Odd tremors. In: Marsden CD, Fahn S, eds. Movement Disorders 3. Oxford: Butterworth-Heinemann; 1994:446.

18. Cogan DG, Norton EWD. Spasmus nutans: a clinical study of twenty cases followed two years or more since onset. Arch Ophthalmol 1965:442-446.

19. Cogan DG. Congenital nystagmus. Can J Ophthalmol 1967;2:4-10.

20. Cogan DG, Chu FC, Reingold DB. Ocular signs of cerebellar disease. Arch Ophthalmol 1982;100: 755-760.

21. Cohen RL, Moore S. Primary dissociated vertical deviation. Am Orthop J 1980;30:106-107.

22. Cotton DG, Newman CGH. Dystonic reactions to phenothiazine derivatives. Arch Dis Child 1966; 41:551-553.

23. Courchesne E, Townsend J, Saitoh O. The brain in infantile autism: posterior fossa structures are abnormal. Neurology 1994;44:214-223.

24. Coventry MB, Harris LE. Congenital muscular torticollis in infancy. J Bone Joint Surg 1959;5:815-822.

25. Crone RA. Visual acuity and torticollis. Neth Ophthalmol Soc 1968;156:6-15.

26. de Decker W. Rotatischer Kestenbaum an geraden Augenmuskeln. Z Prakt Augenheilkd 1990;1:111-114.

27. Dell S. Further observations on the "bobble-headed doll syndrome." J Neurol Neurosurg Psychiatry 1981;44:1046-1052.

28. Dell'Osso LF, Daroff RB. Abnormal head position and head motion associated with congenital nystagmus. In: Keller EL, Zee DS, eds. Adaptive Processes in Visual and Oculomotor Systems. Oxford: Pergamon Press; 1986:473-478.

29. Dell'Osso LF, van der Steen J, Steinman RM, Collewijn H. Foveation dynamics in congenital nystagmus. II: smooth pursuit. Doc Ophthalmol 1992;9:25-49.

30. Deonna T, Dubey B. Bobble-headed doll syndrome. Helv Paediatr Acta 1976;31:221.

31. Dhir SP, Shisku MW, Krewi A. Ocular involvement in histidinemia. Ophthalmic Paediatr Genet 1987;8:175-176.

32. Diamond GR, Katowita JA, et al. Ocular and adnexal complications of unilateral orbital advancement for plagiocephaly. Arch Ophthalmol 1987; 105:381-385.

33. Donnai D. A further patient with the Pitt-Rogers-Danks syndrome of mental retardation, unusual face, and intrauterine growth retardation. Am Med Genet 1986;24:29-32.

34. Dorland's Medical Dictionary. 27th ed. Philadelphia, PA: W.B. Saunders;1988:1734.

35. Duke-Elder ST. System of Ophthalmology, VI. London: Henry Klimpton;1990:680.

36. Feng YK, Liu XQ, Sha Y, Liu PS. Infantile spasms. A retrospective study of 105 cases. Chin Med J 1991;104:416-421.

37. Fenichel GM. Clinical Pediatric Neurology. 2nd ed. Philadelphia, PA: W.B. Saunders;1993:1-43, 285-301.

38. Fishman RA. Neurological aspects of magnesium metabolism. Arch Neurol 1965;12:562-569.

39. Forssman B. A study of congenital nystagmus. Acta Otolaryng 1964;57:429-449.

40. Fredrick DR, Mulliken JB, Robb RM. Ocular manifestations of deformational frontal plagiocephaly. J Pediatr Ophthalmol Strabismus 1990;30:92-95.

41. Gilbert GJ. Familial spasmodic torticollis. Neurology 1977;27:11-13.

42. Göerke W, Pendl G, Pandle CH. Spinal muscular trophy in a boy with head-nodding resulting from a large septum pellucidum cyst. Neuropädiat 1975; 6:190-201.

43. Gote H, Gregersen E, Rindziunski E. Exotropia and panoramic vision compensating for an occult congenital homonymous hemianopia: a case report. Binoc Vis Eye Muscle Surg Q 1993;8:129-132.

44. Gottlob I, Zubcov AA, Wizov SS, et al. Signs distinguishing spasmus nutans (with and without central nervous system lesions) from congenital nystagmus. Ophthalmology 1990;97:1166-1175.

45. Gottlob I, Zubcov AA, Wizov SS, et al. Head nodding is compensatory in spasmus nutans. Ophthalmology 1992;99:1024-1031.

46. Gottlob I, Reinecke RD. Eye and head movements in patients with achromatopsia. Graefe's Arch Clin Exp Ophthalmol 1994;232:392-401.

47. Gresty M, Leech J, Sanders M, Eggars H. A study of head and eye movement in spasmus nutans. Br J Ophthalmol 1976;60:652-654.

48. Gresty MA, Ell JJ. Spasmus nutans or congenital nystagmus? Classification according to objective criteria. Br J Ophthalmol 1981;65:510-511. Letter.

49. Gresty M, Halmagyi GM. Head nodding associated with idiopathic childhood nystagmus. Ann NY Acad Sci 1981;374:614-618.

50. Gresty MA, Barratt NG, Page NGR, Ell JJ. Assessment of the vestibulo-ocular reflexes in congenital nystagmus. Ann Neurol 1985;17:129-136.

51. Guyton DL. Clinical assessment of ocular torsion. Am Orthop J 1983;33:7-15.

52. Halmagyi GM, Brandt TH, Dieterich M, et al. Tonic contraversive ocular tilt reaction due to unilateral meso-diencephalic lesion. Neurology 1990; 40:1503-1509.

53. Hedges TR III, Hoyt WF. Ocular tilt reaction due to an upper brainstem lesion: paroxysmal skew deviation, torsion, and oscillation of the eyes with head tilt. Ann Neurol 1982;11:537-540.

54. Hiatt RL, Cope-Troupe C. Abnormal head positions due to ocular problems. Ann Ophthalmol 1978;10:881-892.

55. Hoefnagel D, Biery B. Spasmus nutans. Dev Med Child Neurol 1968;10:32-35.

56. Horton CE, Crawford HH, et al. Torticollis. South Med J 1967;60:953-958.

57. Hott SR, Pensak ML. Perilymphatic fistula. ENT J 1992;71:568-572.

58. Hough G deN Jr. Congenital torticollis. Surg Gynecol Obstet 1934;58:972-981.

59. Hoyt CS, Good WV. Ocular motor adaptations to congenital hemianopia. Binoc Vis Eye Muscle Surg Q 1993;8:125-126.

60. Hughes AJ, Lees AJ, Marsden CD. Paroxysmal dystonic head tremor. Mov Disord 1991;6:85-86.

61. Hulbert KF. Torticollis. Postgrad Med J 1965;41: 699-701.

62. Hummer CD, MacEwen GD. The coexistence of torticollis and congenital dysplasia of the hip. J Bone Joint Surg 1972;54A:1255-1256.

63. Jan JE, Groenveld M, Connolly MB. Head shaking by visually impaired children: a voluntary neurovisual adaptation which can be confused with spasmus nutans. Dev Med Child Neurol 1990;32:1061-1066.

64. Jan JE. Head movements of visually impaired children. Dev Med Child Neurol 1991;3:645-647.

65. Jensen HP, Pendle G, Göerke W. Head bobbing in a patient with a cyst of the third ventricle. Child Brain 1978;4:235-243.

66. Jones PG. Torticollis in Infancy—Sternomastoid Fibrosis and the Sternomastoid Tumor. Springfield, IL: Charles C. Thomas; 1968:3.

66a. Kalyanaraman K, Jagannathan K, Ramanujam RA, et al. Congenital head nodding and nystagmus with cerebrocerebellar degeneration. J Pediatr 1973;83: 1023-1026.

67. Kinsbourne M. Myoclonic encephalopathy of infants. J Neurol Neurosurg Psychiatr 1962;25:271-276.

68. Kiwak KJ, Deray MJ, Shields WD. Torticollis in three children with syringomyelia and spinal cord tumor. Neurology 1983;33(7):946-948.

69. Knight ME, Roberts RJ. Phenothiazine and butyrophenone intoxication in children. Pediatr Clin North Am 1986;33:299.

70. Kohut RI. Perilymph fistula: clinical criteria. Arch Otolaryngol Head Neck Surg 1992;118:687-692.

71. Kraft SP, O'Donaghue EP, Roarty JD. Improvement of compensatory head postures after strabismus surgery. Ophthalmology 1992;99:1301-1308.

72. Krefman RA, Goldberg MF. Ocular torticollis caused by refractive error. Arch Ophthalmol 1982; 100:1278-1279.

73. Kushner BJ. Ocular causes of abnormal head postures. Ophthalmology 1979;86:2115-2125.

74. Lambert SR, Newman NJ. Retinal disease masquerading as spasmus nutans. Neurology 1993; 43:1607-1609.

75. Leigh JR, Zee DS, eds. The Neurology of Eye Movements. 2nd ed. Philadelphia, PA: F.A. Davis; 1991:246-249.

76. Lidge RT, Bechtol RC, Lambert CN. Congenital muscular torticollis. Etiology and pathology. J Bone Joint Surg 1957;39A:1165-1182.

77. Ling CM. The influence of age on the results of open sternomastoid tenotomy in muscular torticollis. Clin Ortho Rel Res 1976;116:142-148.

78. Marmor MA, Beauchamp GR, Maddox SF. Photophobia, epiphora, and torticollis: a masquerade syndrome. J Pediatr Ophthalmol Strabismus 1990; 27:202-204.

79. McIntosh D, Brown J, Hanson R, et al. Torticollis and bacterial meningitis. Ped Infect Dis J 1993; 12:160-161.

80. McKnight P, Friedman J. Torticollis due to cervical epidural abscess and osteomyelitis. Neurology 1992;42:696-697.

81. Metz HS, Jampolsky A, O'Meara DM. Congenital ocular nystagmus and nystagmoid head movements. Am J Ophthalmol 1974;74:1131-1133.

82. Miller NR, ed. Walsh and Hoyt's Clinical Neuro-ophthalmology, II. 4th ed. Baltimore, MD: Williams and Wilkins; 1985:893-897.

83. Morimoto K, Abekura M, Nil Y, et al. Nodding attacks (infantile spasms) associated with temporal lobe astrocytoma—case report. Neurol Med Chir 1989;29:610-613.

84. Mount LA, Reback S. Familial paroxysmal choreoathetosis. Arch Neurol Psychiatry (Chicago) 1940;44:841-847.

85. Murayama K, Greenwood RS, Rao KW, Aylsworth AS. Neurological aspects of del (1q) syndrome. Am J Hum Genet 1991;40:488-492.

86. Nelhaus G. Abnormal head movements of young children. Dev Med Child Neurol 1983;25:384-398.

87. Newman SA. Spasmus nutans: Or is it? Surv Ophthalmol 1990;34:453-456.

88. Norn MS. Congenital idiopathic nystagmus. Incidence and occupational prognosis. Ophthalmology 1964;42:889.

89. Nutt AB. Abnormal head posture. Br Orthop J 1963;20:18-28.

90. O'Donnell JJ, Howard RO. Torticollis associated with hiatus hernia (Sandifer's syndrome). Am J Ophthalmol 1971;71:1134-1137.

91. Osterberg G. On spasmus nutans. Acta Ophthalmol 1937;15:457-467.

92. Parker W. Migraine and the vestibular system in childhood and adolescence. Am J Otol 1989; 10:364-371.

93. Parks MM. Isolated cyclovertical muscle palsy. Arch Ophthalmol 1958;60:1027-1035.

94. Plager DA. Tendon laxity in superior oblique palsy. Ophthalmology 1992;99:1032-1038.

95. Plagiocephaly and torticollis in young infants. Lancet 1986;2(8510):789-790. Editorial.

96. Prensky AL. An approach to the child with paroxysmal phenomenon with emphasis on nonepileptic disorders. In: Dodson WE, Pellock JM, eds. *Pediatric Epilepsy: Diagnosis and Therapy.* New York: Demos Publications; 1993:63-80.

97. Rajput AH, Rozdilsky B, Ang L, Rajput A. Clinicopathologic observations in essential tremor: report of six cases. Neurology 1991;41:1422-1424.

98. Richards RN, Barnett HJM. Paroxysmal dystonic choreoathetosis. Neurology 1968;18:461-469.

99. Rivest J, Marsden CD. Trunk and head tremor as isolated manifestations of dystonia. Mov Disord 1990;5:60-65.

100. Rubin SE, Wagner RS. Ocular torticollis. Surv Ophthalmol 1986;30:366-376.

101. Rubin SE, Slavin ML. Head nodding associated with intermittent esotropia. J Pediatr Ophthalmol Strabismus 1990;27(5):250-251.

102. Sarnet HB, Morrissy RT. Idiopathic torticollis: sternocleidomastoid myopathy and accessory neuropathy. Muscle Nerve 1981;4:374.

103. Scheffer RN, Zlotogora J, Elpeleg ON, et al. Behr's syndrome and 3-methylglutaconic aciduria. Am J Ophthalmol 1992;114:494-497.

104. Sedwick LA, Burde RM, Hodges FJ. Leigh's subacute necrotizing encephalomyelitis manifesting as spasmus nutans. Ophthalmology 1990;102:1046-1048.

105. Snyder CH. Paroxysmal torticollis of infancy: a possible form of labyrinthitis. AJDC 1969;117:458-460.

106. Spielmann A. Pediatric nystagmus and strabismus. Curr Opin Ophthalmol 1990;1:621-626.

107. Still GF. Head nodding with nystagmus in infants. Lancet 1906;2:207-209.

108. Stone J. Syphilis and the cardiovascular system. In: Schlant RC, Alexander RW, eds. *The Heart.* 8th ed. New York: McGraw-Hill; 1994:1949-1952.

109. Taboas-Perez RA, Rivera-Reyes L. Head tilt: a revisit to an old sign of posterior fossa tumors. Bol Asoc Med PR 1984;76(2):62-65.

110. Taylor D. Disorders of head and eye movements in children. Trans Ophthalmol Soc UK 1980;100:489-494.

111. Tomasovic JA, Nellhaus G, Moe PG. The bobble-headed doll syndrome: an early sign of hydrocephalus. Two new cases and a review of the literature. Dev Med Child Neurol 1975;17:777-792.

112. Urist MJ. Head tilt in vertical muscle paresis. Am J Ophthalmol 1970;69:440-442.

113. Vanasse M, Bedard P, Andermann F. Shuddering attacks in children: an early clinical manifestation of essential tremor. Neurology 1976;26:1027-1030.

114. von Noorden GK. Clinical observations in cyclodeviations. Ophthalmology 1979;86:1451-1461.

115. von Noorden GK, Ruttam M. Torticollis in paralysis of the trochlear nerve. Am Orthop J 1983;33:16-20.

116. von Noorden GK. *Binocular Vision and Ocular Motility.* 4th ed. St. Louis, MO: C.V. Mosby Co; 1990:372-378.

117. von Noorden GK, Jenkins RH, Rosenbaum AL. Horizontal transposition of the vertical rectus muscles for treatment of ocular torticollis. J Pediatr Ophthalmol Strabismus 1993;30:8-14.

118. Walsh FB, Hoyt WF. *Clinical Neuro-ophthalmology.* 3rd ed. Baltimore, MD: Williams and Wilkins; 1969:151.

119. Werlin SL, D'Souza BJ, et al. Sandifer syndrome: an unappreciated clinical entity. Dev Med Child Neurol 1980;22:374-378.

120. Wesson ME. The ocular significance of abnormal head postures. Br Orthop J 1964;21:14-28.

121. Wilson ME, Hoxie J. Facial asymmetry in superior oblique muscle palsy. J Pediatr Ophthalmol Strabismus 1993;30:315-318.

10

Neuro-Ophthalmologic Manifestations of Neurodegenerative Disease in Childhood

Introduction

Neurodegenerative disorders in children pose a unique diagnostic challenge. Unlike many genetic syndromes, the clinical manifestations of childhood neurodegenerative diseases are often nonspecific and show considerable overlap. Pathognomonic clinical signs are rare. Many of these conditions are uncommon, and extensive clinical experience is generally lacking, even in tertiary referral centers. To further complicate matters, these children often present in the early stages of their illness when evidence of progression is lacking and motor or cognitive impairment is relatively mild. It is only with extended observation that both clinical and neuroimaging abnormalities evolve to suggest a limited set of diagnostic possibilities. These children usually require repeated observation by a multidisciplinary team of neurologists, neuroimaging specialists, neuro-ophthalmologists, and geneticists before a specific diagnosis is established.

Children with neurodegenerative diseases often present with a combination of motor and intellectual impairment. Although the definitive diagnosis of many of these disorders is made by testing for biochemical or genetic abnormalities, the differential diagnosis is based on the child's physiognomy, systemic and neurological findings, neuro-ophthalmologic abnormalities, and the results of neuroimaging studies. The neuro-ophthalmologist is frequently called upon to look for ocular motility or retinal signs that suggest a specific diagnosis so that ancillary investigations can be directed appropriately.

It is inappropriate to investigate every child with developmental delay for neurodegenerative disease, and the complex interplay between development and degeneration may make the choice of which patients to investigate a difficult one. In this setting, visual system abnormalities may be among the most quantifiable and reproducible clinical features and therefore figure prominently in the diagnostic decision-making process. In some circumstances, visual system abnormalities will be the presenting sign of a neurodegenerative disease. The neuro-ophthalmological features of these conditions may include optic atrophy, retinal degeneration, cortical visual loss, nystagmus, ophthalmoplegia and other motility disturbances, and cortical visual loss. In particular, the later onset abnormalities (i.e., those occurring after the age of 5 years) may present with visual loss or the new onset of strabismus, ophthalmoplegia with ptosis, or nystagmus.

A traditional framework for categorizing neurodegenerative diseases is to divide them into disorders that involve primarily gray matter versus those that involve primarily white matter. This classification system is useful primarily as a clinical and neuroimaging tool to aid in differential diagnosis. The definitive classification system for neurodegenerative disorders has yet to be established, but it appears that grouping diseases by the effected subcellular organelle—i.e., lysosomal, mitochondrial, and peroxisomal diseases—will be a more appropriate system. In this chapter, a combination of traditional and subcellular organelle classification systems will be used. The classification of each neurodegenerative disease under these systems is summarized in Table 10.1.

TABLE 10.1. Classification systems of neurodegenerative diseases of childhood.

Classification by organelle/biochemical defect

Mitochondrial encephalomyelopathies	Peroxisomal disorders	Lysosomal storage diseases	Aminoacidopathies	Metal metabolism
CPEO (Kearns–Sayre syndrome)	Adrenoleuko-dystrophy	Gangliosidoses (GM$_1$)	Maple syrup urine disease	Wilson disease
MELAS	Zellweger syndrome	Tay–Sachs (GM$_2$) disease	Homocystinuria	Hallervorden–Spatz
MERRF	Infantile Refsum disease	Sandhoff disease		disease
Leigh disease		Fabry disease		
		Gaucher disease		
		Niemann–Pick disease		
		Farber disease		
		Krabbe disease		
		Metachromatic leukodystrophy		
		Mucopolysaccharidoses		
		Mucolipidoses		
		Glycoproteinoses		

Classification by gray versus white matter involvement

Primarily gray matter involvement	Primarily white matter involvement	Mixed gray and white matter involvement
Cortical	Metachromatic leukodystrophy	Zellweger syndrome
Neuronal ceroid lipofuscinosis	Alexander disease	Adrenoleukodystrophy
Tay-Sachs (GM$_2$ type 1) disease	Canavan disease	Leigh disease
Niemann–Pick disease	Pelizaeus–Merzbacher disease	
Gaucher disease	Krabbe disease	
Mucopolysaccharidoses		
Sialidosis		
Deep nuclei and brain stem		
Hallervorden–Spatz disease		
Wilson disease		

The primary involvement of gray versus white matter in neurodegenerative disease is often reflected in the early neurological abnormalities. Gray matter diseases present with intellectual deterioration, seizures, and involuntary movement disorders. Neuro-ophthalmologic abnormalities, when present, are dominated by retinal degeneration and supranuclear oculomotor disturbances (Table 10.2). White matter diseases usually begin with spasticity and optic atrophy (Table 10.3). It

TABLE 10.2. Neurodegenerative conditions associated with prominent ocular motility manifestations.

Disease	Dominant clinical feature	Metabolic defect	Diagnostic test
Pelizaeus–Merzbacher disease	Horizontal jerk nystagmus, head tremor, delayed development	Unknown	Tigroid appears to myelin stain on CNS tissue
Ataxia telangiectasia	Ataxia, defective saccadic initiation, strabismus, erratic vertical movements, immune deficiency	Unknown, possible cellular repair deficiency	Low IgA
Leigh Disease	Ataxia, ophthalmoplegia, nystagmus, seizures, weight loss	Multiple energy pathway abnormalities including cytochrome c oxidase	Enzyme assay on fibroblasts
Kearns–Sayre syndrome	Ptosis, external ophthalmoplegia, pigmentary retinopathy, cardiac conduction defects	Mitochondrial DNA	DNA analysis on leukocytes
Abetalipoproteinemia	Retinal degeneration, internuclear ophthalmoplegia, malabsorption of fat, ataxia	Apo B transport protein deficiency	Serum lipid profile, liver biopsy

TABLE 10.3. Neurodegenerative diseases with optic atrophy as a prominent feature.

Disease	Dominant clinical feature	Metabolic defect	Diagnostic test
Adrenoleukodystrophy			
Neonatal	White matter degeneration in infancy	Peroxisomal disorder (multiple)	Very long-chain fatty acids in serum and cultured skin fibroblasts
X-linked	White matter degeneration in childhood (ages 5 to 15)	Peroxisomal disorder (single)	
Canavan disease	White matter degeneration severe, infancy	Asparto-acylase deficiency	N-Acetyl aspartic acid in urine enzyme assay in fibroblasts
Krabbe disease	Early spasticity, blindness, intellectual deterioration	Galactocerebrosidase B-galactosidase	Enzyme assay on fibroblasts
Menke disease	Seizures, gross motor deterioration, kinky hair	Abnormal copper metabolism	Low serum copper and ceruloplasmin
Metachromatic leukodystrophy	Hypotonia, peripheral neuropathy dementia	Arylsulfatase-A deficiency	Urine or leukocytes
Alexander disease	Severe white matter degeneration, progressive megalencephaly	Unknown	Clinical and neuroimaging diagnosis
Neuronal ceroid lipofuscinosis	Intellectual and motor deterioration, vision loss	Neuronal accumulation of lipofuscin	Leukocytes, conjunctiva
Pelizaeus–Merzbacher disease	Ocular motor abnormalities, head tremor	Unknown	Clinical and neuroimaging
Leigh disease	Ataxia, ocular motor abnormalities, spontaneous remissions	Multiple energy metabolism defects, cytochrome c oxidase deficiency	Fibroblasts
Hallervorden–Spatz	Spasticity, dystonia, intellectual deterioration	Iron storage abnormality	Abnormal cytosomes in lymphocytes, sea blue histiocytes in bone marrow

* Many degenerative syndromes will have optic atrophy as a late consequence of retinal degeneration or diffuse neuronal loss (e.g. spinocerebellar degenerations, MELAS); these diseases are not included in this table.

should be recognized that many gray matter disorders eventually spread to involve white matter and vice versa. Some neurodegenerative disorders involve both gray and white matter primarily.

Immaturity and poor motor control make behavioral evaluation of vision difficult in children with neurodegenerative disease. Accurate assessment of vision can be confounded by the child's ambiguous response to visual stimuli. In this context, ancillary testing in the form of visual physiology and neuroimaging investigations may provide critical objective information.[79] Electroretinography (ERG) is most likely to be abnormal in gray matter diseases, whereas the visual evoked potential (VEP) may provide early evidence of optic atrophy or intracranial white matter tract disturbance.

Neuroimaging findings are frequently nonspecific in neurodegenerative disorders of childhood. The presence of megelencephaly suggests Caravan or Alexander disease. Symmetric changes suggesting edema in the basal ganglia or brain stem are characteristic of Leigh disease. Extensive biooccipital or bifrontal white matter edema with peripheral enhancement is characteristic of x-linked adrenoleukodystrophy with active demyelination. Although rarely diagnostic alone, neuroimaging of children with neurodegenerative diseases can narrow the differential diagnosis and direct genetic or biochemical investigations. Magnetic resonance (MR) imaging is particularly valuable in differentiating white from gray matter disease. These studies should be interpreted by an experienced observer since, even early in the course of gray matter disease, the cerebral white matter may show decreased volume due to Wallerian degeneration, and some white matter disorders have an inflammatory component that can cause a contiguous mass effect on adjacent gray matter.

White matter disorders such as adrenoleukodystrophy (ALD) and Alexander disease may show hypodensity (decreased attenuation) of central white matter on computed tomography (CT) scanning or prolonged T1 and T2 relaxation times on MR imaging (producing low signal on T1-weighted images and high signal on T2-weighted images) before any atrophy is apparent. The site of early white matter involvement may also provide diagnostic information. Neuroimaging specialists divide cerebral white matter into central and peripheral zones. Peripheral white matter is that which immediately underlies the cortex. Because these fibers follow the cortical gyri, they appear in the shape of a "U" on axial imaging of the brain. Disorders where the abnormality is limited to white matter should undergo careful scrutiny of these subcortical "U fibers" since symmetrical involvement in a macrocephalic patient is strongly suggestive of Alexander disease. Bilateral symmetric peripheral white matter disease in a child who is not microcephalic should raise suspicion of galactosemia.[9] Early involvement of deep white matter suggests a different group of disorders. Deep white matter involvement combined with thalamic involvement suggests Krabbe disease, whereas deep white matter involvement combined with corticospinal tracts involvement suggests peroxisomal disorders. A paucity of myelin without evidence of inflammation or injury to myelin is characteristic of Pelizaeus–Merzbacher disease.[9]

Gray matter disease may involve either cortical gray matter or deep gray matter nuclei. Gray matter diseases of the cortex include neuronal ceroid lipofuscinosis, gangliosidoses, and peroxisomal disorders. The MR abnormalities that suggest a peroxisomal disorder include focal migrational derangements combined with hypomyelination, dysmyelination, or demyelination. In addition, the peroxisomal disorders tend to affect the posterior limb of the internal capsule, cerebellar white matter, and brain stem tracts. When the cerebral hemispheres are affected, the occipital white matter may be more severely involved posteriorly. Careful inspection of the subcortical U fibers, gray matter, and the splenium of the corpus collasum may help to differentiate this pattern in peroxisomal disorders from other conditions such as occipital region infarction or the mitochondrial encephalomyelopathies. The peroxisomal disorders spare the subcortical U fibers and gray matter and preferentially involve the splenium of the corpus callosum. The mitochondrial encephalomyelopathies show combined involvement of deep gray matter nuclei and peripheral white matter.[8,162] Other conditions causing primarily cortical gray matter disease early on include the mucopolysaccharidoses and lipid storage disorders.

The differential diagnosis of deep gray matter involvement will depend on which nuclei are principally involved. The thalamus is involved early in

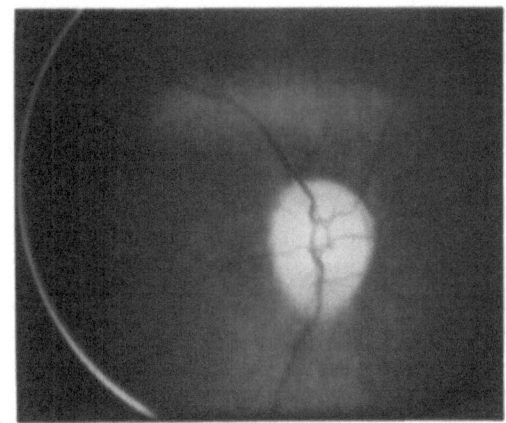
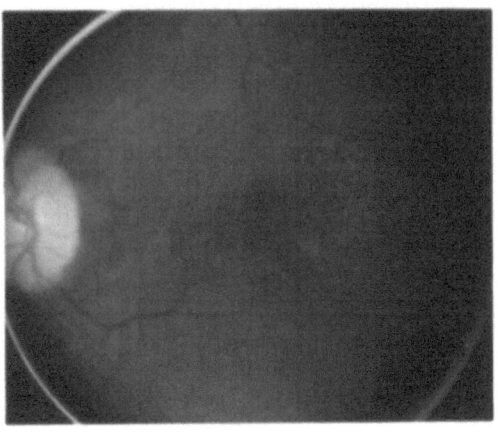

A B

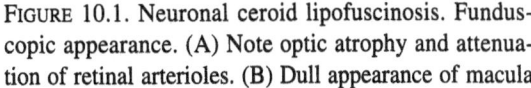

FIGURE 10.1. Neuronal ceroid lipofuscinosis. Fundus-copic appearance. (A) Note optic atrophy and attenua-tion of retinal arterioles. (B) Dull appearance of macula with rippling of internal limiting membrane. (Courtesy of Stephen P. Christiansen MD.)

Krabbe disease and also in the GM2 gangliosi-doses. Globus pallidus involvement is seen in Canavan disease, Kearns–Sayre syndrome (KSS), methyl-malonic and propionic acidemia, and maple syrup urine disease.[9] Involvement of the putamen and caudate (striatal disease) are compat-ible with Leigh disease, MELAS syndrome, or Wilson disease. Hypointensity of the globus pal-lidus on T2-weighted MR imaging suggests the diagnosis of Hallervorden–Spatz disease.[9]

Neuronal Disease

Neuronal Ceroid Lipofuscinosis

The neuronal ceroid lipofuscinoses (NCLs) are a group of disorders with many common features but with enough distinctions to warrant subclassifica-tion. Most reported families of NCL show an auto-somal recessive pattern of inheritance.[20] The enzy-matic defect in this group of disorders is unknown.

All forms of NCL eventually show intellectual and gross motor deterioration, seizures, and visual loss from retinal degeneration and optic atrophy with an abnormal ERG. (Figure 10.1).[87,117] Neu-roimaging reveals evidence of combined white and gray matter atrophy that is most pronounced in the cerebral hemispheres and the brain stem. (Figure 10.2).[125,161]

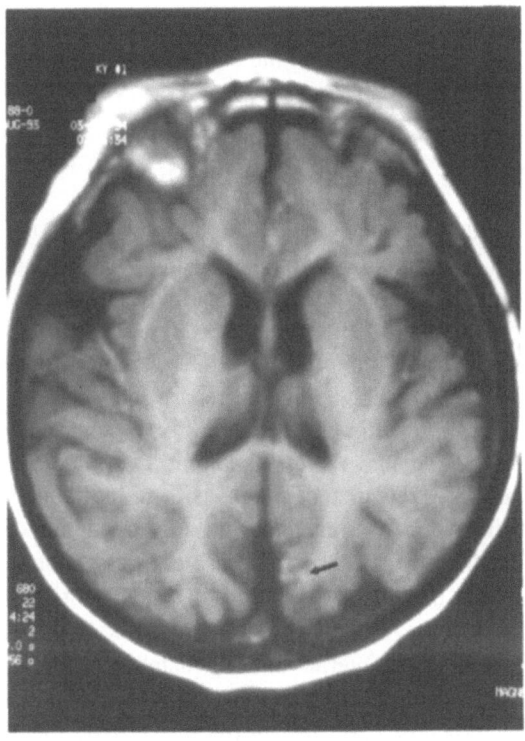

FIGURE 10.2. Neuronal ceroid lipofuscinosis. This T1-weighted MR image shows diffuse atrophy of cortical gray matter combined with diffuse thinning of the cere-bral white matter. A hypointense area is seen in the oc-cipital lobe, possibly representing lipofuscin storage material (arrow).

Infantile (Haltia-Santavuori Disease)

Neurological deterioration with severe visual loss occurs between 8 months and 1 ½ years.[136] Intellectual and gross motor skills are severely affected, myoclonic seizures develop, and death occurs by 4 years of age. The ERG is of low amplitude and ultimately becomes flat,[79] reflecting severe retinal degeneration. Cataracts may also be seen in this condition.[12] Optic atrophy ensues with progression of disease.

Late Infantile (Jansky–Bielschowsky Disease)

These children undergo a similar pattern of deterioration as those with the infantile form, but they gain more skills by the time of onset (age 2 to 4 years), which makes the degenerative aspect of the disease more apparent. The retinal degeneration is most visible in the macula, but the entire retina is involved as reflected by extinction of the ERG early in the disease. Unusual features of this disease are a strikingly enlarged VEP and large photically driven spikes on the electroencephalogram (EEG).[83]

Juvenile NCL (Batten–Mayou Disease)

Visual complaints may be the presenting feature of this disease, occurring between 4 and 10 years of age.[147] "Overlooking" is a common behavioral phenomenon in children with NCL.[155] The child demonstrating this phenomenon appears to look over the top of the object of regard. This strategy has been noted in children with loss of central vision from damage to the papulomacular bundle.[74] Early in the course of the disease, retinal abnormalities may be limited to a striking attenuation of retinal arterioles. As the disease progresses, optic atrophy becomes evident and macular abnormalities develop, including a subtle discoloration and rippling of the internal limiting membrane (Figure 10.1). A coarse pigment granularity or bull's-eye maculopathy may also develop. At first, the b wave of the ERG is selectively attenuated, but progression of the disease leads to extinction of both the a and b waves. The VEP becomes increasingly abnormal as optic atrophy ensues.

The following case description illustrates the evolution of visual and neurological dysfunction in juvenile NCL.

This male patient had a normal prenatal and neonatal course. He walked at 8 to 9 months of age and appeared to have normal vision in early childhood. He went to the Head Start Program at age 4 and did well by the parent's account. At age 5, the child complained of everything being out of focus. His school performance declined and he had difficulties with coordination. Over the next year he developed staring spells and tremors. He was first seen by us at age 11. At that time, his IQ measured 64. His visual acuity was 20/20 in each eye, but the fundus examination showed a pigmentary maculopathy. The neurological examination was remarkable for hyperreflexia and difficulties with tests of coordination. The ERG was unrecordable under both scotopic or photopic conditions. The metabolic screen (including very long-chain fatty acids (VLCFA)) for storage diseases was negative; however, electron microscopy of white blood cells showed irregularly shaped, variably sized, dense osmiophilic granular bodies. Tubular inclusions were commonly seen in several mononuclear cells.

Brain biopsy shows enlargement of most neurons with eccentric nuclei and peripheral displacement of the Nissl substance. The neuronal cytoplasm is filled with granular material that stains pale gray with Sudan black, orange with oil red O, and intensely red or purple with PAS. The neuronal granular material shows a bright yellow autofluorescence. With hematoxylin and eosin, the granules stain pale yellow, resembling lipofuscin. Electron microscopy (EM) of the tissue examined has shown these granules to be cytosomes with curvilinear profiles (Figure 10.3).[15,105] Demon-

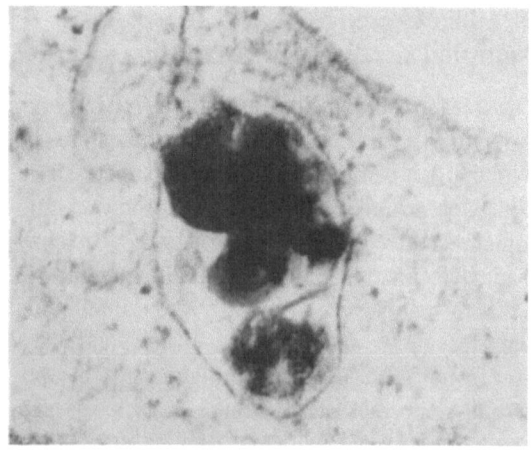

FIGURE 10.3. Electron microscopy of neuron demonstrating characteristic "fingerprint" profile. (Courtesy of Gerald A. Fishman, MD.)

stration of these characteristic findings on electron microscopy is the standard confirmation of diagnosis in all forms of this disease. Tissue for examination is generally obtained via biopsy of conjunctiva, rectum, skin, or muscle.[25,87,88] In some cases, the diagnosis can be established by examining the white blood cell buffy coat and finding: 1) vacuolated lymphocytes or azurophilic hypergranulated neutrophils on light microscopy; or 2) membrane-bound intracellular inclusions and fingerprint profiles or electron microscopy.[87,105] A recently discovered animal model with ultrastructural similarities to NCL may improve our molecular understanding of this condition.[22]

Lysosomal Diseases

Gangliosidoses

The sphingolipidoses, mucopolysaccharidosis, mucolipidoses, glycogen storage diseases, glycoproteinoses, and other storage diseases are the result of an abnormal accumulation of metabolic products within lysosomes. This accumulation is due to a relative deficiency in the activity of hydrolytic enzymes that may be absent or mutated to less effective forms or lacking in activator proteins.[153]

As with most other degenerative diseases the categorization of the gangliosidosis by eponym has been replaced by a system based on biochemistry. The gangliosides are classified by the system of Svennerholm wherein the letter G refers to ganglioside, the number of sialic groups are referred to by M (mono), D (di), or T (trisials), and the number of hexosides in the molecule is given by the subscript 1, 2, or 3 (tetrahexose sides are 1, trihexoside 2, and dihexosides 3).[151] These biochemical categories are then further divided on the basis of age of onset and clinical features. GM_2 gangliosides have the most prominent visual system involvement with rare cases of GM_1 reported with a cherry-red spot.[50]

GM_2 Type I (Tay–Sachs Disease)

This autosomal recessively inherited deficiency of hexosaminidase A causes accumulation of GM_2 ganglioside in the neurons of the central nervous system (CNS) and retinal ganglion cells. In the gangliosidoses, ophthalmoscopy typically shows a macular cherry-red spot (Figure 10.4) that results from the accumulation of opaque gangliosides in the retinal ganglion cell layer surrounding the fovea, with the normal choroidal circulation visible through the ganglion cell-free fovea.[35] Other neurodegenerative diseases associated with a cherry-red-macula sign are summarized in Table 10.4.

The onset is in the first few months of life with blindness, seizures, spasticity, and an exaggerated acoustic response (i.e. a startle response to sound) in the first year of life. The cherry-red macula sign may disappear as retinal ganglion cells are lost.[39,96,118] Electroretinography remains normal throughout the course of the disease.[118] A variety of ocular motor disturbances have been described.[90] Horizontal ocular deviations are an early feature, followed by impaired pursuit and optokinetic responses as the disease progresses. Voluntary saccades are initially impaired, followed by loss of the vestibulo-ocular reflex. Tonic downward ocular deviation may be a persistent sign late in the disease. Death usually ensues by age 4.

CT scanning shows hyperdense areas in the thalamus with white matter attenuation, a small cerebellum and brain stem, and ventricular dilation.[166] Pathological examination of the brain reveals degeneration of cerebral white matter and atrophy of cerebellar hemispheres on gross examination. Neurons are distorted and ballooned and nuclei are displaced to the periphery of the cell. Glial cells are filled with large globules of glycolipid.[153]

GM_2 ganglioside accumulates in large amounts in the central nervous system of patients with Tay–Sachs disease due to a failure of the deficient enzyme

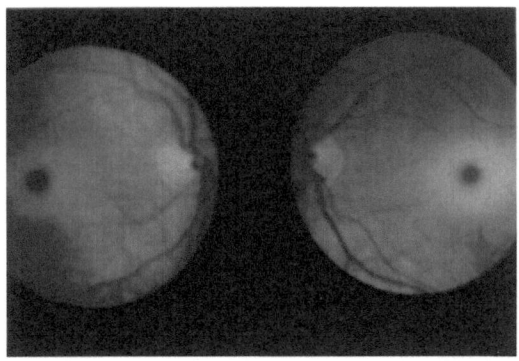

FIGURE 10.4. Tay–Sachs disease. Bilateral macular cherry-red spots.

TABLE 10.4. Pediatric neurodegenerative disorders associated with cherry-red macula.*

Gangliosidosis GM$_2$	Type 1 (Tay–Sachs disease)
	Type 2 (Sandhoff disease)
Sialidosis	Type 1 (Cherry-red spot myoclonus syndrome)
	Type 2 (Cherry-red spot dementia syndrome, Goldberg-Cotlier syndrome)
Niemann–Pick disease	Type A (Typical cherry-red spot)
	Type B (Crystalline macular halo)
	Type C (Variable faint opacification of perimacular area)
Gaucher disease Type II	
Subacate Sclerosing Panencephalitis	
Farber Disease (Disseminated Lipogranulomatosis)	
Krabbe Disease (rare)	
Metachromatic Leukodystrophy (rare)	

* Adapted from Kivlin et al.[96]

hexosaminidase A to cleave n-acetyl-hexosamine from accumulative molecule, thus blocking the normal metabolism of this lipid. The abnormal gene in Tay–Sachs disease is located on chromosome 15 and codes for the alpha chain of the enzyme.[5]

The diagnosis may be suspected on clinical grounds and is confirmed by assaying for the enzymatic activity of hexosaminidase A in leukocytes. Carrier screening and prenatal diagnosis of Tay–Sachs disease has been available for many years, and an analysis of the impact of the screening since 1974 indicates that the instances of laboratory error are extremely low. The identification of couples and pregnancies at risk has resulted in a dramatic decrease in the incidence of Tay–Sachs in the Jewish population.[91]

GM$_2$ Type II (Sandhoff Syndrome)

This condition has similar neuro-ophthalmologic findings to Tay–Sachs disease but differs by virtue of its involvement of visceral tissues. Hexosaminidase A and B activity are both abnormal. Affected children develop hepatosplenomegaly, renal abnormalities, and a cardiomyopathy.[19] Death occurs by 2 to 4 years of age. Biochemical detection of the enzymatic abnormality can be performed on fibroblasts or on leukocytes.[102]

GM$_2$ Type III

These patients experience loss of vision later than those with GM$_2$ types I and II. Ataxia develops between 2 and 6 years of age. Eye movement abnormalities including pursuit deficit and saccadic dysmetria may be seen. Optic demyelination and atrophy are invariable, but rods, cones, and pigment epithelium remain unaffected. In GM$_2$ type III, the ERG is normal, and the VEP is reduced or unrecordable.[71,85] The normal ERG is important in distinguishing this type of gangliosidosis from NCL, which is associated with a severely reduced ERG.

Niemann–Pick Disease

The Niemann–Pick classification includes a group of diseases caused by accumulation of sphingomyelin. These diseases are now divided into two groups with subtypes within each group. Patients in group I have a deficiency of the enzyme sphingomyelinase. Type A sphingomyelin accumulation occurs in both neural and visceral tissue, whereas type B has been characterized as causing visceral accumulation only. Patients with type A disease have a rapidly degenerative neurological course, usually leading to death before 4 years of age. The predominant ophthalmological feature is a classic cherry-red spot in the retina.

Type B is primarily non-neurologic, and patients with type B disease generally live longer than those with type A. However, patients with type B develop massive hepatosplenomegaly, bony changes, and diffuse pulmonary infiltration. Although these children do not develop a classic cherry-red spot, a characteristic *macular halo* has been described consisting of a discreet, white, crystalline-appearing ring surrounding the fovea of each eye.[32] This halo masks macular circulation on fluorescein angiography.

Group II patients with Niemann–Pick disease are not sphingomyelinase deficient but nevertheless have sphingomyelin accumulation. Subgroups are termed types C and D. The D form is rare and occurs only in patients of Nova Scotian descent. Type C disease is also termed the Neville–Lake syndrome or the DAF syndrome (downgaze palsy, ataxia-athetosis, and foamy macrophages).[34] This condition is characterized by an insidious neurologic deterioration occurring between 10 and 12 years of age, often associated with cataplexy. Hepatosplenomegaly may also be present. Neuro-ophthalmological findings figure prominently in this disease with loss of vertical saccades, impaired downgaze, and loss of the fast phase of optokinetic nystagmus (especially downward) in the presence of preserved doll's eye movements. Horizontal saccadic abnormalities may ensue with the development of head thrusts to compensate for the eye movement abnormality.[116] The biochemical abnormality in type C disease is an abnormal esterification of cholesterol that is an abnormality of lipid metabolism with decreased cholesterol esterification leading to the collection of cholesterol in lysosomes. The chain is known to be located on chromosome 18.[60,81] The diagnosis can be made by examining cultured skin fibroblasts.

Gaucher Disease

The three clinically determined types of Gaucher disease all have a defect in glucocerebrosidase. The characteristic accumulation of storage material in the cells has led to a presence of "Gaucher" cells in most tissues. Type I rarely presents in childhood and may cause a pigmented bulbar conjunctival lesion, bringing the patient to ophthalmological attention. These patients may rarely have a macular or perimacular atrophy of the retina.[24] Clusters of foamy macrophages in the retina may form scattered discreet white spots in the posterior pole, especially along the inferior vascular arcades.[33,68]

Type II Gaucher disease presents with seizures and spasticity. Strabismus and horizontal gaze palsies are frequently seen.[58] Some patients develop a cherry-red spot and later show optic atrophy.[155]

Type III Gaucher disease begins in the first decade with organomegaly and growth retardation, progressing to intellectual deterioration and seizures. Cranial nerve dysfunction and an isolated horizontal supranuclear gaze palsy may develop which may be accompanied by horizontal head thrusting and simulate congenital ocular motor apraxia.[34,119]

Mucopolysaccharidoses

Mucopolysaccharidoses are an autosomal recessive group of metabolic disorders characterized by the abnormal accumulation of mucopolysaccharides (glycosaminoglycans) in various tissues. The most obvious defects are intellectual and motor retardation, bone and joint deformities, and a typical coarse facies. Ocular signs include progressive corneal clouding and retinal degeneration varying with subgroups. The early clinical classification of MPS has been supplanted by a biochemical scheme: MPS1H (Hurler syndrome), MPS1S (Scheie syndrome), and MPS1HS (Hunter-Scheie syndrome); MPS2 (Hunter-severe and Hunter-mild) and MPS3 (Sanfilippo A, B, C); MPS4 (Morquio A, B); MPS5 (no longer used); MPS6 (Maroteaux–Lamy); MPS7 (Sly); and MPS8 (diferrante). Retinal degeneration is found in MPS1H, MPS1S, MPS2, MPS3, and MPS7.

MPS1H (Hurler Syndrome)

Children with this condition are normal at birth but begin to develop the characteristic course facies (Figure 10.5) and corneal clouding within the first year of life. Distinct physical characteristics include frontal bossing, saddle nose, short neck, claw-shaped hands, oar-shaped ribs, and bullet-shaped phalanges. Mental retardation becomes obvious during the first few years of life. As motor development progresses, a peculiar stance and gait are noted due to lumbar lordosis, thoracic kyphosis, and flexion contractures at the elbows and knees.[153] The abnormality is progressive and survival beyond 10 years of age is rare. Bone marrow transplantation has resulted in improvement in many clinical features and longer survival; however, cognitive deficits continue to progress.[168,169]

Corneal clouding is the predominant ophthalmological feature in this condition, but these chil-

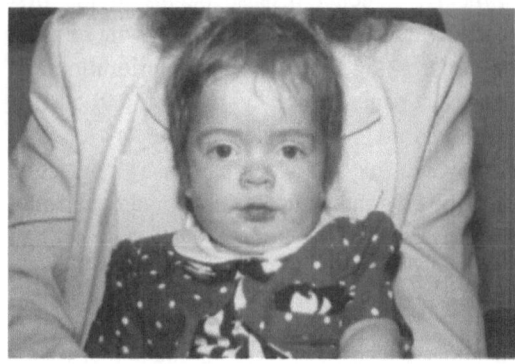

FIGURE 10.5. Hurler syndrome. Characteristic facial appearance includes frontal bossing, saddle nose, coarse features, and short neck.

dren frequently develop glaucoma and have retinal degeneration. Electroretinographic changes show a rod–cone degeneration with the rod function more severely affected.[27] Optic disc abnormalities may include papilledema, pseudopapilledema, and optic atrophy.[16,17,38] Histopathologic examinations have shown that optic disk swelling may result from infiltration of the lamina cribrosa, leading to narrowing of the scleral canal and prelaminar axonal stasis (pseudopapilledema).[16,17] Children with Hurler syndrome may also have papilledema secondary to hydrocephalus.

Although usually not required for the diagnosis of these conditions, ERG can provide valuable objective evidence of retinal function in patients with cloudy corneas. Gills et al described 21 patients with MPS using the older classification. Subnormal ERGs were found in types I (MPS1H), II (MPS2), and III (MPS3).[70] Visual electrophysiologic studies are recommended as part of the pre- and postoperative evaluation for penetrating keratoplasty. With the advent of bone marrow transplantation for these conditions, the ERG and VEP have played an increasing role in the quantification of visual pathway improvement or deterioration during treatment.

Macrocephaly may result from intracranial mucopolysaccharide deposition, hydrocephalus, or a combination of the two.[9] MR imaging shows white matter abnormalities including focal and diffuse areas of prolonged T1 and T2 relaxation times, with focal lesions in the corpus collosum,

basal ganglia, and cerebral white matter.[93] Cerebral atrophy and white matter changes occur earliest in types I, II, III, and VII and may not be seen until the second decade of life in types IV and VI.[99] Imaging of the spine in patients with MPS is often indicated since spinal cord compression is a frequent and serious complication of the disease.[9]

Pathological changes from stored mucopolysaccharide occur in virtually every organ in this condition. The lysosomes of neurons are enlarged with material that resembles lipid. Electromicroscopy shows mucopolysaccharide granular inclusions in lysosomes in tissues throughout the body.[127] The enzymatic defect in MPS1H is an absence of alpha L-iduronidase activity. Large quantities of dermatan sulfate and heparan sulfate accumulate because the alpha L-iduronic acid portions of these compounds are not cleaved. Clinical characteristics will lead to the suspicion of the diagnosis and be confirmed by assaying alpha L-iduronidase activity in leukocytes or cultured fibroblasts.[77] Screening studies can be performed on urine assessing mucopolysaccharide content and dermatan sulfate and heparan sulfate.

MPS1S (Scheie Syndrome)

These patients differ from MPH1H in that the CNS is relatively spared from the condition, corneal clouding is severe, and retinal degeneration may occur. Dermatan sulfate and heparan sulfate are excreted in the urine, and the enzymatic deficiency appears to be similar to MPH1H.[170]

MPS2 (Hunter Syndrome)

Hunter syndrome is an X-linked recessive condition giving a phenotype that is similar to but milder than Hurler syndrome. Hunter syndrome has also been described in females that have mutations of the X chromosome.[21] Corneal clouding is absent or mild, and pigmentary retinopathy and optic disk elevation have been reported.[16,17] Patients may live to the midteens. Iduronate sulfatase activity is deficient, and this enzymatic abnormality can be assayed in leukocytes, fibroblasts, or hair roots.[30]

MPS3 (Sanfilippo Syndrome)

This subgroup has more severe intellectual deterioration, no corneal clouding, and less severe physical changes than types I and II. There are four enzymatic subgroups, inherited as autosomal recessive traits. Electroretinographic changes are more severe than in MPS1H, and examination of retinal pathology shows evidence of rod–cone degeneration with rod degeneration predominating.[27] Characteristic course hair is a singular feature of MPS3A. The biochemical defects can be assayed in leukocytes or fibroblasts.[77]

MPS4 (Morquio Syndrome)

This subcategory is relatively mild compared to the first three groups; however, progressive but mild intellectual deterioration occurs, and characteristic connective tissue abnormalities are noted. There is a characteristic abnormality of tooth enamel leading to discoloration and a rough surface. Corneal opacification is mild. Visual loss is not as severe as in MPS1H.[41]

Two different biochemical syndromes are classified as types A and B. The first is due to a deficiency of N-acetyl-galactose-amine-six-sulfatase and the second is due to beta-galactosidase deficiency. These can be detected on the basis of enzyme assay on leukocytes or fibroblasts.

MPS6 (Maroteaux–Lamy Syndrome)

Children with this form of MPS have similar, physical features to MPS1H. An important feature of Maroteaux-Lamy syndrome is hypoplasia of the odontoid process of the second vertebra, which places these children at risk for spinal cord compression during endotracheal intubation. Intellect may be normal, but skeletal deformities tend to be severe. Corneal clouding is present, and glaucoma may occur. Some children with MPS6 are deaf. The biochemical abnormality is a deficiency in N-acetyl-galactose-amine-four-sulfatase, which is the same enzyme as aryl sulfatase B. The diagnosis can be made by assaying enzyme activity in leukocytes or fibroblasts. The gene is located on chromosome 5.

MPS7 (Beta-Glucuronidase Deficiency)

There is considerable phenotypic variation in this syndrome, but the onset may be in the neonatal period. Intellectual deficiency and motor abnormalities become obvious in the first two or three years of life. Corneal clouding has been reported in some cases. Dysostosis is a prominent feature with notable expansion of the ribs and proximal humerus. The biochemical abnormality is a deficiency of beta glucuronidase. The gene of this enzyme is located on chromosome 7.

Sialidosis

Sialidosis is due to a deficiency of alpha neuraminidase and occurs in two clinical forms. Individuals with type I sialidosis (cherry-red spot myoclonus syndrome) are usually normal into adolescence when they develop visual deterioration and myoclonus. A cherry-red spot in the macula is virtually always present. The visual impairment may be progressive, and intellectual deterioration occurs. Cultured fibroblasts demonstrate a deficiency of alpha neuraminidase. A concomitant deficiency of beta galactosidase has been described. These patients may have angiokeratoma corporis diffusum, which is also seen in Fabry disease and fucosidosis.[153] Type II sialidosis has also been termed Goldberg-Cotlier syndrome and cherry-red spot dementia syndrome; it is the same as mucolipidosis type I. Children become symptomatic between 8 and 15 years of age with Hurler facies, decreased visual acuity, ataxia, myoclonus, mental retardation, corneal clouding, and cherry-red spots.[44a,72a] Enlarged viscera and vacuolated blood cells are not found.

Subacute Sclerosing Panencephalitis

Subacute sclerosing panencephalitis (SSPE) is a rare sequela of measles virus infection. It usually occurs in children who were infected prior to the age of 4. Symptoms of SSPE do not develop for many years following the primary infection. Early signs are often subtle and include personality changes, behavioral abnormalities, and declining school performance (phase 1).[48] Phase II begins with the onset of involuntary movements, usually an axial myoclonus. Phases III and IV of the disease are characterized by progressive neurological deterioration, severe EEG abnormalities, and usually coma and death. Rare cases of prolonged survival, stabilization, and improvement have been noted.[48,128–130] Neuro-ophthalmologic abnormalities are found in a large number of these patients and include cortical blindness, homonymous hemianopia, visual hallucinations, and impaired visual spatial function.[18,65,131,134] Oculor motor abnormalities are also seen, including nystagmus, supranuclear palsies, and cranial nerve palsies.[80,131] Retinal examination may show focal white retinal lesions in the posterior pole that cause loss of central vision. These may produce a cherry-red spot appearance when they involve the macula[76,80,98,131] These white lesions resolve into areas of retinal pigment epithelium (RPE) atrophy with gliotic scarring of the retina and radiating retinal folds (Figure 10.6). There is no evidence of vitreous inflammation during this process. Histopathologically, retinal necrosis is evident with minimal inflammation, and Cowdry type A and Cowdry type B intranuclear inclusions have been recovered from retinal tissue.[63,66,98]

Since the neuro-ophthalmologic findings may be the only clinical signs to accompany the behavioral changes early in the disease, recognition of the full spectrum of potential neuro-ophthalmologic dysfunction is important. Neuroimaging is nonspecific, with CT scanning showing diffuse atrophy and MR imaging showing patchy areas of prolonged relaxation time in the cerebral and cerebellar white matter.[9]

White Matter Disorders

Metachromatic Leukodystrophy

Metachromatic leukodystrophy is the commonest white matter degeneration of childhood. This autosomal recessive abnormality begins as a gait abnormality, usually in early childhood (1 to 2 years of age in the late infantile form and 5 to 10 years in the juvenile form). These children become progressively weak, and ultimately bedridden and demented, with death usually occurring by age 10. A prominent feature of this condition is peripheral nerve involvement leading to decreased deep tendon reflexes.[103,121]

Neuro-ophthalmologic abnormalities include optic atrophy, leading to delayed VEPs, and strabismus.[36,173] Rarely, nystagmus[101] and a cherry-red macula are seen.[13] CT scanning reveals generalized atrophy and diffuse white matter lesions with no enhancement after contrast.[4,93] MR imaging demonstrates high-signal intensity lesions in the periventricular white matter on T-2 weighted images.[126] The peripheral white matter is spared until late in the disease[93] (Figure 10.7).

This condition is named for the appearance of the pathologically stored lipid material on light microscopy when stained with toluidine blue. Un-

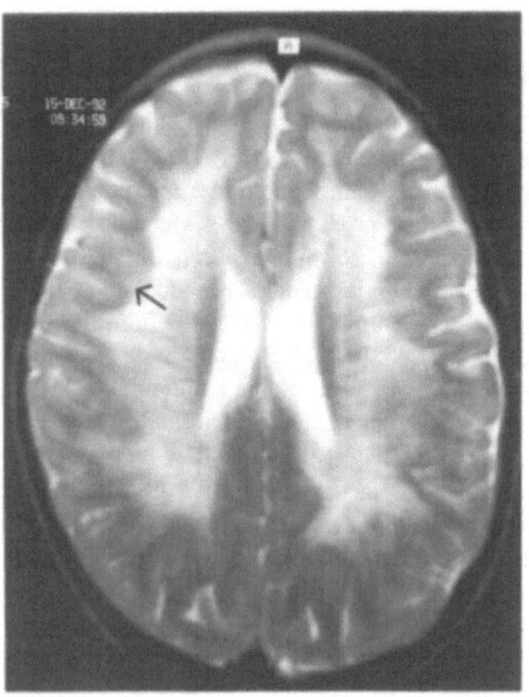

FIGURE 10.7. Metachromatic leukodystrophy. This T2-weighted MR image shows prolongation of the T2 relaxation time throughout the cerebral white matter. Sparing of the peripheral white matter (subcortical U fibers) is seen (arrow).

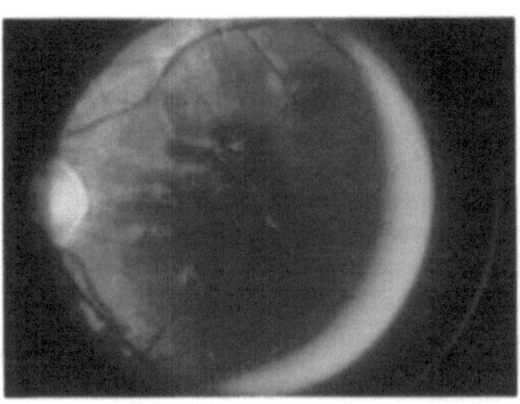

FIGURE 10.6. Subacute sclerosing panencephalitis. Note macular pigmentary changes and folds in internal limiting membrane.

der these circumstances, the accumulated material stains brown or gold and demonstrates a birefringent character in samples of cerebral white matter.[153] In addition to white matter involvement, some stored material is found in the cortex. The accumulation occurs within both neurons and glial cells. The condition also involves the deep cerebral nuclei and the spinal cord. The biochemical abnormality is an accumulation of sulfatides due to deficiency of arylsulfatase-a activity.[150] The deficiency of this enzyme results in failure to break down and reutilize myelin. Several molecular forms of arylsulfatase-a exists and may account for the different phenotypes of metachromatic leukodystrophy.[53]

The enzyme activity can be assayed in urine or leukocytes. Ancillary studies may disclose elevated spinal fluid protein and a nonfunctioning gall bladder as assessed by cholecystogram.[153] The heterozygous state (carriers) can be characterized by the enzymatic activity in white blood cells or fibroblasts.[11]

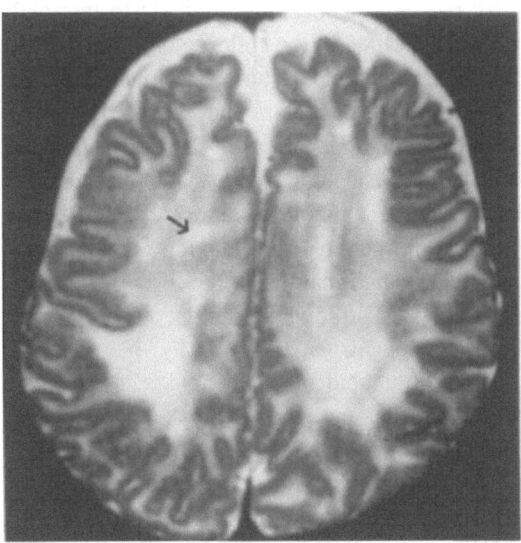

FIGURE 10.8. Canavan disease. T2-weighted MR image shows diffuse increased signal intensity in the deep white matter with multifocal round areas of higher signal intensity, suggesting vacuolar changes (arrow). (Courtesy of Charles M. Glasier, MD.)

Canavan Disease—Spongy Degeneration of the Cerebral White Matter

This entity has been characterized in the past by the common finding of a spongiform degeneration of cerebral white matter. Three clinical variants are described, differing mainly in the age of onset. Most children fall into the infantile form. These infants develop poorly in the first few months of life with slow development of motor control. Head and neck control is especially lacking. Motor deterioration accelerates causing spasticity and ultimately decorticate posturing. Most children are noted to have a concomitant deterioration in visual functioning. As optic atrophy develops and vision loss progresses, nystagmus may be seen. Progressive megalencephaly develops in these children and in those with Alexander disease. The pathologic sine qua non of Canavan disease is vacuolization of the deep cortical layers and subcortical white matter. As tissue is lost, the ventricles may become enlarged (Figure 10.8). Myelin sheaths are decreased in size, and in the later stage, axonal loss is noted. Cortical neurons appear normal early in the course of the disease but neuronal loss may be seen in long-standing cases.[56]

Canavan disease, like the other spongy myelopathies such as Kearns–Sayre syndrome and myoclonic epilepsy with ragged red fibers (MERRF), shows preferential involvement of the subcortical white matter on pathological studies. This distinguishes it from Krabbe disease and metachromatic leukodystrophy, which spare peripheral white matter until late in the disease.[9] Unlike other spongiform myelopathies, Canavan disease does not show pathological involvement of gray matter. This condition was once thought to be a mitochondrial disorder because of its clinical similarities to other mitochondrial encephalomyopathies.[145] However, in Canavan disease, there is a deficiency of the enzyme aspartoacylase.[106]

Krabbe Disease

This autosomal recessive disease is evident in early infancy. Infants initially demonstrate overresponsiveness to stimulation such as touch, light, or noise. This progresses to increasing degrees of spasticity with flexed arms, clenched fists, and scissored legs. Generalized seizures develop, and optic atrophy ensues.[23,78] On rare occasion, a cherry-red spot has been reported.[114] In terminal stages of this illness, the children are blind, deaf, and have opisthotonic posturing. Computerized tomography shows periventricular hyperdensity.[29,55] The most common locations of these densities are the thalamus, caudate nucleus, and corona radiata. They occur concomitantly with decreased attenuation in white matter.[9] MR imaging demonstrates white matter abnormalities in the form of nonspecific T1 and T2 prolongation in deep cerebral and cerebellar white matter (Figure 10.9).[7,52]

Clumps of globoid and epithelioid cells and cerebral white matter are the characteristic pathological abnormality in Krabbe disease. Cortical atrophy and overall loss of brain mass may also be noted.

The lipid accumulation in this disease is due to deficiency of the enzyme galactocerebroside beta galactosidase, resulting in the storage of large amounts of galactocerebroside (galactosyl ceramide).[153]

Other White Matter Disorders

Pelizaeus–Merzbacher Disease

This syndrome has not yet been characterized biochemically or genetically; therefore, it is described on the basis of clinical findings and

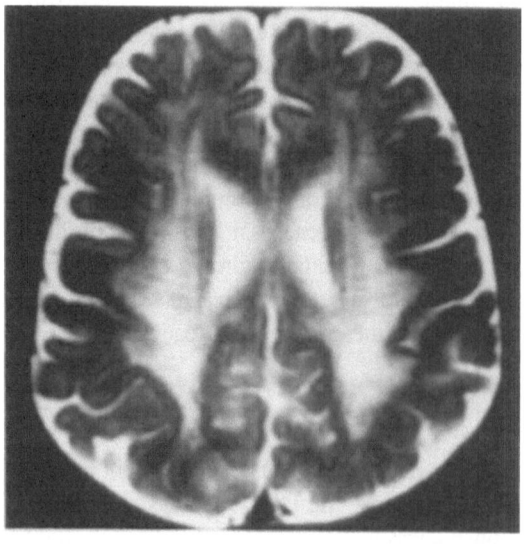

FIGURE 10.9. Krabbe disease. T2-weighted MR image showing diffusely increased signal intensity in deep white matter. (Courtesy of Charles M. Glasier, MD.)

pathology. Seitelberger recommended division of the disease into six variants, depending primarily on age of onset and rapidity of progression.[143] The sixth variant is also known as Cockayne syndrome; however, this appears to be a multisystem disease and will be described separately. The common features of all clinical types of Pelizaeus–Merzbacher disease include involuntary movements, spasticity, and nystagmus. The pathological hallmark is patchy demyelination with preservation of islands of normal myelin resulting in a tigroid appearance of stained sections of white matter on light microscopy.

Pelizaeus–Merzbacher disease has its onset in the first few months, beginning with nystagmus[154] and head tremor and progressing to ataxia limb tremor and choreoathetosis. Trobe et al[158] have described distinctive electro-oculographic characteristics of the nystagmus in this condition, consisting of an elliptical pendular nystagmus that may be superimposed or interposed with upbeating nystagmus.[158] Early in the course of this disease, nystagmus may be associated with head nodding and simulate spasmus nutans. Optic atrophy and seizures occur later. Intellectual function is relatively preserved, but a mild dementia may occur. Most of these patients die in the second decade or during early adulthood, and most are male. This type appears to have an X-linked recessive pattern of inheritance; however, some cases are sporadic. The connatal form is more severe with death in the first few years of life.[139]

Neuroimaging in Pelizaeus–Merzbacher disease shows a lack of myelination without evidence of a white matter destructive process (Figure 10.10).[9,146,148,163] The finding of white matter abnormalities in a child thought to have spasmus nutans should raise suspicion of this disorder.

Cockayne Syndrome

This condition is sometimes classified as type VI Pelizaeus–Merzbacher disease because of the presence of patchy demyelination and preserved island of myelin seen at autopsy. However, in Pelizaeus–Merzbacher disease, pathology is limited to the CNS, whereas Cockayne syndrome involves multiple organs. Cockayne syndrome has been reported to be inherited in an autosomal recessive fashion in some families.

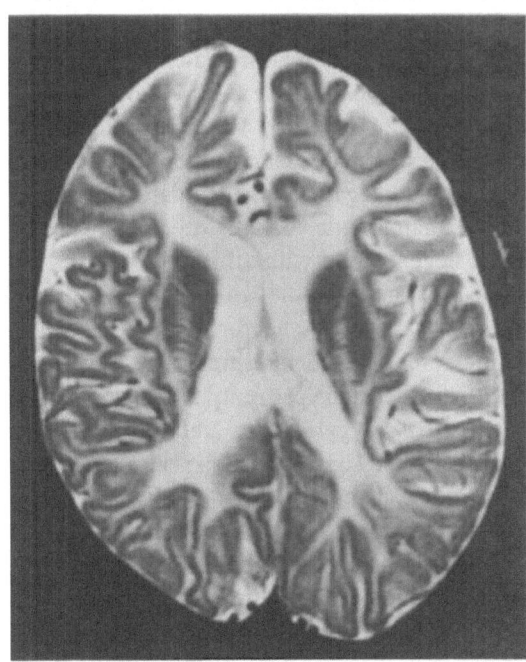

FIGURE 10.10. Pelizaeus–Merzbacher disease. This T2 MR image in a 7-year-old child shows severe loss of myelin. Myelin should appear dark in this image. (Courtesy of A. James Barkovich, MD.)

The earliest evidence of this condition is often a photosensitive dermatitis in the first few months of life, followed by growth retardation, bony abnormalities, and characteristic facial appearance in the first few years. Progressive cerebellar dysfunction and motor deterioration ensue. Ophthalmologic features include retinitis pigmentosa and optic atrophy with cataracts, corneal opacities, and impaired lacrimation noted in some patients.[111]

A CT shows calcifications in basal ganglia and dentate nucleus of the cerebellum along with cerebral atrophy.[43] MR imaging demonstrates delayed myelination and T2 prolongation in periventricular white matter, basal ganglia, and dentate.[43] The subcortical U fibers may be involved early, but more often they are preserved until later.[9,40] Some children have been noted to have normal pressure hydrocephalus and have benefitted from shunting.[61]

Neuropathologic changes resemble those of Pelizaeus–Merzbacher disease, showing patches of nonmyelination with preserved islands of nor-

mal myelin. In addition, globus pallidus and cerebellum may show calcifications. No biochemical abnormality has yet been identified for this syndrome, and diagnosis is made on clinical grounds.

Alexander Disease

This sporadic neurodegenerative disorder occurs in an infantile and juvenile form. The infantile form begins in the first year of age with intellectual and motor retardation, spasticity, seizures, and progressive megalencephaly without hydrocephalus. The head enlargement is progressive, and hydrocephalus may be superimposed in later stages.[61] The prominent neuro-ophthalmologic feature in the infantile form is optic atrophy. The juvenile form is rare and has its onset between 7 and 14 years of age. Bulbar or pseudobulbar dysfunction occurs, including difficulty swallowing, abnormal speech, nystagmus, ptosis, facial diplegia, and atrophy of the tongue. Mentation appears to be normal.[72] The possibility of an adult form has been suggested with a clinical picture resembling multiple sclerosis. On pathological examination of the brain, the characteristic finding is refractile cyanophilic bodies related to astrocytes around blood vessels. These occur throughout gray and white matter and in the optic nerves and tracts.[133] Loss of myelin is marked in the infantile cases. The brain stem may be predominantly involved in the juvenile form.

Imaging studies show abnormalities in the white matter beginning in the frontal areas and gradually proceeding posteriorly. CT scanning shows low-density lesions in the frontal lobes with contrast enhancement near the tips of the frontal horns.[54] MR imaging shows a similar pattern of abnormality with prolonged T1 and T2 relaxation times progressing from anterior to posterior white matter. Peripheral white matter is affected early.[9]

No biochemical defect has yet been defined in this disorder, and there is no specific therapy.

Peroxisomal Disorders

Peroxisomes are subcellular organelles that were first recognized in 1954 in the proximal tubule of the kidney. They are found in all eukaryotic species and in almost every cell. The name was chosen because these organelles produce and reduce hydrogen peroxide. They also contain enzymes needed for the oxidation of amino and dicarboxylic acids. In this process, H_2O_2 is formed and then detoxified by catalase, another peroxisomal enzyme.[49,120] In 1973, Goldfischer discovered that peroxisomes were absent in liver and renal tubular epithelial cells of patients with Zellweger syndrome.[73] Various peroxisomal functions were found to be absent. Incomplete deficiency of peroxisomal functions has been found in other conditions.

Inherited diseases of peroxisomes can be divided into two classes: those in which only a single peroxisomal function is impaired—such as X linked ALD and the adult form of Refsum disease—and those in which more than one peroxisomal function is impaired—such as the cerebrohepatorenal (Zellweger) syndrome, the infantile form of Refsum disease, the neonatal form of ALD, the rhizomelic type of chondrodysplasia punctata, and hyper-pipecolic acidemia.[62]

Abnormal retinal pigmentation occurs in Zellweger syndrome, neonatal ALD, hyper-pipecolic acidemia, and infantile Refsum disease. These children may have abnormal ERGs early in the course of the disease. Optic disc pallor has been reported in Zellweger syndrome, neonatal ALD, and hyperpipecolic acidemia.[26,122]

MR imaging studies in children with peroxisomal disorders have shown the following general abnormalities: (1) neuronal migrational disturbances in combination with hypomyelination, dysmyelination, or demyelination; (2) symmetrical demyelination of the posterior limb of the internal capsule, cerebellar white matter, and brain stem tracts with a variable affection of the cerebral hemispheres; and (3) symmetrical demyelination—exhibiting two zones: the first starting in the occipital area and spreading outward and forward, and the second involving the brain stem tracts.[9,162]

Zellweger Syndrome

Zellweger syndrome is an autosomal recessive disease characterized by unique facies, failure to thrive, and visual impairment. The characteristic facial abnormality includes shallow orbits, epicanthal folds, flattened nasal bridge, high forehead, and high arched and malformed ears. Psychomotor retardation and failure to thrive occur in the early weeks of life, and severe hypotonia and seizures ensue rapidly. Other systemic features include organomegaly and hypoplastic genitalia. The ophthalmologic features are dominated by retinal degeneration with a flat ERG in early infancy. Most children die within the first year of life. The characteristic neuronal migration abnormalities are easily demonstrated by MR imaging.[162] These include periventricular neuronal heterotopias, pachygyria, and polymicrogyria. A severe deficiency of myelination is also noted.

The gross pathologic abnormalities relate to neuronal migration abnormalities and polymicrogyri. Microscopically, there is evidence of gliosis and accumulation of lipids; however, unlike storage diseases, the lipid droplets in Zellweger syndrome are in the astrocytic cytoplasm rather than in macrophages.[1] The severe lack of myelin noted histologically in the brains of these infants may be due to a combination of disturbed myelination and accelerated demyelination.[2]

Zellweger cerebrohepatorenal syndrome is a severe form of diffuse peroxisomal deficiency. Initially, the syndrome was attributed to the absence or a decrease in the number of peroxisomes; however, peroxisomal membrane ghosts have now been identified in cells, indicating that Zellweger syndrome and other conditions like it may in fact be due to peroxisomal assembly abnormalities.[137] Plasma levels of VLCFAs, pipecolic acid, phytanic acid, and bile acid intermediates are all elevated in this syndrome.

Homozygotes also have characteristic lens abnormalities consisting of a dense cortex producing a cortical-nuclear interface that is visible at the slit lamp through a dilated pupil. Hittner et al have shown that the heterozygous parents of four infants with Zellweger syndrome had lens changes consisting of curvilinear condensations in the cortical region in the same location as the lens changes in the homozygous state.[83] No electrophysiological studies were done on these patients. The combination of neuronal and white matter disease is reflected in retinal ganglion cell abnormality and optic atrophy.

Adrenoleukodystrophy

The original description of ADL by Siemerling and Creutzfeldt emphasized adrenal insufficiency and cerebral demyelination. The clinical features have since been defined as including visual defects,[138] hypoadrenalism,[86] hypogonadism,[59] and gross motor and intellectual deterioration. This disease has since been defined as a peroxisomal disorder of VLCFA oxidation. There are several phenotypes, and multiple organs are affected.[113]

X-linked ALD is associated with a deficiency of a single peroxisomal function. This condition differs from the newly recognized neonatal ALD in which there is impairment of multiple peroxisomal functions, including deficiencies in VLCFA oxidation by phytanic acid oxidase and plasmalogen synthesizing enzymes.[140] Several phenotypes of X-linked ALD have been described, including progressive cerebral disease in young boys, progressive spinal cord degeneration in young men, and an intermediate form with both spinal cord and cerebral involvement in males and mild spinal cord disease or multiple sclerosis–like features in female carriers.[59,149] X-linked ALD usually presents between 4 and 8 years of age. Initial manifestations include increased skin pigmentation, decreased school performance, and "dementia-type" changes in memory and emotional expression. Motor disturbances may be prominent, with a stiff-legged spastic gait. Visual disturbances are common, and occasionally they occur early. Homonymous hemianopia, visual agnosia, decreased visual acuity, and cerebral blindness have all been reported. Optic atrophy eventually develops.[156,172]

Infants with ALD (neonatal form) have severe hypotonia and seizures at birth, and later they exhibit growth and mental retardation. Other neurological features include macrocephaly, large fontanels, nystagmus, optic atrophy, pigmentary retinopathy, and abnormal vision and hearing. Most children die before 5 years of age. A few have survived until age 10.

The biochemical hallmark of ALD is excess VLCFA, which can be measured in cultured skin fibroblasts, white cells, red blood phospholipids, or total plasma lipids. The concentration of C26:0 is elevated to approximately five times normal. Analysis of VLCFA appears to be a reliable way of diagnosing ALD.

Electrophysiological findings in two cases of neonatal ALD were reported by Verma et al.[164] One child was examined at age 1 year, and the other, at age 3 ½ years. Neither child demonstrated visual-following responses, and both had severe seizures and long-tract signs. Both had nonrecordable or extremely diminished ERG responses and no consistent, identifiable positivity in VEP responses except for the right eye of the 1-year-old, which showed a delayed positive wave with a mean latency of 137 ms. Ophthalmological examination of the younger patient showed normal media, normally reactive pupils, full extraocular movements, intermittent fine jerk nystagmus on horizontal gaze, and unremarkable fundi other than mild temporal pallor in each eye. The older child had sluggishly reactive pupils, pendular nystagmus, clear media, bilateral optic atrophy, and retinitis pigmentosa, suggesting a degeneration of photoreceptors and accumulation of lipids in the ganglion cells.

Battaglia et al[14] have studied the EEG, ERG, and flash VEP in 14 boys with X-linked ALD and in two siblings of affected boys. These siblings had adrenocortical deficiency but were neurologically normal. All 14 affected boys had EEG abnormalities characterized by irregular, large-amplitude, slow activity. Similar EEG findings were seen in the two siblings of affected patients. The ERG was normal in all cases. The VEP was abnormal in 4 of 12 cases. The recording deteriorated over a short time frame in two cases and was low or unrecordable when first measured in two others. The VEPs in two siblings were normal.[14] Detection of the carrier state of X-linked ALD by VEP has been reported.[110]

Neuroimaging studies are normal prior to the onset of symptoms. X-linked adrenal leukodystrophy classically involves the occipital white matter bilaterally. Areas of active demyelination may show intense contrast enhancement at the periphery of the lesions. These lesions are usually symmetric and may affect the posterior occipital region most severely. White matter lesions in the occipital region also characteristically involve the splenium of the corpus callosum early on. Occipi-

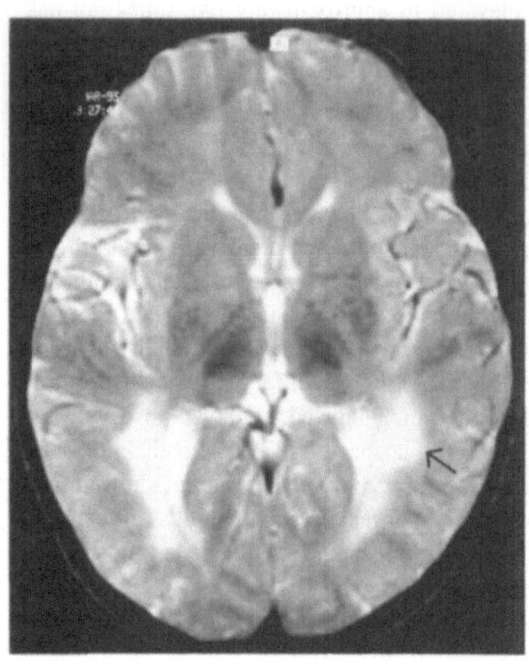

FIGURE 10.11. Adrenoleukodystrophy. This T2-weighted MR image shows symmetrical hyperintense hemispheric lesions primarily involving occipital white matter (arrow).

tal U fibers are relatively spared (Figure 10.11). With time the lesions extend forward to involve the lateral and medial geniculate bodies, the thalamus, and posterior limb of the internal capsule bilaterally. Cerebellar and brain stem white matter are relatively spared. Lesions are usually symmetric and may effect the posterior occipital region most severely with the anterior occipital region affected to a lesser extent.[162]

Basal Ganglia Disease

Hallervorden–Spatz Disease

The basic pathophysiology of Hallervorden–Spatz syndrome remains unknown, however, its clinical manifestations, recessive genetic transmission, and characteristic iron deposition in the globus pallidus and substantia nigra seen on neuroimaging establish the diagnosis. The typical clinical findings include an onset in early childhood of motor disorders of an extrapyramidal type, characterized by dystonic posturing, difficulty walking, and muscular rigidity. As the disease progresses, involuntary movements of a choreoathetoid type appear along with progressive intellectual deterioration. Most patients die in early adulthood. Although optic atrophy is rare in degenerations of the extrapyramidal system, it has been described as the presenting symptom in Hallervorden–Spatz disease.[28,171] Retinitis pigmentosa has been described in some children.[46,152] Although the metabolic abnormality in Hallervorden–Spatz syndrome is unknown, it is likely to involve abnormal iron binding within the basal ganglia. Iron may play a role in modulating dopamine binding to postsynaptic receptors, and abnormal iron storage may interrupt these mechanisms, as well as disrupting oxidation and peroxidation reactions, leading to cellular damage within the basal ganglia.[152]

MR imaging may show abnormalities early in the course of this disease, characterized by an overall low signal on T2-weighted images in the globus pallidus and substantia nigra with a central zone of high signal within the globus pallidus[57,123,144] (Figure 10.12). This MR pattern is

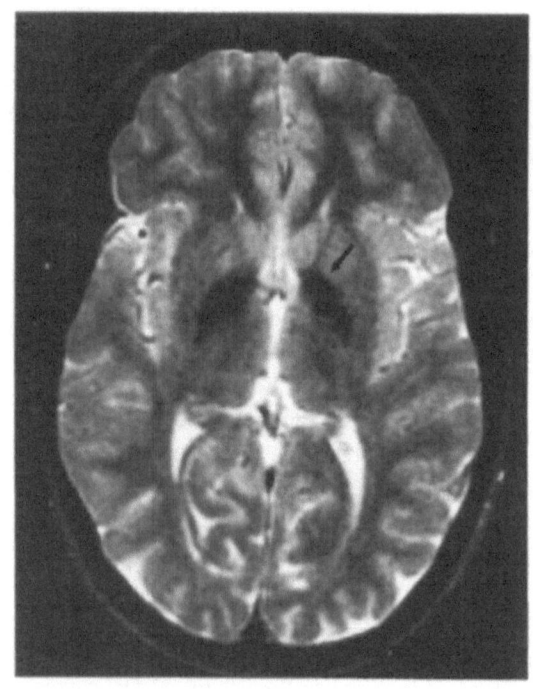

FIGURE 10.12. Hallervorden-Spatz disease. This axial T2-weighted MR image shows markedly hypointense signal in the inferior globus pallidus bilaterally (arrow). (Courtesy of Dr. A. James Barkovich.)

not characteristic of other extrapyramidal-type movement disorders, such as Parkinson disease, Wilson disease, and Leigh disease, thus allowing a fairly confident diagnosis when this imaging pattern is seen in a child with characteristic clinical findings.

Wilson Disease

The symptoms of Wilson disease are caused by an abnormal accumulation of copper, primarily in the liver but subsequently in many other organs including the CNS. This disease is inherited in an autosomal recessive fashion and is due to the presence of an abnormal protein in the liver that binds copper much more strongly than liver proteins in normal individuals. The copper-storing capacity is exceeded, and unbound copper increases in the circulation with deposition in other tissues.

Although patients are usually diagnosed in the second and third decade, they may become symptomatic as early as 5 years of age, usually with signs of liver failure. Patients who are diagnosed in adolescence and in later life more frequently have neurological signs predominating, such as loss of fine motor skills, progressive clumsiness, and dysarthria.

The principal ophthalmological sign in Wilson disease is the Kayser–Fleischer ring. Ophthalmologists are frequently asked by the internal medicine and pediatrician consultants to examine patients with liver disease or unexplained neurological degeneration for Kayser–Fleischer rings, as this will establish the diagnosis of Wilson disease. A slit lamp examination is required for this evaluation, even though advanced Kayser–Fleischer rings can be seen by the naked eye. These rings reflect copper deposition in Descemet's membrane, leading to a brownish-green discoloration of the membrane, seen most easily near the limbus of the cornea. Patients with Wilson disease may also have "sunflower cataracts." Neuro-ophthalmologic features of Wilson disease include supranuclear gaze palsies, difficulty initiating saccades, and cogwheel pursuit.[95,100]

The laboratory confirmation of Wilson disease includes serum levels of ceruloplasmin (less than 20 mg per dL) and increased urinary excretion of copper (greater than 100 mg per 24 hours). Treatment of the condition includes a low-copper diet and D-penicillamine (a chelator of copper), which increases urinary excretion.

The CNS damage in Wilson disease is associated with increased tissue copper content. Copper interferes with cellular metabolism and enzymatic activity, leading to cellular death. Toxic levels of copper are found throughout the brain in this disease; however, the main pathological findings are in the basal ganglia, thalamus, and brain stem. These changes include degeneration of neurons, increased numbers of astrocytes with neurofibrillary plaques and tangles, and ultimately spongy degeneration and cavitation of the structures.

Several studies have shown good correlation between neurological features and MR abnormalities in Wilson disease. The correlation is particularly good with moderate to advanced disease, whereas asymptomatic patients with biochemically proven Wilson disease have no MR imaging findings.[3,104] Most symptomatic patients demonstrate lesions of the putamen. The characteristic lesion is a peripheral high signal area on T2-weighted imaging surrounding a central area of low signal. Pathological correlation of this finding has not been clarified. Patients with MR abnormalities limited to the putamen usually show dystonia. Patients with involvement of the putamen and the caudate may show Parkinsonian features, as will patients with abnormal MR findings in the substantia nigra.

Aminoacidopathies and Other Biochemical Defects

Maple Syrup Urine Disease

This disease is named after the smell of urine that contains increased amounts of the three branched-chain amino acids: valine, leucine, and isoleucine. The enzymatic defect is one of oxidative decarboxylation of the ketoacids of these aminoacids and can be demonstrated in leukocytes. This disease becomes manifest in the neonatal period with difficulties in feeding, hypoglycemia, metabolic acidosis, and a severe progressive neurological deterioration.

Supranuclear gaze palsies are frequent findings in this condition, including paralysis and paresis of upward gaze[108,175] or a combination of vertical and horizontal gaze palsies.[31,141] Ptosis is also frequently seen, and nystagmus commonly accompanies the recovery phase after the institution of dietary measures. This nystagmus frequently occurs in bursts, and associated bursts of flutter-like movement of the eyelids may also occur in the recovery phase.[45,141,175] Untreated cases die within the first few months of life. Treatment consists of a diet limited in the branched-chain amino acids, and this can arrest the progressive deterioration of the condition. There are several variants of this condition, one of which shows responsiveness to a supplement with Vitamin B[1] (thiamine).[115]

Homocystinuria

Homocystinuria is an inborn error of metabolism involving methionine metabolism. Clinical features of the untreated condition involve progressive intellectual deficiency, tall stature, arachnodactyly, malar flush, fair hair, and dislocated lenses. Affected patients are also at an increased risk of thromboembolic episodes, frequently involving the cerebral vasculature and sometimes brought on by anesthesia.[112]

Several enzymatic deficiencies may result in a similar phenotype. Type I homocystinuria (classic) is due to a deficiency of cystathionine-beta synthetase and results in high blood levels of homocystine and methionine.

Neuro-ophthalmological abnormalities such as visual field defects, papilledema, and optic atrophy may arise from cerebral thromboembolic events.

Abetalipoproteinemia

Abetalipoproteinemia is a rare autosomal recessive condition characterized by malabsorption of fat, neurological degeneration, progressive pigmentary retinopathy, and a strikingly abnormal plasmolytic and lipoprotein profile.[124]

The condition was first described in a patient with atypical retinitis pigmentosa, malformed erythrocytes, ataxia, and intestinal malabsorption which had led to the misdiagnosis of celiac disease. The authors of this paper correctly identified this as a new condition with a genetic basis, and the disease became known as Bassen–Kornzweig syndrome.[10] A more specific abnormality of low-density lipoproteins, or beta lipoproteins, established the biochemical hallmark of this disease.[135]

A lipoprotein called apo-lipoprotein B (apo b) is found to be completely absent in the plasma of patients with abetalipoproteinemia, and it was thought that a molecular defect in the apo b gene may be responsible for this condition; however, the apo b gene was proven to be normal by genetic studies.[97] Rather, a protein responsible for intracellular assembly and secretion of apo b containing lipoproteins has been found to be deficient in abetalipoproteinemia.[92,167] This defect leads to deficient fat absorption from the intestine interfering with the absorption of all fat soluble vitamins. The defect profoundly affects the metabolism of vitamin E, which relies upon this lipoprotein not only for absorption from the intestine but also for transport to peripheral tissues from the liver.[98] The other fat soluble vitamins have their own transport and metabolism systems from the liver to peripheral tissues.

Vitamin A and K supplements can adequately increase the plasma and tissue levels of these vitamins; however, very large oral doses of vitamin E are required to achieve adequate tissue levels of vitamin E. The recommended dosage is 150 to 200 mg/kg per day. Adults may require up to 20,000 mg per day (the recommended dietary allowance for normal people for vitamin E is 15 mg/d.

Children with pigmentary retinopathy and neurological degeneration, and infants with malabsorption or failure to thrive, should be screened for abetalipoproteinemia by performing a plasma cholesterol level. A level lower than 1.5 mmol/L (60 mg/dL) is suspicious for abetalipoproteinemia. Most patients who have very low cholesterol will not have abetalipoproteinemia but will have one of the more common syndromes, such as familial hypobetalipoproteinemia. Treatment with high doses of vitamin E can retard or halt progression of the neurological disease and possibly the retinal disease.[132]

Neurological symptoms usually begin in the second decade with loss of deep-tendon reflexes, progressing to decreased distal lower extremity vibratory and proprioreceptive senses, and spasticity may develop by the third or fourth decade. Neuropathology reveals axonal degeneration of the spinocerebellar tracts and demyelination of the fasciculus cuneatus and gracilis.[124] Evidence is accumulating that shows high-dose vitamin E therapy can halt or retard the progression of neurological disease.[92,124]

The most prominent ophthalmological finding in abetalipoproteinemia is a pigmentary retinal degeneration. (Figure 10.13) A clinicopathologic correlation in a patient with abetalipoproteinemia dying of unrelated causes showed that the pigmentary retinal degeneration was accompanied by loss of photoreceptors in the posterior pole, loss or attenuation of pigment epithelium, excessive accumulation of lipofuscin in the submacular pigment epithelium, and invasion of the retina by macrophage-like pigment and cells.[37] Retinal degeneration is associated with waxy pallor of the optic disc, narrowing of the retinal vessels, and clump or spot RPE pigmentation rather than the bone corpuscle pigmentation usually seen in retinitis pigmentosa.[67] Abetalipoproteinemia may also be complicated by subretinal neovascularization associated with retinal angioid streaks.[47] Ocular motor abnormalities are also prominent. Yee et al[174] first described an unusual form of internuclear ophthalmoplegia in which the adducting rather than the abducting eye, showed nystagmus on sidegaze. Absence of adduction was accompanied by convergence insufficiency in these patients.[89,174]

Mitochondrial Encephalomyelopathies

Several neurodegenerative syndromes are caused by disorders of mitochondrial metabolism. These abnormalities produce defects in the energy cycle of susceptible cells causing abnormal function and ultimately death of the cell. Nerve tissue and striated muscle are most commonly affected. The conditions included in this group of disorders are Alpers disease, Menkes disease, and Leigh disease, all manifesting their abnormalities in early childhood. A group of disorders with progressive neurological symptoms occurring later in life include chronic progressive external ophthalmoplegia {CPEO}, KSS, mitochondrial encephalomyopathy with lactic acidosis and strokelike syndrome (MELAS), and myoclonic epilepsy with ragged red fibers (MERRF).

Several unique features of mitochondrial functioning account for the genetic and clinical features of these syndromes. The mitochondrial encephalomyopathies have only recently begun to be understood on a molecular level, and a detailed classification system has yet to be worked out.[84] A thorough understanding of these conditions is made difficult by the complexity of mitochondrial energy metabolism, which is controlled by both nuclear DNA and mitochondrial DNA, and by the characteristics of mitochondrial inheritance and deterioration of mitochondrial function with aging.[165] Mitochondria are the major supplier of adenosine triphosphate for cellular energy metabolism. The mitochondrial metabolism itself can be disturbed in any of four major steps.[8] The complexity of the interplay between these steps of mitochondrial metabolism and other cellular functions can be illustrated by the fact that abnormalities of the different steps in the mitochondrial energy chain can result in the same phenotype, whereas identical

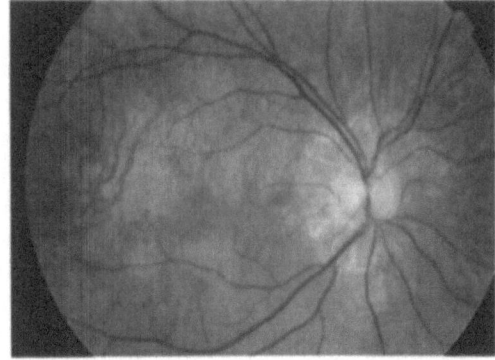
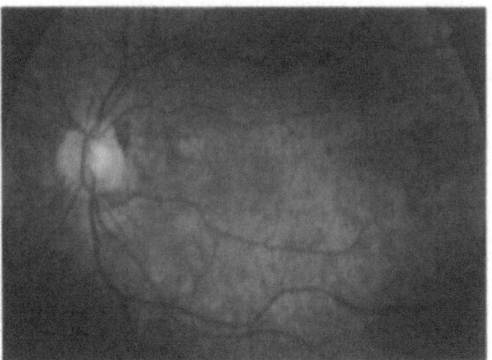

FIGURE 10.13. Kearns–Sayre syndrome. Note bilateral retinal pigmentary changes and discrete ring of peripapillary pigment atrophy OD. (A) Right retina. (B) Left retina.

genetic defects can cause different phenotypic expression.[84,159,160,165] The complexity of mitochondrial diseases becomes more readily apparent when one considers that the circular mitochondrial DNA containing 16,500 base pairs work in concert with nuclear DNA to build and execute the energy-producing function of the subcellular organelle. Each circular mitochondrial DNA has 37 genes encoding 22 transfer RNAs, two ribosomal RNAs, and 13 proteins essential to oxidative phosphorylation. Nuclear DNA encodes for 56 subunits of the mitochondrial electron transport chain, and the expression of the mitochondrial DNA genes requires replication, transcription, and translation, most of which is encoded by nuclear DNA. Oxidative phosphorylation alone requires hundreds of nuclear, mitochondrial, and cytoplasmic genes.[8]

Mitochondria are the only subcellular organelles to have their own DNA, and this DNA differs from nuclear DNA in several important ways. First, it is circular and has no enterons (the noncoding sequences common to nuclear DNA). The genetic code used by mitochondrial DNA is also different from the nuclear DNA code. Mitochondria divide in a manner similar to the budding of bacteria. Upon cell division, mitochondria are randomly divided into each daughter cell. During fertilization, the human sperm cytoplasm has very few mitochondria and does not contribute significantly to the mitochondrial content of the zygote; therefore, all offspring inherit the female parent's mitochondrial genotype. While nuclear DNA is inherited in a Mendelian fashion, mitochondrial DNA is entirely maternally inherited. The mitochondrial function is not controlled exclusively by the mitochondrial DNA present in the organelle, but rather, most mitochondrial functions are still under the control of nuclear DNA. However, mitochondrial DNA encodes for 13 components of the electron transport chain, most importantly, complex I, III, IV, and V. Ribosomal and transfer RNA are also encoded by the mitochondrial DNA. Abnormalities in these RNAs produce multiple defects in oxidative phosphorylation.

The clinical recognition of mitochondrial disorders as a group has been impeded by the variability in phenotypic expression of mitochondrial encephalomyopathies. There are hundreds of mitochondria per cell and thousands of copies of mitochondrial DNA, which leads to a mixture of normal mitochondrial DNA and mutant DNA, a phenomenon called heteroplasmy. Furthermore, a cell may drift toward the expression of more normal or more mutant DNA with cell replication, a phenomenon called mitotic segregation. Whether a cell's energy metabolism reflects the abnormal DNA present in a cell may be influenced by a threshold effect where a certain percentage of abnormal DNA is required before energy metabolism is affected. Finally, the degree to which a particular cell depends on mitochondrial energy metabolism may vary, thus explaining why muscle, brain, and heart, with their very high energy demands, may be particularly vulnerable to these abnormalities.

Chronic Progressive External Ophthalmoplegia (CPEO)

Chronic progressive external ophthalmoplegia has been divided into many subsets according to clinical findings. The most well known of the syndromes considered to be a subset of CPEO is Kearns–Sayre syndrome. Its unique phenotype not withstanding, Kearns–Sayre syndrome may be one particular manifestation of a larger group of abnormalities, all caused by deletions of mitochondrial DNA. These deletions lead to similar biochemical abnormalities that are found to produce clinical syndromes that differ because of the phenomena previously noted. Mitochondrial DNA deletions of varying sizes have been demonstrated in patients with CPEO, but to date, no correlation between the size of the deletion and the severity of symptomatology has been described.

Complete Kearns–Sayre syndrome is characterized by onset of clinical abnormalities in the first or second decade of life with progressive ptosis and external ophthalmoplegia. A characteristic retinal abnormality occurs in patients with Kearns–Sayre syndrome consisting of widespread salt-and-pepper retinal pigment epithelial mottling, seen most strikingly in the macula, together with a discrete halo associated with peripapillary pigmentary atrophy[69] (Figure 10.13). Cardiac conduction defects due to degeneration of the HIS Purkinje system beginning with partial block but leading to complete heart block with or without an associated cardiomyopathy. The CSF protein is found to be elevated to greater than 100 mg/dL, and many patients demonstrate cerebellar ataxia.

Current criteria for diagnosis include two obligatory features: early-onset CPEO (prior to age 20) and retinal pigmentary degeneration, plus one of the following three: heart block, CSF protein greater than 100 mg/dL, or cerebellar syndrome.[42] However, a large number of systemic, neurologic, and laboratory abnormalities have been noted in Kearns–Sayre syndrome (Table 10.5). The use of systemic corticosteroids in these patients can precipitate hyperglycemic acidotic coma and death.[6]

The characteristic MR imaging abnormalities in CPEO include abnormal hyperintensities in the deep gray matter nuclei (particularly the thalamus and globus pallidus) on T2-weighted images, and patchy white matter involvement.[8,93] The white matter involvement is predominantly peripheral with early involvement of the subcortical U fibers sparing of the periventricular fibers (Figure 10.14). Other disorders involving myelin, such as lysosomal disorders and peroxisomal abnormalities, tend to spare this subcortical myelin and effect the older central myelin first.[9]

TABLE 10.5. Associated manifestations of Kearns–Sayre syndrome.

Hypoparathyroidism with hypocalcemia
Hypomagnesemia
Diabetes
Short stature
Delayed sexual maturation
Hypogonadism
Subnormal intelligence
Slow EEG
Pyramidal tract signs
Sensory-neuro hearing loss
Vestibular dysfunction on caloric testing
Past history of aseptic meningitis
Basal ganglionic calcifications

The brain ultimately undergoes a spongy degeneration affecting both gray and white matter, and these patients may eventually become demented. Muscle biopsy shows ragged red fibers as it does in patients with the other mitochondrial encephalomyopathies.

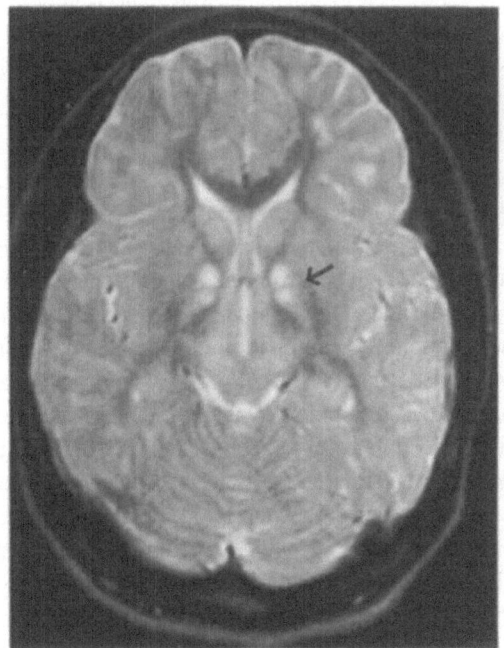
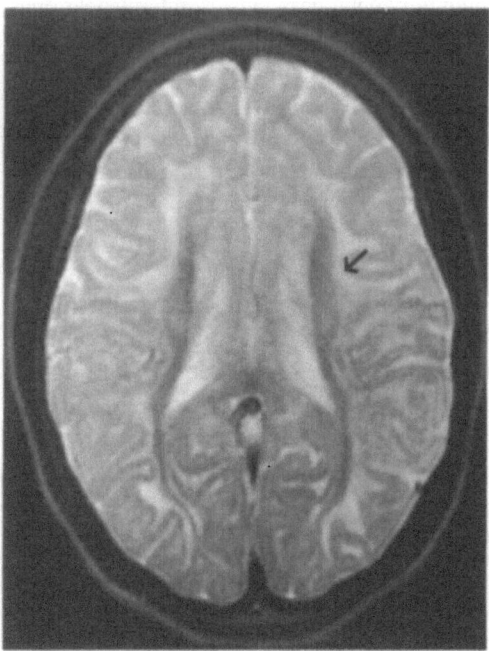
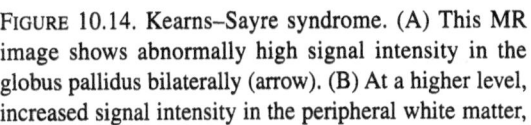

FIGURE 10.14. Kearns–Sayre syndrome. (A) This MR image shows abnormally high signal intensity in the globus pallidus bilaterally (arrow). (B) At a higher level, increased signal intensity in the peripheral white matter, including the subcortical U fibers is evident (arrow), while the periventricular white matter is spared. (Courtesy of A. James Barkovich, MD.)

The biochemical defects have been localized to complex I, complex III, and complex IV in the respiratory chain, all of which are linked to proteins encoded by mitochondrial DNA.

Leigh Subacute Necrotizing Encephalomyelopathy

Leigh disease is an autosomal recessively inherited abnormality that leads to widespread degeneration of neural tissue without accumulation of a storage material. A waxing and waning course of vomiting, weight loss, stupor, and seizures reflect a pathological process that is distributed around the third ventricle, aqueduct of Sylvius, and fourth ventricle. There is a striking resemblance to the pathological abnormalities of thiamine deficiency (Wernecke encephalopathy). These abnormalities have lead to the suggestion that Leigh disease is secondary to an inborn error of thiamine metabolism. However, a variety of energy metabolism abnormalities have been found, including cytochrome c oxidase deficiency.[94]

Children with Leigh disease may develop a variety of unusual brain stem motility abnormalities, including horizontal gaze palsies, internuclear ophthalmoplegia, dorsal midbrain syndrome, and a condition initially resembling spasmus nutans.[142] Although primarily a gray matter disease, white matter is eventually involved, and optic atrophy may develop late in the course of the disease.

A characteristic symmetrical pattern of neuroimaging abnormalities is now known to be highly characteristic for Leigh disease. MR imaging shows prolonged T1 and T2 relaxation times in the basal ganglia, periaqueductal region, and cerebral peduncles. Involvement of cerebral white matter may also occur[9,109] (Figure 10.15). Serum and CSF lactate levels may be elevated. Proton spectroscopy may be useful in delineating Leigh disease from other diseases primarily affecting basal ganglia, as it is the only disorder to date to show elevated lactate levels in these areas by this study.[44]

Encephalomyopathy, Lactic Acidosis, and Stroke-Like Episodes (MELAS)

Initial symptoms in the MELAS condition begin in early childhood and include headache (which may be indistinguishable from complicated migraine),

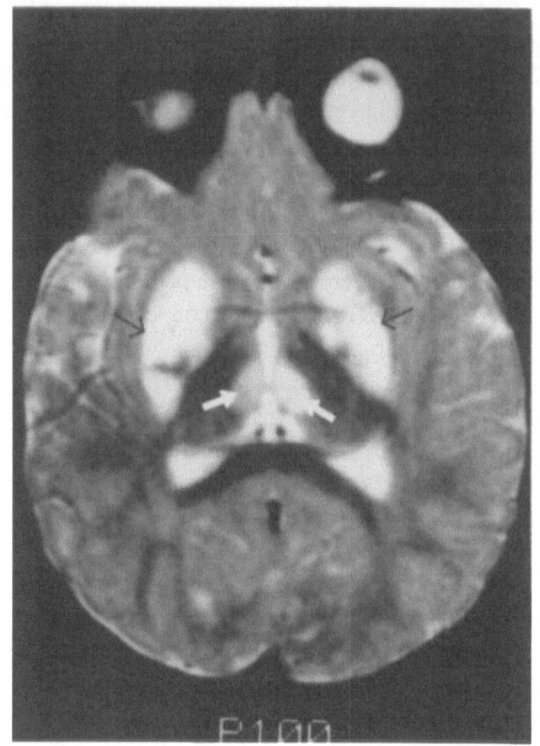

FIGURE 10.15. Leigh disease. This T2-weighted MR image shows increased signal intensity in the lentiform nuclei (large arrows) and medial thalamic nuclei (small arrows) bilaterally. (Courtesy of Charles M. Glasier, MD.)

vomiting, seizures, and reversible neurological deficits, including visual disturbances.[82] The recovery following the strokelike events may be surprisingly good, but recurrences of neurologic deficits occur, ultimately leaving patients with hemiparesis, hemianopia, or complete blindness. Patients with otherwise characteristic MELAS syndrome may have ptosis and external ophthalmoplegia suggestive of CPEO.[51] Angiographic studies have failed to demonstrate significant vascular occlusions, leading to the hypothesis that these are metabolic strokes caused by an area of brain exceeding its respiratory ability rather than by thromboembolism. MR imaging studies in this condition show edema in affected areas that are not restricted to specific vascular distributions.[107] Patients with MELAS have been described as showing parietooccipital hypodensity on CT scan and T2 prolongation on MR.[8] On pathologic examination, spongiform changes are primarily in the gray matter.

A point mutation in mitochondrial transfer RNA at position 3,243 can be identified in most patients with this syndrome.[75] The resulting biochemical abnormalities include decreased respiratory activity in complexes I, III, and IV. There are no clinical differences between patients who have the point mutation in mitochondrial DNA and those with MELAS syndrome who do not have the mutation.[75] This finding illustrates the heterogeneity of mitochondrial energy metabolism abnormalities noted earlier.

Myoclonic Epilepsy and Ragged Red Fibers (MERRF)

This relatively uncommon condition consists of myoclonic epilepsy, generalized epilepsy, ataxia, proximate weakness, fatigability, spasticity, sensory loss, dysarthria, optic atrophy, and dementia. Onset and progression are variable even within families. Muscle biopsy shows ragged red fibers seen in the other conditions. Optic atrophy may develop; however, there is no ophthalmoplegia or retinal abnormality in this disease. This condition has a point mutation in mitochondrial transfer RNA encoded by a mutation of mitochondrial DNA at the 8344 nucleotide pair.

References

1. Agamanolis DP, Patre S. Glycone accumulation in the central nervous system in the cerebral-pararenal syndrome. J Neurologic Sci 1979;41: 325-342.
2. Agamanolis DP, Robinson HB, Timmons GD. Cerebral-pararenal syndrome. A report of a case with histochemical and ultrastructural observations. J Neuropathol Experiment Neurol 1976;35: 226-246.
3. Aisen AM, Martel W, Gabrielson TO, Glazer GM, et al. Wilson disease of the brain: MR imaging. Radiology 1985;157:137-141.
4. Alves D, Pires MM, Guimaraes A, Miranda MC. Four cases of late onset metachromatic leukodystrophy in a family: clinical, biochemical, and neuropathological studies. J Neurol Neurosurg Psychiatry 1986;49:1417-1422.
5. Arpaia E, Dumbrille-Ross A, Maler T, Neote K, et al. Identification of an altered splice site in Ashkenazi Tay-Sachs disease. Nature 1988;333:85-86.
6. Bachynski BN, Flynn JT, Rodrigues MM, Rosenthal S, et al. Hyperglycemic acidotic coma and death in Kearns-Sayre syndrome. Ophthalmology 1986;93:391-396.
7. Baram TZ, Goldman AM, Percy AK. Krabbe disease: specific MRI and CT findings. Neurology 1986;36:111-115.
8. Barkovich AJ, Good WV, Koch TK, Berg BO. Mitochondrial disorders: analysis of their clinical and imaging characteristics. Am J Neuroradiol 1993; 14:1119-1137.
9. Barkovich AJ. Pediatric Neuroimaging. 2nd ed. New York: Raven Press; 1995:55-105.
10. Bassen FA, Kornzweig AL. Malformation of the erythrocytes in the case of atypical retinitis pigmentosa. BLOOD 1950;5:381-387.
11. Bass NH, Witmer EJ, Dreifuss FE. A pedigree study of metachromatic leukodystrophy: biochemical identification of a carrier state. Neurology 1970;20:52-62.
12. Bateman JB, Philippart M. Ocular features of the Hagberg-Santavuori syndrome. Am J Ophthalmol 1986;102:262-271.
13. Bateman JB, Philippart M, Isenberg SJ. Ocular features of multiple sulfatase deficiency and a new variant of metachromatic leukodystrophy. J Pediatr Ophthalmol Strabismus 1984;21:133-140.
14. Battaglia A, Harden A, Pampiglione G, Walsh PJ. Adrenoleukodystrophy: neurophysiological aspects. J Neurol Neurosurg Psychiat 1981;44:781-785.
15. Baumann RJ, Markesbery WR. Santavuori disease: diagnosis by leukocyte ultrastructure. Neurology 1982;32:1277-1281.
16. Beck M. Papilloedema in association with Hunter's syndrome. Br J Ophthalmol 1983;67:174-177.
17. Beck M, Cole G. Disc oedema in association with Hunter's syndrome: ocular histopathological findings. Br J Ophthalmol 1984;68:590-594.
18. Begeer JH, Haaxma R, Snoek JW, Boonstra S, le Coultre R. Signs of focal posterior cerebral abnormality in early subacute sclerosing panencephalitis. Ann Neurol 1986;19:200-202.
19. Blieden LC, Desnick RJ, Carter JB, Krivit W, et al. Cardiac involvement in Sandhoff's disease: inborn error of glycosphingolipid metabolism. Am J Cardiol 1974;34:83-88.
20. Boehme DH, Cottrell JC, Leonberg SC, Zeman W, et al. A dominant form of neuronal ceroid-lipofuscinosis. Brain 1971;94:745-760.
21. Broadhead DM, Kirk JM, Burt AJ, Gupta V, et al. Full expression of Hunter's disease in a female with an x-chromosome deletion leading to nonrandom inactivation. Clin Genet 1986;30:392-398.
22. Bronson RT, Lake BD, Cook S, Taylor S, Davisson MT. Motor neuron degeneration of mice is a model of neuronal ceroid lipofuscinosis (Batten's disease). Ann Neurol 1993;33:381-385.
23. Brownstein S, Meagher-Villemure K, Polomeno RC, Little JM. Optic nerve and globoid leukodystrophy (Krabbe's disease). Arch Ophthalmol 1978;96:864-870.

24. Carbone AO, Petrozzi CF. Gaucher's disease: case report with stress on eye findings. Henry Ford Hosp Med J 1968;16:55-60.

25. Carpenter S, Karpati G, Andermann F. Specific involvement of muscle, nerve, and skin in late infantile and juvenile amaurotic idiocy. Neurology 1972;22:170-186.

26. Carr RE, Siegel IM. Visual electrodiagnostic testing: a practical guide for the clinician. Baltimore, MD: Williams & Wilkins; 1982:1-33.

27. Caruso RC, Kaiser-Kupfer MI, Muenzer J, Ludwig IH, et al. Electroretinographic findings in the mucopolysaccharidoses. Ophthalmology 1986;93: 1612-1616.

28. Casteels I, Spillers W, Swinnen T, et al. It is optic atrophy as the presenting sign in Hallervorden-Spatz syndrome. Neuropediatrics 1994;25:265-267.

29. Cavanagh N, Kendall B. High density on computed tomography in infantile Krabbe's disease: a case report. Dev Med Child Neurol 1986;28:799-802.

30. Chase DS, Morris AH, Ballabio A, Pepper S, et al. Genetics of Hunter syndrome: carrier detection, new mutations, segregation and linkage analysis. Ann Hum Genet 1986;50:349-360.

31. Chabria S, Tomasi LG, Wong PWK. Ophthalmoplegia and bulbar palsy in variant form of maple syrup urine disease. Ann Neurol 1979;6:71-72.

32. Cogan DG, Chu FC, Barranger J, Gregg RE. Maculo halo syndrome. Variant of Niemann-Pick disease. Arch Ophthalmol 1983;101:1698-7000.

33. Cogan DG, Chu FC, Gittinger J, Tychsen L. Fundal abnormalities of Gaucher's disease. Arch Ophthalmol 1980;98:2202-2203.

34. Cogan DG, Chu FC, Reingold D, Barranger J. Ocular motor signs in some metabolic diseases. Arch Ophthalmol 1981;99:1802-1808.

35. Cogan DG, Kawabora T. Histochemistry of the retina in Tay-Sachs disease. Arch Ophthalmol 1959;61:414-423.

36. Cogan DG, Kawabora T, Moser H. Metachromatic leukodystrophy. Ophthalmologica 1970;80:2-17.

37. Cogan DG, Rodrigues M, Chu FC, Schaefer AJ. Ocular abnormalities in abetalipoproteinemia: a clinicopathologic correlation. Ophthalmology 1984;91:991-998.

38. Collins ML, Traboulsi EI, Maumenee IH. Optic nerve head swelling and optic atrophy in the systemic mucopolysaccharidoses. Ophthalmology 1990;97:1445-1449.

39. Copenhaver RM, Goodman G. The electroretinogram in infantile, late infantile, and juvenile amaurotic familial idiocy. Arch Ophthalmol 1960;63: 559-566.

40. Dabbagh O, Swaiman KF. Cockayne syndrome: MRI correlates of hypomyelination. Pediatr Neurol 1988;4:113-116.

41. Dangel ME, Tsou BH. Retinal involvement in Morquio's syndrome (MPS IV). Ann Ophthalmol 1985;17:349-354.

42. Daroff R. CPEO in Kearns-Sayre syndrome: an update. North American Neuro-ophthalmology Society Meeting, 1989, Cancun, Mexico.

43. Demaerel P, Kendall BE, Kingsley D. Cranial CT and MRI in diseases with DNA repair defects. Neuroradiology 1992;34:117-121.

44. Detre JA, Wang ZY, Bogdan AR, et al. Regional variation in brain lactate in Leigh syndrome by localized 1H magnetic resonance spectroscopy. Ann Neurol 1991;29:218-221.

44a. Deutsch JA, Asbell PA. Sialidosis and Galactosialidosis. In Gold DH and Weingeist TA (eds): *The Eye in Systemic Disease.* Philadelphia, PA: J.B. Lippincott, 1990. 376-377.

45. Dickinson JP, Holton JB, Lewis GM, Littlewood JM, Steel AE. Maple syrup urine disease: four years' experience with dietary treatment of a case. Acta Pediatr Scand 1969;58:341-351.

46. Dooling EC, Schoene WC, Richardson EP Jr. Hallervorden-Spatz syndrome. Arch Neurol 1974; 30:70-83.

47. Duker JS, Belmont J, Bosley TM. Angioid streaks associated with abetalipoproteinemia. Case Report. Arch Ophthalmol 1987;105:1173-1174.

48. Dyken PR. Subacute sclerosing panencephalitis. Current Status. Neurol Clin 1985;3:179-196.

49. Ek J, Kase BF, Reith A, Bjorkhem I, Pedersen JI. Peroxisomal dysfunction in a boy with neurologic symptoms and amaurosis (Leber disease): clinical and biochemical findings similar to those observed in Zellweger syndrome. J Pediatr 1986;108:19-24.

50. Emery JM, Green WR, Wyllie RG, Howell RR. GM^1-gangliosidosis. Ocular and pathological manifestations. Arch Ophthalmol 1971;85:177-187.

51. Fang W, Huang CC, Lee CC, Cheng SY, et al. Ophthalmologic manifestation in MELAS syndrome. Arch Neurol 1993;50:977-980.

52. Farley TJ, Ketonen LM, Bodensteiner JB, Wang DD. Serial MRI and CT findings in infantile Krabbe disease. Pediatr Neurol 1992;8:455-458.

53. Farrell DF, MacMartin MP, Clark AF. Multiple molecular forms of arylsulfatase A in different forms of metachromatic leukodystrophy (MLD). Neurology 1979;29:16-20.

54. Farrell K, Chuang S, Becker LE. Computed tomography in Alexander's disease. Ann Neurol 1984;15:605-607.

55. Feanny SJ, Chuang SH, Becker LE, Clarke JT. Intracerebral paraventricular hyper densities: a new CT sign in Krabbe globoid cell leukodystrophy. J Inherit Metabol Dis 1987;10:24-27.

56. Feigin I, Pena CE, Budzilovich G. The infantile spongy degenerations. Neurology 1968;18:153-166.

57. Feliciani M, Curatolo P. Early clinical and imaging (high-field MRI) diagnosis of Hallervorden-Spatz disease. Neuroradiology 1994;36:247-248.

58. Fenichel GM. *Clinical Pediatric Neurology: A Symptom and Sign Approach,* 2nd ed. Philadelphia, PA: W.B. Saunders and Company; 1993.

59. Fettes I, Killinger D, Volpe R. Adrenoleukodystrophy: report of a familial case. Clin Endocrinol 1979;11:151-160.
60. Fink JK, Filling-Katz MR, Sokol J, Cogan DG, et al. Clinical spectrum of Niemann-Pick disease type C. Neurology 1989;39:1040-1049.
61. Fishman MA. Disorders primarily of white matter. In: Swaiman KF, ed. *Pediatric Neurology, Principles and Practice*. Vol. II, St. Louis, MO: C.V. Mosby Co.; 1994;II:999-1017.
62. Folz SJ, Trobe JD. The peroxisome and the eye. Surv Ophthalmol 1991;35:353-368.
63. Font RL, Jenis EH, Tuck KD. Measles maculopathy associated with subacute sclerosing panencephalitis: immunofluorescent and immuno-ultrastructural studies. Arch Pathol 1973;96:168-174.
64. Francke U. The human gene for beta glucuronidase is on chromosome 7. Am J Hum Genet 1976; 28:357-362.
65. Gardner-Thorpe C, Kocen RS. Subacute sclerosing panencephalitis presenting as transient homonymous hemianopia. J Neurol Neurosurg Psychiatry 1983;46:186-187.
66. Gass, J, Donald M, eds. Inflammatory diseases of the retina and choroid. In: *Stereoscopic Atlas of Macular Diseases. Diagnosis and Treatment*. St. Louis, MO: C.V. Mosby; 1987;2:455-549.
67. Gass, J, Donald M, eds. Heredodystrophic disorders affecting the pigment epithelium and retina. In: *Stereoscopic Atlas of Macular Diseases. Diagnosis and Treatment*. St. Louis, MO: C.V. Mosby; 1987;2:312.
68. Gass, J, Donald M, eds. Heredodystrophic disorders affecting the pigment epithelium and retina. In: *Stereoscopic Atlas of Macular Diseases. Diagnosis and Treatment*. St. Louis, MO: C.V. Mosby; 1987;2:316.
69. Gass, J, Donald M, eds. Heredodystrophic disorders affecting the pigment epithelium and retina. In: *Stereoscopic Atlas of Macular Diseases. Diagnosis and Treatment*. St. Louis, MO: C.V. Mosby; 1987;2:310.
70. Gills JP, Hobson R, Hanley WB, McKusick VA. Electroretinography and fundus oculi findings in Hurler's disease and allied mucopolysaccharidoses. Arch Ophthalmol 1965;74:596-603.
71. Godel V, Blumenthal M, Goldman B, et al. Visual functions in Tay-Sachs diseased patients following enzyme replacement therapy. Metab Ophthalmol 1978;2:27-32.
72. Goebel HH, Bode G, Caesar R, Kohlschutter A. Bulbar palsy with Rosenthal fiber formation in the medulla of a 15-year-old girl. Localized form of Alexander's disease? Neuropediatrics 1981;12: 382-391.
72a. Goldberg MF, Cotlier E, Fischenscher LG, et al. Macular cherry-red spot, corneal clouding, and betagalactosidase deficiency. Arch Int Med 1971; 128:387.
73. Goldfischer S, Collins J, Rapin I, Coltoff-Schiller B, et al. Peroxisomal defects in neonatal-onset and X-linked adrenoleukodystrophies. Science 1985; 227:67-70.
74. Good WV, Crain LS, Quint RD, Koch TK. Overlooking: a sign of bilateral central scotomata in children. Dev Med Child Neurol 1992;34:69-73.
75. Goto Y, Horai S, Matsuoka T, Koga Y, et al. Mitochondrial myopathy, encephalopathy, lactic acidosis and stroke-like episodes [MELAS]: a correlative study of the clinical features in mitochondrial DNA mutation. Neurology 1992;42:545-550.
76. Green SH, Wirtschafter JD. Ophthalmoscopic findings in subacute sclerosing panencephalitis. Br J Ophthalmol 1973;57:780-787.
77. Hall CW, Liebars I, Dinatale P, Neufeld EF. Enzymatic diagnosis of the genetic leuco-polysaccharide storage disorders. Meth Enzymol 1978;50: 439-456.
78. Harcourt B, Ashton N. Ultrastructure of the optic nerve in Krabbe's leukodystrophy. Br J Ophthalmol 1973;57:885-891.
79. Harden A, Adams GG, Taylor DS. The electroretinogram. Arch Dis Child 1989;64:1080-1087.
80. Hiatt RL, Grizzard HT, McNeer P, Jabbour JT. Ophthalmologic manifestations of subacute sclerosing panencephalitis. Trans Am Acad Ophthalmol Otolaryngol 1971;75:344-350.
81. Higgins JJ, Patterson MC, Dambrosia JM, Pikus AT, et al. A clinical staging classification for type C Niemann-Pick disease. Neurology 1992;42: 2286-2290.
82. Hirano M, Pavlakis SG. Mitochondrial myopathy, encephalopathy, lactic acidosis, and stroke-like episodes [MELAS]: current concepts. J Child Neurol 1994;9:4-13.
83. Hittner HM, Ketzer FL, Mehta RS. Zellweger syndrome: lenticular opacities indicating carrier status and lens abnormalities characteristic of homozygotes. Arch Ophthalmol 1981;99:1977-1982.
84. Holt IJ, Harding AE, Cooper JM, Schapira AH, et al. Mitochondrial myopathies: clinical and biochemical features of 30 patients with major deletions of muscle mitochondrial DNA. Ann Neurol 1989;26:699-708.
85. Honda Y, Sudo M. Electroretinogram and visually evoked cortical potential in Tay-Sachs disease: a report of two cases. J Pediatr Ophthalmol 1976;13: 226-229.
86. Hormia M. Diffuse cerebral sclerosis, melanoderma and adrenal insufficiency (adrenoleukodystrophy). Acta Neurol Scand 1978;58:128-133.
87. Jaben S, Flynn JT. Neuronal ceroid lipofuscinosis (Batten-Vogt's disease). In: *Neuro-Ophthalmology*. 1982:chap. 27.
88. Jaben SL, Flynn JT, Parker JC. Neuronal ceroid lipofuscinosis. Diagnosis from peripheral blood smear. Ophthalmology 1983;90:1373-1377.

89. Jampel RS, Falls HF. Atypical retinitis pigmentosa, acanthocytosis and herido degenerative neuromuscular disease. Arch Ophthalmol 1958;59:818-820.

90. Jampel RS, Quaglio ND. Eye movements in Tay-Sach's disease. Neurology 1964;14:1013-1019.

91. Kaback M, Lim-Steele J, Dabholkar D, Brown D, et al. Tay-Sachs disease—carrier screening, prenatal diagnosis, and the molecular era. An international perspective, 1970 to 1993. JAMA 1993; 270:2307-2315.

92. Kayden HJ, Traber MG. Absorption, lipoprotein transport, and regulation of plasma concentrations of vitamin E in humans. J Lipid Res 1993;34:343-358.

93. Kendall BE. Disorders of lysosomes, peroxisomes, and mitochondria. Am J Neuroradiol 1992;13:621-653.

94. Keppler K, Cunniff C. Variable presentation of cytochrome c oxidase deficiency. Am J Dis Child 1992;146:1349-1352.

95. Kirkham TH, Kamin DF. Slow saccadic eye movements in Wilson's disease. J Neurol Neurosurg Psychiatry 1974;37:191-194.

96. Kivlin JD, Sanborn GE, Myers GG. The cherry-red spot in Tay-Sachs and other storage diseases. Ann Neurol 1985;17:356-360.

97. Lackner KJ, Monge JC, Gregg RE, et al. Analysis of the apolipoprotein B gene and messenger ribonucleic acid in abetalipoproteinemia. J Clin Invest 1986;78:1707-1712.

98. Landers MB III, Klintworth GK. Subacute sclerosing panencephalitis (SSPE). A clinicopathologic study of the retinal lesions. Arch Ophthalmol 1971;86:156-163.

99. Lee C, Dineen TE, Brack M, Kirsch JE, Runge VM. The mucopolysaccharidoses: characterization by cranial MR imaging. Am J Neuroradiol 1993;14:1285-1292.

100. Leigh RJ, Zee DS. The Neurology of Eye Movements: Contemporary Neurology Series. 2nd ed. Philadelphia, PA: F.A. Davis Company; 1991.

101. Libert J, Van Hoof F, Toussaint D, Roozitalab H, et al. Ocular findings in metachromatic leukodystrophy. Arch Ophthalmol 1979;97:1495-1504.

102. Lowden JA. Evidence for a hybrid hexosaminidase isoenzyme and heterozygotes for Sandhoff disease. Am J Hum Genet 1979;31:281-289.

103. MacFaul R, Cavanagh N, Lake BD, Stephens R, Whitfield AE. Metachromatic leukodystrophy: review of 38 cases. Arch Dis Child 1982;57:168-175.

104. Magalhaes AC, Caramelli P, Menezes JR, Lo LS, Bacheschi LA, Barbosa ER, Rosemberg LA, Magalhaes A. Wilson's disease: MRI with clinical correlation. Neuroradiology 1994;36:97-100.

105. Markesbery WR, Shield LK, Egel RT, Jameson HD. Late infantile neuronal ceroid-lipofuscinosis: an ultrastructural study of lymphocyte inclusions. Arch Neurol 1976;33:630-635.

106. Matalon R, Michals K, Sebesta D, Deanching M, et. al. Aspartoacylase deficiency and N-acetylas-partic aciduria in patients with Canavan disease. Am J Med Genet 1988;29:463-471.

107. Matthews PM, Tampieri D, Berkovic SF, Andermann F, et al. Magnetic resonance imaging shows specific abnormalities in the MELAS syndrome. Neurology 1991;41:1043-1046.

108. MacDonald JT, Sher PK. Ophthalmoplegia as a sign of metabolic disease in the newborn. Neurology 1977;27:971-973.

109. Medina L, Chi TL, DeVivo DC, Hilal SK. MR findings in patients with subactue necrotizing encephalomyelopathy (Leigh syndrome): correlation with biochemical defect. Am J Neuroradiol 1990; 11:379-384.

110. Moloney JB, Masterson JG. Detection of adrenoleukodystrophy carriers by means of evoked potentials. Lancet 1982;2:852-853.

111. Moossy J. The neuropathology of Cockayne's syndrome. J Neuropathol Exp Neurol 1967;26:654-660.

112. Mudd SH, Skovby F, Levy HL, Pettigrew KD, et al. The natural history of homocystinuria due to cystathionine beta-synthase deficiency. Am J Hum Genet 1985;37:1-31.

113. Naidu S, Moser H. Peroxisomal disorders. In: Swaiman KF, ed. Pediatric Neurology. Principles and Practice. 2nd ed. St. Louis, MO: C.V. Mosby; 1994:1357-1383.

114. Naidu S, Hofmann KJ, Moser HW, Maumenee IH, Wenger DA. Galactosylceramide-beta-galactosidase deficiency in association with cherry red spot. Neuropediatrics 1988;19:46-48.

115. Naughten ER, Jenkins J, Francis DE, Leonard JV. Outcome of maple syrup urine disease. Arch Dis Child 1982;57:918-921.

116. Neville BG, Lake BD, Stephens R, Sanders MD. A neurovisceral storage disease with vertical supranuclear ophthalmoplegia and its relationship to Niemann-Pick disease: a report of nine patients. Brain 1973;96:97-120.

117. Pampiglione G, Harden A. So-called neuronal ceroid lipofuscinosis: neurophysiological studies in 60 children. J Neurol Neurosurg Psychiatry 1977;40:323-330.

118. Pampiglione G, Privett G, Harden A. Tay-Sachs disease: neurophysiological studies in 20 children. Dev Med Child Neurol 1974;16:201-208.

119. Patterson MC, Horowitz M, Abel RB, Currie JN, et al. Isolated horizontal supranuclear gaze palsy as a marker of severe systemic involvement in Gaucher's disease. Neurology 1993;43:1993-1997.

120. Peachey NS, Sokol S, Moskowitz A. Recording the contralateral PERG: effect of different electrodes. Invest Ophthalmol Vis Sci 1983;24:1514-1516.

121. Percy AK, Brady RO. Metachromatic leukodystrophy: diagnosis with samples of venous blood. Science 1968;161:594-595.

122. Plant GT, Hess RF. The electrophysiological assessment of optic neuritis. In: Hess RF, Plant GT,

eds. *Optic Neuritis.* Cambridge, MA: University Press; 1986:208-214.

123. Porter-Grenn L, Silbergleit R, Mehta BA. Hallervorden-Spatz disease with bilateral involvement of globus pallidus and substantia nigra: MR demonstration. J Comput Assist Tomogr 1993;17:961-963.

124. Rader DJ, Brewer HB Jr. Abetalipoproteinemia. New insights into lipoprotein assembly and vitamin E metabolism from a rare genetic disease. JAMA 1993;270:865-869.

125. Raininko R, Santavuori P, Heiskala H, Sainio K, Palo J. CT findings in neuronal ceroid lipofuscinosis. Neuropediatrics 1990;21:95-101.

126. Reider-Grosswasser I, Bornstein N. CT and MRI in late-onset metachromatic leukodystrophy. Acta Neurol Scand 1987;75:64-69.

127. Renteria VG, Ferrans VJ, Roberts WC. The heart in the Hurler syndrome: gross histologic and ultrastructural observations in five necropsy cases. Am J Cardiol. 1976;38:487-501.

128. Resnick JS, Engel WK, Sever JL. Subacute sclerosing panencephalitis. Spontaneous improvement in a patient with elevated measles antibody in blood and spinal fluid. N Engl J Med 1968;279:126-129.

129. Risk WS, Haddad FS, Chemali R. Substantial spontaneous long-term improvement in subacute sclerosing panencephalitis. Six cases from the Middle East and a review of the literature. Arch Neurol 1978;35:494-502.

130. Robertson WC Jr, Clark DB, Markesbery WR. Review of 38 cases of subacute sclerosing panencephalitis: effect of amantadine on the natural course of the disease. Ann Neurol 1980;8:422-425.

131. Robb RM, Watters GV. Ophthalmic manifestations of subacute sclerosing panencephalitis. Arch Ophthalmol 1970;83:426-435.

132. Runge P, Muller DP, McAllister J, Calver D, Lloyd JK, Taylor D. Oral vitamin E supplements can prevent the retinopathy of abetalipoproteinemia. Br J Ophthalmol 1986;70:166-173.

133. Russo LS Jr, Aron A, Anderson PJ. Alexander's disease. A report and reappraisal. Neurology 1976;26:607-614.

134. Salmon JF, Pan EL, Murray AD. Visual loss with dancing extremeties and mental disturbances. Surv Ophthalmol 1991;35:299-306.

135. Salt HB, Wolff OH, Lloyd JK, Fosbrooke AS, Cameron AH, Hubble DV. On having no betalipoprotein: a syndrome comprising abetalipoprotein, acanthocytosis, and steatorrhoea. Lancet 1960;2:325-329.

136. Santavuori P, Haltia M, Rapola J, Raitta C. Infantile type of so-called neuronal ceroid lipofuscinosis. 1: a clinical study of 15 patients. J Neurol Sci 1973;18:257-267.

137. Santos MJ, Imanaka T, Shio H, Small GM, Lazarow PB, et al. Peroxisomal membrane ghosts in Zellweger syndrome—aberrant organelle assembly. Science 1988;239:1536-1538.

138. Schaumberg HH, Powers JM, Raine CS, Suzuki K, Richardson EP Jr. Adrenoleukodystrophy: a clinical and pathological study of 17 cases. Arch Neurol 1975;32:577-591.

139. Scheffer IE, Baraitser M, Wilson J, Harding B, Kendall B, Brett EM. Pelizaeus Merzbacher disease: classical or connatal? Neuropediatrics 1991; 22:71-78.

140. Schutgens RB, Heymans HS, Wanders RJ, van den Bosch H, Tager JM. Peroxisomal disorders: a newly recognized group of genetic diseases. Eur J Pediatr 1986;144:430-440.

141. Schwartz JF, Kolendrianos ET. Maple syrup urine disease. A review with a report of an additional case. Dev Med Child Neurol 1969;11:460-470.

142. Sedwick LA, Burde RM, Hodges FJ III. Leigh's subacute necrotizing encephalomyelopathy manifesting as spasmus nutans. Arch Ophthalmol 1984;102:1046-1048.

143. Seitelberger F. Pelizaeus Merzbacher disease. In: Viken P, Bruyn G, eds. *Handbook of Clinical Neurology.* Amsterdam: Elsevier North Holland; 1970:150-202.

144. Sethi KD, Adams RJ, Loring DW, el Gammal T. Hallervorden-Spatz syndrome: clinical and magnetic resonance imaging correlations. Ann Neurol 1988;24:692-694.

145. Shapira Y, Harel S, Russell A. Mitochondrial encephalomyopathies: a group of neuromuscular disorders with defects in oxidative metabolism. Isr J Med Sci 1977;13:161-164.

146. Shimomura C, Matsui A, Choh H, Funahashi M, et al. Magnetic resonance imaging in Pelizaeus Merzbacher disease. Pediatr Neurol 1988;4:124-125.

147. Spalton DJ, Taylor DS, Sanders MD. Juvenile Batten's disease: an ophthalmological assessment of 26 patients. Br J Ophthalmol 1980;64:726-732.

148. Statz A, Boltshauser E, Schinzel A, Spiess H, et al. Computed tomography in Pelizaeus Merzbacher disease. Neuroradiology 1981;22:103-105.

149. Stockler S, Millner M, Molzer B, Ebner F, et al. Multiple sclerosis-like syndrome in a woman heterozygous for adrenoleukodystrophy. Eur Neurol 1993;33:390-392.

150. Suzuki K. Biochemical pathogenesis of genetic leukodystrophies: comparison of metachromatic leukodystrophy and globoid cell leukodystrophy (Krabbe's disease). Neuropediatrics 1984;15:32-36.

151. Svennerholm L. The gangliosides. J Lipid Res 1964;5:145-155.

152. Swaiman KF. Hallervorden-Spatz syndrome in brain iron metabolism. Arch Neurol 1991;48:1285-1293.

153. Swaiman KF. Lysosomal diseases. In: Swaiman KF, ed. *Pediatric Neurology, Principles and Prac-*

tice, 2nd ed. St. Louis, MO: C.V. Mosby Company; 1994;II:1275-1334.

154. Taylor D. Ophthalmological features of some human hereditary disorders with demyelination. Bull Soc Belge Ophthalmol 1983;208:405-413.

155. Taylor D. Neurometabolic disease. In: *Pediatric Ophthalmology.* London, Edinburgh, Melbourne: Blackwell Scientific Publications, Inc.; 1990:525-544.

156. Traboulsi EI, Maumenee IH. Ophthalmologic manifestations of X-linked childhood adrenoleukodystrophy. Ophthalmology 1987;94:47-52.

157. Tripp JH, Lake BD, Young E, Ngu J, Brett EM. Juvenile Gaucher's disease with horizontal gaze palsy in three siblings. J Neurol Neurosurg Psychiatry 1977;40:470-478.

158. Trobe JD, Sharpe JA, Hirsh DK, Gebarski SS. Nystagmus of Pelizaeus-Merzbacher disease: a magnetic search-coil study. Arch Neurol 1991; 48:87-91.

159. Tulinius MH, Holme E, Kristiansson B, Larsson NG, Oldfors A. Mitochondrial encephalomyelopathies in childhood. I. biochemical and morphologic investigations. J Pediatr 1991;119: 242-250.

160. Tulinius MH, Holme E, Kristiansson B, Larsson NG, Oldfors A. Mitochondrial encephalomyopathies in childhood. II. clinical manifestations and syndromes. J Pediatr 1991;119:251-259.

161. Valavanis A, Friede RL, Schubiger O, Hayek J. Computed tomography in neuronal ceroid lipofuscinosis. Neuroradiology 1980;19:35-38.

162. van der Knapp MS, Valk J. The MR spectrum of peroxisomal disorders. Neuroradiology 1991;33: 30-37.

163. van der Knapp MS, Valk J. The reflection of histology in MR imaging of Pelizaeus-Merzbacher disease. Am J Neuroradiol 1989;10:99-103.

164. Verma NP, Hart ZH, Nigro M. Electrophysiologic studies in neonatal adrenoleukodystrophy.

Electroencephalogr Clin Neurophysiol 1985; 60:7-15.

165. Wallace D. Mitochondrial genetics: a paradigm for aging and degenerative diseases? Science 1992; 256:628-632.

166. Watanabe K, Mukawa A, Muto K, Nishikawa J, Takahashi S. Tay-Sachs disease with conspicuous cranial computerized tomographic appearances. Acta Pathal Jpn 1985;35:1521-1532.

167. Wetterau JR, Aggerbeck LP, Laplaud PM, McLean LR. Structural properties of the microsomal triglyceride-transfer protein complex. Biochemistry 1991;30:4406-4412.

168. Whitley CB, Below KG, Chang PN, et. al. Long term outcome of Herler syndrome following bone marrow transplantation. Am J Med Genet 1993; 46:209-218.

169. Whitley CB, Ramsay NK, Kersey JH, Krivit V. Bone marrow transplantation for Hurler syndrome: assessment of metabolic correction. Birth Defects 1986;22:7-24.

170. Weismann U, Neufeld EF. Scheie and Hurler syndromes: apparent identity of the biochemical defect. Science 1970;169:72-74.

171. Wolpert Sir Stewart, Elder Duke, Scott George I. System of ophthalmology. In: *Neuro-ophthalmology.* London: Henry Kimpton; 1971;12:222.

172. Wray SH, Cogan DG, Kuwabara T, Schaumberg HH, Powers JM. Adrenoleukodystrophy with disease of the eye and optic nerve. Am J Ophthalmol 1976;82:480-485.

173. Wulff CH, Trojaborg W. Adult metachromatic leukodystrophy: neurophysiologic findings. Neurology 1985;35:1776-1778.

174. Yee RD, Cogan DG, Zee DS. Ophthalmoplegia and dissociated nystagmus in abetalipoproteinemia. Arch Ophthalmol 1976;94:571-575.

175. Zee DS, Freeman JM, Holtzman NA. Opthalmoplegia in maple syrup urine disease. J Pediatr 1974;84:113-115.

11

Neuro-Ophthalmologic Manifestations of Systemic and Intracranial Disease

Introduction

Recent advances in neuroimaging have improved our understanding of intracranial diseases in children. An integrated understanding of these diseases has also emerged from the proliferation of multidisciplinary clinics and programs combining expertise in pediatric neurology, neurosurgery, neuropathology, neuroradiology, neuro-oncology, and neuro-ophthalmology. Genetic defects are increasingly implicated in the pathogenesis of various intracranial disorders, and basic research is elucidating many of these diseases at the molecular level. Refinement in neurosurgical management will undoubtedly continue to play a significant role in the treatment of these disorders, but the future holds promise as preventative measures are expected to arise from molecular genetic research.

The Phakomatoses

In 1920, van der Hoeve, a Dutch ophthalmologist, first used the term "phakoma" to describe retinal astrocytic hamartomas in tuberous sclerosis and myelinated retinal nerve fibers in neurofibromatosis. Noting that the retinal astrocytic hamartomas resembled dried lentils ("phaki"), he assumed that tuberous sclerosis and neurofibromatosis were related conditions and coined the term "phakomatosis" as an umbrella term to describe congenital disorders that produce benign growths in the central nervous system (CNS).[342] He later expanded this concept to include other conditions character-

ized by CNS, cutaneous, and often ocular involvement.[342] In its present usage, phakomatosis is a loosely defined and somewhat arbitrary term that has evolved to include a heterogeneous group of multisystem disorders that share a predisposition to develop hamartomas within the CNS, often in association with cutaneous, ocular, or visceral lesions. Approximately 20 to 30 disorders have now been classified as phakomatoses, and rare patients may display features found in more than one phakomatosis. All are congenital in origin, but their inheritance patterns vary, and some do not appear to be genetically transmitted. The phakomatoses of neuro-ophthalmologic significance in children are discussed below.

Neurofibromatosis (NF-1)

von Recklinghausen neurofibromatosis (NF-1) is an autosomal dominant disorder that affects numerous organ systems, including the eye.[363] Only 50% of patients have afflicted relatives,[334] and it has been stated that this disorder has one of the highest mutation rates in humans.[363] Having no known racial, ethnic, or geographic predilection, NF-1 is estimated to occur once in every 2500 to 3300 births.[363] It is one of several autosomal diseases that are associated with advanced paternal age. The responsible gene for NF-1 is located in the pericentromeric region of the long arm of chromosome 17.[22] To account for the high mutation rate, Barker[22] hypothesized that the defect in NF-1 may involve an unusually large gene on chromosome 17.[363] It has recently been cloned and characterized[299]. The characteristics of neurofibromin, the NF-1 gene product, are complex and still being defined, but there is increasing evidence to suggest that it acts primarily as a tumor suppressor gene.[299]

The numerous dysgenetic, hamartomatous, and neoplastic lesions that arise in NF-1 have been attributed to a disturbance in neural crest migration brought about by the NF-1 mutation so that abnormal aggregations of Schwann cells or melanoblast precursors occur during the migratory phase of neural crest development.[52] Because many of the disparate findings in NF-1 relate to a common neural crest origin, Bolande[52] has termed NF-1 "the quintessential neurocristopathy." This hypothesis may account for the fact that malignancies of neural crest–derived cells, such as malignant schwannoma, pheochromocytoma, medullary carcinoma of the thyroid, neuroblastoma, and malignant melanoma, occur more commonly in NF-1 patients.[52,363] However, many features of NF-1 such as short stature, intellectual impairment, macrocephaly, speech impediment, pseudoarthrosis, and malignancies of non-neural crest origin—such as Wilms tumor, myelogenous leukemia, and rhabdomyosarcoma, cannot be reconciled with the notion of a neural crest origin.[363]

The cardinal pathologic features of NF-1 are the café au lait spots of the skin and a variety of neural hamartomas, known collectively as neurofibromas, that develop in the peripheral, autonomic, and central nervous system.[52,303–305] Café au lait spots are pigmented macules of the skin that result from aggregation of heavily pigmented melanoblasts in the basal layers of the epidermis.[52] They are present in the majority of children with NF-1 at birth and become prominent by the end of the first decade of life. Children with NF-1 may also have diffuse skin hyperpigmentation or innumerable freckles. Axillary freckling in NF-1 tends to be congenital, whereas diffuse freckling or freckling at points of friction (e.g., inguinal or other intertriginous zones) is often acquired.[299]

Pathologically, neurofibromas consist of an overgrowth of Schwann cells variably admixed with tortuous nerve fibers and perineural fibroblasts.[52] The proportion and growth pattern of these constituents account for the morphologic differences, so that plexiform neurofibromas, pure schwannomas, and neuromas are described.[52]

Neurofibromas occurring as subcutaneous nodules near the terminations of peripheral nerves in the dermis comprise the most conspicuous feature of neurofibromatosis, but neurofibromas may also arise within the central and autonomic nervous systems.[52] Cutaneous neurofibromas develop toward the end of the first decade, just before puberty. They are initially sessile but often become pedunculated.[299] Enlarging neurofibromas may produce intense pruritis that may respond to mast cell stabililzers (e.g., oral Ketotifen). The histology of neurofibromas is typically hypocellular, and the cytology is indolent.[52] However, if a skin neurofibroma is being constantly traumatized by friction with clothing, it is generally recommended that it be removed, because of the potential risk of malignant transformation.[299] Large patches of cutaneous hyperpigmentation in patients with neurofibromatosis tend to overlie large plexiform neuromas that have an unusually high incidence of degeneration to neurofibrosarcoma. When the hyperpigmentation overlying a plexiform neurofibroma extends to midline, it may signify underlying spinal cord involvement.[299]

The most common ocular feature of neurofibromatosis is the Lisch nodule of the iris.[231,232,299,363] Lisch nodules are tan to brown avascular dome-shaped lumps in the anterior iris (Figure 11.1). Pathologically, they are melanocytic hamartomas with a compact plaque of spindle cells overlying a loose stromal accumulation of melanocytes.[393] In blue and green irides, they appear pale to medium brown with feathery margins, and in dark brown irides, they are cream colored, dome-shaped, and extremely well-defined (Figure 11.1).[299] When present in young children, they tend to be glassy and translucent in appearance. Ragge et al[298] recently combined data from six large studies of Lisch nodules in different age groups. The authors found that, while they are probably not visible at birth, prevalence of Lisch nodules in neurofibromatosis gradually increases to about 50% at age 5 years, 75% at age 15 years, and 95% to 100% of adults over age 30.[298] Despite the absence of Lisch nodules in many young children, the diagnosis of neurofibromatosis can usually be established on the basis of other criteria.[277] Unlike neurofibromas, there is no acceleration in the rate of appearance of Lisch nodules associated with puberty.[226] Lisch nodules are highly

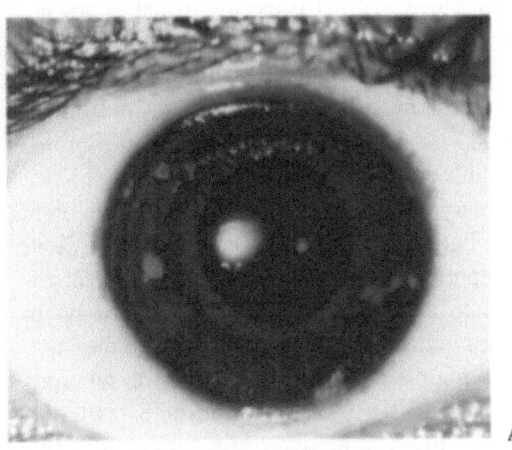

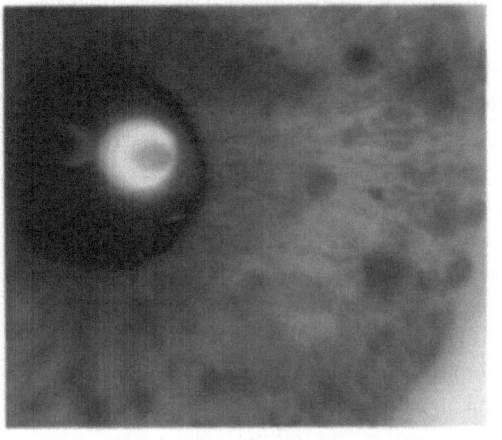

FIGURE 11.1. Neurofibromatosis-1. Lisch nodules on the surface of the iris may be few (A) or numerous (B).

occurring in patients with a multiple endocrine neoplasia syndrome.[255]

Cutaneous involvement of the face is relatively uncommon in NF-1, but plexiform neurofibroma of the upper lid tends to be associated with ipsilateral dysgenesis of the globe and orbit. Plexiform neurofibroma of the upper lid classically produces the "swan neck" or "lazy S" deformity (Figure 11.2). While only 50% of children with plexiform lid neurofibromas have congenital glaucoma, congenital glaucoma in neurofibromatosis occurs only in association with plexiform lid neuofibroma. In addition to congenital glaucoma and buphthalmos, children with plexiform neurofibroma of the upper eyelid may have ipsilateral orbital enlargement, ipsilateral sphenoid dysplasia (absence of the sphenoid wing and anterior clinoid, with or without pulsating exophthalmos), and progressive facial hemihypertrophy (Francois syndrome).[21,182] These changes may be associated with prolapse of the temporal lobe into the orbit or lateral expansion of the middle cranial fossa (termed orbitotemporal neurofibromatosis).[189] Some children with NF-1 have buphthalmos in the absence of congenital glaucoma.[191] Weiner[385] and Hoyt and Billson[182] have suggested that buphthalmos in neurofibromatosis may sometimes represent a generalized hyperplasia of the orbit and its contents (i.e., an expression of regional giantism) rather than a consequence of uncontrolled intraocular pressure. Prior to neu-

suggestive but not pathognomonic of NF-1. Rarely, they have been reported to occur in patients with segmental neurofibromatosis,[386] NF-2,[79] and Cushing disease.[54]

Caucasians with neurofibromatosis frequently have choroidal pigment hamartomas in the posterior pole, which tend to be flat and hyperpigmented or silvery gray. These easily overlooked lesions are probably the next most common ocular finding in neurofibromatosis following Lisch nodules. Choroidal and ciliary body neurofibromas are well-recognized but uncommon manifestations of NF-1.[108] Although myelinated nerve fibers are said to be more common in children with neurofibromatosis, this association may be fortuitous. The purported association between enlargement of the corneal nerves and neurofibromatosis is also dubious, with previously described cases possibly

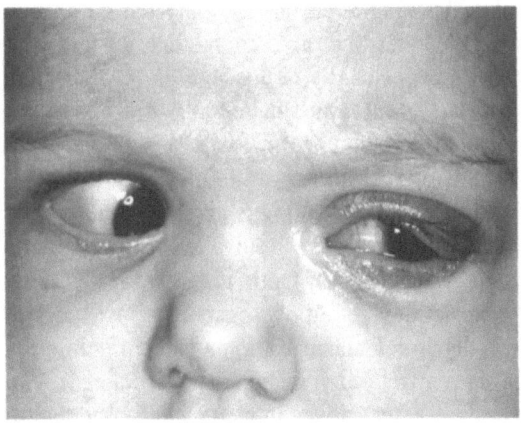

FIGURE 11.2. Neurofibromatosis-1. Plexiform neurofibroma of the left eyelid in a child with NF-1 who had ipsilateral glaucoma and absence of the sphenoid wing.

roimaging, the combination of unilateral proptosis and poor vision in such cases was often incorrectly attributed to orbital optic glioma.

The incidence of CNS disorders in NF-1 is about 15%. The most common primary brain lesion is optic pathway glioma.[227] The prevalence of optic pathway glioma on computed tomography (CT) scanning in neurofibromatosis has been estimated to be 15%.[225] Westerhof et al[389] have claimed that the finding of hypertelorism in a child with NF-1 heralds the presence of optic glioma. The clinical features and controversies surrounding the management of optic glioma in NF-1 are detailed in Chapter 4.

Children with NF-1 may also display a variety of disparate CNS manifestations unrelated to tumor formation. Macrocephaly is common and does not seem to correlate with intellectual performance, seizures, or electroencephalographic abnormalities.[255,305] Aqueductal stenosis also occurs more commonly. Most cases appear to reflect a structural alteration of the aqueduct rather than tumor compression.[255] Intracranial arachnoid cysts may also occur.[62,189,244] Seizures are more common and may occur without a structural lesion.[255] Headaches are particularly common in patients with NF-1. Intellectual impairment, learning disability, or hyperactivity are seen in approximately 40% of children with NF-1.

The major neuro-ophthalmologic manifestations in children with NF-1 are proptosis, optic disc swelling, optic atrophy, ptosis, strabismus, and amblyopia. Pulsating proptosis may occur when the sphenoid wing is absent and only the dura separates the brain and orbit. Enophthalmos may also be seen occasionally in this setting. Nonpulsating proptosis occurs most commonly with ipsilateral orbital optic glioma but may also result from a localized or plexiform orbital neurofibroma.[255] When optic disc swelling is accompanied by ipsilateral proptosis, the causative lesion is usually an orbital optic glioma. Optic disc swelling without proptosis may herald hydrocephalus secondary to hypothalamic/chiasmal glioma extending into the third ventricle, hydrocephalus associated with aqueductal stenosis, an intracranial arachnoid cyst, a spinal ependymoma, or some other NF-1–associated spinal tumor. Optic atrophy may occur primarily with optic glioma or pursuant to prolonged optic disc swelling from any of the above-mentioned

causes. Ptosis in NF-1 is usually S-shaped and associated with an upper lid plexiform neurofibroma. Strabismus and amblyopia may result from nonaxial proptosis due to orbital optic glioma, or from visual depriva-tion when a plexiform neurofibroma of the lids or buphthalmos are present.

Primary retinal involvement is more common in NF-2, but may occasionally occur in NF-1. Several reports of retinal dialysis and detachment adjacent to a peripheral astrocytic hamartoma in children with NF-1 suggest that, unlike the visually benign astrocytic hamartomas of tuberous sclerosis, NF-1–associated astrocytic hamartomas are more likely to produce retinal traction, dialysis, and ultimately detachment.[108,245] Retinal vascular disease is another occasional finding.[108,259] Children with NF-1 have been described with bilateral capillary hemangiomatosis[108] as well as retinal vascular occlusive disease,[259] which may be similar in etiology to the vascular ischemic manifestations that have been described in the aortic, cerebral, and renal vasculature.[326]

Certain features on magnetic resonance (MR) imaging are now felt to be highly suggestive of NF-1 (Figure 11.3).[299] These include (1) bilateral optic gliomas; (2) tubular expansion with lengthening and kinking of one or both optic nerves; (3) a double-intensity signal to the orbital optic nerve, with a bright outer signal on T2-weighted images corresponding to the perineural tumor and the dark central core corresponding to the optic nerve;[62,186,332] (4) chiasmal glioma extending into both optic tracts; and (5) high-signal intensity foci in the brain parenchyma on T2-weighted images, especially in the globus pallidus, basal ganglia, and cerebellar white matter.[113] The latter lesions progress and regress on serial studies in children but are distinctly rare in adults with NF-1.[299,342]

Once diagnosed, optic pathway tumor progression in children with NF-1 is uncommon. In one study, no child found to have a tumor confined to the optic nerve by neuroimaging screening developed decreased vision or other evidence of progression.[227a] Children with chiasmal involvement incurred more complications such as visual loss and precocious puberty. Long-term survival is reduced in patients with NF-1, primarily due to their propensity to develop malignant neoplasms and benign CNS tumors; however, this effect is less so for affected relatives.

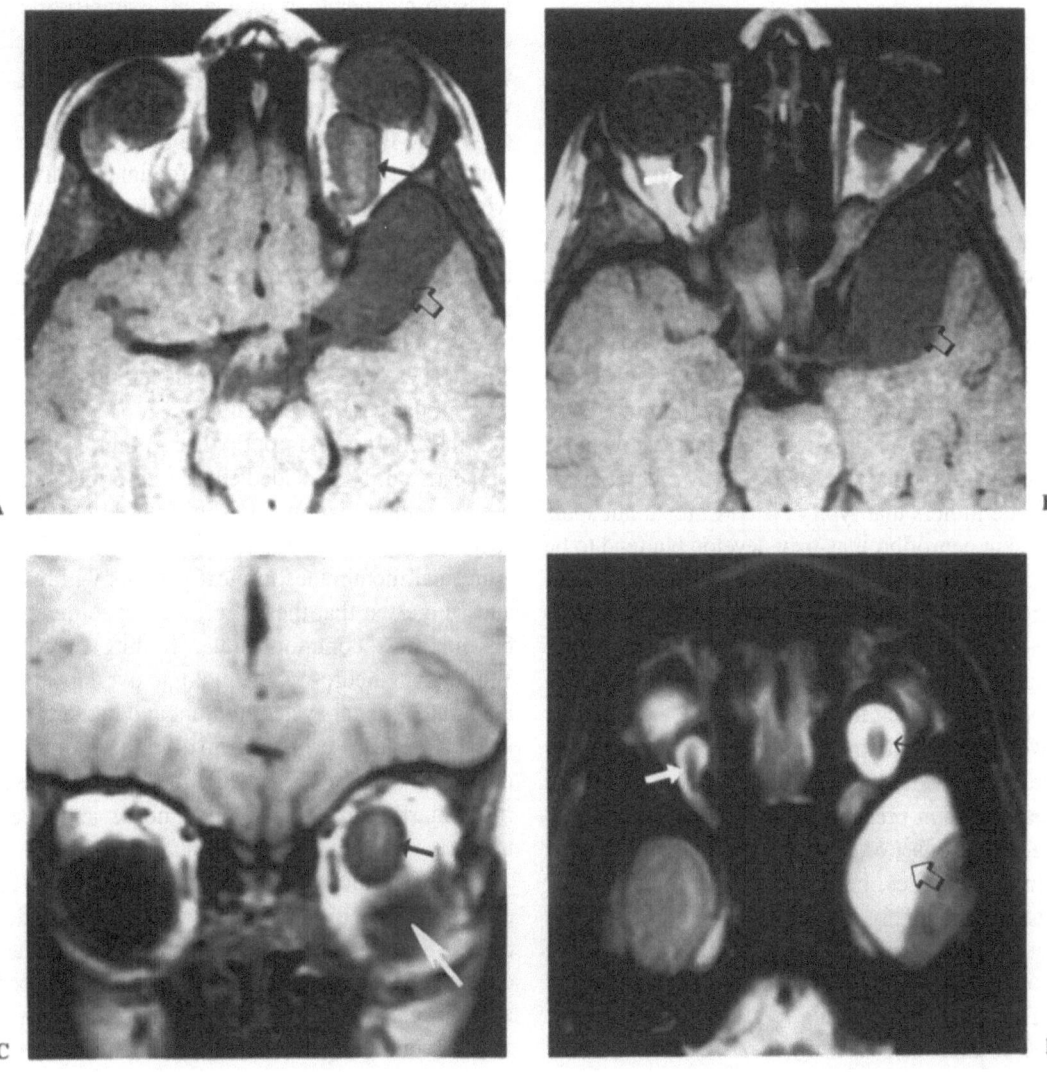

FIGURE 11.3. Distinctive MR imaging characteristics of orbital optic glioma in NF-1. (A) T1-weighted axial MR image of left orbital glioma. A fusiform area of low intensity (closed arrow) surrounds a central core of high signal intensity. An arachnoid cyst (open arrow) occupies the left anterior temporal fossa. Note that the peripheral (outer) tumor signal is isointense to the CSF contained within the arachnoid cyst. The tumor is kinked posteriorly. (B) T1-weighted MR image of right orbital glioma showing linear enlargement of the right optic nerve with circumferential zone of low signal intensity (closed arrow) surrounding a central core of higher signal intensity. Open arrow denotes CSF within the arachnoid cyst that is hypointense to brain on T1-weighted images. (C) T1-weighted coronal MR image of the left orbital glioma. There is marked enlargement of the optic nerve with a ring of low signal intensity (dark arrow) surrounding a core of higher signal inten-

sity. The large area of low signal intensity inferior and lateral to the optic nerve (white arrow) corresponds to the anterior extent of the arachnoid cyst. (D) T2-weighted axial MR image through the superior aspect of both optic gliomas. In the left orbit, there is a donut-shaped area of high signal intensity (dark arrow) surrounding an inner circle of low signal intensity. This image represents a tangential cut through the superior aspect of the upwardly kinked tumor. In the right orbit, a linear area of high signal intensity surrounds a central core of low signal intensity. Note that the outer signal within both tumors remains isointense to CSF. (Open arrow denotes CSF within the arachnoid cyst that is hyperintense to brain on T2-weighted images.) (From Brodsky MC. The "pseudo-CSF" signal of orbital optic glioma on magnetic resonance imaging: A signature of neurofibromatosis. Surv Ophthalmol 1993;38:213–218. With permission.)

Neurofibromatosis-2 (NF-2)

The hallmark of NF-2 (formerly known as central neurofibromatosis) is the presence of bilateral vestibular schwannomas (a more accurate term than acoustic neuroma).[290,299,365] According to National Institutes of Health (NIH) criteria,[267] the diagnosis can also be made if there is a first-degree relative with NF-2 together with either a unilateral eighth nerve mass or any two of the following: neurofibroma, meningioma, glioma, schwannoma, or posterior subcapsular or capsular lens opacity of adolescent onset. Patients with NF-2 tend to develop acoustic and visual pathway tumors arising from neural coverings (meningiomas, schwannomas, ependymomas) in contrast to the neural or astrocytic tumors that typify NF-1. Café au lait spots and skin neurofibromas may develop but tend to be fewer in number, and Lisch nodules are absent.[216,299] The main features that distinguish NF-2 from NF-1 are bilateral vestibular schwannomas, cutaneous schwannomas, spinal schwannomas, lack of Lisch nodules (with rare exceptions), fewer café au lait spots, and the presence of juvenile-onset cataracts.[299] Bilateral hearing loss is the most common presenting symptom.[200] The average age of onset of hearing loss in NF-2 is in the teens or twenties, but the age at presentation (or detection) is highly variable.[299] The genetic defect that produces NF-2 has been localized to the long arm of chromosome 22.[314,388]

The spectrum of ocular and neuro-ophthalmological manifestations in NF-2 has only recently received attention.[306] Kaiser-Kupfer et al[197] described juvenile posterior subcapsular cataracts in children with NF-2 and noted that they were not a feature of NF-1. These characteristic "posterior subcapsular cataracts" are actually central posterior cortical opacities that extend posteriorly to the lens capsule.[54,55] Some children with NF-2 also have cortical cataracts near the lens equator.[197,204] The genetic sequence that codes for the beta-crystalline component of the human lens has also been localized to chromosome 22, which raises the possibility that these juvenile cataracts may result from a structural defect in this protein.[178]

Optic nerve sheath meningiomas may develop in children with NF-2, and this finding in a child should prompt medical evaluation for NF-2.[96,204]

These tumors behave in a more invasive and aggressive manner than their adult counterparts as evidenced by the intraocular extension of an optic nerve sheath meningioma in a 13-year-old girl with NF-2 described by Cibis et al.[83] Landau et al[215] were the first to recognize the association of combined retinal pigment epithelial hamartoma with NF-2. Numerous reports of this association have followed.[162,204] Dossetor et al[115] reviewed the two previous reports of optic disc glioma along with an additional case and found that all three documented cases occurred in patients with NF-2. These cases, along with an additional report of a similar case by Landau and Gloor,[216] suggest that the finding of an optic disc glioma is highly suggestive of NF-2. Good et al[162] described multiple epiretinal glial opacities in a child with NF-2. Kaye et al[204] and Landau and Yasargil[214] found epiretinal membranes in most patients with NF-2 and suggested that these preretinal opacities may be the most common ocular finding in NF-2. While some neuro-ophthalmologic overlap exists, associated visual system tumors and hamartomas in NF-2 tend to primarily involve the retina and optic disc (Figure 11.4), while those of NF-1 tend to primarily involve the optic nerve and uveal tract.

Medical evaluation of the child with NF-2 includes a detailed family history with examination of first-degree relatives, slit lamp examination, audiogram, MR imaging of the brain and spinal cord, and chromosome analysis to look for a deletion of chromosome 22q11. Children and affected relatives should be warned not to swim without supervision, as several deaths from drowning have been reported in patients with NF-2.[299]

Although vestibular schwannomas may be detected on neuroimaging in children with NF-2 (Figure 11.5), they often remain asymptomatic until young adulthood.[248] While decreased vision secondary to a retinal or optic nerve lesion may not be amenable to treatment, some children show visual improvement following treatment of cataract, exposure or neurotrophic keratopathy, strabismus, or amblyopia. Since many children with NF-2 eventually become deaf, even moderate degrees of visual loss can be devastating, and attempts at visual rehabilitation may have a significant positive impact on their future independence and quality of life.

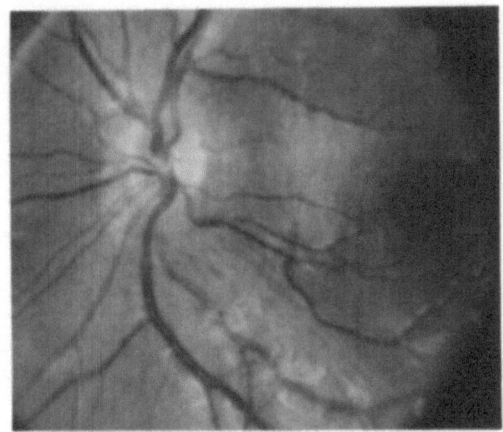

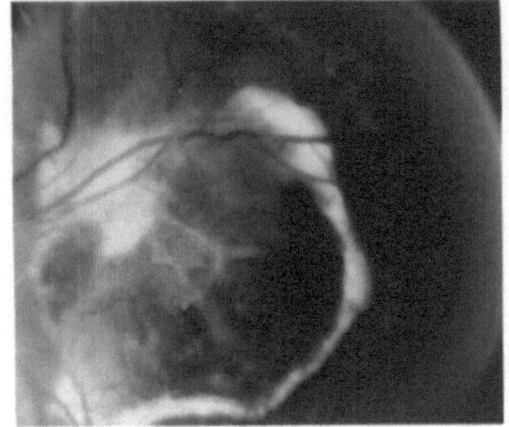

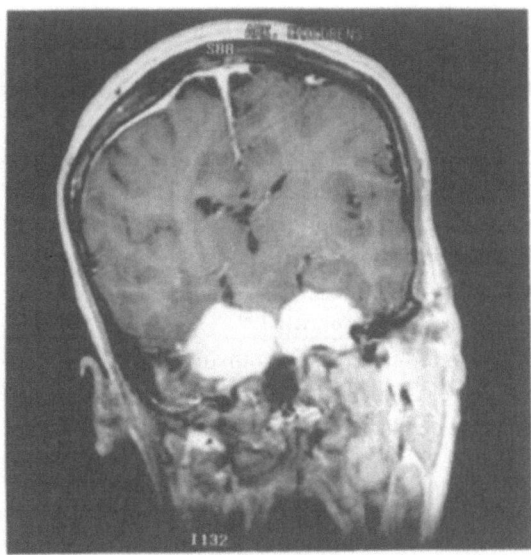

FIGURE 11.5. Neurofibromatosis-2. Coronal MR image shows kissing schwannomas.

FIGURE 11.4. Neurofibromatosis-2. Combined hamartoma of the retina and RPE. (A) Early lesion resembling epiretinal membrane with macular pucker. (B) Advanced lesion.

Tuberous Sclerosis

Tuberous sclerosis is an autosomal dominant disorder with no racial or sexual predilection. The rate of spontaneous mutation approaches 60%, and many affected individuals have no family history.[342] As with neurofibromatosis, tuberous sclerosis has been associated with advanced paternal age. Linkage analysis has recently demonstrated unexpectedly that the tuberous sclerosis complex is genetically heterogeneous with approximately one-third of cases linked to a site on chromosome 9q34,[140] and the remaining two-thirds linked to chromosome 16p13 near the locus for adult polycystic kidney disease.[198] These are probably tumor suppressor genes that, when deleted, predispose to various tumorous growths.[342]

Although tuberous sclerosis was originally defined by the classic clinical triad of adenoma sebaceum, epilepsy, and mental retardation, the complete triad occurs in less than one-third of cases diagnosed by modern criteria, and some patients with tuberous sclerosis have none of the three classic features.[175,342] Gomez[161] divided the diagnostic criteria of tuberous sclerosis into primary criteria (adenoma sebaceum, ungual fibroma, cerebral cortical tuber, subependymal nodule, fibrous forehead plaque) and secondary features (infantile spasms, hypopigmented macules, shagreen patch, retinal hamartoma, bilateral renal cysts or angiomyolipomas, cardiac rhabdomyoma, a first-degree relative with tuberous sclerosis). The diagnosis of tuberous sclerosis, according to this classification, can be established when a patient exhibits one primary criterion or two or more secondary criteria.[309] Separate neuroimaging criteria have also been established. A definitive diagnosis of tuberous sclerosis can be assigned when computed tomography (CT) scanning or MR imaging demonstrate multiple subependymal nodules (especially with calcification) or when multiple cortical abnormalities with calcification and subcortical white matter edema are

present.[342] A presumptive diagnosis can be established when there is (1) an intraventricular tumor
consistent with a subependymal giant cell astrocytoma, (2) focal wedge-shaped calcifications in the
cerebral or cerebellar cortex, or (3) multiple corti-
cal/subcortical foci of edema.[342] The availability
of specific molecular markers may soon permit
tuberous sclerosis to be diagnosed even in patients
with minimal clinical manifestations and perhaps
lead to prenatal diagnosis.[199]

Systemic manifestations involve primarily skin
and viscera. Adenoma sebaceum are angiofibro-
mas that occur in a butterfly distribution over the
nose and cheeks. The rash eventually develops in
80% to 90% of cases and is pathognomonic for
tuberous sclerosis.[391] However, it is typically absent in children younger than 2 years of age,
which may delay the diagnosis. When it develops
late in the first decade of life, it is sometimes mistaken for prepubertal acne. Other cutaneous lesions include ash-leaf spots, which are whitish hypopigmented lesions seen best with ultraviolet
light (Wood's lamp). The light is selectively absorbed by skin melanin, causing the hypopigmented lesions to stand out more conspicuously.
Histopathologically, ash-leaf spots contain a normal number of melanocytes, but the melanosomes
are smaller and contain subnormal amounts of
melanin. Shagreen patches (yellowish plaques located on the eyelids or lumbosacral regions) and
periungual or subungual fibromas are also characteristic of the syndrome. Some children also have
café au lait spots and nevi.

The most common ocular manifestation of
tuberous sclerosis is the astrocytic hamartoma (the
original "phakoma" of van der Hoeve, which is
present in most cases but is easily overlooked
(Figure 11.6).[374] These angiogliomatous hamartomas may appear early in infancy[337] as flat,
translucent, noncalcified superficial retinal lesions
that have a slushy appearance reminiscent of cotton in water. These lesions are sometimes vascu-
larized and, rarely, may be associated with vitreous hemorrhage or seeding.[17,104,208] Since they
arise from the retinal nerve fiber layer, they are
usually situated near the optic disc. Over time,
they calcify and enlarge into raised tumors with a
"mulberry-like" appearance that resemble optic
disc drusen in consistency but are much larger.
Small calcified astrocytic hamartomas of the optic

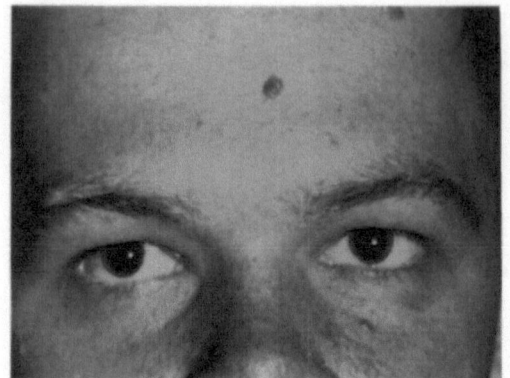

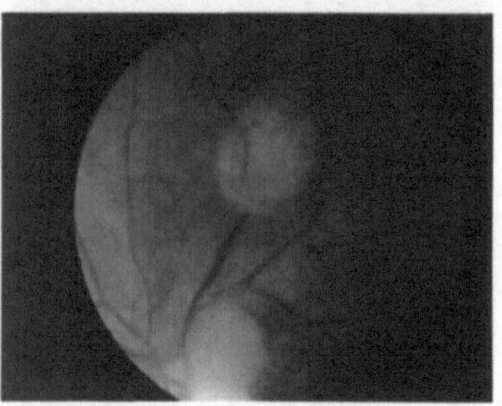

FIGURE 11.6. Tuberous sclerosis. (A) Adenoma sebaceum. (B) Retinal astrocytic hamartomas. The lesion
next to the optic disc is gelatinous in appearance, while
the lesion above it shows scattered focal calcific areas.

disc may be impossible to distinguish from disc
drusen. Uncalcified astrocytic optic disc hamartomas appear as a focal elevated mass of whitish,
gray or yellowish tissue that obscures visualization of the underlying disc.[253] Astrocytic hamartomas may be confused with a variety of other
retinal lesions caused by retinoblastoma, toxoplasmosis, and toxocara. They rarely compromise vision (unless they are situated in the macula or a vitreous hemorrhage occurs), and the importance of
their recognition lies primarily in establishing the
diagnosis of tuberous sclerosis. However, these
lesions must be distinguished from the rare solitary retinal astrocytoma that is unassociated with
phakomatosis, prominently vascular, and causes severe intraocular damage.[13] Approximately one-
third of children with tuberous sclerosis will have
discrete achromic patches in the peripheral retina
that are analogous to ash-leaf spots. These white

lesions that can be focal, linear, circular, or "paint brush" in configuration are often dismissed as peripheral chorioretinal scars.

The brain lesions in tuberous sclerosis are almost always benign hamartomas. They have been variously described as low-grade benign neoplasms, clusters of heterotopic neurons within the white matter, and regions of gliosis or abnormal myelin (destruction/dysplasia).[44,51,342] Bender and Yunis[43] have suggested that the same cellular components are present in all the parenchymal brain lesions, that they represent a combination of both neuronal and astrocytic features, and that they result from disordered migration and differentiation. These hamartomas occur in two prominent locations: on the surface as superficial cerebral cortical "tubers" and as deep subependymal nodules. The cortical tubers are typically large and pale compared with the surrounding normal gyri.[342] They lack the normal six-layered lamination of cortical gray matter and may contain giant neurons. On CT scanning, they appear as an enlarged gyrus with a central hypodensity. They show a central hyperintensity on T2-weighted imaging (termed a "gyral core") and a central hypointensity surrounded by a hyperintense rim (termed a "sulcal island") on T1-weighted imaging (Figure 11.7).[342] Cortical tubers are associated with seizures (which are often the presenting sign of tuberous sclerosis) and mental retardation. The seizures often manifest as infantile spasms, which consist of sudden flexion and extension movements of the extremities that may occur numerous times daily and evolve into grand mal seizures as the child becomes older. Mental retardation, once thought to be an invariable association, is only present in 60% of cases.[391]

The subependymal nodules are usually located along the lateral borders of the ventricles (Figure 11.7) in the striothalamic groove between the caudate nucleus and the thalamus.[342] They are sharply circumscribed, do not spread through the periventricular tissue, and are covered by intact ependyma. They may be calcified or uncalcified and, as with retinal lesions, their degree of calcification increases with age.[375] Due to their mixed signal characteristics, the nodules are more easily visualized on CT than on MR imaging.[342] These subependymal nodules may give rise to subependymal giant cell astrocytomas in 5% to 15% of indi-

viduals with tuberous sclerosis. This transition tends to occur within the first two decades of life. The distinction between subependymal nodules and giant cell astrocytoma is one of size and position rather than histology.[116] Although histologically benign and slow growing, giant cell astrocytomas cause major visual and neurological morbidity by enlarging to obstruct the foramina of Monro, leading to hydrocephalus, chronic papilledema, and eventually optic atrophy.[116]

Visceral involvement, which is also prominent in tuberous sclerosis, may include renal cysts, renal angiomyolipomas, cardiac rhabdomyomas, and cystic lesions of the lungs. The skeletal system is affected in 40% of patients, with sclerotic areas occurring in the calvarium and the spine and with phalangeal cysts in the hands and feet.[391] The shortened life span in some patients with tuberous sclerosis is attributable to a combination of causes, including status epilepticus, renal failure from extensive angiomyolipomas, cardiac failure, pulmonary complications from lung involvement, and hydrocephalus or hemorrhage from intraventricular lesions or their surgical complications.[342]

Sturge–Weber Syndrome (Encephalotrigeminal Angiomatosis)

Encephalotrigeminal angiomatosis is a misleading label for the Sturge–Weber syndrome since it fails to reflect the underlying neuropathology as we now understand it. The term angioma refers to a mass of plump endothelial cells with high mitotic activity. An angioma involves capillaries that are actively proliferating and that appear histopathologically as a tumor.[69] A typical facial hemangioma in children is the capillary hemangioma, that is not present at birth and that proliferates for about a year before it involutes. This lesion differs from the "port-wine stain" or nevus flammeus of Sturge–Weber that is present at birth and consists of a venous dilatation with no capillary proliferation.[69] The port-wine color of the facial lesion is due to the presence of deoxygenated blood within the vascular spaces. Although the embryogenesis is unknown, some have recently attributed the venous malformation of Sturge–Weber to a congenital deficiency of autonomic innervation to the in-

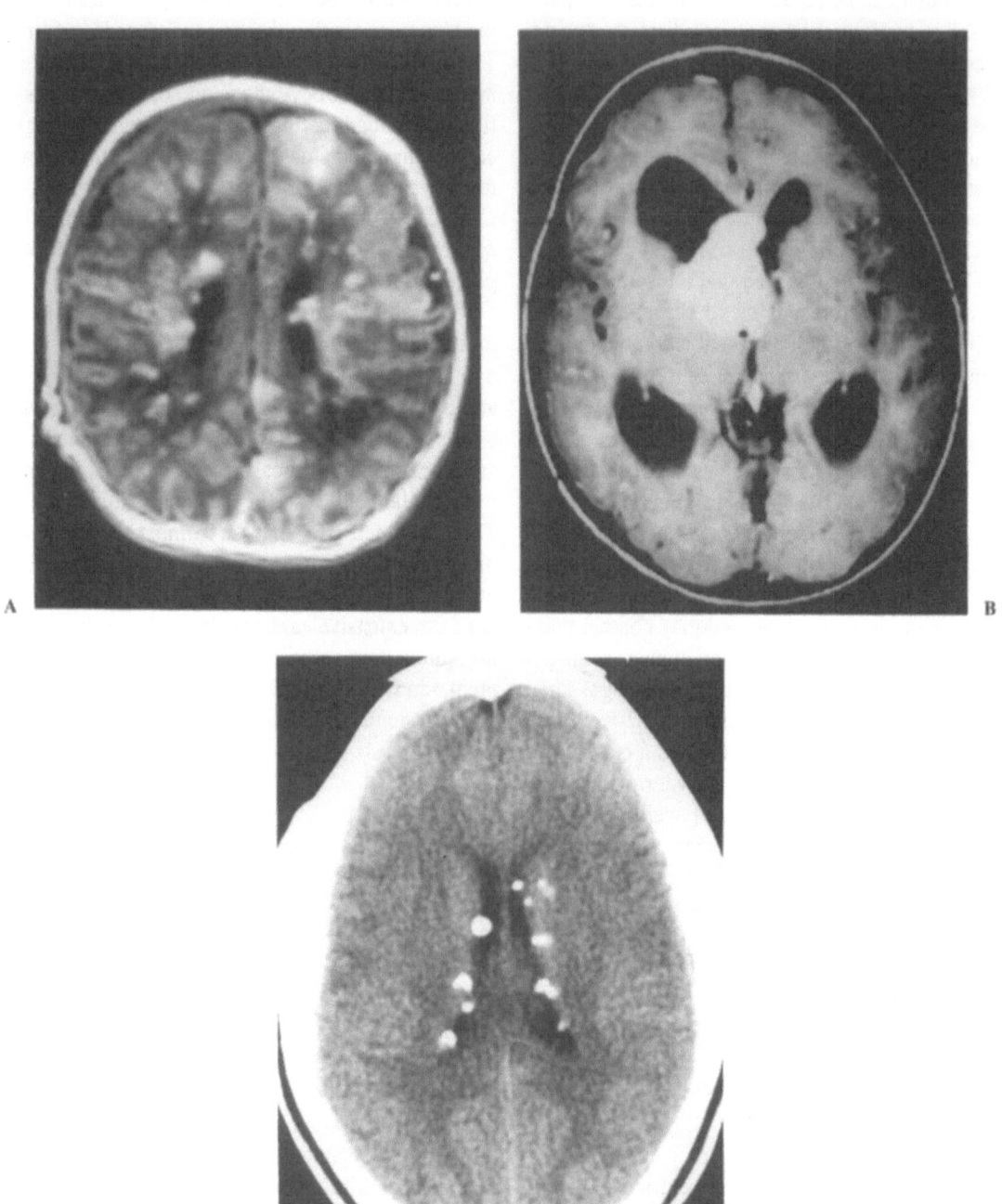

FIGURE 11.7. Tuberous sclerosis. (A) MR image in an infant demonstrating multiple subependymal nodules and cortical tubers. (B) MR image in an older child demonstrating a giant cell astrocytoma with associated hydrocephalus. (C) CT scan shows characteristic multiple nodular calcific lesions in the subependymal regions. (Upper figures courtesy of Charles M. Glasier, MD.)

volved venous bed.[318,345] Waner et al[381] postulate that the port-wine stain occurs in an area that has an absolute or relative deficiency of autonomic in-nervation. When the deficiency is absolute, progressive ectasia will occur more rapidly, and CNS sequela will be more severe.

The adjective *encephalotrigeminal* is also inaccurate since the location of the port-wine stain may coincidentally have a dermatomal distribution but is in no way dictated by trigeminal innervation. The facial telangiectasia is primarily unilateral, but it may cross the midline slightly and may extend to involve the mucosa of the hard palate and the linings of the paranasal sinus along with the conjunctiva, episclera, and choroid of the ipsilateral eye.[342,354] Glaucoma involves the eye on the affected side in at least 30% of cases and may lead to buphthalmos, anisometropia, and amblyopia if present within the first two years of life.[82,380] Although glaucoma in Sturge–Weber syndrome is generally attributed to elevated episcleral venous pressure, isolated trabeculodysgenesis may play a dominant role in infant eyes.[83,188,354] Sturge–Weber syndrome is nonhereditary, and medical management involves laser therapy for treatment of the nevus flammeus and medical and/or surgical treatment of seizures and glaucoma. Most children with facial port-wine stains will not have ocular or pial involvement (i.e., no Sturge–Weber syndrome). Those that develop glaucoma almost invariably have involvement of both the upper and midface.[36]

The intracranial lesion of Sturge–Weber syndrome is a leptomeningeal vascular malformation that is similar to and ipsilateral to the facial lesion.[342] It typically overlies the occipitoparietal region but may extend anteriorly in some children. This leptomeningeal malformation lies along the surface of the brain in the subarachnoid space between the pia and the arachnoid membrane but does not involve the brain itself (Figure 11.8). Over time, the underlying cerebral cortex becomes dysfunctional, progressively atrophic, and calcified.[342] As unilateral cerebral atrophy occurs, the skull develops asymmetrically, and the calvarium thickens on the side of the lesion with increased diploic space, increased pneumatization of the paranasal sinuses, elevation of the petrous ridge, and elevation of the lesser wing of the sphenoid.[342]

Infants with Sturge–Weber syndrome are often neurologically intact at birth, but there is a high incidence of focal or generalized seizure activity that usually begins within the first year of life.[342] Focal neurological deficits, such as spastic hemiparesis with or without atrophy or hemianopia, or mental retardation are thought to be secondary to

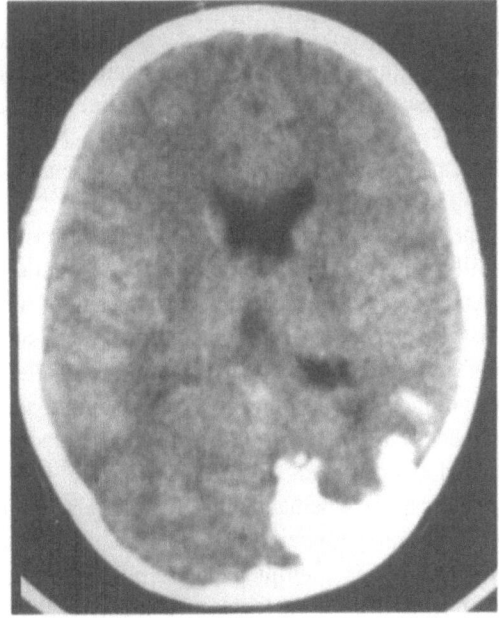

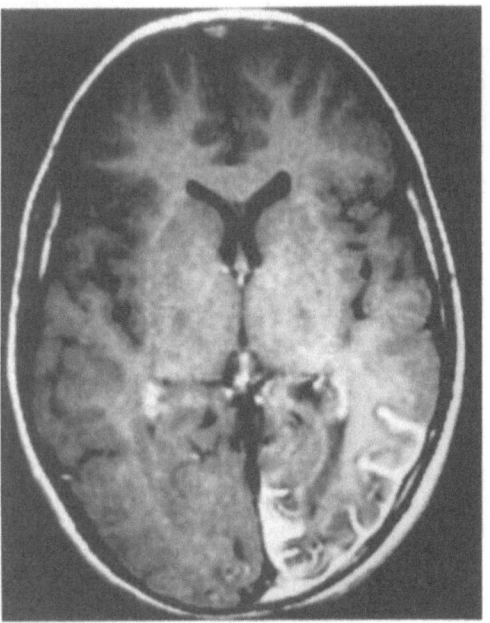

FIGURE 11.8. Sturge-Weber Syndrome (A) Noncontrast axial CT scan demonstrating dense cortical calcifications. (B) T1-weighted gadolinium-enhanced demonstrating enhancing leptomeningeal vascular malformation and mild cerebral hemiatrophy. (Courtesy of Charles M Glasier, MD.)

atrophy of the involved cortex.[10] Computed tomography scanning shows the three Cs: cerebral atrophy, calvarial thickening, and cortical calcifications (Figure 11.8).[342] The MR imaging often shows superficial enhancement of the cerebral hemispheres. Although the leptomeningeal malformation alone is sufficient to establish the diagnosis,[10,95] it is important to distinguish this vascular lesion from meningoepithelial angiomatosis that occurs in some patients with neurofibromatosis. Unlike the leptomeningeal malformation of Sturge–Weber syndrome, meningoepithelial angiomatosis tends to be more focal and it infiltrates into the underlying brain.[342]

Neuro-ophthalmologic complications in Sturge–Weber syndrome are generally limited to homonymous hemianopia from occipital lobe involvement, positive visual phenomena due to seizures, and glaucomatous optic atrophy. Strabismus and anisometropic amblyopia are also common in children with glaucoma and buphthalmos.

Seizures in Sturge–Weber syndrome are often difficult to control with medication. Bilateral intracranial involvement, although rare, is associated with seizure onset at an earlier age and with seizures that are more difficult to control.[276] The presence of seizure activity within the first year of life seems to be predictive of a poor outcome.[276] Surgical lobectomy or hemispherectomy with resection of the involved cortex in children with intractable seizures has produced encouraging results.[276,342]

von Hippel–Lindau Disease

von Hippel–Lindau disease is a familial disorder with an autosomal dominant pattern of inheritance.[270] There is no racial or gender predilection. The responsible gene is linked to DNA markers that map to the short arm of chromosome 3.[333] Unlike neurofibromatosis and tuberous sclerosis, von Hippel–Lindau disease has a low mutation rate. Most affected children have inherited the disease, and each family member should also be thought of as having the disease.

Affected patients develop a variety of ocular, CNS, and visceral tumors, including retinal angiomatosis, CNA hemangioblastoma (50%), renal cell carcinoma (22%), pheochromocytoma (approximately 14%), and epididymal cystadenoma.[173,236,268,269] The retinal lesions tend to become symptomatic earlier than the CNS lesions, which tend to become symptomatic earlier than the visceral tumors.[173,185,255] Cysts of the lungs, kidneys, bones, pancreas, adrenal glands, and omentum have also been described. The CNS hemangiomas are found in approximately 50% of gene carriers and differ from sporadic hemangioblastoma in their tendency for multiple occurrence and their tendency to develop at a younger age.[269] Approximately 75% are cystic versus solid, and 75% develop intracranially versus intraspinally.[269,325] Most intracranial hemangioblastomas are located within the cerebellum and often in the midline.[255] Cerebellar hemangioblastomas generally present in the mid-thirties with signs of increased intracranial pressure (headache, nausea, vomiting) and, less commonly, signs of cerebellar dysfunction (ataxia, clumsiness, nystagmus).[185] A small number of patients with von Hippel–Lindau syndrome have a syrinx of the brain stem, spinal cord, or both.[255] The associated polycythemia in some cases probably relates to the extremely high levels of erythropoietin found within the hemangioblastoma tumor cyst. Huson et al[185] have suggested that patients carrying the diagnosis and those at risk should undergo an annual retinal examination starting at 5 years of age and biennial neuroimaging of the head, spine, and abdomen and urinary VMA and meta-adrenaline testing starting at age 10, since life-threatening CNS and visceral tumors can remain clinically occult for long periods of time.[173]

The characteristic ocular lesion is the retinal capillary hemangioblastoma, which is generally detected within the second or third decade of life. This vascular tumor is a reddish retinal mass supplied by a single, dilated, tortuous feeder artery extending from the optic disc to the tumor and drained by a similarly engorged vein extending from the tumor back to the disc (Figure 11.9). Retinal capillary hemangiomas tend to develop in the temporal periphery or midperipheral retina, may be single or multiple, and are bilateral in approximately half of cases. Occasionally, exudative hemangiomas may be situated within the disc substance and simulate neuroretinitis or juxtapapillary choroidal neovascularization.[146] These posterior tumors differ from the peripheral ones in that

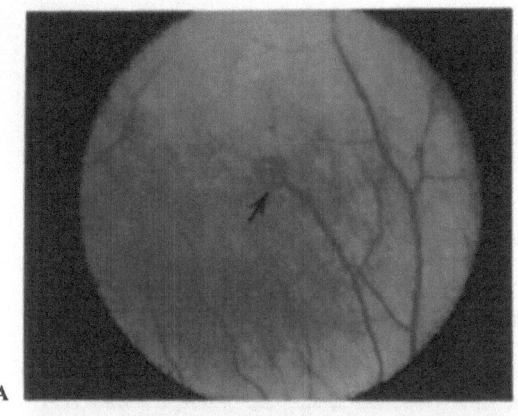

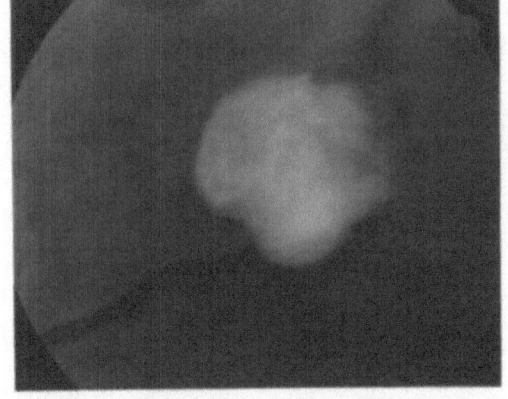

FIGURE 11.9. von Hippel-Lindau disease—retinal hemangioblastoma may be subtle (A; arrow) or large (B). (Upper figure courtesy of William F. Hoyt, MD.)

they typically lack the dilated feeder vessels.[255] Retinal capillary hemangioblastomas are histopathologically identical to cerebellar hemangioblastomas, showing an extensive network of capillaries with intertwined plump stromal cells. Their capillaries are fenestrated, explaining their proclivity to cause massive retinal exudation that, if left untreated, may lead to total exudative retinal detachment and permanent visual loss. The exudative retinopathy in this condition may be mistaken for Coats disease if the underlying hemangioma is not recognized. These retinal angiomas are treatable with a combination of retinal cryotherapy or laser photoablation depending upon their size and location, but careful follow-up is mandatory since they tend to recur. Solitary capillary hemangiomas may be seen in older adults with no other signs of von Hippel–Lindau disease and no evidence of familial involvement. These tumors generally lack

the markedly dilated and tortuous feeder vessels but otherwise resemble those of von Hippel–Lindau syndrome.[339]

Retinal examination can often provide confirmation of the disorder long before CNS hemangiomas develop. de Jong et al[103] found that twin retinal vessels provide a reliable retinal marker for von Hippel–Lindau disease. Unlike normal retinal arterioles and venules, twin vessels are separated by less than one venule width and run a parallel and sometimes overlapping course. In children with a family history of von Hippel–Lindau disease, a careful search should be made for incipient retinal lesions that are most frequently located in the equatorial or pre-equatorial retina. Incipient lesions resemble diabetic microaneurysms and are not associated with dilation of the major vascular channels leading to and from them.[195] Aside from their obvious diagnostic significance, incipient lesions can be easily photocoagulated and obliterated.[195]

Ataxia-Telangiectasia (Louis–Bar Syndrome)

Ataxia-telangiectasia is a rare autosomal recessive neurocutaneous disease characterized by combinations of telangiectasia of the skin and eye, cerebellar ataxia, various immune deficiencies, frequent sinus and pulmonary infections, and a predilection to develop malignancies. Linkage analysis has localized a gene for ataxia telangiectasia to chromosome region 11q22 to 11q23, but more than one gene locus may be present.[149] It is classified with the "breakage syndromes," which are diseases with a high frequency of chromosome breaks and rearrangement and an elevated risk of leukemia and other neoplasms. Cutaneous telangiectasias are most often first noted in the conjunctiva then in the malar area, ears, palate, and across the bridge of the nose. The conjunctival telangiectasia is generally confined to the area of the palpebral fissure. Mottled hypo- and hyperpigmented skin regions may also be seen. The major neurological findings arise from characteristic progressive degeneration of the cerebellar cortex which is readily demonstrable on neuroimaging. Progressive cerebellar ataxia usually develops by the time the affected child begins walking. In contrast, the telangiectatic lesions develop later, usually around 3 to 7 years of age. The ataxia is followed by progressive neurological deterioration that leaves the patients confined to a wheelchair. Dysarthria, choreoathetosis, myoclonic jerks, and endocrine abnormalities usually develop.

The characteristic ophthalmologic finding is bilateral bulbar conjunctival telangiectasis which becomes apparent during childhood (Figure 11.10). The telangiectatic conjunctival vessels are confined to the area of the palpebral fissure, have numerous sausage-shaped aneurysmal dilatations, and take frequent abrupt turns. Patients later develop abnormalities in ocular motility disturbances described as ocular motor apraxia, due to defective saccadic initiation. Head thrusts may be less conspicuous or absent in this setting, however. Nystagmus and other cerebellar eye signs may also be present.

Patients develop a variety of immunological abnormalities that include both defective cellular and humoral immunity. The thymus is absent or rudimentary. Patients are prone to developing frequent sinopulmonary infections, skin infections, and T-cell lymphoproliferative disorders (lymphomas and leukemias). Persistent elevated levels of alpha fetoprotein are present in almost all patients.[307] Pulmonary failure due to frequent infections and resulting bronchiectasis is the most common cause of death.

The most important neuropathologic abnormality in ataxia-telangiectasia is cerebellar degeneration, with reduced number of Purkinje, granular and basket cells in the cerebellar cortex, and neurons in the vermian and deep cerebellar nuclei. Magnetic resonance is the preferred neuroimaging modality and typically shows vermian atrophy with an enlarged fourth ventricle and cisterna magna. A lesser degree of cerebellar hemispheric atrophy may also be present (Figure 11.10).[321]

Aicardi et al[1] recently described a slowly progressive syndrome that mimics ataxia-telangiectasia by showing indistinguishable neurological signs (ocular motor apraxia, spinocerebellar degeneration, choreoathetosis) but with a later onset and with no associated telangiectasias or multisystemic involvement. They excluded other causes of supranuclear ophthalmoplegia, such as Gaucher

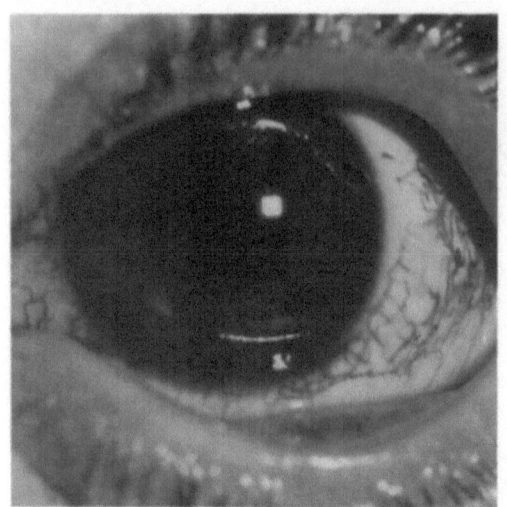

A

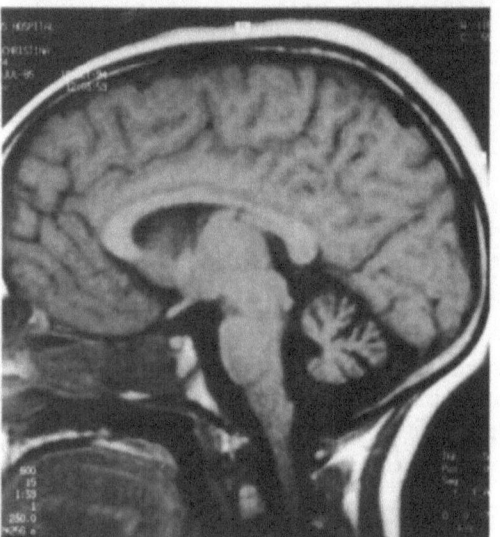

B

FIGURE 11.10. Ataxia-telangiectasia. (A) Conjunctival telangiectasias consisting of dilated vessels within the palpebral fissure. (Courtesy of William F. Hoyt, MD.) (B) T1 weighted MR scan shows diffuse atrophy of the cerebellum.

disease, Niemann–Pick disease, or Huntington chorea, by clinical features, by family history, and when appropriate, by enzymatic and skin biopsy studies. They suggested that this syndrome represents an unusual form of spinocerebellar degeneration.

Linear Sebaceous Nevus Syndrome

In 1963, Feuerstein and Mims described two patients with a neurocutaneous disorder consisting of the triad of a midline facial skin lesion (linear sebaceous nevus of Jadassohn), seizures, and mental retardation.[132,213] Affected children display a nondermatomal linear pigmented nevus that is elevated and plaquelike in appearance and is present at birth.[132] Since its original description, numerous descriptions of associated ophthalmological findings have been reported,[67,203,213] and its underlying brain malformation has been more clearly defined.[76]

Linear sebaceous nevus syndrome is now recognized as one of several "coloboma syndromes" with multisystem involvement. In addition to optic disc coloboma, a variety of other optic disc anomalies, including optic nerve hypoplasia[203] and peripapillary staphyloma,[67] may be present. This syndrome should be included in the differential diagnosis of conjunctival or corneal dermoids, along with Goldenhar syndrome and encephalocranial lipomatosis (discussed later). Other ocular choristomas such as choroidal osteoma have also been described.[213] A variety of ophthalmological findings have been noted including lid colobomas, ptosis, and Coats disease.[67] These children generally have severe neurological impairment, with seizures and severe mental retardation as the predominant neurological findings. Neuroimaging has shown that the majority of these children have hemimegalencephaly (discussed later), which accounts for their poor neurological prognosis.[76]

Klippel–Trenauney–Weber Syndrome

Klippel–Trenauney–Weber syndrome is a rare congenital angiodysplasia of uncertain etiology consisting of cutaneous vascular malformations, varicosities, and boney and soft tissue hypertrophy of the involved parts that appear in childhood on the affected side.[68,255] Only one side of the body is usually affected, but occasionally, both sides are involved.[255] The upper extremity is affected in 60% of cases, the lower extremity in 30%, and the head and trunk exclusively in the remaining

10%.[255] While hypertrophy is the most common abnormality of bone and soft tissue, atrophy may also occur. This condition is inherited as an autosomal dominant trait with variable expressivity. Ocular and neurological abnormalities are more common when the cutaneous vascular malformations involve the face.[68]

Unlike in Sturge–Weber, seizures and mental retardation may occur but are infrequent. A number of intracranial vascular malformations, including leptomeningeal vascular malformations, arteriovenous malformations, and aplasia of the internal carotid artery have been described.[255] Hemimegalencephaly has also been described in several patients with Klippel–Trenauney–Weber syndrome.[68,246] One child had ipsilateral facial hypertrophy and high myopia, suggesting an overgrowth syndrome involving both brain and eye.[68]

Neuro-ophthalmologic abnormalities in Klippel–Trenauney–Weber syndrome include optic disc anomalies, which include tilted disc with telangectatic vessels;[275] optic nerve hypoplasia;[301] optic nerve sheath meningioma;[348] and orbital optic nerve enlargement in the absence of visual dysfunction,[163] Horner syndrome,[255] ptosis,[255] afferent pupillary defect,[255] strabismus,[255] and nystagmus.[68] Additional ophthalmological findings include conjunctival and retinal varicosities, choroidal angiomas, orbital varices iris colobomas, iris heterochromia, strabismus, ptosis, and enophthalmos.[68] Glaucoma occurs but with less frequency than in the Sturge–Weber syndrome.[163] Although this disorder shares cutaneous features with the Sturge–Weber syndrome, the relationship, if any, between the two disorders is not known.

Brain Tumors

Primary brain tumors are the most common solid neoplasms in children and are second only to leukemia in overall frequency during childhood.[30,293] Childhood brain tumors differ considerably from the adult variety in incidence, location, histology, morphology, and natural history. Common adult tumors such as meningiomas, schwannomas, pituitary tumors, and metastasis are rare in children. The predilection of adult neoplasms to affect the cerebral hemispheres differs markedly from childhood tumors wherein approximately 50% of tumors in children older than 1 year are infratentorial.

Within the pediatric age group, the distribution of brain tumors differs between infants and older children. Although posterior fossa tumors are generally more common than supratentorial tumors in children, supratentorial tumors (suprasellar gliomas, teratomas, primitive neuroectodermal tumors, choroid-plexus tumors) predominate in infants. In the first six months of life, the tumors are more commonly supratentorial than infratentorial; in the second six months of life, the incidence is about equal in both locations, and thereafter, a posterior fossa predominance emerges. The younger the child, the more likely is the tumor to be supratentorial.

Brain tumors in infants have protean clinical manifestations that include irritability, listlessness, lethargy, vomiting, failure to thrive, and hydrocephalus with increasing head circumference and bulging fontanelles.[5,9,151,181] Focal neurologic deficits are generally absent because of the immaturity of the brain and the expansile nature of the cranium. Increased intracranial pressure is caused by obstruction of the ventricular system by the mass or less commonly by the sheer bulk of a supratentorial mass without ventricular obstruction.[297] Vomiting is the most common presenting symptom of infants with brain tumors (as in all age groups). It may result from increased intracranial pressure or from neoplastic involvement of the floor of the fourth ventricle where the vomiting center is located. In the absence of papilledema, such children may initially be misdiagnosed as having gastrointestinal disease.

Infants with cerebral hemispheric tumors and hemiparesis may be misdiagnosed as having static encephalopathy with hemiparetic cerebral palsy. Seizures are most commonly partial, with elementary symptoms and with or without generalization, but infantile spasms may occur. In some infants with brain tumors, infantile spasms show a favorable response to ACTH therapy prior to diagnosis of the tumors.[316]

Infants with midline tumors may show failure to thrive, endocrine dysfunction, and visual disorders. The diencephalic syndrome may also be found. This is characterized by profound failure to thrive despite good appetite. Affected children are alert and energetic despite severe emaciation. If the tumor involves the chiasm, decreased vision and nystagmus may be present.

Older children are more likely to show localizing neurological findings (cranial nerve palsy, hemiparesis, clumsiness, ataxia) and often present with recurrent headaches, nausea, vomiting, and visual complaints, which may be ascribed to nonspecific causes, delaying the diagnosis of underlying hydrocephalus and associated tumor. Tumors in the region of the hypothalamus often cause endocrine dysfunction (decreased appetite, failure to thrive), bitemporal hemianopia, or abnormal eye movements (seesaw nystagmus, spasmus nutans–like syndrome). Seizures are generally less common in children with posterior fossa tumors than in children with supratentorial tumors. In a study involving 3291 children with brain tumors, supratentorial tumors were associated with seizures in 22% of children younger than 14 years of age and 68% of older teenagers. Among children with infratentorial tumors, the prevalence of seizures was approximately 6% in all age groups. The tumor location with the highest incidence of seizures was the superficial cerebrum, with seizures occurred in more than 40% of cases.[154] Headaches occur very frequently in children with brain tumors and are commonly, but not exclusively, associated with increased intracranial pressure.

A significant portion of the clinical signs and symptoms in children with brain tumors involves the visual system either due to direct involvement of related structures in the neoplastic process or due to the mass effect of the tumor with associated hydrocephalus or secondary compression, deformation, or parenchymal shifts. Occasionally, children present initially to an ophthalmologist with visual signs and symptoms. Neuro-ophthalmologic evaluation is also a significant component of the clinical follow-up of these children.

Signs and symptoms of brain tumors can be nonlocalizing, falsely localizing, or localizing. Tumors are the most common cause of noncommunicating hydrocephalus (obstruction of cerebrospinal fluid (CSF) flow within the ventricular system) in children. The associated increased intracranial pressure gives rise to most of the nonlocalizing signs that include headache, papilledema, and sixth nerve palsy. This constellation of signs and symptoms does not provide specific clues regarding the tumor location. Falsely localizing signs are exemplified by the presence of bitemporal hemianopia in a child with posterior fossa tumor. The field defect results not from direct chiasmal infiltration but rather from compression by an enlarged third ventricle due to tumor-associated hydrocephalus. Once nonlocalizing and falsely localizing signs are excluded, the remaining symptoms and signs are generally related to the location of the tumor. Although skew deviation is usually listed with nonlocalizing disorders, it has been suggested that the presence of alternating skew on lateral gaze in a child with brain tumor suggests a lesion in the lower brain stem or the cerebellum.

Acute changes in intracranial pressure associated with brain tumors may cause a variety of herniation syndromes characterized by displacement of brain tissue either downward or, less commonly, upward. These syndromes include uncal, transtentorial, and falcial herniation. Uncal herniation results when a lateralized tumor in the frontal or temporal lobe causes a shift of structures through the tentorial notch into the midbrain. Pupillary-involving oculomotor palsy results from entrapment of the nerve by the herniated uncus on the free edge of the tentorium. Downward displacement of the cerebellar tonsils may result in compression of the medulla. Early signs of tonsilar herniation may include head tilt and a stiff neck, presumably arising from irritation of the cervical roots by the herniated mass.

Although children with posterior fossa tumors often develop paralytic strabismus, some may present with acute comitant esotropia.[392] Therefore, the finding of comitancy in acute esotropia is no guarantee that there is no underlying intracranial mass. Acute comitant esotropia that does not fit the classic profile of accommodative esotropia should prompt a search for other neuro-ophthalmologic signs, such as papilledema or nystagmus. The failure to fuse despite satisfactory postoperative ocular alignment in this setting should also raise concern about an underlying brain tumor.[392] Acute comitant esotropia may also occur in the setting of Chiari malformation. Associated gaze-evoked nystagmus or downbeat nystagmus in such a child should suggest this possibility. Acute comitant esotropia in children may also follow minor head trauma or be cryptogenic, and such cases generally lack associated neurologic findings, such as papilledema or nystagmus.[84] Children with posterior fossa tumors may rarely develop spasm of the near reflex[100] or signs and symptoms reminiscent of myasthenia gravis.[300,353]

Suprasellar Tumors

Suprasellar tumors in children include optic pathway gliomas, craniopharyngiomas, germinomas, pituitary adenomas, and others.[317] Due to the proximity of these tumors to the various structures that comprise the anterior visual pathway, these tumors have a high propensity to cause various neuro-ophthalmologic symptoms and signs. These include optic atrophy, chiasmal syndrome, papilledema, spasmus nutans, seesaw nystagmus, and bobble-headed doll syndrome. The clinical and neuroimaging features of suprasellar tumors in the pediatric age group are detailed in Chapter 4.

Hemispheric Tumors

Hemispheric Astrocytomas

Astrocytomas are the most common supratentorial tumors in childhood, constituting approximately 30% of such tumors. There is no gender predilection. Most cases in children are benign, but more malignant grades (e.g., glioblastoma multiforme) can occasionally occur. In general, the duration of symptoms before diagnosis is longer with supratentorial than with infratentorial astrocytomas. Supratentorial tumors are often large at the time of presentation.[46,251]

The clinical signs of cerebral hemispheric astrocytomas are generally determined by the tumor location. Signs and symptoms of increased intracranial pressure, seizures, and focal neurologic deficits predominate. Headaches may be focal or diffuse; persistent focal headaches may have a localizing value. Seizures are relatively common, presenting abnormalities of hemispheric tumors, ranging in incidence from 30% to 60% of cases. It should be emphasized, however, that the incidence of tumors in children with epilepsy is quite low in general. They tend to occur more frequently in the slow-growing astrocytoma than in the rapidly growing glioblastoma multiforme and, in this respect, can be considered a good prognostic sign. Seizures are more likely when tumors involve the sensory-motor strips of the cortex or the temporal lobes. Ataxia may be present with tumors of the frontal lobes or thalamus, presumably due to involvement of the frontopontine pathway, and this may lead to the incorrect diagnostic suspicion of a posterior fossa process.

Neuro-ophthalmologic abnormalities may arise from direct involvement of the geniculostriate pathways or from hydrocephalus. Visual field abnormalities and papilledema are the most common neuro-ophthalmologic signs. Involvement of the frontal gaze center causes inability to look volitionally to the contralateral side while retaining reflexive eye movements to that side. If the lesion is irritative rather than paralytic (as in tumor-associated seizure activity), there may be tonic conjugate deviation of the eyes toward the side contralateral to the lesion. Tumors involving the deep parieto-occipital regions may be associated with defects in conjugate horizontal pursuit to the side of the lesion in association with contralateral homonymous hemianopia.

Cerebral astrocytomas may appear on CT scanning as solid, with a central necrotic area, or cystic, with an enhancing mural nodule. The tumors are typically found deep within the cerebral hemispheres but can occur in the centrum semiovale or in the cortex. It is usually impossible to differentiate benign from malignant astrocytomas of the cerebrum with MR imaging, although low-grade tumors tend to be homogeneous, whereas higher-grade tumors show considerable heterogeneity. No definitive MR criteria exist to differentiate cerebral astrocytomas from ependymomas or oligodendrioglioma.

The best prognosis is attained by patients with benign cystic astrocytomas resembling their infratentorial counterparts.[251] These can be cured by total excision and may show prolonged symptom-free survival, even after subtotal resection. The therapeutic role of radiation in these tumors is under current debate. In contrast, children with glioblastoma multiforme or anaplastic astrocytoma require radiation and potentially chemotherapy.[118]

Gangliogliomas and Ganglioneuromas

These tumors differ from most CNS tumors in that both neuronal and glial elements are involved in the neoplastic process. They are labeled as gangli-ogliomas when the glial elements predominate and as ganglioneuromas when the neuronal elements predominate. There is no gender predilection.[344,355]

These tumors are slow growing and frequently present in the second decade of life or beyond with a long history of focal neurological deficits. The specific clinical manifestations depend on the location of the tumor. If the motor cortex or the temporal lobe is affected, patients present with a long history of focal seizures.[358] If the occipital lobe is affected, homonymous hemianopia may result. The treatment is surgical resection.

Supratentorial Ependymomas

Supratentorial ependymomas are histologically identical to their infratentorial counterparts and tend to peak in incidence between the ages of 1 and 5 years. These is a slight male preponderance. The presenting clinical features depend upon the location of the tumor, with focal seizures and signs and symptoms of increased intracranial pressure being most common.[125,159,160,372]

Primitive Neuroectodermal Tumors

Primitive neuroectodermal tumors (PNETs) are a group of highly malignant tumors found primarily in the cerebral hemispheres of children and young adults. They represent a pathologic quagmire in that there is considerable confusion regarding their differention on pathologic grounds from other neuroectodermal tumors, such as neuroblastomas, medulloblastomas, and pinealoblastomas. They are uncommon and occur most often in children under 5 years of age. In general, the duration of symptoms to diagnosis is short, with an average of 3 months.[141,364]

The PNETs are sharply delineated from surrounding brain tissue and are cystic with hemorrhagic features on gross inspection. Microscopically, they are highly cellular tumors composed of very poorly differentiated small cells (90% to 95%) with a high nuclear-to-cytoplasmic ratio. Focal areas of differentiation along neural or glial lines and a prominent mesenchymal component may be present. Their cell of origin is impossible to identify with certainty, but ultrastructural studies show resemblance to the developing cortical plate of the fetus, suggesting an origin from primitive undifferentiated neuroectoderm of the cerebrum.

The clinical presentation depends upon the location and growth rate of the tumor. The most common presentations include signs and symptoms of increased intracranial pressure, seizures, and long tract signs. Strikingly, some children may be relatively asymptomatic despite a huge tumor mass and may be spared severe neurological symptoms and signs (with the exception of papilledema and an inappropriate affect) until death.[88] Motor deficits such as hemiparesis or paraparesis are common. Visual field abnormalities and papilledema are the most common neuro-ophthalmologic findings.

The MR reveals a sharply-defined tumor due to relative lack of edema and the presence of enhancement.[134] Because the tumors may sometimes show extensive calcification, CT scanning without contrast may be a useful adjunct to MR imaging.

Although aggressive treatment with surgery, radiation, and chemotherapy has been attempted, the prognosis remains poor irrespective of treatment modality. The average 5-year survival is at best 20%.

Posterior Fossa Tumors

Medulloblastoma

Medulloblastomas are otherwise known as the PNETs of the posterior fossa.[139] They are the most common posterior fossa tumor in childhood, comprising 30% to 40% of all such tumors. The incidence peaks around 5 years of age. Boys are affected somewhat more frequently than girls in most series.

Children are usually diagnosed shortly after the onset of symptoms. Cushing's[97] description of the clinical course of a child with cerebellar medulloblastoma provides a graphical portrait of this disease:

"A pre-adolescent child previously in good health begins to complain of headaches, or of sub-occipital discomfort and to have occasional attacks of vomiting without preliminary nausea, usually on first arising in the morning. Attendance at school meanwhile may continue but the teacher soon notices that the child is listless, inattentive, and the character of his work notice-

ably falls off. Ere long it is apparent that there is some unwanted clumsiness in movement and awkwardness in gait. The mother may find that the child quickly outgrows its caps and she thinks the head enlarges unduly fast. In course of time it is noticed, at home or in school, that the child's sight is impaired; or a beginning squint of one eye may be detected, even in the absence of any complaint of double vision. The family doctor, who has previously suspected some gastrointestinal disorder, may then have the eye grounds examined and to the surprise and shock of everyone a choked disc is found. Three or four months, on the average, have elapsed, and at about this stage of the malady many cases come under hospital care."

The most common presenting symptoms are nausea, vomiting, and headaches due to increased intracranial pressure. This arises as the tumor grows and impinges on the roof of the fourth ventricle causing obstruction to CSF flow. Vomiting is the most common presenting sign of cerebellar tumors and may also arise independent of intracranial pressure by direct tumor pressure on the area postrema (vomiting center) located near the inferior aspect of the fourth ventricle. Other abnormalities include papilledema, diplopia, and nystagmus. Unilateral and bilateral internuclear ophthalmoplegia have been reported, arising either from brain stem neoplastic infiltration or compression.[12] In addition, older children and adults may initially present with ataxia, while infants may initially present with increasing head size due to hydrocephalus.

Most medulloblastomas are located in the midline of the cerebellum. They are putatively considered to be congenital in nature, deriving from remnants of the fetal external granular layer of the cerebellum or the medullary velum. Medulloblastomas are highly cellular tumors composed of primitive, undifferentiated, small round cells with abundant mitoses. Homer–Wright pseudorosettes are typically found. They are highly malignant tumors, showing local invasiveness as well as a high tendency, perhaps more than any other tumor, to seed the subarachnoid space. Extraneural metastasis to bone, lymph nodes, or viscera may arise as a result of tumor manipulation or shunting. The putative congenital origin of medulloblastoma has led some authors to use Collins' rule in predicting its course.[50] This rule predicts that the period of risk for recurrence of a tumor of embryonal origin after treatment is the patient's age at the time of diagnosis plus 9 months.

CT scanning classically reveals a well-defined, hyperdense tumor of the vermis. Isolated hemispheric involvement is rare in children.[320] The hyperdensity of the tumor arises from its composition by small, round cells with high nuclear-to-cytoplasmic ratio. The tumor enhances diffusely with contrast. Unlike cerebellar astrocytomas, cysts are uncommonly seen, and unlike cerebellar ependymomas, calcification is seen in less than 10% of cases. The MR appearance is variable and nonspecific (Figure 11.11). The T2-weighted are hypointense or isointense to gray matter,[252] which reflects the tumor composition of increased nuclear-to-cytoplasmic ratio and, hence, reduced water content. The heterogeneity of the MR signal results from cysts and calcification within the tumor mass.

The management is complex and includes various combinations of surgical excision, irradiation, and chemotherapy.[128] However, in comparison with all malignant brain tumors, the outlook has improved most dramatically for children with

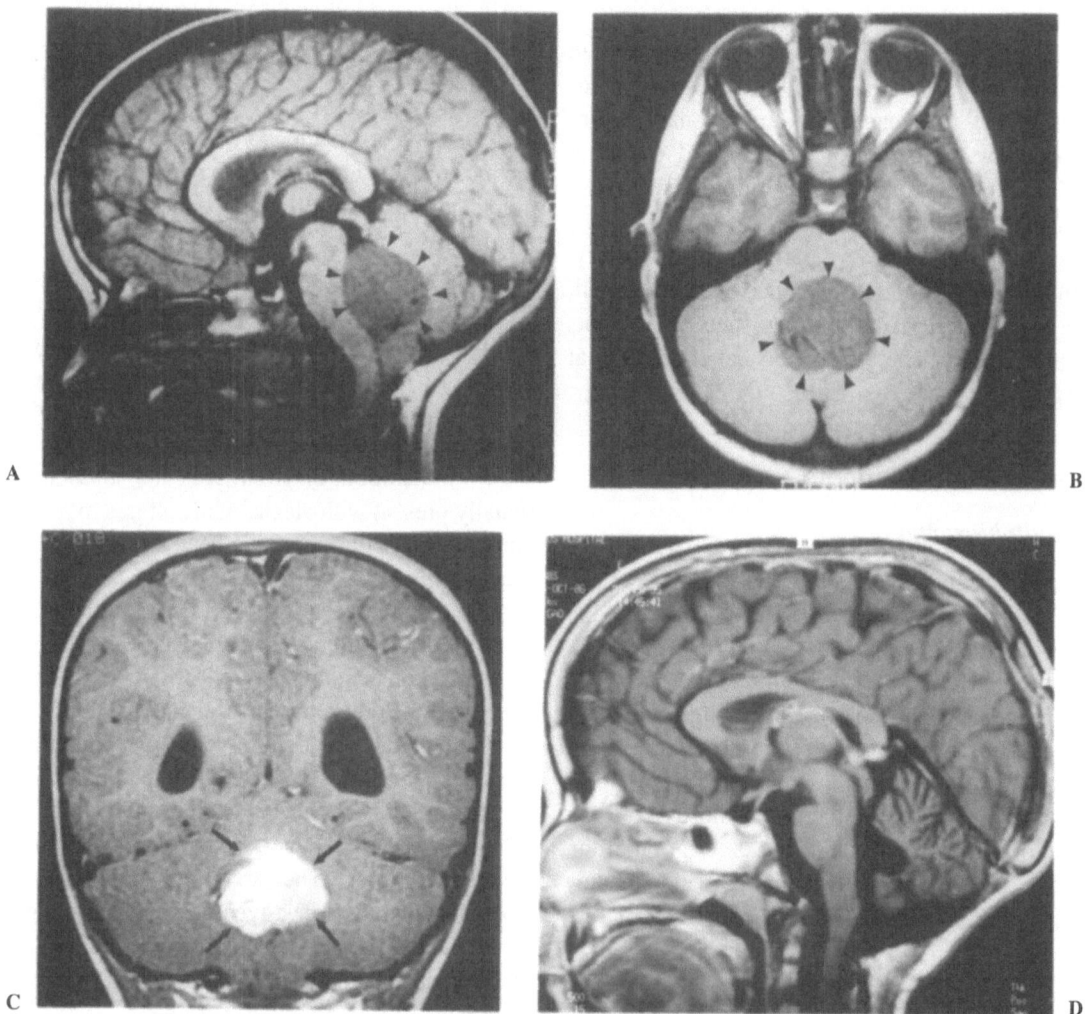

A

B

C

D

FIGURE 11.11. Cerebellar medulloblastoma. (A) Sagittal T1-weighted MR image shows a mass with lower intensity than the brain parenchyma (arrowheads). The mass occupies the fourth ventricle. (B) Axial T1-weighted image shows the mass filling the fourth ventricle (arrowheads). (C) Coronal T1-weighted MR image shows uniform tumor enhancement (arrows). (D) Sagittal T1-weighted MR image of the same patient after treatment consisting of surgical excision, radiation, and chemotherapy.

medulloblastomas. This is largely due to the use of craniospinal rather than local radiotherapy, with the addition of chemotherapy in selected patients. Because leptomeningeal dissemination is common, a staging workup of the neuroaxis is now advocated for guiding postoperative management.[109] The average 5-year survival rate using modern multimodality treatment is approximately 50% to 70%.

Cerebellar Astrocytoma

Astrocytomas are the most common brain tumors in children. They tend to occur in various locations both infratentorially and supratentorially. Cerebellar astrocytomas may occur anywhere in the cerebellum, including the vermis, the hemispheres, or both. Cerebellar astrocytomas show no gender predilection and tend to develop in a slightly older age group than medulloblastomas, generally peaking in incidence in the latter half of the first decade.[102,143]

The early presentation of affected children consists of early morning headaches and vomiting due to increased intracranial pressure. Vomiting generally occurs in the morning and may occur without nausea. After vomiting, the child may feel well for the rest of the day, with a repeat performance the following morning. Because the symptoms are recurrent, the child may undergo gastrointestinal evaluation before a correct diagnosis is finally made. As the tumor enlarges, the headaches become persistent. Neurologic symptoms may help predict the location of the tumor. The child with a midline cerebellar tumor will present with truncal ataxia, whereas the child with cerebellar hemispheric tumor will show appendicular signs (e.g., dysdiadochokinesia, dysmetria). Children may show apathy, irritability, and neck stiffness and pain and may develop attacks of unconsciousness, so-called "cerebellar fits." Because of the insidious nature of the symptoms, some children have little or no complaints until late in the disease, despite the presence of a large tumor, with papilledema as the only abnormal finding. The average duration of symptoms before diagnosis is approximately 18 months as compared to only 5 months in medulloblastoma.

The most common neuro-ophthalmologic abnormalities are papilledema, diplopia, and nystagmus.

Coarse nystagmus to the side of the lesion is of localizing value and should be distinguished from vestibular nystagmus, which is directed to the side opposite the lesion. The presence of a sixth nerve palsy may be a false localizing sign indicating increased intracranial pressure or may signal neoplastic invasion of the brain stem, the latter usually accompanied by hyperreflexia and Babinski responses. Children may have torticollis if brain stem involvement results in fourth nerve palsy.

Cerebellar astrocytomas are generally noninvasive, well-demarcated tumors.[329] Mitoses are conspicuously absent and, when present, suggest a malignant astrocytoma. Approximately 80% of cerebellar astrocytomas are cystic, showing either a large cyst with a solid mural nodule or multiple smaller cysts. Microscopic or gross calcification is present in up to 25% of cases. At least two histologic types exist. The most common form (termed the juvenile variety) consists of areas of compact, fibrillated cells with abundant Rosenthal fibers alternating with loose spongy areas composed of microcysts. Rosenthal fibers are eosinophilic, beaded, or cigar-shaped swellings of astrocytes that represent a benign degenerative process. The second type is a diffuse form, consisting of fibrillated stellate or piloid cells, identical to that encountered in cerebral astrocytomas. The juvenile form has a considerably better prognosis than the diffuse form. Early recurrence and poor survival is also associated with brain stem invasion and onset before 4 years of age.

The presence on CT scanning of a low-density mass, typically within the cerebellar hemispheres, often with a cystic component, is suggestive of a cerebellar astrocytoma. The presence of an enhancing nodule on CT scanning adjacent to the cyst is compelling evidence for the diagnosis. On MR imaging the tumor signal is nearly always hypointense to surrounding cerebellum on T1-weighted imaging and hyperintense and generally homogenous in appearance on proton density and T2-weighted imaging (Figure 11.12).

Cerebellar astrocytomas have the best overall prognosis of any childhood brain tumor.[357] The preferred treatment of cerebellar astrocytomas is complete surgical resection.[218,371] If this is accomplished, the 10-year survival rate exceeds 90%. If only incomplete excision is possible due to invasion of critical surrounding brain stem

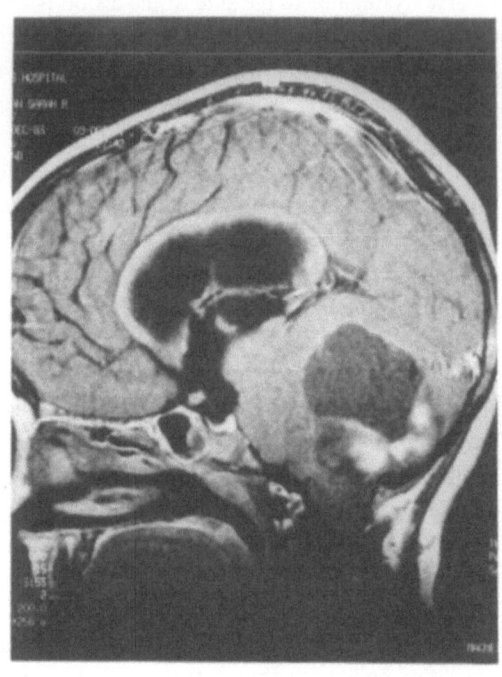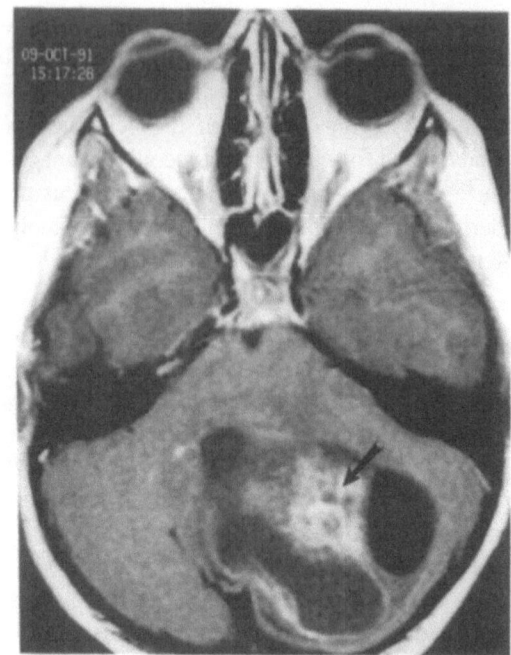

A   B

FIGURE 11.12. (A) Sagittal MR image shows a large cystic cerebellar mass. Note enhancing portion inferiorly. (B) Axial scan shows involvement of the left cerebellar hemisphere and midline structures. Note enhancing mural nodules (arrow).

parenchyma, patients may be observed expectantly for tumor progression before radiotherapy is considered.

Ependymoma

Intracranial ependymomas may arise from any region of the ventricular system, but the majority of childhood ependymomas are located in the posterior fossa.[210] The average age at diagnosis is 5 to 6 years. Unlike medulloblastomas, the diagnosis is usually delayed as a result of the insidious onset of symptoms.[93]

Posterior fossa ependymomas arise from differentiated ependymal cells that line the roof, floor, or lateral recesses of the fourth ventricle. Most are solid in nature, but some are very soft and deformable. Therefore, in contrast with most other brain tumors that grow as steadily enlarging masses, ependymomas can wrap themselves around various structures in their vicinity and become quite adherent to the adjacent brain. They also have a tendency to exit through the foramena of Magendie and Luschka into the subarachnoid space.[235]

In general, posterior fossa ependymomas present with signs and symptoms of increased intracranial pressure (due to obstruction of the fourth ventricle) and unsteady gait. The growth characteristics of these tumors render them more likely to present with neuro-ophthalmologic manifestations than other posterior fossa tumors. Invasion of the cerebellum, brain stem, or cerebellopontine angle produce corresponding neurological abnormalities that include nystagmus, ocular motor nerve palsies, and internuclear ophthalmoplegia. Torticollis may result from involvement of the trochlear nerve or may accompany neck pain and stiffness resulting from enchroachment of the tumor on the upper cervical nerve roots. Spinal cord ependymomas are a well-recognized but readily overlooked cause of papilledema.[247]

Ependymomas are cellular tumors with regular histologic pattern. Ependymal rosettes are diagnostic and are composed of tumor cells lined around a central lumen. Perivascular pseudorosettes are common, and cilia may be present. Two grades of ependymomas are recognized: a benign or differentiated ependymoma and a malignant or anaplastic variety. The anaplastic variety have typical features of ependymomas but in addition have pleomorphism, necrosis, increased cellularity, mitoses, and giant cells. Anaplastic ependymomas are more common in the supratentorial regions.

A posterior fossa ependymoma appears on CT scanning as a hyperdense or isodense fourth ventricular mass with punctate calcifications, small cysts, and moderate enhancement with contrast.

Extension of the mass through the fourth ventricular foramina or the foramen magnum further supports the diagnosis. The MR imaging signals may be heterogeneous or homogenous depending upon the presence of calcification, hemorrhage, and cysts (Figure 11.13).[349]

Posterior fossa ependymomas are quite difficult to surgically excise in their entirety and show a high recurrence rate after surgery.[6,174] This is compounded by the tendency of the tumor to seed

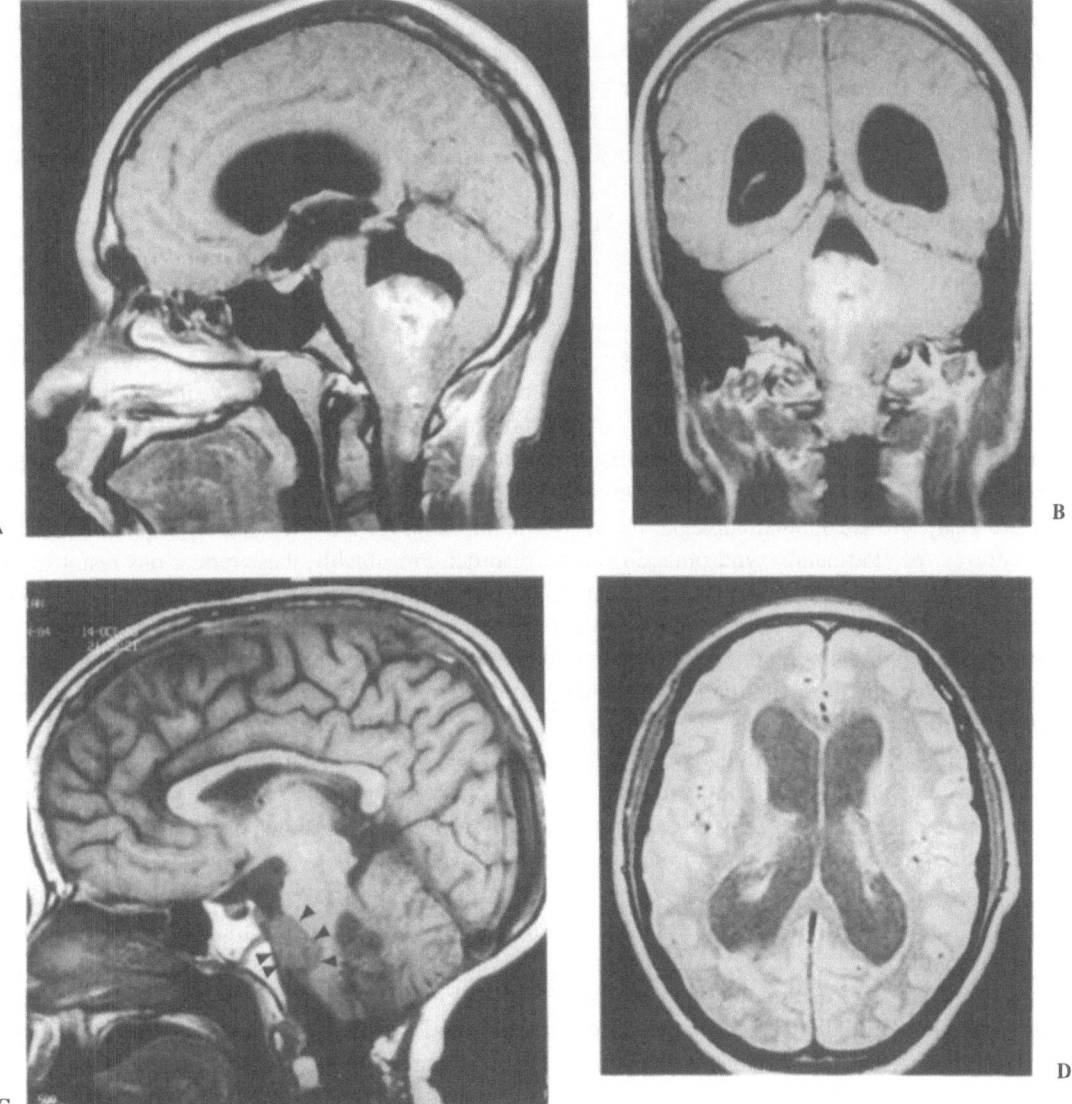

FIGURE 11.13. Posterior fossa ependymoma. (A) Sagittal and (B) coronal MR images show extension of the tumor through the fourth ventricular foramina. (C) Note extension of tumor anteriorly (arrowheads). (D) MR imaging shows associated hydrocephalus.

the CSF pathways, including the spinal subarachnoid space. Postoperative irradiation is recommended as adjunctive therapy of all posterior fossa ependymomas.

Brain Stem Tumors

Brain stem gliomas represent about 15% of pediatric CNS tumors. They show no gender predilection. These tumors show a variable clinical presentation but a uniformly poor outcome by virtue of their location. The pons is the most common site of origin of brain stem gliomas, followed by the midbrain and the medulla.[243,285]

Brain stem tumors are suggested by the triad of long tract signs, cranial neuropathies, and ataxia. In addition, brain stem gliomas should be considered in the differential diagnosis of an infant with failure to thrive who has facial paresis, absent cough reflex during suctioning, or a depressed gag reflex. The cranial nerves most commonly affected are the sixth and seventh nerves, and the two are often present together. The most common neuro-ophthalmologic symptom is diplopia due to involvement of the ocular motor nerves.

Seesaw nystagmus in a patient with brain stem tumor localizes the tumor to the region of the diencephalon. The presence of a third or fourth cranial nerve palsy, diffuse ophthalmoplegia, the various features of Parinaud syndrome in any combination, or profound hydrocephalus suggests a mesencephalic component to the tumor. Occasionally, diffuse ophthalmoplegia due to mesencephalic involvement may simulate myasthenia gravis both clinically as well as by showing a false-positive response to Tensilon. Convergence palsy may accompany midbrain tumors or tumors of the pineal region. Primary position upbeat nystagmus has been observed in tumors at the pontomesencephalic junction.[367] Horizontal eye movement abnormalities (horizontal gaze paresis due to involvement of the abducens nuclei or the paramedian pontine reticular formation, internuclear ophthalmoplegia, one-and-a-half syndrome) are features of pontine involvement.[86] Pontine horizontal gaze abnormalities may be associated with ipsilateral facial palsy and contralateral hemiparesis. Pontine gliomas have been reported to cause chronic isolated sixth nerve palsy.[142] An associated sixth nerve palsy may also occasionally show

spontaneous improvement. Asymmetry of the palate, absent gag reflex, atrophy of the tongue, and various other bulbar signs, including swallowing and feeding abnormalities, indicate medullary involvement. Vomiting, unaccompanied by headache, may occur due to direct infiltration of the emesis center in the medulla. Ataxia may result from direct cerebellar involvement or, more likely, from compromise of cerebellar pathways passing through any of the cerebellar peduncles. Rarely, brain stem tumors have been associated with congenital ocular motor apraxia.[404]

In contrast with the cerebellar tumors discussed, hydrocephalus and signs and symptoms of increased intracranial pressure are quite uncommon in pontine glioma until late, despite significant enlargement of the brain stem and even bulging of the enlarged brain stem into the fourth ventricle. However, tectal and tegmental gliomas may present with headaches and increased intracranial pressure due to compression and obstruction of the sylvian aqueduct.

Duration of symptoms until diagnosis varies widely from several weeks to several years. Although the natural history is one of inexorable progression, there are a few reports of brain stem tumors showing a remitting and exacerbating course.[322] This presentation may understandably be mistaken for a demyelinating or parainfectious disorder. Presumably, these remissions result from resolution of edema or necrosis in the area of the tumor.

Most brain stem gliomas are fibrillary astrocytomas similar to those found in the cerebral hemispheres; only a small minority are pilocytic in nature. The tumor cells are seen to intermingle with neurons and nerve fibers on histopathologic examination, infiltrating along these structures rather than destroying them. This may explain the relative preservation of various neural functions within the brain stem despite apparent diffuse involvement of the brain stem structures. It is not unusual for the child with a pontine glioma to present initially to the ophthalmologist for evaluation of a horizontally incomitant esotropia or a face turn resulting from a sixth nerve palsy. If such a child has an initially negative neuroimaging study, reimaging for a possible pontine glioma is indicated if the palsy fails to completely resolve within 6 months.

Brain stem tumors are much more easily identified with MR imaging than CT scanning (Figure 11.14).[28,71] CT scanning typically shows an expanded brain stem that is hypodense or isodense to the surrounding brain stem.[48] MR imaging shows a brain stem mass that is hypointense on T1-weighted images and hyperintense on T2-weighted images. T2-weighted images are especially useful for detecting tumor infiltration into surrounding structures.[135] Diffuse tumors enlarge the brain stem smoothly, without focal areas of exophytic growth, and have a worse prognosis.

The treatment of brain stem tumors by either surgery, radiotherapy, or chemotherapy alone or in various combinations has been disappointingly ineffective.[124,192] Most of these tumors are infiltrative, malignant intrinsic tumors that are not amenable to resection. Their diffuse nature is readily demonstrable on T2-weighted MR images, obviating the need for biopsy. The prognosis of brain stem gliomas is generally poor, with an average 5-year survival rate of approximately 10% to 30% and a median survival of less than a year. Particularly bad prognostic signs include: (1) history suggestive of onset before 6 months of age, (2) long tract signs, (3) ataxia, (4) diffusely infiltrative lesion, (5) involvement of two-thirds or more of the pons. Generally, pontine gliomas, which tend to be diffuse and infiltrative, have a poorer prognosis than mesencephalic or medullary gliomas. In contrast, low-grade tumors located in the medulla or midbrain, exophytic tumors, and those that are associated with neurofibromatosis are associated with improved survival.

Tumors of the Pineal Region

Tumors of the pineal region are relatively rare but disproportionately important from the neuro-ophthalmologic standpoint by virtue of their location. Pineal region tumors are classified into those that are derived from the pineal gland parenchyma, those that are of germ cell origin, and those representing other histological types not related to the previous two.[39,106,121,194] Pineal gland tumors include pineocytomas and pinealoblastomas.[130] Germ cell tumors include germinomas, choriocarcinomas, embryonal cell carcinomas, endodermal sinus tumors, and teratomas. Tumors derived from contiguous structures include quadrigeminal plate gliomas, gangliogliomas, ganglioneuromas, and meningiomas. Dermoids and epidermoids as well as other tumors also occur in this region.[293] The diversity of tumor histology reflects the diversity of anatomic sites from which the neoplasm may arise (e.g., the pineal gland, brain parenchyma, and dura).

The most common tumors in this location are germ cell tumors, which arise from midline rests of multipotential germinal cells.[131,193,400] Germ cell tumors thus occur primarily in the midline and are

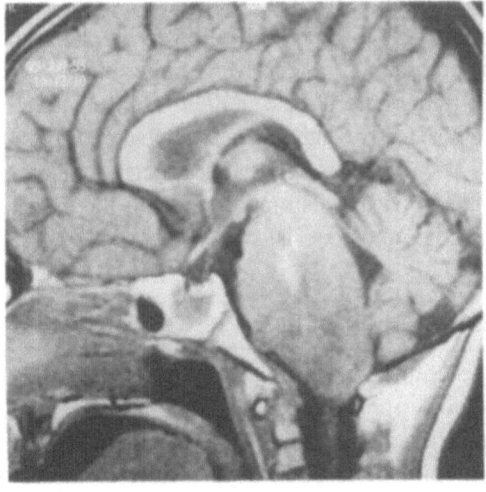

A

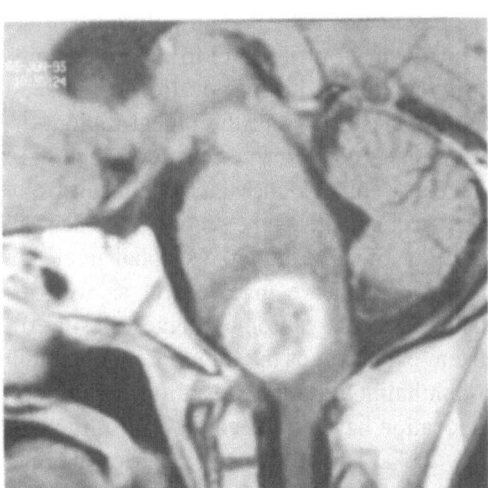

B

FIGURE 11.14. Brain stem glioma. (A) MR scan of large pontomedullary glioma. (B) Pontomedullary glioma with gadolinium enhancement of the largely medullary mass.

found in the pineal region, cistern, or both. Germinomas and teratomas are the least malignant and have the best overall prognosis. Teratomas consist of elements derived from all three germinal layers, usually present within the first six months of life and occasionally present at birth. Choriocarcinomas, embryonal carcinomas, and endodermal sinus tumors are more malignant tumors.

Germinomas represent at least 50% of all pineal region tumors. They are identical histologically to those found in the gonads, abdomen, and chest. Germinomas usually occur in the second decade of life and show slight male predominance. When germinomas occur in the suprasellar area, no gender predilection is noted. Microscopically, germinomas consist of two cell types, large vesicular cells and small cells resembling lymphocytes. Mitotic activity is confined to the larger cell type. Germinomas may contain elements of other germ cell tumors and are then referred to as mixed germ cell tumors.

The clinical presentation of pineal region tumors is variable and depends upon the location of the tumor at the time of diagnosis. The most common presentations of tumors in this location are hydrocephalus due to compression of the sylvian aqueduct,[294] and the dorsal midbrain syndrome (Parinaud syndrome) due to compression of the dorsal mesencephalon. The dorsal midbrain syndrome manifests as lid retraction, pupillary light-near dissociation, impaired upward gaze, and convergence-retraction nystagmus. Visual loss, bitemporal hemianopia, diabetes insipidus, precocious puberty, and failure to thrive imply involvement of the anterior hypothalamus by a primary tumor in this location or as secondary to metastasis from the pineal region.[220] Pineal tumors are one of the few neuro-ophthalmologic causes of *myopia*, which can result from increased accomodative tone secondary to central disinhibition of the Edinger–Westphal nucleus. Multiple cranial nerve involvement as well as various brain stem syndromes suggest basilar or brain stem extension of the tumor. Less common neuro-ophthalmologic manifestations of tumors in this location have also been described, including skew deviation and bilateral superior oblique palsy due to compression of the decussating fourth cranial nerves. Pineal germinomas may also cause visual loss by direct seeding of the optic nerve or chiasm.[240]

The germ cell tumors often produce biological markers that are detectable in the blood or the CSF. Endodermal sinus tumors elaborate Alpha-fetoprotein, choriocarcinomas produce the beta subunit of human chorionic gonadotropin, and embryonal carcinoma produce both markers.[196] Germinomas and teratomas are generally devoid of markers. These markers are helpful in establishing the diagnosis and monitoring of treatment response (markers decrease or disappear) and tumor recurrence (markers re-emerge).

The neuroimaging modality of choice for this region is contrast-enhanced MR imaging (Figure 11.15);[362] however, the histologic diagnosis is difficult to infer by neuroimaging alone. Germinomas tend to be well defined and to show homogeneous enhancement, while pinealoblastomas and pineocytomas tend to have a mixed signal on T1-weighted images, hyperintense signal on T2-weighted images, and variable enhancement. The definitive diagnosis is made only after tumor resection and histopathologic examination although the diagnosis can be inferred by neuroimaging if positive markers are also present.

The treatment of pineal region tumors depends to a large measure on the tumor histology. Benign teratomas, dermoid cysts, and pineocytomas can be cured with surgery alone. Because of their exquisite chemosensitivity and radiosensitivity, pure germinomas are associated with at least an 80% long-term survival rate.[156] The treatment of other germ cell tumors entails surgical debulking and shunting if needed, followed by staging of the tumor. This is generally followed by chemotherapy and radiation. However, nongerminoma germ cell tumors are largely neither radiosensitive nor chemosensitive and generally have a poor prognosis. The overall prognosis of affected patients depends upon the histologic type and the extent of the tumor at diagnosis.

Epidermoids and Dermoids

These tumors occur relatively more frequently in the posterior fossa. As the name implies, epidermoids are derived from epidermal elements (squamus epithelium with keratin) while dermoids are derived from epidermal as well as dermal components (have additional pilosebaceous structures). They represent congenital rests of tissue that are

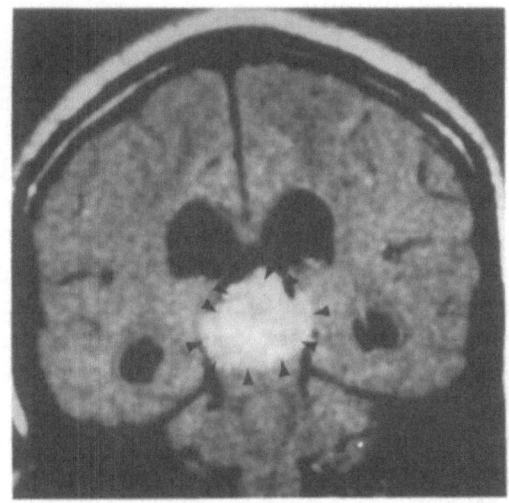

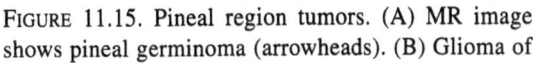

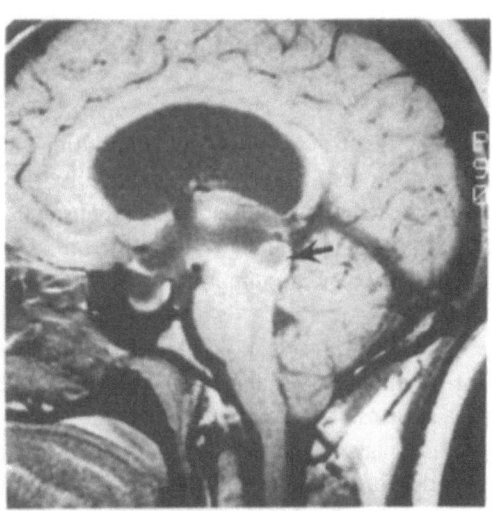

FIGURE 11.15. Pineal region tumors. (A) MR image shows pineal germinoma (arrowheads). (B) Glioma of the quadrigeminal plate (arrow) causing aqueductal occlusion and hydrocephalus.

retained intracranially due to incomplete separation of neuroectoderm from surface ectoderm during neural tube closure.

The clinical presentation of these tumors varies with their location. The most common location of epidermoids is the cerebellopontine angle, followed by the pineal region, the suprasellar area, and the middle cranial fossa. Epidermoids in the cerebellopontine angle usually present with cranial neuropathies, suprasellar epidermoids tend to present with hydrocephalus, whereas middle cranial fossa epidermoids often present with aseptic meningitis secondary to leakage of epidermoid contents into the subarachnoid space. Dermoids are less common than epidermoids within the intracranial cavity and tend to occur in the posterior fossa (within the vermis or the fourth ventricle).

Metastasis

Unlike adult tumors, extracranial tumors rarely metastasize to the intracranial compartment in children. However, seeding of certain brain tumors in children occurs often along the CSF pathways, causing invasion of the leptomeninges.[350] "Drop metastasis" to the spinal subarachnoid space and cauda equina can occur. Seeding and spinal drop metastasis occur most commonly in medulloblastoma (one-third of cases) but also in other tumors such as ependymomas, germinomas, pinealoblastmas, and anaplastic gliomas.

Complications of Treatment of Intracranial Tumors in Children

One of the key concerns in the treatment of brain tumors in children is the adverse effect of irradiation on the developing brain. The glial and vascular endothelial cells are more radiosensitive than neurons, explaining the nature of the delayed brain response to radiation, namely, vascular occlusion. The parameters that increase the extent and likelihood of irradiation damage include a younger age of the patient, deeper path of radiation, a larger overall volume of brain irradiated, the presence of hydrocephalus, and the overall dose of radiation administered as well as its fractionation. Reduced radiation dose is particularly necessary in very young children because of the immaturity of the brain and the predisposition to develop postirradiation vaso-occlusive disease. Concurrent administration of chemotherapy (e.g., methotrexate) may potentiate the adverse effects of radiation on the brain. Trials of preradiation chemotherapy are now used in infants and young children to obviate or delay subsequent radiation therapy.

One of the most significant delayed effects of radiation is a reduction of the level of cognitive function in both the neuropsychologic and intellectual spheres.[157,217] A significant proportion of these children show a significant diminution in their IQ, which may appear many years after the conclusion of radiotherapy. Endocrine abnormalities and cranial neuropathies can result from cranial radiation. Secondary tumors may also arise or near the site of irradiation.

One particular presentation of postirradiation damage in children is Moyamoya disease. Moyamoya, a Japanese word meaning "something hazy like a puff of cigarette smoke drifting in the air," is a descriptive name applied to the angiographic finding of an abnormal network of collateral vessels at the base of the brain in the region of the basal ganglia. Most authors consider occlusive vasculopathy of the internal carotid artery and/or the proximal portion of the anterior or middle cerebral arteries to be the primary condition and the abnormal network of vessels to be a result of it. Moyamoya disease is a progressive disorder that has been described with basal meningitis, tumor, neurofibromatosis, atherosclerosis, connective tissue disease, sickle cell disease, Fanconi anemia, Down syndrome, and following radiation of the brain between 6 months and 12 years of age.[280] Children with Moyamoya disease usually present with recurrent transient cerebral ischemic attacks and infarctions (hemiplegia, paresthesia, seizures). Actions requiring hyperventillation, such as crying, running, and inflating balloons, are known to precipitate cerebral ischemia in patients with Moyamoya disease. neuro-ophthalmologic features of Moyamoya disease are more common in children with Moyamoya disease than in adults and usually arise from involvement of the posterior cerebral circulation. These include visual field defects (most commonly homonymous hemianopia), decreased visual acuity, blurred vision, episodic blindness, and scintillating scotomata.[258] In one series of 178 patients, visual symptoms were found in 43 (24.1%) of cases.[258] Children at risk of Moyamoya disease who present with a suggestive history such as scintillating scotomata or other transient visual disturbances should undergo prompt evaluation since cerebral vascular bypass may forestall or prevent permanent visual loss.[258]

Hydrocephalus

Hydrocephalus, in the broadest sense, denotes an increased amount of CSF in the cerebral ventricles, as opposed to local fluid accumulation in subdural hygromas, arachnoid cysts, or within tissue defects (e.g., porencephalic cyst). It results from impaired CSF circulation, reabsorption, or hypersecretion. Most of the CSF is produced within the ventricular system by the choroid plexus. The flow of CSF may be traced as it leaves the lateral ventricles passing through the foramina of Monro to the third ventricle, then through the sylvian aqueduct to the fourth ventricle. The CSF then exits the ventricular system by passing through the foramina of Magendie and Luschka into the cisterna magna and the basilar cistern. Most of the fluid then enters the cisternal system (suprasellar cistern, cistern of the lamina terminalis, ambient cistern, superior cerebellar cistern) before flowing into the cerebral subarachnoid space. The remainder of the fluid enters the spinal subarachnoid space but also eventually flows into the cerebral subarachnoid space.

The drainage of CSF occurs via absorption through the arachnoid villi, which are evaginations of the subarachnoid space into the lumina of the dural and cerebral venous sinuses. Alternate pathways of absorption most likely also exist, such as absorption through cerebral lymphatics or capillaries.

The extent of ventricular enlargement as a result of increased CSF pressure partially depends on the age of the patient (and hence the distensibility of the ventricular system). Except for the rare occurrence of choroid plexus papilloma,[123] hydrocephalus generally results from impaired CSF flow and absorption (obstructive hydrocephalus). Impaired drainage may occur as a result of blockage within the ventricles, the cisterns, the cerebral convexities, or the arachnoid villi. Thus, obstructive hydrocephalus is divided into communicating hydrocephalus, in which there is either extraventricular obstruction of CSF flow or diminished absorption of CSF, and noncommunicating hydrocephalus, in which the obstruction is within the ventricles, including the outlet foramina of the fourth ventricle.

Several terms pertaining to hydrocephalus warrant clarification. *Normal pressure hydrocephalus* is a form of hydrocephalus in which signs of progressive hydrocephalus exist despite the fact that the CSF pressure is within the normal range. It is most commonly encountered as a sequelae of meningitis or perinatal asphyxia. Intermittent spikes of high pressure may be responsible, requiring intracranial pressure monitoring. The term *arrested hydrocephalus* describes a disorder in which the hydrocephalus has spontaneously resolved, although some residual clinical signs may persist (e.g, enlarged head size). The term *hydrocephalus ex vacuo* is used to describe the situation where enlarged ventricles result from periventricular white matter destruction rather than actual hydrocephalus. *Hydranencephaly* refers to a situation where most of the brain has been destroyed in utero and resorbed, being replaced by a CSF-filled sac. It should be emphasized that these mechanisms of ventricular dilation are not mutually exclusive. For example, long-standing hydrocephalus due to increased intracranial pressure eventually causes periventricular tissue damage and hemispheric atrophy. Conversely, hydranencephaly may become complicated by secondary impairment of CSF circulation, causing increased intracranial pressure.

Hydrocephalus due to CSF Overproduction

This is exclusively produced by choroid plexus papilloma, which is a rare neoplasm, accounting for 2% to 4% of childhood intracranial tumors. Nearly half of these tumors occur within the first decade of life with many occurring in infancy. These papillomas occur in infants, most frequently in the lateral ventricles, occasionally in the third, and rarely in the fourth ventricle. This distribution pattern is reversed in older patients. These papillomas can produce huge amounts of CSF and present during infancy with signs of intracranial hypertension. The tumors most commonly originate within the trigones of the lateral ventricles. Resection of the tumor is curative for the hydrocephalus.

Noncommunicating Hydrocephalus

Noncommunicating hydrocephalus arises from a variety of lesions that cause blockage of CSF flow within the ventricular system at any level from the foramena of Monro to the foramina of Magendie and Luschka. Underlying disorders include tumors, aqueductal stenosis, aqueductal gliosis, arachnoid cysts, congenital anomalies, and isolated fourth ventricle. Tumors are the most common cause of this type of hydrocephalus.

Communicating Hydrocephalus

Communicating hydrocephalus results from extraventricular obstruction of CSF flow or reabsorption. After the CSF exits the ventricular system through the foramina of the fourth ventricle, it enters the cisterna magna and basilar cisterns then flows into the subarachnoid space. CSF drainage may be impaired within the cisterns, or when the arachnoid villi are obstructed. Causative disorders include intraventricular hemorrhage, meningitis, CSF seeding of tumor, cerebral venous sinus thrombosis, and normal pressure hydrocephalus.

From the neuro-ophthalmologic standpoint, noncommunicating hydrocephalus is much more likely to cause impaired upgaze and the various features of the dorsal midbrain syndrome than the communicating variety, with most of these cases being due to developmental or acquired aqueductal stenosis.[356]

Common Causes of Hydrocephalus in Children

The common causes of hydrocephalus in the pediatric age group are summarized in Table 11.1 according to the age of onset.

Aqueductal Stenosis

Normally, the sylvian aqueduct in the newborn measures 3 mm in length and an average of 0.5 mm in cross section. The cerebral aqueduct is the most common site of ventricular obstruction of CSF flow, being the longest and narrowest passage. Complete obstruction of the aqueduct is re-

TABLE 11.1. Common causes of hydrocephalus in the pediatric age group.

Before the age of 2 years
Aqueduct stenosis
Aqueductal gliosis (infection or hemorrhage)
Chiari malformations (+/– myelomeningocele)
Dandy-Walker malformation
Perinatal asphyxia, hemorrhage (premature infants)
Intrauterine infection
Neonatal meningoencephalitis
Congenital midline tumors
Choroid plexus papilloma
Vein of Galen malformation
Congenital idiopathic
After the age of 2 years
Posterior fossa neoplasms
Aqueductal stenosis, gliosis, obstruction
Chiari I malformation
Intracranial hemorrhage
Intracranial infections
Idiopathic

ferred to as atresia, incomplete obstruction as stenosis. In aqueductal stenosis, focal narrowing generally occurs either at the level of the superior colliculi or the intercollicular sulcus. Aqueductal stenosis occurs as a developmental abnormality or an acquired lesion due to obstruction of the sylvian aqueduct most often by tumor (e.g., tumors of the pineal gland or midbrain).[294] When the aqueduct is obstructed after perinatal hemorrhage, meningitis, or other inflammatory disorder, the term aqueductal gliosis is used. The developmental variety of aqueductal stenosis accounts for approximately 20% of cases of hydrocephalus. Less common causes of aqueductal stenosis or obstruction include systemic viral infections (e.g., mononucleosis, mumps),[92,278] intracranial toxoplasmosis,[387] basilar dolichoectasia,[56] and mesencephalic venous malformations.[279] Nontumoral aqueductal stenosis may occur in patients with NF-I.[150] A rare X-linked, genetic syndrome combines the features of aqueductal stenosis with hydrocephalus, macrocephaly, adducted thumbs, spasticity, mental retardation, and cerebral malformations (usually agenesis of corpus callosum).[336] This is usually diagnosed at birth or prenatally by ultrasound and is regularly lethal.[335] A rarer form of aqueductal stenosis inherited as an autosomal recessive disorder has also been described.[35]

The onset of symptoms in both aqueductal stenosis and gliosis is usually insidious. Patients may become symptomatic at any age from birth to adulthood.[310] Neuroimaging shows dilation of the lateral and third ventricles but a normal-sized fourth ventricle.

Aqueductal stenosis is often accompanied by aqueductal forking, or branching of the aqueductal channel. Developmental aqueductal stenosis may be associated with fusion of the quadrigeminal bodies, fusion of the oculomotor nuclei, peaking of the tectum, and spina bifida cystica and occulta.

One rare cause of hydrocephalus due to obstruction of the sylvian aqueduct in children is an arteriovenous aneurysm involving the great vein of Galen (vein of Galen "aneurysm") (Figure 11.16).[405] This malformation arises from a congenital connection between intracranial vessels (usually thalamoperforator, choroidal, and anterior cerebral artery) and a vein in the region of the vein of Galen. This abnormal vascular communication produces aneurysmal dilatation of the short vein of Galen, located just behind the posterior wall of the third ventricle. The most common presenting symptom in children below 2 years of age is hydrocephalus. Neonates may present with congestive heart failure and loud intracranial bruits.

Tumors

Tumors are the most common cause of noncommunicating hydrocephalus (obstruction of CSF flow within the ventricular system) in children. The sites of obstruction are most commonly those where the ventricular pathways are narrowest: the foramina of Monro, the sylvian aqueduct, the fourth ventricle, and the foramina of Magendie and Luschka. The location and size of the tumor are significant determinants for the development of hydrocephalus, but tumor size alone is less important. For example, large pontine gliomas are only infrequently associated with hydrocephalus, but tectal gliomas uniformly present with hydrocephalus. Tumors may also cause increased intracranial pressure by causing brain edema and swelling and by compression of the cerebral venous sinuses.

Intracranial Hemorrhage

Intraventricular hemorrhage arising from the subependymal germinal matrix, with subsequent rupture into the lateral ventricle, is the most com-

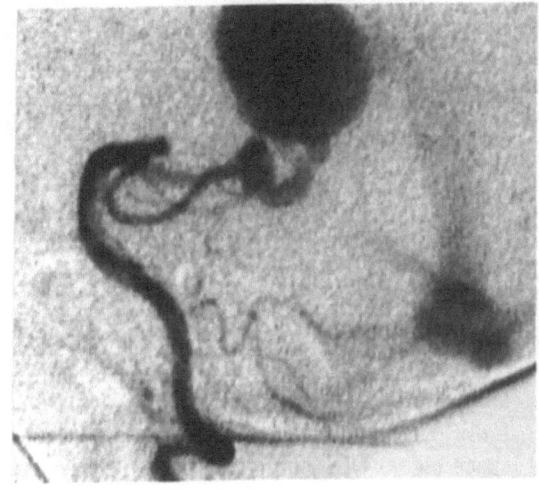
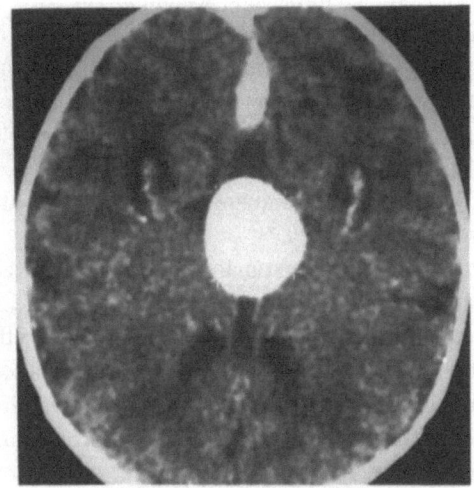

FIGURE 11.16. Vein of Galen malformation. (A) Cerebral angiography in a 4-day-old female infant with a prenatal diagnosis of vein of Galen malformation. (B) Computed tomography scan in the same infant.

mon variety of intracranial hemorrhages and are characteristic of premature infants. This form of hemorrhage usually arises postnatally, less commonly perinatally, and rarely prenatally.[376,377] The subependymal germinal matrix, a cellular structure located immediately ventrolateral to the lateral ventricle, is a source of cerebral neuroblasts between 10 and 20 weeks of gestation as well as a source of glioblasts (progenitors of cerebral oligodendroglia and astrocytes) in the third trimester. The numerous thin-walled blood vessels within the germinal matrix are a ready source of bleeding. The most common site of bleeding is just posterior to the foramen of Monro. The blood spreads from one or both lateral ventricles into the third and fourth ventricles and the basal cisterns. It enters the cerebral and spinal subarachnoid space where it may incite an obliterative arachnoiditis with obstruction of CSF flow. Impaired CSF dynamics may also occur at the level of the sylvian aqueduct and the arachnoid villi.

This form of intracranial hemorrhage is responsible for an increasing proportion of pediatric hydrocephalus, as advances in neonatology enable us to salvage an increasingly number of premature infants. Hydrocephalus is considered the main complication of intraventricular hemorrhage, with periventricular hemorrhagic infarction and germinal matrix destruction being additional common complications. The likelihood of and the rapidity of progression of hydrocephalus after intraventricular hemorrhage are directly related to the quantity of intraventricular blood.[378] Large hemorrhages lead to hydrocephalus within days, while smaller hemorrhages lead to hydrocephalus over weeks. Acute obstructive hydrocephalus may arise from hematoma clogging the basal cisterns or the arachnoid villi. Later, an adhesive arachnoiditis develops that perpetuates the hydrocephalus long after the red blood cells break down. Another mechanism is organization of an intraventricular hematoma with reactive gliosis of the ventricular wall.

The pathogenesis of germinal matrix hemorrhage and subsequent intraventricular hemorrhage in premature children is multifactorial and is related to intravascular, vascular, and extravascular factors.[376] Intravascular factors pertain to control of blood flow and pressure within the germinal matrix and include fluctuations of cerebral blood flow, abrupt increases or decreases of flow, increased cerebral venous pressure, and in selected infants disturbances of platelet function. Vascular factors pertain to the microcirculation of the germinal matrix and include vulnerability of the matrix vessels to ischemic injury. Extravascular factors include the mesenchymal and glial support for the germinal matrix vessels and the local fibrinolytic activity in the germinal matrix.[376,377]

The imaging procedure of choice to detect intraventricular hemorrhage in a premature infant is real-time cranial ultrasound scanning. The severity of intraventricular hemorrhage may be graded by ultrasound criteria. Grade I denotes a germinal matrix hemorrhage with intraventricular hemorrhage involving less than 10% of the ventricular area on parasagittal views, grade II involves 10% to 50% of that area, and grade III involves greater than 50% of that area.[377]

Periventricular leukomalacia is a frequent accompaniment of intraventricular hemorrhage in premature infants but is not causally related to the hemorrhage. Their occurrence in the same patient complicates the clinical picture, especially if hydrocephalus also exists, since both processes are characterized by enlarged ventricular size, in hydrocephalus due to elevated CSF pressure and in periventricular leukomalacia due to ischemic dropout of periventricular white matter.

In full-term infants, intracranial hemorrhage occurs most frequently after trauma. Intraventricular hemorrhage is less common than in premature infants, and the incidence of hydrocephalus due to this complication is therefore much less in the full-term infant. It may arise from extension of a hemorrhagic cerebral infarction or a thalamic hemorrhage, vascular malformation, tumor, trauma, residual germinal matrix, or a choroid plexus hemorrhage.

Intracranial Infections

Various infectious processes involving the intracranial compartment may result in hydrocephalus. Bacterial, viral, and fungal meningitis and various protozoan and parasitic infections of the brain may be associated with or followed by hydrocephalus. Brain abscesses may occasionally cause hydrocephalus and/or homonymous hemianopia. Congenital infections of the CNS (congenital toxoplasmosis, cytomegalovirus, varicella, and herpes simplex virus) may occasionally manifest with hydrocephalus.

The hydrocephalus may result from more than one mechanism in any given infection. For instance, neurocysticercosis (infestation of the brain by the larval form of Taenia solium) may cause hydrocephalus by obstruction of the CSF pathways with cysts, by leptomeningitis, or by the mass effect and associated edema of intraparenchymal cysts.[399] Intracranial hydatid cysts

due to Echinococcus granulosus infections often manifest with signs and symptoms of hydrocephalus in endemic areas.[126] Granulomatous meningitis (e.g., tuberculous meningitis) is more likely to cause hydrocephalus than bacterial meningitis, which is more likely to cause it than viral meningitis. Meningitis causes hydrocephalus acutely by a combination of blockage of the CSF pathways by purulent exudates and by involvement of the arachnoid granulations in the infectious process. Cerebral abscesses and cerebral venous sinus thrombosis may complicate meningitis and contribute to the production of hydrocephalus. Later, fibrosis and scarring of the subarachnoid space blocks CSF outflow. Clogging of the arachnoid granulations by debris may play a role. Subclinical virus infections may cause "noninflammatory" aqueductal stenosis and hydrocephalus. Rarely, neurosarcoidosis may underlie the manifestation of hydrocephalus in children.[384]

Two other infectious diseases are particularly noteworthy, namely, AIDS and Lyme disease. Lyme disease, a multisystem disease caused by *Borrelia burgdorferi,* a tick-borne spirochete, commonly affects children.[43] The disorder causes various ophthalmic manifestations, including cranial neuropathies, iridocyclitis, vitritis, pars planitis, orbital myositis, keratitis, episcleritis, conjunctivitis, and optic neuritis.[15] The disease may manifest as a meningitis, a meningoencephalitis, or an isolated cranial neuropathy. In some patients, the disorder may resemble pseudotumor cerebri.[43] AIDS also occurs in children and can present with increased intracranial pressure due to various underlying lesions (lymphomas, infections), but these intracranial lesions tend to be rare in children with AIDS as compared to adults.[295]

Chiari Malformations

Chiari malformations are characterized by herniation of the posterior fossa contents below the level of the foramen magnum. They are categorized into three types based upon the degree of herniation.[119] The treatment is generally directed at the posterior fossa pathology and includes decompression of the cervicomedullary junction, posterior decompressive procedures (e.g., opening of outlet foramina of the fourth ventricle, fourth ventricular shunting), and ventriculoperitoneal shunting.

Generally, the major presenting symptoms of the Chiari malformations are weakness, pain, dissociative sensory loss, and headache. The symptoms and signs of Chiari malformations are largely a result of impaction of the posterior fossa contents at the foramen magnum, abnormal CSF dynamics at the craniocervical junction, as well as the associated hydrocephalus and syringomyelia.

Chiari I

This malformation is characterized by protrusion of the cerebellar tonsils below the level of the foramen magnum (Figure 11.17). It may be observed in several clinically different settings: (1) Some infants may develop herniation of the cerebellar tonsils as a result of intrauterine hydrocephalus. These cases are usually diagnosed with hydrocephalus in infancy or early childhood. (2) Some patients may have craniocervical dysgenesis (e.g., Klippel–Feil anomaly). This group often have concurrent platybasia and cervical vertebral abnormalities and usually present during childhood with headaches when straining and with cranial nerve palsies. (3) Some

patients may have acquired deformities of the foramen magnum (e.g., basilar invagination). They are generally asymptomatic during childhood but present during adulthood with symptoms and signs similar to group 2 above. (4) Some patients develop Chiari I as a result of lumbo-peritoneal shunting and may show resolution of the abnormalities after shunt removal.

In Chiari malformations, hydrocephalus generally results from lack of communication between the spinal subarachnoid space and the cranial subarachnoid space. The herniated fourth ventricle communicates with the spinal subarachnoid space, but the latter does not communicate with the cranial subarachnoid space. The two subarachnoid compartments are separated by the impacted cerebellar tissue.

Approximately 50% of patients with Chiari I malformation have concurrent syringomyelia. Symptoms of Chiari I may be intermittent and may simulate those of multiple sclerosis. The diagnosis of Chiari I malformation should be suspected in any patient with intermittent sensorineural hearing loss, headache, vertigo, oscillopsia, ataxia, disequilibrium, or dysphagia, especially if these symptoms coexist with other more characteristic symptoms of the disorder such as cervical pain or weakness.[331]

Neuro-ophthalmologic abnormalities reported in Chiari I malformation include the various disorders associated with increased intracranial pressure (if it coexists). An acquired downbeat nystagmus is the classical neuro-ophthalmologic finding associated with Chiari I malformation, but other types of nystagmus may occur (discussed later). It should be noted that some of the abnormalities associated with Chiari I malformation may be intermittent, causing a diagnostic quandary. Intermittent abnormalities include symptoms of increased intracranial pressure,[379] oscillopsia, and downbeat nystagmus.[401] A case of convergence nystagmus has been reported wherein the nystagmus was provoked by a Valsalva maneuver with neck flexion or extension; the nystagmus diminished on deep inspiration.[264] Precipitation of nystagmus by Valsalva maneuver or neck movements suggests intermittent rise in intracranial pressure as the cause, as was documented by intraventricular monitoring in one patient.[379] Although downbeat nystagmus is the most common cause of oscillop-

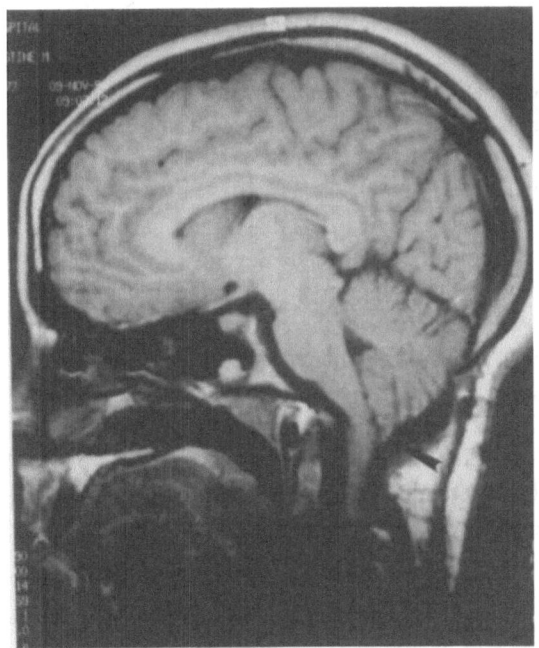

FIGURE 11.17. Chiari I malformation. MR image shows that the cerebellar tonsils extend 1 cm below the level of the foramen magnum.

sia in this disorder, oscillopsia can also occur in the absence of nystagmus.[155]

The various eye movement disorders in Chiari I malformation largely result from cerebellar ectopia and lower brain stem distortion. Periodic alternating nystagmus, which also localizes a lesion to the level of the foramen magnum,[20] has been reported. Interestingly, seesaw nystagmus (which usually localizes to the diencephalon or parasellar region)[406] and convergence retraction nystagmus (which localizes to the pretectal area of the midbrain) have also been described. Another case with signs localizing to the midbrain was reported by Cogan who described a patient in whom neck extension regularly induced spasm of the near reflex and an exacerbation of the downbeat nystagmus that lasted several seconds after the head was returned to the primary position.[87] Another patient with a Chiari I malformation and spasm of the near reflex has since been reported.[100]

Other neuro-ophthalmologic disorders include Horner syndrome (due to associated spinal cord syringomyelia),[352] comitant strabismus, fourth nerve palsy, skew deviation, ocular dysmetria, ocular flutter, and various neuro-otologic abnormalities also occur.[383]

Acquired, nonparalytic esotropia is a rare presentation of Chiari I malformation. Bixenman and Laguna[49] described a 13-year-old girl who developed comitant esotropia that was successfully treated with strabismus surgery. Three years later, downbeat nystagmus developed and Chiari I malformation was diagnosed with MR imaging. The nystagmus resolved, and the eyes remained aligned after neurosurgical decompression. Passo et al[289] described a similar patient who was initially treated with strabismus surgery. After recurrence of esotropia and development of downbeat nystagmus, Chiari I malformation was diagnosed. In this patient, neurosurgical decompression of the posterior fossa restored ocular alignment and single binocular vision. Before diagnosis of comitant esotropia in this setting, subtle bilateral fourth nerve palsy should be ruled out.

In addition to comitant vertical strabismus, posterior fossa disease may also precipitate comitant strabismus that is purely horizontal. In its current usage, the rubric *skew deviation* is a descriptive term that is applied only to certain forms of acquired vertical strabismus which are precipitated by posterior fossa disease. The term connotes no specific pathophysiological mechanism. In light of recent reports, it would seem appropriate to expand our concept of skew deviation to include horizontal cases of acquired comitant esotropia that are increasingly recognized to accompany the Arnold–Chiari malformations and posterior fossa tumors in some children. Like its vertical counterpart, *horizontal skew deviation* may be precipitated by a supranuclear perturbance of the ocular motor system, neurological disruption of fusion, or a combination of the two.

Neuro-ophthalmologic symptoms and signs associated with Chiari I malformation often stabilize, improve, or resolve after suboccipital craniotomy.[347,406]

Chiari II

Chiari II malformation, the Arnold–Chiari malformation, is the most common of the Chiari malformations in the pediatric age group. It is a highly complex malformation that is almost exclusively present in children with myelomeningocele. It can show any of the infratentorial features of Chiari I malformation but it differs by involving supratentorial structures as well (Figure 11.18). Ninety percent of cases of Chiari II malformation occur in association with myelomeningocele and hydrocephalus. Conversely, all patients with myelomeningocele and hydrocephalus harbor a Chiari II malformation.

Patients are usually diagnosed at birth with myelomeningocele and develop hydrocephalus shortly after its repair. After the repair of the myelomeningocele, the clinical presentation to be expected from the underlying Chiari II malformation as well as the associated hydrocephalus, lower cranial nerve palsies, and syringomyelia may differ according to the age of the child. Patients younger than 6 months tend to present with stridor, apnea, and/or dysphagia (feeding difficulty) while children older than 3 years of age tend to present with hemiparesis, quadriparesis, oscillopsia, nystagmus, or opisthotonos.[41,42,180] Chiari II malformation accounts for approximately 40% of all hydrocephalic children, and hydrocephalus develops in approximately 85% of patients with myelomeningoceles.[111]

The cause of the myelomeningocele and associated Chiari II malformation is theorized to be lack

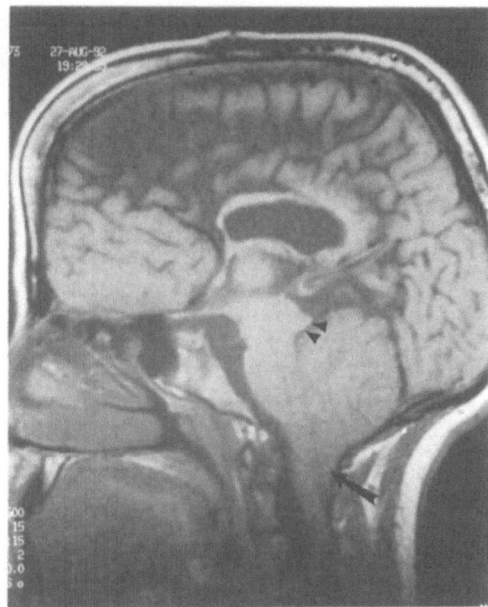
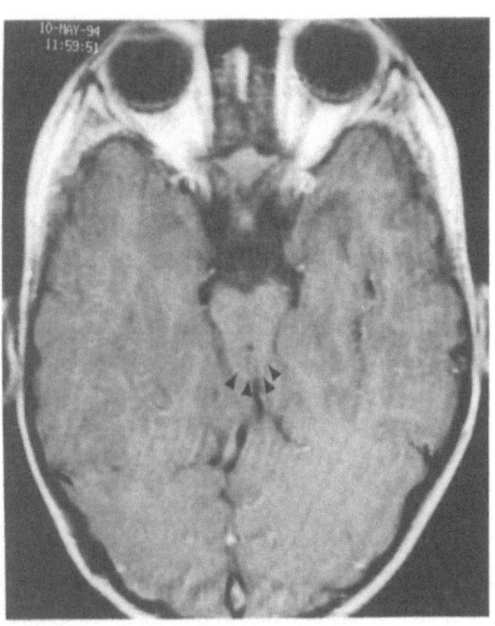

FIGURE 11.18. Chiari II malformation. (A) Sagittal MR scan shows extension of the cerebellar tonsils below the level of the foramen magnum (arrow) as well as tectal beaking (arrowheads). (B) Axial MR scan shows tectal beaking (arrowheads).

of expression of carbohydrate molecules on the surface of neural cells in the developing neural tube.[249] These surface molecules are required for neural tube closure as well as expansion of the central canal that eventually leads to formation of the cerebral ventricles. The absence or incorrect expression of these molecules leads to failure of closure of the posterior neuropore and failure of expansion of the cerebral ventricles, which in turn leads to the formation of an abnormally small posterior fossa. This causes the normally developing cerebellum to be squeezed out of the posterior fossa as it grows, getting indented in the process by the tentorium superiorly and the foramen magnum inferiorly. Hydrocephalus in Chiari II malformation is presumed to result from abnormal location of the foramina of the fourth ventricle below the foramen magnum, and associated poor communication between the cerebral and lumbar subarachnoid space.

Affected patients show a wide constellation of abnormalities that vary in severity. Mild cases show only minimal hindbrain abnormalities and may be confused with Chiari I malformation, but the concurrent myelomeningocele and supratentorial abnormalities are not features of Chiari I. The mesencephalic tectum is often distorted, being stretched posteriorly and inferiorly. This appears as tectal "beaking" on CT or MR scans. The pons, medulla, and cervical spinal cord are stretched inferiorly. There is a high incidence of associated syringomyelia that may lead to the formation of a characteristic cervicomedullary kink. The cerebellum may extend anteriorly to encircle the brain stem. The cerebellar vermis usually herniates into the cervical spinal canal and may subsequently degenerate, leading in severe cases to nearly total absence of the cerebellum on neuroimaging. The fourth ventricle is usually small, low-lying, narrow, and vertically-oriented. It may become encysted or isolated. Supratentorial abnormalities include an absent rostrum and an absent or hypoplastic splenium of the corpus callosum, prominent occipital horns, and abnormal gyral pattern in the medial aspect of the occipital lobes on MR imaging.

Neuro-ophthalmologic abnormalities described in Chiari II malformation include the various signs and symptoms related to the associated hydrocephalus, myelomeningocele, and syringomyelia.[47,133,148] These patients have a propensity to develop A-pattern strabismus with superior oblique overaction,[222,223] probably representing a form of alternating skew deviation on lateral gaze.[169–172] Pathological studies on patients with myelomeningocele and Chiari II malformation have shown disorganized brain stem nuclei,[153] a feature that may explain the propensity of these children to show this type of skew deviation. Other reported abnormalities include internuclear ophthalmoplegia,[14,273,397] defective smooth pursuit and optokinetic nystagmus, and Horner syndrome. Staudenmaier and Buncic[351] described a 4-year-old boy with Chiari II who had periodic alternating gaze deviation.

Chiari III

This is an exceedingly rare malformation in which the contents of the posterior fossa (cerebellum +/– brain stem) herniate through a cervical spina bifida cystica at the level of C1-C2. Hydrocephalus is a regular feature of this malformation.

The Dandy–Walker Malformation

The disorders called Dandy–Walker malformation, Dandy–Walker variant, and mega cisterna magna are considered to represent a continuum of developmental anomalies and are collectively designated as the Dandy–Walker complex by Barkovich et al (Figure 11.19).[25] The Dandy–Walker malformation is classically characterized by the neuropathologic triad of (1) complete or partial agenesis of the cerebellar vermis, involving the cortex and deep cerebellar nuclei; (2) a greatly expanded, cystic, fourth ventricle; and (3) an enlarged posterior fossa with upward displacement of the lateral sinuses, tentorium, and torcula.[221,283,288] An occipital encephalocele is also occasionally present. The Dandy–Walker malformation accounts for 2% to 4% of cases of hydrocephalus in children. The Dandy–Walker *variant* shows the above findings but with a normal-sized posterior fossa. It is more common than the true Dandy–Walker malformation and comprises about a third of posterior fossa malformations. Hydrocephalus occurs in the majority of cases but is not required to make the diagnosis. Mega cisterna magna (retrocerebellar arachnoid pouch) refers to a cystic malformation of the posterior fossa wherein the posterior fossa is enlarged secondary to enlarged cisterna magna, but

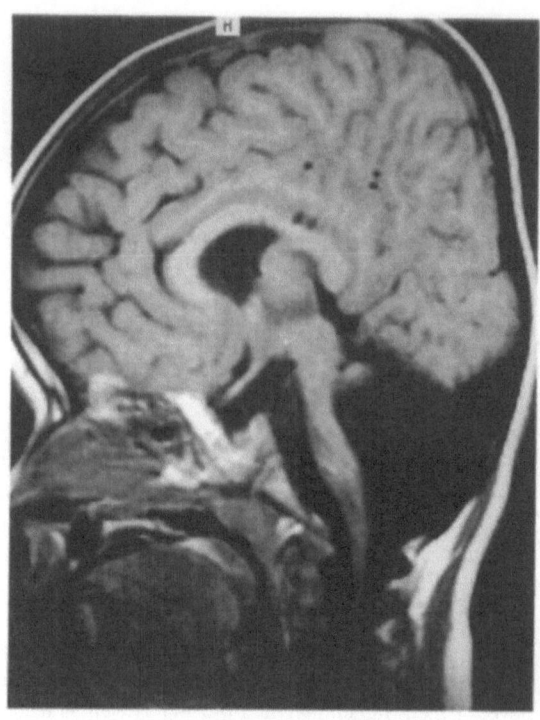

FIGURE 11.19. Dandy–Walker cyst. MR image shows replacement of most of the posterior fossa contents with a large cyst. Note attenuation of the brain stem.

the cerebellar vermis and the fourth ventricles are normal.

The majority of cases of the Dandy–Walker malformation are diagnosed within the first year of life, and most of these are diagnosed at birth. The major signs and symptoms are those of hydrocephalus as well as associated developmental delay and failure to thrive. Some features are more characteristic of Dandy–Walker malformation than other causes of hydrocephalus, such as a large occiput with a higher-than-normal inion and the predisposition of patients to show recurrent attacks of pallor, ataxia, and occasionally sudden respiratory arrest. Hydrocephalus is infrequently present at birth but appears by 3 months of age in over 75% of patients. Some patients may remain asymptomatic throughout life. Dandy–Walker syndrome must be distinguished from arachnoid cysts of the fourth ventricular roof. Although the cerebellum is essential in adults for control of many aspects of ocular motility, eye movement abnormalities in children with Dandy–Walker syndrome are often mild or absent, suggesting that other parts of the brain may be capable of taking over these roles in the developing nervous system.[221]

The Dandy–Walker malformation was originally thought to result from developmental occlusion of the exit foramina of the fourth ventricle (Magendie and Luschka) and hence classified as one of the causes of noncommunicating hydrocephalus. It is now known, however, that the foramina of the fourth ventricle are patent in many cases. More recently, this malformation has been attributed to a developmental insult to the embryonic fourth ventricle and cerebellum.[25] Most often, the Dandy–Walker malformation occurs as an isolated finding with low risk of occurrence in subsequent siblings. The risk to siblings is higher when the malformation occurs with Mendelian disorders such as Warburg syndrome, Aicardi syndrome, or with various chromosomal anomalies such as duplications of 5p, 8p, and 8q and trisomy of chromosomes 9, 13, and 18.

Oculocutaneous hypopigmentation in a child with Dandy–Walker syndrome should suggest the diagnosis of Cross syndrome (oculocutaneous hypopigmentation resembling albinism, mental retardation, spastic tetraplegia, abnormalities of the tongue and gingivae, microdontia, and generalized osteoporosis). This rare autosomal disorder is often seen in children of consanguineous parents.[224] The Dandy–Walker malformation may also be associated with hypoplasia of the corpus callosum, polymicrogyria, gray matter heterotopia, porencephaly, low set ears, malformed pinna, polydactyly, syndactyly, Klippel–Feil syndrome, Cornelia de Lange syndrome, Sjögren–Larsson syndrome[136] and cleft palate. Doubling of the optic disc has been described in one patient with a Dandy–Walker cyst.[282] Various cardiac anomalies have been reported including ventricular septal defects, patent ductus arteriosus, tetralogy of Fallot, and atrial septal defect.[283]

Congenital, Genetic, and Sporadic Disorders

In addition to the aforementioned major causes of hydrocephalus, it should also be noted that hydrocephalus occurs as a feature in numerous genetic, metabolic, neurodegenerative, and sporadic syndromes. In some syndromes, hydrocephalus is presumed to result from diminished venous out-

flow through the jugular foramena. Syndromes in which this is thought to be the underlying mechanism include the craniosynostosis (Apert syndrome, Carpenter syndrome, Pfeiffer syndrome, Crouzon syndrome),[272] achondroplasia,[215] and the Marshall–Smith syndrome (a syndrome of accelerated osseous maturation and CNS malformations).[286,319] Other disorders occasionally reported to be associated with hydrocephalus include the Walker–Warburg syndrome,[73] osteopetrosis,[338] gestational cocaine exposure, Aicardi syndrome, ring chromosome 22, the various phakomatoses, Meckel–Gruber syndrome, focal dermal hypoplasia syndrome,[8] the immotile cilia syndrome,[105,403] and numerous others. The immotile cilia syndrome is an autosomal recessive disorder with variable clinical manifestations that include recurrent respiratory infections, situs inversus, and sterility characterized by live but immotile spermatozoa. It has been occasionally reported in association with hydrocephalus. The pathogenesis of the associated hydrocephalus has not been elucidated, but some investigators believe that dysmotility of the ependymal cilia lining the ventricular system adversely affects the CSF circulation, leading to hydrocephalus in some patients. In most of the aforementioned syndromes described, the other associated anomalies lead to the correct diagnosis, but the hydrocephalus should be treated in the usual expeditious manner.

Clinical Features of Hydrocephalus

Symptoms of hydrocephalus are generally dependent upon the cause, the rate of increase in intracranial pressure, and the age of the patient at the time of onset. The presenting clinical features of hydrocephalus are legion. Although most children present with the classic signs and symptoms of intracranial hypertension, some may present only with gradual intellectual deterioration or behavioral changes or signs that suggest brain stem compression from associated Chiari malformations or spinal cord dysfunction due to tethering or syringomyelia.

The age at which hydrocephalus develops in relation to the status of the cranial sutures determines whether enlargement of the head is a presenting sign. Thus, the most notable clinical finding in hydrocephalus prior to the age of 2 years is a rapid rate of head growth. Frontal bossing, separated skull sutures, tense anterior fontanelle with occasional intercalate bones, dilated scalp veins, and sparse hair are present. In severe cases (usually aqueductal stenosis) remolding of the anterior fossa can significantly reduce orbital volume and lead to bilateral proptosis. Irritability, failure to thrive, and developmental delay are often noted. After 2 years of age, the most common presenting signs and symptoms involve focal deficits resulting from the primary lesion or nonlocalizing ones associated with increased intracranial pressure. These usually appear before any significant change in head size. Head size shows significant progressive enlargement only if the hydrocephalic process started before functional suture closure (usually 2 years of age), in which case the hydrocephalus prevents suture fusion.

The neuro-ophthalmologic manifestations of hydrocephalus have been detailed in previous chapters and are summarized in Table 11.2.[47,133,148,222,223,370] Children can present with various combinations of these findings, which may complicate the clinical picture. For example, a child may show poor vision due to both bilateral optic atrophy and cortical visual impairment, posing some difficulty in determining the weighted contribution of each to the visual deficit. Also, a patient may show dorsal midbrain syndrome and bilateral sixth nerve palsy, the latter serving to reduce or mask coexisting convergence-retraction nystagmus. Light-near dissociation is difficult to ascertain in the presence of severe bilateral optic atrophy, and other signs of the dorsal midbrain syndrome should be sought before making the diagnosis. Neuro-ophthalmologic complications are most commonly encountered in the setting of aqueductal obstruction and enlargement of the third ventricle; however, they do occur in children with communicating hydrocephalus. It is useful but not always possible to differentiate the neuro-ophthalmologic signs arising due to the hydrocephalic process itself from those caused by associated tumors, malformations, infections, etc.

Ocular Motility Disorders in Hydrocephalus

Hydrocephalus can cause horizontal diplopia by producing either unilateral or bilateral sixth nerve palsy or comitant horizontal strabismus. These findings are nonlocalizing. The sixth nerve paresis may result from a variety of causes: (1) a nonspecific response to the increased intracranial pressure, (2) traction at Dorello's canal, or (3) a result of shunt placement. Divergence paralysis, defined as comitant esotropia larger at distance than at near, has been reported as an early sign of aqueductal stenosis.[179] In the setting of increased intracranial pressure, divergence paralysis may represent mild bilateral sixth nerve palsy, but damage to a putative divergence center cannot usually be ruled out.

Unilateral or bilateral fourth nerve palsy occurs much less frequently and may be due to compression of the trochlear nerve by the tentorial margin. Bilateral fourth nerve palsy may also result from involvement of the superior medullary velum (the site of decussation of the trochlear nerves) either by tumor or by other changes brought about by the hydrocephalus itself. When

TABLE 11.2. Neuro-ophthalmologic manifestations of hydrocephalus.

Motility abnormalities
  Setting sun sign (young infants)
  Dorsal midbrain syndrome (older children)
  Comitant horizontal strabismus (esotropia, exotropia)
  Sixth cranial nerve palsy
  Fourth cranial nerve palsy
  Third cranial nerve palsy
  Skew deviation
  A-pattern esotropia
  Bilateral superior oblique muscle overaction
  Fixation instability
  V-pattern pseudobobbing
  Bobble-headed doll syndrome
  Bilateral internuclear ophthalmoplegia
Pupillary abnormalities
  Light-near dissociation
  Afferent pupillary defect
Anterior visual pathways abnormalities
  Papilledema
  Optic atrophy
  Strabismic amblyopia
  Chiasmal syndrome (dilated third ventricle)
  Optic tract syndrome (damage during shunt placement or hippocampal herniation)
  Optociliary shunt vessels
Cortical/cerebral abnormalities
  Cortical visual impairment
  Homonymous hemianopia, other visual field changes
  Higher cortical function disorders (e.g., constructional apraxia, dyscalculia, etc.)

bilateral fourth nerve palsy is found in the setting of nonneoplastic hydrocephalus, it may be a localizing sign of involvement of the superior medullary velum due to compression by a dilated aqueduct and/or downward pressure from an enlarged third ventricle. Such children typically show other neuro-ophthalmologic signs indicative of dorsal midbrain syndrome.[166]

Third nerve palsy rarely results from hydrocephalus independent of underlying causes such as tumors or infections.[370] Exotropia in hydrocephalic children more commonly results from poor vision due to optic atrophy. Both comitant esotropia and exotropia are more common in children with hydrocephalus and neurodevelopmental abnormalities.

The dorsal midbrain syndrome in hydrocephalus usually occurs with aqueductal stenosis and results from secondary dilation of the third ventricle or enlargement of the suprapineal recess with pressure on the posterior commissure.[85,284] It is also an early sign of shunt failure. The dorsal midbrain syndrome may begin with light-near dissociation with little limitation of upgaze. The pupils are moderately enlarged and contract poorly to light stimulation but more fully to a near effort. Gaze paretic upbeat nystagmus then supervenes, followed by upgaze paralysis.[91] The upgaze paralysis typically affects upward saccades more than upward pursuit, but complete paralysis of all volitional upward movements sometimes occurs. Vertical vestibulo-ocular movements are usually preserved, except in severe cases.

The exact pathophysiology of the dorsal midbrain syndrome in hydrocephalus is unknown, but plausible explanations have been detailed by Corbett.[91] The overriding factor appears to be increased periaqueductal tissue water content, due to aqueductal dilation, which results in decreased blood flow. Stretching of neural fibers may also play a role. Pupillary light-near dissociation results from dysfunction of the brachium of the superior colliculus and pretectal oculomotor fibers. Pathologic lid retraction (Collier sign) results from compression of levator inhibitory neurons within the posterior commissure by a dilated third ventricle. Paresis of upgaze results from stretching of nerve fibers and diminished blood supply to the ventral posterior commissure (upgaze center), which in turn result from increased aqueductal

size and increased periventricular water, with attendant decrease in blood flow. Convergence retraction nystagmus probably results from impairment of recurrent inhibition within the oculomotor subnuclei, which results in cofiring of the rectus muscles. It is not true nystagmus and is composed of opposing adducting saccades.

A variant of convergence-retraction nystagmus that may be mistaken for ocular bobbing has been described in patients with acute obstructive hydrocephalus. This has been termed V-pattern, pretectal pseudobobbing. The typical features consist of arrhythmic, repetitive, fast downward and inward movements of the eyes (hence the V pattern designation) at a rate of 0.5 to 2 movements per second. The fast downward movement and the slower return render the condition readily mistakable for ocular bobbing due to pontine dysfunction, but it can be readily distinguished by the accompanying pretectal signs (e.g., abnormal pupillary light reaction, lid retraction), the intact horizontal eye movements, and a mute or stuperous (rather than comatose) patient.[205] This constellation of findings occurs in acute obstructive hydrocephalus and warrants prompt neurosurgical intervention.

The setting sun sign may be thought of as representing an exaggerated form of the dorsal midbrain syndrome and is unique to infants and young children. The setting sun sign is suggestive of congenital hydrocephalus and is usually diagnosed before closure of the anterior fontanelle.[370] In addition to lid retraction and upgaze palsy, the eyes are conjugately deviated downward, a finding apparently unique to hydrocephalus in this age group. This suggests a specific susceptibility of the neonatal brain to the mass effect of hydrocephalus on the downgaze center of the midbrain or a higher sensitivity of the pretectal area in infants to hydrocephalus, leading to a more profound upgaze palsy (causing the eyes to deviate downward).

Various other ocular motility signs are often associated with specific disease processes underlying the hydrocephalus. For example, both unilateral and bilateral internuclear ophthalmoplegia have been described in patients with Chiari malformations (previously discussed). Downbeat nystagmus commonly suggests Chiari malformation, although it may rarely be a nonlocalizing sign of communicating hydrocephalus.[292]

Infants and children who develop hydrocephalus as a result of arachnoid cysts of the third ventricle may develop the bobble-headed doll syndrome. This consists of vertical head titubations (head nodding) that are slower (1 to 2 cycles per second) and larger in amplitude than those in spasmus nutans. Nystagmus is usually absent. Children with this syndrome are usually found to have a chiasmal syndrome by the time the diagnosis is made. They may also show nonparalytic horizontal strabismus. The head nodding resolves when the ventricular cyst is removed and the hydrocephalus is shunted.

Visual Loss in Hydrocephalus

Hydrocephalus may have profound effects on the visual pathways, both anteriorly and posteriorly. A variety of visual field defects have been described in patients with hydrocephalus.[207] Anterior visual pathway damage can result in unilateral or bilateral optic nerve damage, chiasmal syndrome, or optic tract injury. Many mechanisms of optic nerve damage in hydrocephalus have been reported, but the major mechanism is postpapilledema optic atrophy. A component of strabismic amblyopia may also be present.

Papilledema is infrequently encountered in infants with hydrocephalus. Only 12% of 200 consecutive infants with hydrocephalus examined before shunt placement were found to have papilledema in one series.[152] This paucity of papilledema has been explained by the presence of open sutures, permitting cranial enlargement which reduces the rate of rise of intracranial pressure. However, an acute rapid elevation of the intracranial pressure in an infant may overwhelm the compensatory effect of the open sutures and result in papilledema. After shunt placement, the cranial sutures fuse and subependymal fibrosis reduces ventricular compliance so that intracranial pressure increases and papilledema readily develops as a response to shunt malfunction. The papilledema that may accompany repeated bouts of shunt malfunction can eventually cause visual loss and visual field defects due to axonal attrition. The majority of postpapilledema optic atrophy and visual loss are bilateral, often asymmetric, but can be unilateral.[72]

In addition to postpapilledema atrophy, the anterior visual pathways can be damaged by distortion of normal intracranial relationships by dilated ventricles and by compression of the pathways by a dilated third ventricle, adjacent arteries and veins, and adjacent basal bones. A chiasmal syndrome may result from compression of the optic chiasm by a dilated third ventricle. The anterior optic tracts are supplied by small arteries lying over bone. Pressure on these arteries has been suggested as one mechanism of visual loss.[16] Downward herniation of the hippocampal gyrus into the tentorial notch may be another mechanism.

Posterior visual pathway damage arises from posterior cerebral artery circulatory compromise, often presumably due to bilateral compression of the arteries on the tentorial edge (most common); from damage to the optic radiations associated with white matter loss as the posterior occipital horns enlarge; from neurosurgical damage; and from edema and swelling associated with hypoxia, meningitis, septicemia, surgical trauma, and seizures.[148,343] Posterior visual pathway damage probably occurs more commonly after shunt failure than as a primary result of the hydrocephalus.[16] Many children with hydrocephalus show evidence of mixed anterior and posterior visual pathway damage.

Effects and Complications of Treatment

Untreated hydrocephalus inevitably leads to tissue damage and hemispheric atrophy. The brunt of the atrophy is borne by the white matter. Hydrocephalus is usually treated by placement of a ventriculoperitoneal shunt or a ventriculoatrial shunt to divert the CSF. Timely treatment of hydrocephalus is essential in order to minimize the permanent neurological and ophthalmic adverse consequences. Ventricular dilation can regress completely upon early shunting. Certain neurologic abnormalities are quickly reversible upon shunting of the hydrocephalus. In some hydrocephalic children with cortical visual impairment, revision or placement of a shunt may be followed within several hours[89] to a few months[77] by visual improvement, possibly resulting from improved circulatory hemodynamics within the visual cortex. The setting sun sign and the various components of the dorsal midbrain syndrome ordinarily resolve shortly after shunt placement.

Various electronystagmographic abnormalities continue to be detected in shunt-treated hydrocephalic children.[229]

Despite treatment, hydrocephalic children continue to perform below average in various neurologic and visual spheres. Rabinowicz[296] examined visual perception in 100 hydrocephalic patients and found that the presence of constructional apraxia, dyscalculia, and homonymous field defects in some of the patients suggested disorder of the posterior visual pathway and the parietal lobe. The setting sun sign usually improves quickly after shunting, but some upgaze paresis often persists.

Mechanical malfunction and infection are the major complications of ventriculoperitoneal shunts.[328] Ventricular shunt obstruction continues to represent a significant problem in the management of hydrocephalus, despite advances in materials, catheter design, new valves, and neurosurgical techniques.[382] Shunt failure is usually associated with recurrence of symptoms and signs of increased intracranial pressure (severe headache, nausea, vomiting, depressed consciousness). In some children, it may manifest either as a new seizure or as recurrent seizure activity.[129] Some patients may exhibit akinetic mutism and parkinsonian symptoms.[45] Shunt malfunction is most commonly caused by occlusion of the lumen of the ventricular catheter by choroid plexus or glial tissue. The ventricles typically show enlargement upon shunt occlusion, but occasionally, increased intracranial pressure may be associated with little or no ventricular enlargement. Rarely, chronic papilledema can occur as the sole manifestation of shunt failure and cause permanent visual loss if undetected.[203a] Therefore, clinical signs of increased intracranial pressure suggest shunt blockage even if the neuroimaging is unremarkable.[271] Shunt dysfunction with increased intracranial pressure but small or normal-sized ventricles, termed the "slit ventricle syndrome," is thought to arise from considerable scar tissue formation in the ventricular walls, decreasing their compliance.[110]

Shunt obstruction may cause acute rise in intracranial pressure and acute papilledema with rapid loss of vision. Loss of ventricular and cranial elasticity as the infant gets older contributes to the acute nature of symptoms and signs. Rapid shifts in intracranial compartment may also occur, with compression of the posterior cerebral arteries and occipital infarction.

The onset of an acute headache with or without nausea and vomiting in a child with a shunt may pose a diagnostic quandary. Misinterpretation of signs and symptoms of a shunt obstruction as migraine attack delays proper revision of the shunt, and the converse leads to unnecessary surgical intervention. It is important to evaluate such a child promptly for shunt obstruction. If signs of shunt obstruction and increased intracranial pressure such as papilledema, fourth nerve palsy, or enlarging ventricular size on neuroimaging are absent, alternative diagnosis should be entertained.[274] These include (1) intermittent shunt malfunction, (2) intracranial hypotension (overshunting syndrome), (3) intermittent episodes of increased intracranial pressure in the presence of normal shunt function, and (4) migraines.[65]

A family history of migraine, which is usually positive in up to 90% of cases of childhood migraines, should be carefully sought in such a child. If adequate shunt function can be demonstrated in such children, treatment for possible migraines should preempt operative intervention.[190]

Precipitous drop in intracranial pressure after shunting may rarely be associated with acute visual loss.[40] This is thought to arise from as yet incompletely understood vascular insufficiency at the optic disc,[40] possibly related to changes in the autoregulation of the optic nerve blood flow. Intracranial hypotension secondary to overdrainage of CSF in patients with shunted hydrocephalus may be associated with symptoms and signs nearly identical to those associated with intracranial hypertension (intermittent headaches, nausea, emesis, lethargy, diplopia, strabismus, and paresis of upward gaze). However, the symptoms are usually brought about by standing and are relieved by lying down,[137] which is the opposite of that observed in intracranial hypertension or blocked shunts. This disorder is usually seen shortly after shunt placement or revision and is often self-correcting within a few days.[274]

Although rare, neuro-ophthalmologic deficits can arise as a result of direct injury to the brain during insertion of intraventricular shunts. Shults et al[340] reported four such cases that showed homonymous hemianopia due to optic tract damage, esotropia and residual bilateral facial paresis (bilateral sixth and seventh nerve palsy) from dorsal pontine injury at the level of the facial colliculi, monocular blindness from optic nerve damage, and dorsal midbrain syndrome from catheter compression in the region of the posterior commissure. Two cases of chiasmal syndrome with bitemporal hemianopia due to compression by a catheter placed in the third ventricle[90] or the suprasellar cistern[341] have been reported. In the latter case, the visual field loss progressed slowly over approximately 1 year. A malpositioned shunt may rarely cause reversible quadrantic visual field loss due to intracerebral edema surrounding the ventricular end of the shunt.[80] Direct damage to the visual pathways should always be considered in the differential diagnosis of neuro-ophthalmologic deficits found in patients with intracranial shunts.

Patients may also develop sixth nerve palsy after shunt placement. This is thought to be analogous to sixth nerve palsy arising after lumbar puncture, myelography, or spinal anesthesia. Headache and nausea may precede the onset of esotropia and double vision. Most cases are transient, but some are permanent, requiring extraocular muscle surgery.[127]

Strokes in Children

The advent of modern neuroimaging has led to the appreciation that childhood neurovascular disorders are more common than previously thought, perhaps approaching or exceeding in incidence childhood brain tumors.[70,308] Strokes may be classified by the pathophysiologic mechanisms of the vascular dysfunction into cerebral embolism, arterial embolism, venous thrombosis, intraparenchymal hemorrhage, and subarachnoid hemorrhage. Unlike adults, in whom hypertension and atherosclerosis are the major risk factors for stroke, children have a wide array for risk factors and a wide variety of stroke etiologies (Table 11.3). The neuro-ophthalmologic complications of strokes in children are the same as those in adults, with the caveat that children tend to show greater recovery of function and superior abilities to compensate for their deficits.

Vascular Lesions

Arteriovenous Malformations

Arteriovenous Malformations (AVMs) are the most common cause of spontaneous intracranial hemorrhage in children.[184] Although the generally ac-

TABLE 11.3. Risk factors for pediatric cerebrovascular disease.

Congenital heart disease
  Ventricular or atrial septal defects
  Patent ductus arteriosus
  Valvular stenosis
  Cardiac rhabdomyoma
Acquired heart disease
  Rheumatic heart disease
  Infectious endocarditis
  Cardiomyopathy
  Arrhythmia
  Kawasaki disease
  Atrial myxoma
Systemic vascular disease
  Systemic hypertension, hypotension
  Diabetes
  Progera
  Superior vena cava syndrome
Vasculitis
  Meningitis, sepsis, varicella
  Systemic lupus erythematosis
  Polyarteritis nodosa, granulomatous angiitis
  Takayasu arteritis
  Drug abuse (Cocaine)
Vasculopathies
  Homocystinuria, Fabry disease, pseudoxanthoma elasticum
  Moyamoya syndrome
  MELAS syndrome
Vasospastic disorders
  Migraine
  Vasospasm due to subarachnoid hemorrhage
Hematologic disorders/hypercoagulopathies
  Sickle cell diseases
  Platelet disorders
  Neoplasms (e.g., leukemia)
  Protein C deficiency, protein S deficiency
  Lupus anticoagulant, anticardiolipin antibodies
  Antiphospholipid antibody syndrome
Cerebrovascular structural anomalies
  Fibromuscular dysplasia
  Intracranial aneurysms
  Arteriovenous malformations
  Sturge-Weber syndrome
Trauma
  Shaken baby syndrome
  Penetrating intracranial trauma

cepted view is that they are congenital lesions, the age of presentation is usually between 20 to 40 years, suggesting a latency in the malformation's evolution. Fewer than 10% of AVMs become symptomatic in the first decade of life. The classic AVM is presumed to represent a structural defect in the formation of the primitive arteriolar-capillary network normally interposed between brain arteries and veins.[184] Histopathologically, surface AVMs appear as a conglomeration of turgid vessels covered by opacified and thickened arachnoid on the brain's surface. The nearby cerebral convolutions show variable degrees of atrophy. Some AVMs are situated subcortically or hidden in a sulcus.[184] Because of their low resistance, the tangled arteriovenous communications attract exaggerated blood flow. Over years, many AVMs gradually enlarge by increasing the size and tortuosity of their feeding and drainage channels but the number of fistulous connections probably does not increase.[184]

Clinical Features of AVMs in Children

Arteriovenous malformations are well known to produce the triad of hemorrhage, seizures, and recurrent headaches. A greater percentage of children than adults experience hemorrhage as the initial symptom, while adults are more likely to display symptoms of headache, dementia, or slowly progressive neurological dysfunction, which are presumed to be ischemic in origin.[184] The prognosis in children with AVMs is less favorable than that in adults, because of a higher mortality rate in younger patients due to hemorrhage.[263] This discrepancy may be related to several factors: (1) there is some evidence that smaller AVM are more likely to hemorrhage than giant ones (the larger the lesion, the longer it has been present, and the less likely it is to rupture);[261] (2) some believe that hemorrhage in pediatric AVM is associated with more violent and massive bleeding than in adults;[78] and (3) children have a higher incidence of AVM location in the posterior fossa, where the effects of hemorrhage are more critical.[184] Because bleeding may originate on the venous side of the malformation, it tends to be less torrential than with aneurysmal rupture. Terson syndrome, which may result from hyperacute elevation of intracranial pressure following aneurysmal rupture, is uncommon following hemorrhage from an AVM.

AVMs can also shunt blood from adjacent brain parenchyma, resulting in relative underperfusion of the adjacent brain and in focal or generalized seizures. Cerebrovascular steal symptoms are inferred to be present when surgical excision or embolization of the AVM leads to clinical improvement in neurological function corresponding to sites that are remote from the AVM.[261]

Seizures are presumed to result from gliosis of brain because of chronic ischemia adjacent to the arteriovenous shunt. Estimates of the incidence of seizures as the presenting sign of AVM vary from 28% to 67%.[261] These may be focal, generalized, or psychomotor, and they tend to show more variation in type and frequency than in cryptogenic or traumatic epilepsy. Many patients experience resolution of seizures following excision of the AVM.

Headaches occurring in association with AVMs may be the result of dilation of the feeding arteries and possibly of the draining veins that involve the adjacent dura, particularly the tentorium.[233] The notion that the recurrent headache associated with AVM can be differentiated from migraine by the fact that it always occurs on the same side (i.e., ipsilateral to the lesion) is deeply entrenched in the literature, with scant data to support it.[261] There is some controversy as to whether AVMs may also potentiate migraine in some patients since their surgical resection sometimes leads to resolution of classic migraine headaches.[302,366]

Natural History

Ondra et al[281] prospectively studied the natural history of AVMs of the brain. They observed 160 unoperated symptomatic patients with brain AVMs for a mean follow-up period of 23.7 years. The mean interval between initial presentation and subsequent hemorrhage was 7.7 years. The rate of major rebleeding was 4.0% per year and the mortality rate was 1.0% per year. The combined morbidity and mortality rate was 2.7% per year, and this rate remained constant over the entire period of the study. Initial presentation with or without hemorrhage did not change the incidence of rebleeding or death.

Treatment

If AVM of the brain is surgically accessible, surgical resection is the treatment of choice. Small or modest AVMs located in the frontal or polar regions are routinely treated with surgical resection since they carry significant risk of recurrent hemorrhage or progressive neurological deficit and have a low surgical morbidity and mortality.[261] Larger lesions, lesions located in or around the motor or speech areas, lesions with arterial supply from all three vascular trees, and lesions involving the diencephalon, basal ganglia, or brain stem are associated with a higher risk of surgical complications. Such lesions are often treated with preoperative endovascular embolization of particulate matter into the feeding channels of AVMs prior to surgical resection to decrease the size and prevent intraoperative hemorrhage.[184,261] Deep AVMs that are less than 2 cm in size can now be treated with stereotactic radiosurgery.[184,234] This treatment involves focusing a collimated radiation beam on the AVM, which leads to a radiation-induced vasculitis, endarteritis obliterans, and thrombosis of the AVM in approximately 80% of cases.

Neuro-ophthalmologic manifestations of AVMs are protean (Table 11.4). Band atrophy and congenital homonymous hemianopia are associated with congenital arteriovenous malformations that occupy the occipital lobe.[183] Although arteriovenous malformations in this location are generally believed to be congenital in origin and to produce optic atrophy via transsynaptic degeneration, some occipital AVMs have abnormal deep venous drainage remote from the nidus that directly involves the lateral geniculate nucleus and posterior optic tract, which could recruit blood from arteries near the optic tract and could progressively injure pregeniculate axons postnatally.[211]

Papilledema may be associated with AVMs that (1) produce subarachnoid hemorrhage, (2) produce obstructive hydrocephalus by their mass effect, or (3) shunt large volumes of arterial blood into a venous sinus, resulting in venous sinus hypertension and decreased CSF absorption.[64,212,256,315] Papilledema is most common in dural AVMs that drain directly into the venous si-

nuses[202] and occur primarily in adults but may occasionally be seen in children.[64] In some cases, chronic papilledema associated with AVMs can lead to progressive visual field loss.[202]

Proptosis in children can be the presenting manifestation of an arteriovenous malformation involving the galenic system.[120] Remote supratentorial AVMs can also rarely produce unilateral or bilateral proptosis, presumably from direct shunting of blood into the cavernous sinus and its resultant hemodynamic changes within the orbit.[239]

The syndrome of unilateral retinocephalic AVM was first described by Bonnet, Dechaume, and Blanc in 1937.[53] Six years later, Wyburn-Mason[398] added his report. Although Bonnet-Dechaume-Blanc syndrome is generally classified with the phakomatosis, cutaneous manifestations are usually subtle when present, consisting of a faint facial blush with scattered punctate red spots.[57,361] In some cases, the retinocephalic malformation may also extend into the ipsilateral nasopharynx, maxilla, and mandible and produce severe epistaxis or life-threatening hemorrhage during dental extraction.[60,361] The location of the AVM may lead to congenital or acquired neuro-ophthalmologic dysfunction. *Homonymous hemianopia* and *cranial nerve palsies* may result from hemorrhage, ischemia, or congenital replacement of neural tissue when the AVM involves the ipsilateral hemisphere or the brain stem. Ipsilateral *optic atrophy* occurs when the optic nerve is either replaced or honeycombed by a tangle of dilated vascular channels. Angiomatous involvement of the chiasm can cause *band atrophy with a temporal hemianopia in the fellow eye*.[60] The orbital component of the retinocephalic malformation can lead to proptosis and dilation of conjunctival vessels.[361,398] Over time, the retinal component of the AVM (Figure 11.20) can progressively compromise vision by enlarging, hemorrhaging, sclerosing, or thrombosing.[327] Effron et al[122] described a 4-year-old girl with Bonnet-Dechaume-Blanc syndrome who developed a central retinal vein occlusion and neovascular glaucoma in the involved eye.

Occipital AVMs can act as irritative epileptic foci and produce *photopsias* that can mimic the visual aura of migraine. These photopsias differ from those of classic migraine in that they begin and end abruptly, and they remain stationary

TABLE 11.4. Neuro-ophthalmologic complications from arteriovenous malformations.

Acquired visual field defects
Congenital homonymous hemianopia
Congenital or acquired band atrophy
Papilledema
Ocular motility deficits
Proptosis
Unformed visual hallucinations (occipital lobe epilepsy)
Arteriovenous malformation of the optic nerve and retina (Bonnet-Dechaume-Blanc syndrome)
Cerebral ptosis

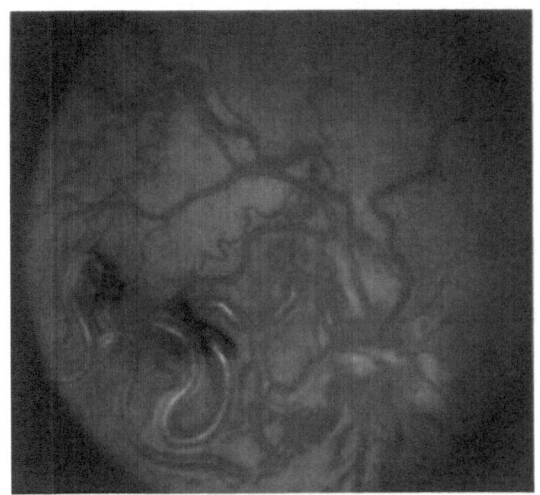

FIGURE 11.20. Retinal photograph from a patient with Bonnet–Dechaume–Blanc syndrome.

rather than enlarging in a crescendo-like fashion.[368]

Supranuclear or infranuclear ocular motility deficits may be secondary to elevated intracranial pressure or to direct brain stem involvement.[257] Dorsal midbrain syndrome can occur primarily from intrinsic midbrain involvement or secondary to compressive hydrocephalus.[257] Other supranuclear disorders (gaze paresis, skew deviation, and internuclear ophthalmoplegia) may also be seen.[257]

Acquired progressive unilateral ptosis can be a rare manifestation of a contralateral hemispheric AVM. Lowenstein et al[230] documented "cerebral ptosis" in two children who showed resolution of the ptosis following surgical removal of the AVM. They speculated that disruption of efferent fibers from the posterior frontal cortex by hemorrhage and edema surrounding the AVM may have produced this reversible phenomenon.

Cavernous Angiomas

Cavernous angiomas are congenital blood vessel hamartomas composed of irregular venous sinusoidal channels separated by fibrous septae.[238] They are often referred to as *cryptic* or *occult* vascular malformations because they are difficult to identify with angiography; however, they are now detected much more readily with MR imaging. Patients with cavernous angiomas may remain asymp-

tomatic or present with seizures, intracerebral hemorrhage, or symptoms of an intracerebral mass lesion. Although rare in children, cavernous angiomas of the optic nerve and chiasm have been reported to produce visual loss.[238] Chiasmal cavernous angiomas may present with insidious visual loss or acute visual loss associated with a throbbing headache (termed chiasmal apoplexy).[237,238] Cavernous angiomas are now initially diagnosed by MR imaging and confirmed by biopsy. Some cavernous hemangiomas of the CNS occur in conjunction with cavernous hemangiomas of the retina and skin.[145,147] When the diagnosis is established, other family members should also be examined since the conditions are often familial.[238]

Intracranial Aneurysms

Intracranial aneurysms are uncommon in children. When they occur, aneurysms in the pediatric population are more commonly of the giant type (greater than 2.5 cm in size), and they more commonly arise peripheral to the circle of Willis than in the adult population.[32,291] In a joint study of pediatric aneurysms, Roche et al[311] found a marked sex predilection, with 70% of aneurysms arising in males. Several studies have noted an unequal topographic incidence in the circle of Willis, with 50% arising from the internal carotid bifurcation, 25% from the anterior cerebral artery, and 12.5% from the posterior cerebral artery in one study.[187] Subarachnoid hemorrhage is the most common clinical presentation, which may produce severe headache, vomiting, and obtundation, sometimes progressing to coma.[32] Surgical treatment, consisting of removal of the aneurysmal sac, produces more favorable results than in adults, presumably due to cerebral plasticity and tolerance to vasospasm in children.[311]

Neuro-ophthalmologic signs of aneurysm in children usually result from subarachnoid hemorrhage (i.e., papilledema and sixth nerve palsy, rather than neural compression). In some cases, hyperacute elevation in intracranial pressure associated with aneurysmal rupture results in Terson syndrome (papilledema with retinal and vitreous hemorrhage). Children with giant intracranial aneurysms (which constitute 20% to 40% of pediatric cases) may present with focal neurological symptoms and signs as a result of compression of the surrounding brain by the aneurysm.[32] Posterior communicating artery aneurysms are particularly rare in children, but because of their immediate proximity to the third nerve, their enlargement may allow them to be diagnosed before rupture and subarachnoid hemorrhage occur, unlike other intracranial aneurysms that must reach giant size before producing signs of compression without subarachnoid hemorrhage.[138] There have been only a handful of documented cases of acute third nerve palsy in children with posterior communicating artery aneurysms, all within the second decade of life.[18,254,396] The question of whether to obtain cerebral angiography in children with acute third nerve palsy with pupillary involvement and headache but no signs of subarachnoid hemorrhage remains controversial.[138]

Most pediatric aneurysms are surgically clipped, but endovascular obliteration of the aneurysm can be performed in cases where surgery is unsuccessful or when the aneurysm has no definable neck.[32,168]

Cerebral Dysgenesis and Intracranial Malformations

Optic disc anomalies, cortical visual loss, and homonymous hemianopia in children frequently reflect a primary dysgenesis or intrauterine injury of the developing brain. The availability of MR imaging has enhanced our ability to identify dysgenetic anomalies and CNS malformations in vivo and to correlate them with their associated neuro-ophthalmologic findings.[34] Congenital or perinatal brain injury may affect the developing visual system at multiple levels. As discussed in Chapter 2, many midline or hemispheric brain malformations directly or secondarily involve the developing visual system and produce congenital visual loss associated with small optic nerves. Other brain malformations are associated with additional malformations of one or both optic nerves at the junction with the globe, as in the morning glory disc anomaly, optic disc coloboma, and the Aicardi syndrome. The type of optic disc malformation can often be predicted from the associated brain anomalies.[63] Conversely, the appearance of the

anomalous optic disc may be used in conjunction with other associated systemic and neurological abnormalities to predict that a specific constellation of CNS abnormalities will be found on neuroimaging. While considerable progress has been made in correlating malformations of the brain with those of the optic discs, little is known about the pathogenesis of each malformation complex.

Intrauterine or perinatal brain injury can precipitate congenital nystagmus when the following criteria are met: (1) anterior visual pathway development is disrupted, (2) vision is decreased bilaterally, and (3) a functioning occipital cortex is present. Children with cortical visual loss or congenital homonymous hemianopia do not generally develop nystagmus (even when bilateral optic nerve dysfunction coexists). Children with primary anterior visual pathway dysfunction tend to gradually become esotropic, while those with cortical visual loss or congenital homonymous hemianopia may have straight eyes initially but tend to gradually become exotropic.

Ocular motility disturbances such as nystagmus, strabismus, or ocular motor apraxia may reflect structural malformations within the posterior fossa, such as the Arnold–Chiari malformation or Joubert syndrome. Ischemic injury to the developing brain stem in the intrauterine or perinatal period can occasionally be associated with a congenital ocular motor nerve palsy. While congenital third nerve palsy may be the presenting sign of intrauterine or perinatal brain stem injury,[19,162] congenital fourth nerve palsy and congenital sixth nerve palsy (including Duane syndrome) rarely portend associated brain malformations.

Lissencephaly

The term lissencephaly, or agyria-pachygyria, is applied to several disorders of neuronal migration that result in a smooth cortex with absent sulci (agyria) or in a paucity of broad cortical gyri (pachygyria) (Figure 11.21).[3] In this condition, the architectonics of the cortical plate is severely disturbed as a result of altered or arrested neuronal migration during corticogenesis.[3] Type I, or classic lissencephaly, is characterized histologically by a thick, four-layered cortex and is associated clinically with mental retardation, diplegia, and seizures.

Type II, or Walker lissencephaly, is an autosomal recessive disorder that is of neuro-ophthalmologic interest primarily because of its association with hydrocephalus and optic disc anomalies and because of its overlap with septo-optic dysplasia.

Ophthalmologic abnormalities in Walker–Warburg syndrome may involve both the anterior and posterior segments and include coloboma, Peters anomaly, persistent hyperplastic primary vitreous, retinal dysplasia with rosette formation, retinal de-

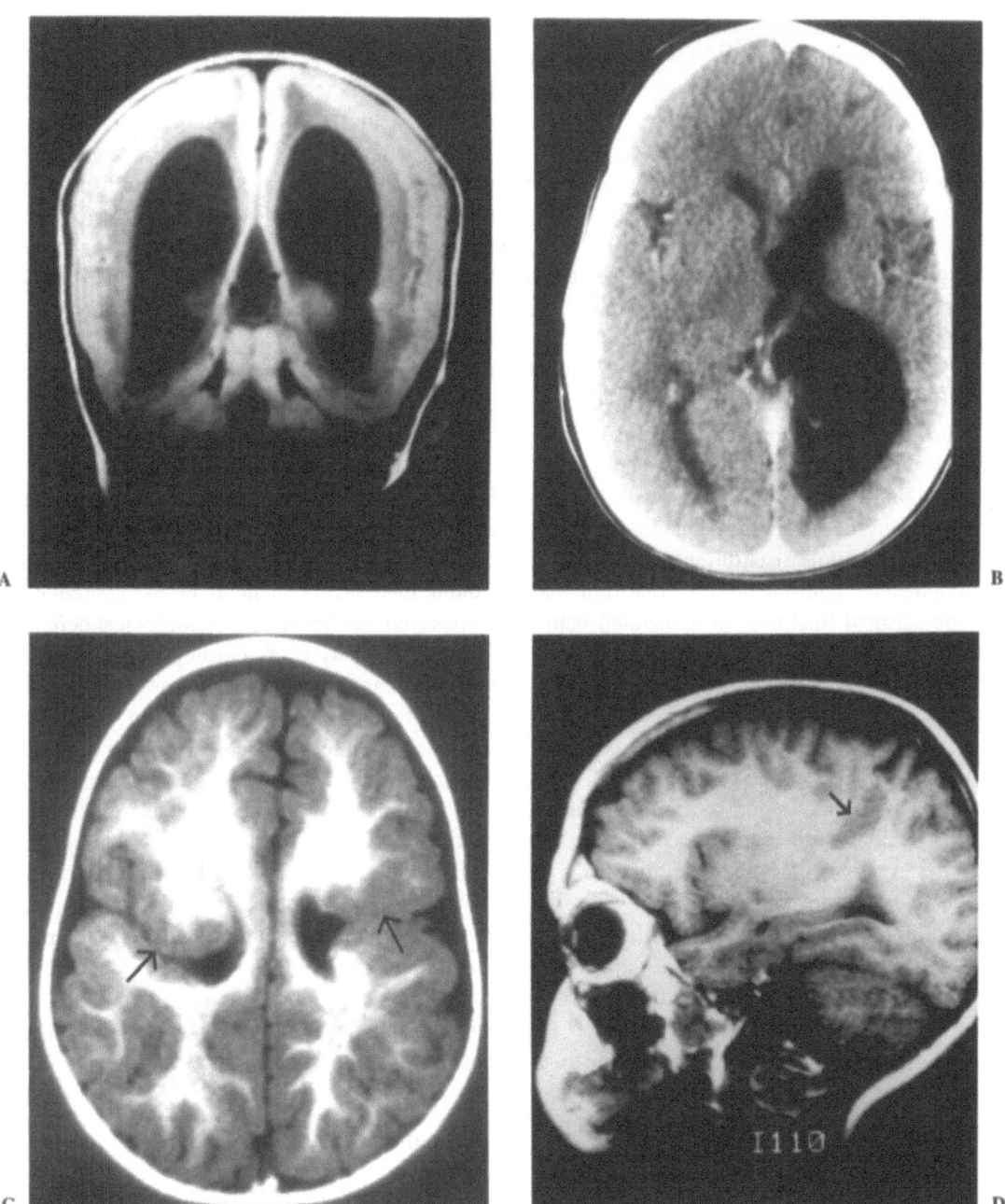

FIGURE 11.21. Cerebral dysgenesis: (A) lissencephaly; (B) porencephaly; (C) bilateral schizencephaly (arrows)—note gray matter lining schizencephalic cleft; (D) isolated cortical heterotopia (arrow).

tachment, optic nerve coloboma, and optic nerve hypoplasia.[3] Histologically, it is characterized by an unlayered, totally anarchic cortical architecture, together with proliferation of glio-mesenchymal tissue in the leptomeninges, especially around the brain stem, to the point that the subarachnoid space is often totally obliterated, resulting in hydrocephalus.

MR imaging shows a smooth cerebral surface and a cortex that is abnormally thick with absent white matter interdigitations.[114] The cerebellum is hypoplastic and usually lacks a posterior vermis. Although most cases lack a cerebellar vermis, the posterior fossa is not enlarged, which is one feature that distinguishes Walker–Warburg syndrome from the Dandy–Walker syndrome.[3] The corpus callosum and septum pellucidum are frequently absent or hypoplastic.[114] Aqueductal stenosis and posterior encephalocele are variable findings. The white matter is severely hypomyelinated with a paucity of oligodendrocytes and axons. Signs of congenital muscular dystrophy are usually present; these include pathological changes, myopathic changes on electromyography, and elevated creatinine kinase levels.[114] Children with Walker–Warburg syndrome are severely hypotonic, usually from birth.[3] Since most children survive only a few months, recognition of this condition may preclude surgical treatment of associated ocular malformations such as PHPV, Peters anomaly, glaucoma, or retinal detachment.

Porencephaly

The term porencephaly refers to a smooth-walled, fluid-filled cavity that communicates with the ventricular system, the subarachnoid space, or both.[24,31] The finding of porencephaly signifies localized brain injury during the first half of gestation, when the brain has limited capacity to mount a glial reaction and necrotic tissue is completely reabsorbed by liquefaction necrosis.[31] On MR imaging, porencephalic cysts appear as smooth-walled cavities that are isointense to CSF on all pulse sequences (Figure 11.21). When posterior porencephalic cysts involve the optic radiation or occipital cortex, affected patients have congenital homonymous hemianopia with homonymous hemioptic hypoplasia.[183,359] Davidson et al[101] recently documented porencephaly and op-

tic nerve hypoplasia in four infants who were found to have neonatal isoimmune thrombocytopenic purpura.[101]

Schizencephaly

Schizencephaly refers to an abnormal gray matter–lined cleft that extends through the cerebral hemisphere from the lateral ventricle to the cortical surface (Figure 11.21).[32] The gray matter lining the cleft is usually abnormal in the form of polymicrogyria (small, irregular gyri without intervening sulci). Unlike porencephaly, schizencephaly is believed to result from destruction of a portion of the germinal matrix before the hemispheres form.[32] Schizencephaly occurs most commonly in the parasylvian region and in the precentral and postcentral gyri.[11] Pathological studies suggest that schizencephaly results from a hemispheric injury early in the second trimester.[27] The specific mechanism of injury may vary from case to case. Clinically, children with schizencephaly often have seizures, focal neurological deficits, and variable degrees of mental retardation.[11] Barkovich and Kjos[26] reviewed neurodevelopmental records from 20 patients with schizencephaly and found bilaterality, large cleft size, and frontal lobe involvement to be associated with more severe intellectual and neurological deficits.

Schizencephaly is of neuro-ophthalmologic interest primarily because of its association with septo-optic dysplasia.[23,29,58,81,209] In some cases, this association may reflect a disruption of normal guidance mechanisms involved in the migration of both neurons and optic nerve axons in utero, preventing them from forming appropriate connections at their target sites. Alternatively, a prenatal hemispheric injury or malformation that directly involves the optic radiations will lead to transsynaptic degeneration and homonymous hemioptic hypoplasia. In some children with both midline and hemispheric CNS anomalies, these two mechanisms undoubtedly coexist.

Cortical Heterotopia

Cortical heterotopias are masses of normal neurons in abnormal locations, presumably resulting from an arrest of normal neuronal migration along radial glial fibers. Heterotopias have been associated with a wide array of genetic, vascular, and environmental causes, and they may be subcortical, diffuse, or subependymal in location.[24] Magnetic resonance diagnosis of cortical heterotopias is based on the finding of heterotopic gray matter that is isointense with orthotopic gray matter on all pulse sequences and that does not enhance with contrast (Figure 11.21).[24] Children with heterotopic gray matter usually present with seizures.[31] The degree and type of associated neurodevelopmental deficits are related to size, extent, and location of the heterotopias.

Polymicrogyria (Cortical Dysplasia)

The term polymicrogyria refers to an abnormal ophthalmoscopic appearance of brain gyration that is characterized by too many abnormally small convolutions (Figure 11.22). It is believed to result from a midcortical ischemic necrosis predominating in layer 5 of the developing cortex.[24] Polymicrogyria is a disorder that is recognized with increased frequency with the advent of MR imaging. Polymicrogyria is a common manifestation of congenital CMV infection.[31] It may be accompanied by other cerebral migration anomalies and callosal agenesis in the Aicardi syndrome.[31,75] The clinical manifestations depend primarily on the location and extent of cortical involvement. Children with focal unilateral polymicrogyria involving the frontal cortex may present with congenital unilateral hemiplegia while focal occipital polymicrogyria may result in congenital homonymous hemianopia.[369] Bilateral cases involving the occipital lobe may cause cortical visual impairment.[164] Diffuse polymicrogyria is associated with microcephaly, hypotonia with subsequent appendicular spasticity, seizures (usually infantile spasms), and developmental delay.[33]

Absence of the Septum Pellucidum

Absence of the septum pellucidum may accompany a variety of cerebral malformations,[2, 29,262] however, its frequent association with optic nerve hypoplasia has given it widespread attention in neuro-ophthalmologic circles (Figure 11.22). Despite its numerous neuroanatomical connections with subcortical regions,[324] congenital absence of the septum pellucidum in humans appears to be of

no neurodevelopmental or endocrinological consequence unless concurrent abnormalities of the cerebral hemispheres (e.g., schizencephaly, periventricular leukomalacia) or pituitary infundibulum (i.e., posterior pituitary ectopia) are present.[58,390] The ability of MR imaging to detect the presence or absence of these other clinically relevant anomalies now enables the neuro-ophthalmologist to predict the likelihood that hormone supplementation will be required or that additional neurodevelopmental deficits will complicate the clinical course in the infant with optic nerve hypoplasia.[58]

Hypoplasia, Agenesis, or Partial Agenesis of the Corpus Callosum

The corpus callosum is the major white matter tract concerned with interhemispheric transfer and integration of information.[29] Dysgenesis of the corpus callosum may occur as part of a midline malformation syndrome (e.g., in association with Dandy–Walker syndrome or transsphenoidal encephalocele). More commonly, however, it results from a wide variety of gestational or perinatal insults to the cerebral hemispheres, which secondarily affect early formation or myelination of the corpus callosum.[29] Because the corpus callosum forms in an anterior-to-posterior direction with the rostrum forming last, a partially-formed corpus callosum will always have a genu and less commonly a body, while the splenium and rostrum will frequently be absent.[29,31] This concept is useful in distinguishing a dysgenetic corpus callosum from secondary callosal destruction that may result in a small or absent genu or body in the presence of a normal splenium or rostrum.[31]

Although primary agenesis of the corpus callosum has been documented, high-resolution MR imaging has demonstrated that callosal anomalies (Figure 11.22) almost always occur in the setting of additional CNS anomalies, such as migration anomalies (schizencephaly, lissencephaly, cortical heterotopia), transsphenoidal encephalocele, holoprosencephaly, or the Dandy–Walker malformation.[29] In the child with optic nerve hypoplasia, thinning of the corpus callosum is commonly seen, but complete callosal agenesis is rare.[58] In this context, thinning of the corpus callosum is predictive of neurodevelopmental problems only

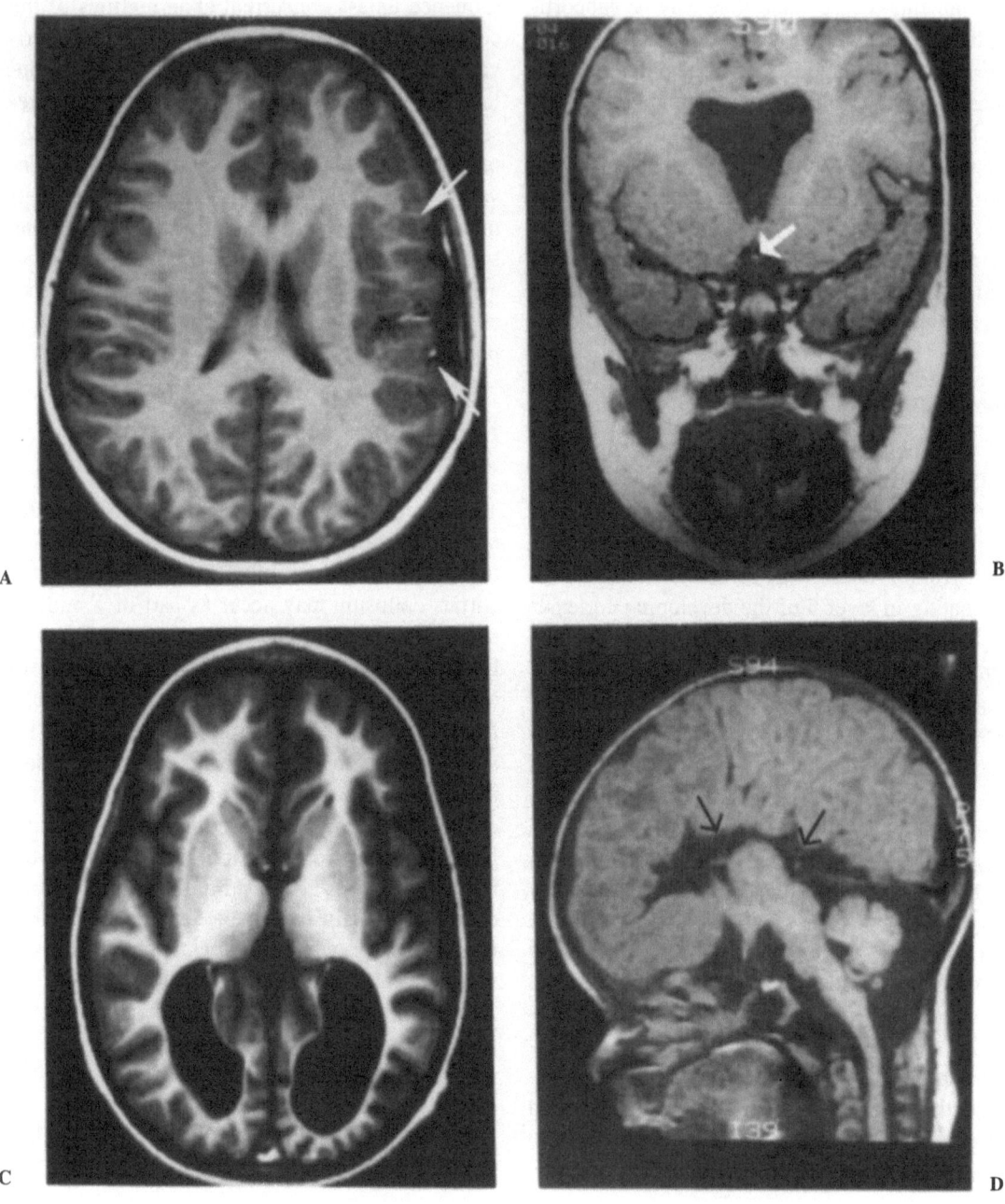

FIGURE 11.22. Cerebral dysgenesis: (A) polymicrogyria (arrows denote region of anomalous cortical migration); (B) absence of the septum pellucidum (arrow denotes associated chiasmal hypoplasia); (C) colpocephaly; (D) agenesis of the corpus callosum (arrow denotes position of the normal corpus callosum).

by virtue of its frequent association with cerebral hemispheric abnormalities. The finding of callosal anomalies on MR imaging therefore necessitates a careful search of cerebral hemispheric abnormalities, which appear to be the most direct neuro- imaging correlate of neurodevelopmental impairment.[58] The complete callosal agenesis in Aicardi syndrome and in some of the coloboma syndromes may also reflect the severity of the associated CNS anomalies.[75]

Colpocephaly

Colpocephaly is an anatomic finding in the brain manifested by occipital horns that are disproportionately enlarged in comparison to other parts of the lateral ventricles (Figure 11.22).[176] It is a secondary finding with no inherent diagnostic significance. Although most often discussed in association with agenesis of the corpus callosum, colpocephaly can accompany a variety of degenerative or encephaloclastic insults to the developing brain.[176] It is often associated with seizures, spasticity, and mental retardation, but some children are neurodevelopmentally normal.[176] Colpocephaly and associated callosal agenesis accompany a variety of congenital optic disc anomalies, most notably optic nerve hypoplasia, the morning glory disc anomaly, and other optic disc dysplasias in children with transsphenoidal encephalocele and Aicardi sydnrome.[75] It has also been described with bilateral cortical visual loss and with congenital homonymous hemianopia.[144]

Posterior Pituitary Ectopia

Posterior pituitary ectopia is seen in approximately 15% of children with optic nerve hypoplasia. It is a highly sensitive and highly specific neuroimaging marker for anterior pituitary hormone deficiency in children with optic nerve hypoplasia.[58] Posterior pituitary ectopia refers to the constellation of (1) absence of the normal posterior pituitary bright spot, (2) absence of the pituitary infundibulum, and (3) an abnormal focus of hyperintense tissue at or near the tuber cinereum on T1-weighted MR images (Figure 11.23). Posterior pituitary ectopia is believed to result from an ischemic injury to the hypophyseal portal system that causes necrosis of the infundibulum. Normally, the posterior lobe of the pituitary gland is hyperintense on T1-weighted MR images, probably because of the chemical composition of the phospholipid vesicles contained within it. It is speculated that, following injury to the infundibulum, the trophic influence of continued antidiuretic hormone/neurophysin secretion at the median eminence causes an abnormal collection of posterior pituicytes to form where the upper infundibulum is normally located. This ectopic cluster of cells seems to function as a normal posterior pituitary gland. The finding of posterior pituitary ectopia in MR images implicates the infundibulum as the primary site of structural derangement in patients with optic nerve hypoplasia and endocrine deficiency. Posterior pituitary ectopia may also be seen in patients with pituitary dwarfism without optic nerve hypoplasia, transection of the pituitary infundibulum, compression or destruction of the posterior lobe of the pituitary gland, and rarely as a normal variant.[58]

Holoprosencephaly

The term holoprosencephaly refers to a failure of differentiation and cleavage of the prosencephalon, so that the cerebrum fails to cleave laterally into distinct cerebral hemispheres and transversely into a diencephalon and telencephalon (Figure 11.23). Severe cases are associated with facial dysmorphism, particularly hypotelorism and midline facial clefts.[31] Affected areas of brain show no definable interhemispheric fissure and no falx cerebri. Holoprosencephaly is the only nondestructive condition in which one may see presence of the splenium of the corpus callosum and absence of the rostrum, body, and genu.[31] Although the terms *alobar, semilobar,* and *lobar* are often applied to describe the extent of involvement, the holoprosencephalies represent a continuum of forebrain malformation with the anterior portions of the brain most severely affected and the posterior portions least severely affected, and no clear distinction between these categories exists.[31] Holoprosencephaly may be seen in children with trisomy 13 and, less commonly, trisomy 18.[31] Barkovich has questioned whether some forms of septo-optic dysplasia with a central holoventricle, and no hemispheric malformations fall within the mildest end of the spectrum of holoprosencephaly.[23]

Hemimegalencephaly

Hemimegalencephaly is a rare brain malformation characterized by congenital hamartomatous overgrowth of one cerebral hemisphere with increased white matter volume and dilation of the lateral ventricle on the larger side (Figure 11.23). MR imaging and histopathological examination show a wide array of migration anomalies, including pachygyria, polymicrogyria, and cortical heterotopias in the enlarged hemisphere.[31] Hemimegalencephaly may accompany a number of neurocu-

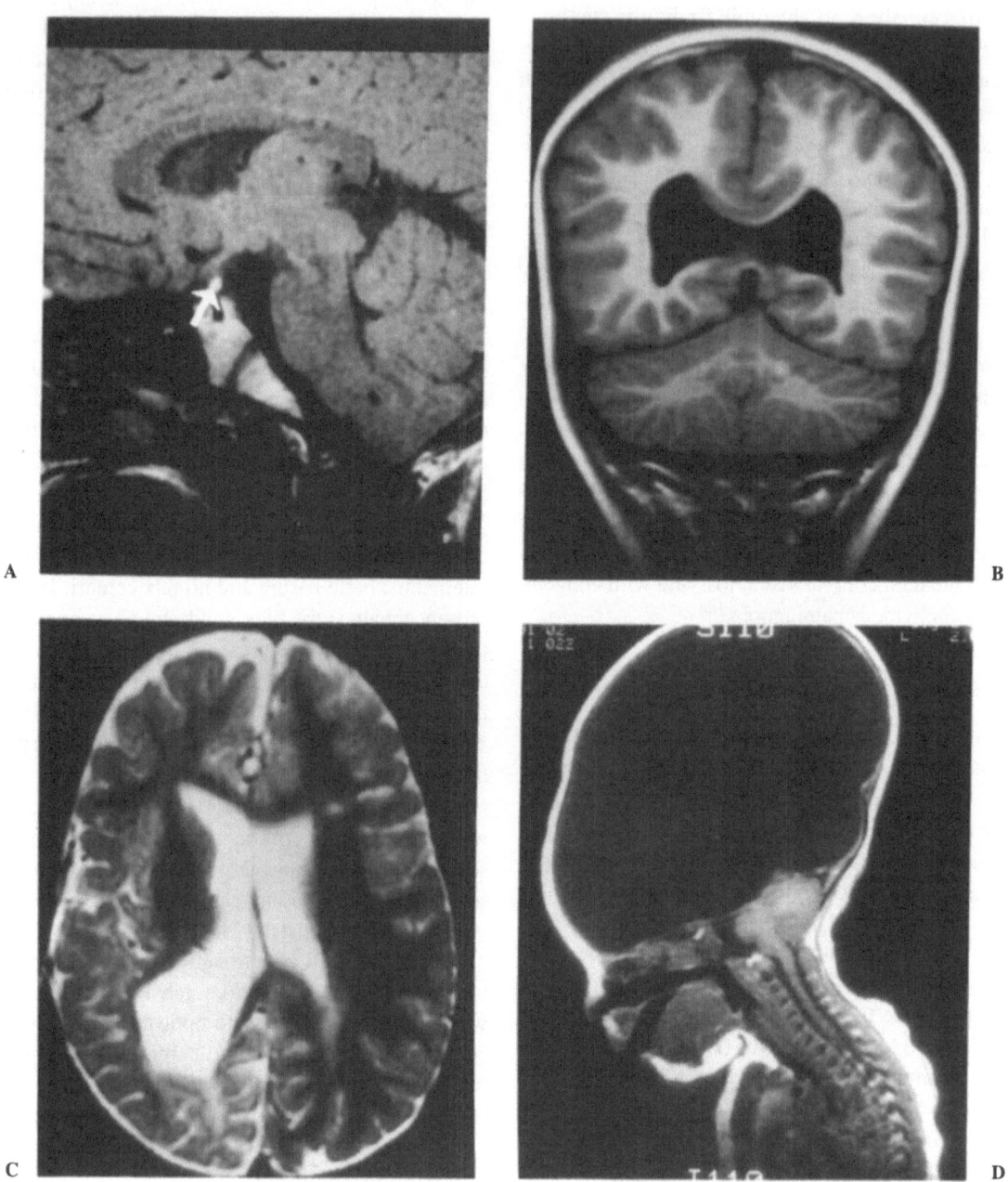

FIGURE 11.23. Cerebral dysgenesis: (A) posterior pituitary ectopia (arrow); (B) mild holoprosencephaly in a child with septo-optic dysplasia—note anomalous interdigitations of cerebral gray and white matter just above the dilated lateral ventricles; (C) hemimegalencephaly—note larger right hemisphere with ipsilateral ventriculomegaly; (D) hydranencephaly.

taneous disorders of neuro-ophthalmologic interest; however, its frequency in the linear sebaceous nevus syndrome is particularly high.[167,323] It has been occasionally reported in neurofibromatosis,[98] Klippel–Trenauney–Weber syndrome,[68] and hypomelanosis of Ito.[99] Clinical features include early-onset seizures, severe encephalopathy, and hemiplegia or hemianopia.[99] Since the affected hemisphere has essentially no function, partial or complete hemispherectomy may be indicated in children with intractable seizures and a normal contralateral hemisphere.[31]

Hydranencephaly

Hydranencephaly is a condition in which the cerebral hemispheres are almost completely replaced by CSF (Figure 11.23). The brain stem is usually atrophic, but the thalami and cerebellum are relatively well preserved.[31] Severe hydrocephalus may produce extreme thinning of the cortical mantle and simulate hydranencephaly. The optic nerves are formed but severely hypoplastic. Neurologically, children with hydranencephaly are severely developmentally delayed from birth and may be macrocephalic, normocephalic, or microcephalic, depending upon the degree of associated hydrocephalus.[31] When hydranencephaly is associated with hydrocephalus, shunting does not improve intellectual development but may prevent the development of a grotesquely enlarged head.[31]

Encephaloceles

Cephaloceles are congenital malformations consisting of a defect in the cranium and dura mater with extracranial herniation of any intracranial structure. *Meningoceles* are cephaloceles in which the protruding structures contain only leptomeninges and CSF. *Meningoencephaloceles* are cephaloceles in which the protruding structure contains leptomeninges, brain, and CSF.[266] The terms *meningoencephalocele* and *encephalocele* are often used interchangeably. The most common anatomical location of encephaloceles varies according to geographic distribution, with occipital encephaloceles most common in Europe and North America and frontoethmoidal encephaloceles most common in Russia and southeast Asia.[112,266] Most encephaloceles occur in a sporadic basis and are not associated with syndromes.[112] The embryology is complex and may vary according to location.[373]

Orbital Encephalocele

Orbital encephalocele is a rare congenital abnormality caused by a defect of the cranio-orbital bones that usually manifests soon after birth as a soft, cystic fullness in the superomedial canthal area with associated exophthalmos.[360] The globe may pulsate synchronously with the heartbeat, and crying or coughing may increase the degree of proptosis. The encephalocele can herniate through a bony orbital defect or, in some cases, through a natural opening such as the optic foramen or orbital fissures. Surgical treatment usually requires a combined orbital and intracranial approach, with use of dural flaps and bone grafts to close the defect. Most orbital encephaloceles are isolated anomalies that do not preclude normal mental and physical development; however, posterior orbital encephaloceles may be associated with neurofibromatosis.[360]

Transsphenoidal Encephalocele

Transsphenoidal encephalocele is a rare midline congenital malformation in which a meningeal pouch, often containing the chiasm and adjacent hypothalamus, protrudes inferiorly through a large round defect in the sphenoid bone (Figure 11.24). Children with this occult basal meningocele have a wide head, a flat nose, a mild hypertelorism, a midline notch in the upper lip, and sometimes a midline cleft in the soft palate. The meningocele protrudes into the nasopharynx, where it may obstruct the airway. Associated brain malformations include agenesis of the corpus callosum and posterior dilatation of the lateral ventricles. Most affected children have no overt intellectual or neurological deficits, but panhypopituitarism is

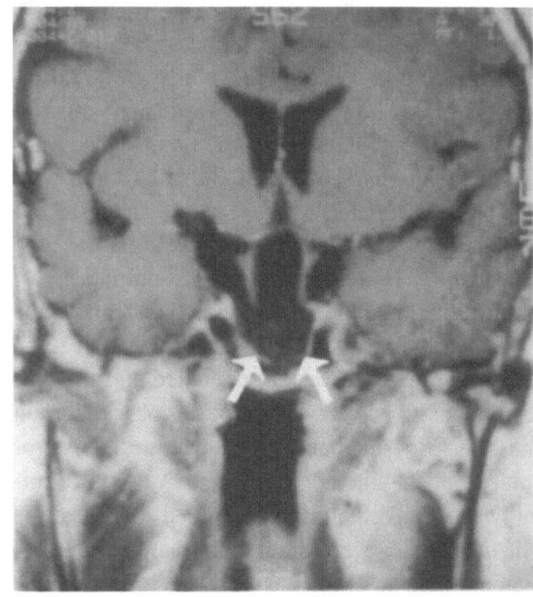

FIGURE 11.24. Transsphenoidal meningocele. Arrow denotes lower margin of the meningeal pouch just above the hard palate. The optic chiasm is split and herniated downward into the defect.

common. Surgery for transsphenoidal encephalocele is considered by many authorities to be contraindicated, since herniated brain tissue may include vital structures, such as the hypothalamic-pituitary system, optic nerves and chiasm, and anterior cerebral arteries, and because of the high postoperative mortality reported, especially in infants.[402]

A variety of optic disc dysplasias, particularly the morning glory disc anomaly, occur in association with transsphenoidal encephalocele.[66,74] The combination of a V- or tongue-shaped zone of infrapapillary retinochoroidal depigmentation with optic disc dysplasia may be a retinal marker for transsphenoidal encephalocele.[61]

Occipital Encephalocele

Occipital encephaloceles account for 80% of encephaloceles in the white population of Europe and North America.[31] Occipital encephalocele may be associated with callosal anomalies, cerebral migration anomalies, Chiari malformation, and Dandy–Walker malformation.[31] The size of the defect is highly variable, ranging from a few millimeters in diameter to encephaloceles that contain most of the brain.[112] Hydrocephalus may affect the entire ventricular system or may be limited to the extracranial portion of the ventricles.[266] The occipital lobes and cerebellar hemispheres may be included partially or totally in the herniated sac and show extensive vascular lesions in the form of old and recent infarction.[201] The finding of meningomyelocele in 7% of children with occipital encephalocele suggests that occipital encephaloceles are related to defects in neural tube closure.[266] Histopathological examination of brains with large, herniate occipital encephalocele reveals atrophic anterior visual pathways. In some cases, the optic nerves are stretched and the chiasm is postfixed, suggesting posterior traction on the anterior visual pathways as one mechanism of injury.[201] The diagnosis is usually obvious clinically, and MR imaging is obtained to determine whether other severe brain abnormalities are present and whether the dural venous sinuses course within the encephalocele.[31] The clinical outcome depends upon the size, presence, or absence of brain herniation and the presence or absence of associated brain malformations.[266] Children with small occipital meningomyeloceles do well, while those with larger lesions associated with brain herniation are totally dependent.[250] Surgical correction is performed to protect the child from ulceration of the sac that could lead to infection or hemorrhage, to prevent the sac from expanding, and to improve the cosmetic appearance.[266]

Miscellaneous

Proteus Syndrome

In an older child with cutaneous manifestations of NF-1, the absence of Lisch nodules raises the rare possibility of Proteus syndrome, which can also produce skeletal, visceral, and cutaneous abnormalities.[54] The macrocephaly, hemihypertrophy, and cutaneous tumors of Proteus syndrome can simulate neurofibromatosis, but children with Proteus syndrome lack the other neuro-ophthalmologic manifestations of neurofibromatosis. Periorbital exostosis, epibulbar tumors, and "eye enlargement" are considered to be the most characteristic ophthalmologic signs in Proteus syndrome.[54]

Goldenhar Syndrome (Oculoauriculovertebral Dysplasia)

The Goldenhar syndrome comprises a complex of hemifacial microsomia, preauricular appendages, auricular abnormalities, vertebral anomalies, and epibulbar dermoids.[241] Patients with Goldenhar syndrome show a phenotypic spectrum ranging from mild facial asymmetry to severe hypoplasia of one side of the face with ipsilateral macrostoma.[177,242] As a minimal sign, microtia must be present.[330] Auricular abnormalities are usually unilateral and, in addition to microtia, may include malpositioning of the ear and hypoplasia of the external auditory canal, with or without hearing loss.[265] Additional features are cardiac and renal anomalies, cleft lip/palate, CNS, cervical, and radial limb anomalies.[330] Colobomas and focal upper lid defects may also be present. The eye on the involved side may be microphthalmic or anophthalmic in severe cases. Gorlin et al[165] now use the term oculo-auriculo-vertebral spectrum (OAVS) because of the extreme heterogeny of the condition. This nonhereditary spectrum affects males more than females, and right-sided involvement is more common and more severe.[312]

Neuro-ophthalmologic abnormalities include unilateral or bilateral fourth nerve palsy,[7,177] congenital corneal anesthesia,[260] unilateral and bilateral Duane syndrome,[7,241] sixth nerve palsy,[177] optic nerve hypoplasia and coloboma on the affected side,[242] and ptosis.[37] Amblyopia may also result from associated strabismus or anisometropia.[177] The association of Goldenhar syndrome with predominantly ipsilateral cranial nerve palsies is explained by the occurrence of aplasia of the cranial nerve nuclei in this condition.[7,241,260] Intelligence is usually normal, but mental retardation is more likely to be present in severe cases that are associated with ipsilateral microphthalmia or anophthalmia.[242]

Goldenhar syndrome may be associated with a broad array of CNS abnormalities, including hydrocephalus, Arnold–Chiari malformation, unilateral arhinencephaly, occipital and frontal encephalocele, intracranial arachnoid cyst, intracranial lipoma, holoprosencephaly, callosal hypoplasia, lissencephaly, and intracranial lipoma.[330] An intracranial dermoid cyst has also been reported in a patient with Goldenhar syndrome.[265] Various bony defects may also be present, including microcephaly, cranial asymmetry, platybasia, hypoplasia of the petrous and ethmoid bones, and absence of the internal auditory canals.[330,394]

The Wildervanck (cervico-oculo-acoustic) syndrome may be difficult to distinguish from the Goldenhar syndrome. It consists of sensorineural deafness, Klippel–Feil anomaly, and Duane syndrome. It is much more common in women. As Duane syndrome is much more common in the Wilderwanck than the Goldenhar syndrome, its presence necessitates a search for the associated Klippel–Feil anomaly.[38,94] Since many patients have overlapping features, the syndromes of Goldenhar and Wilderwanck may represent different ends of a spectrum.[94]

Delleman (Oculocerebrocutaneous) Syndrome

In 1981, Delleman and Oorthuys described two children with multiple intracranial cysts, orbital cysts, agenesis of the corpus callosum, periorbital skin appendages, punchlike skin defects, and skin atrophy or hypoplasia.[107] Numerous cases have since been described as the Delleman or oculocerebrocutaneous syndrome. Additional anomalies in this condition include seizures, generalized asymmetry, skull defects, rib anomalies, and mental retardation.[4,395] Unilateral anophthalmos with ipsilateral orbital hypoplasia and hypoplasia of the corresponding intracranial optic nerve may also be seen.[59] In some children, the clinical features of Delleman syndrome overlap those of Goldenhar spectrum, making the clinical distinction between these two entities difficult.[59]

Encephalocraniocutaneous Lipomatosis

Encephalocraniocutaneous lipomatosis is a rare neurocutaneous syndrome characterized by lipomas of the cranium and CNS, alopecia of the scalp, and a broad range of CNS abnormalities including unilateral intracranial cysts, cerebral migration anomalies, and cortical atrophy.[206,228] Affected children have seizures, spasticity, and mental retardation. Epibulbar choristomas and small skin nodules are the most common ophthalmologic manifestations, but neuro-ophthalmologic findings including papilledema and optic disc pallor have also been reported.[206] Encephalocraniocutaneous lipomatosis should be considered along with Goldenhar syndrome and linear sebaceous nevus syndrome in the differential diagnosis of conditions with epibulbar choristomas.[206]

Incontinentia Pigmenti (Bloch–Sulzberger Syndrome)

Incontinentia pigmenti is a rare neurocutaneous disease that affects the skin, bones, teeth, CNS, and eyes. Its almost exclusive occurrence in females is attributed to an X-linked dominant mutation, which is lethal in males. Linear lesions appear at birth or soon afterward. These lesions subsequently resolve to leave a linear pattern of pigmentation. Retinal abnormalities most commonly involve the temporal equator and include vascular dilation, arteriovenous anastamosis, preretinal fibrosis, vascular proliferation, and nonperfusion of the retina temporal to the vascular abnormalities.[147] These vascular changes, which resemble those of retinopathy of prematurity and sickle cell disease, may lead to retinal detachment. Dragging of the retinal vessels, macular heterotopia, retinal folds, foveal hypoplasia, and RPE mottling may also occur.[147,158] Other ophthalmologic abnormalities may include cataract, optic atrophy, retinal dysplasia, a retrolental mass (termed pseudoglioma) secondary to extensive retinal detachment, nystagmus, and esotropia.[313]

Pascual-Castroviejo et al[287] found MR abnormalities including focal atrophy of the cerebrum, cerebellum, and hypoplasia of the corpus callosum in four of eight patients with incontinentia pigmentia. The MR abnormalities were only seen in those patients who had neurological abnormalities. The CNS manifestations in incontinentia pigmenti may be ischemic in origin secondary to intracranial small vessel disease.[219] Lee et al[219] found the severity of retinal vascular occlusions to correlate with the degree of CNS involvement on MR imaging and suggested that retinal vascular occlusions may eventually prove to be a marker for CNS disease. The finding of optic atrophy in some children with incontentia pigmentia may also reflect ischemic white matter injury.[158]

References

1. Aicardi J, Barbosa C, Andermann E, et al. Ataxia-ocular motor apraxia: a syndrome mimicking Ataxia-Telangiectasia. Ann Neurol 1988;24:497-502.
2. Aicardi J, Goutieres F. The syndrome of absence of the septum pellucidum with porencephalies and other developmental defects. Neuropediatrics 1981;12:319-328.
3. Aicardi J. The lissencephaly syndromes. Int Pediatr 1989;4:118-126.
4. Al-Gazali LI, Donnai D, Berry SA, et al. The oculocerebrocutaneous (Delleman) syndrome. J Med Genet 1988;25:773-778.
5. Albright AL. Brain tumors in neonates, infants, and toddlers. Contemp Neurosurg 1985;7:1-6.
6. Aleksic S, Budzilovich G, Choy A, et al. Congenital ophthalmoplegia in oculoauriculovertebral dysplasia-hemifacial microsomia (Goldenhar-Gorlin syndrome). A clinicopathological study and review of the literature. Neurology 1976;26:638-644.
7. Almeida L, Anyane-Yeboa K, Grossman M, Rosen T. Myelomeningocele, Arnold-Chiari anomaly and hydrocephalus in focal dermal hypoplasia. Am J Med Genet 1988;30:917-923.
8. Ambrosino MM, Hernanz-Schulman M, Genieser NB, et al. Brain tumors in infants less than a year of age. Pediatr Radiol 1988;19:6-8.
9. Andriola M, Stolfi J. Sturge-Weber syndrome. Report of an atypical case. AJDC 1972;123:507-510.
10. Aniskiewicz AS, Frumkin NL, Brady DE, et al. Magnetic resonance imaging and neurobehavioral correlates in schizencephaly. Arch Neurol 1990;47:911-916.
11. Arnold A. Bilateral internuclear ophthalmoplegia in a young adult. Presented at the 18th Annual Frank B. Walsh Society Meeting, Seattle, Washington, February 21-22, 1986.
12. Arnold AC, Hepler RS, Yee RW, et al. Solitary retinal astrocytoma. Surv Ophthalmol 1985;30: 173-181.
13. Arnold AC; Baloh RW; Yee RD; et al. Internuclear ophthalmoplegia in the Chiari type II malformation. Neurology 1990;40:1850-1854.
14. Arnold RW, Schriever G. Lyme amaurosis in a child. J Pediatr Ophthalmol Strabismus 1993;30: 268-270.
15. Arroyo HA, Jan EJ, McCormick AQ, et al. Permanent visual loss after shunt malfunction. Neurology 1985;35:25-29.
16. Atkinson A, Sanders MD, Wang V. Vitreous haemorrhage in tuberous sclerosis: report of two cases. Br J Ophthalmol 1973;57:773-779.
17. Bagianelli EB, Klingele TG, Burde RM. Acute oculomotor nerve palsy in childhood: Is arteriography necessary? J Clin Neuro-ophthalmol 1989; 9(1):33-36.
18. Balkan R, Hoyt CS. Associated neurologic abnormalities in congenital third nerve palsies. Am J Ophthalmol 1984;97:315-319.
19. Baloh RW, Honrubia V, Konrad HR. Periodic alternating nystagmus. Brain 1976;99:11-26.
20. Bardelli AM, Hadjistilianou T. Buphthalmos and progressive elephantiasis in neurofibromatosis. A report of three cases. Ophthal Paediatr Genet 1989;10:279-286.
21. Barker D, Wright E, Nguyen K, et al. Gene for von Recklinghausen neurofibromatosis is in the pericentromeric region of chromosome 17. Science 1987;236:1100-1102.
22. Barkovich AJ, Fram EK, Norman D. Septo-optic dysplasia: MR imaging. Radiology 1989;171:189-192.
23. Barkovich AJ, Gressens P, Evrard P. Formation, maturation, and disorders of brain neocortex. AJNR 1992;13:423-446.
24. Barkovich AJ, Kjos BO, Norman D, et al. Revised classification of posterior fossa cysts and cyst-like malformations based on results of mutiplanar MR imaging. AJNR 1989;10:977-988.
25. Barkovich AJ, Kjos BO. Nonlissencephalic cortical dysplasias: correlation of imaging findings with clinical deficits. AJNR 1992;13:95-103.
26. Barkovich AJ, Kjos BO. Schizencephaly: correlation of clinical findings with MR characteristics. AJNR 1992;13:85-94.
27. Barkovich AJ, Krischer J, Kun LE, et al. Brain stem gliomas: a classification system based on magnetic resonance imaging. Pediatr Neurosurg 1991;16:73-83.

28. Barkovich AJ, Norman D. Absence of septum pellucidum: a useful sign in the diagnosis of congenital brain malformations. AJNR 1988;9:1107-1114.

29. Barkovich AJ, Norman D. Anomalies of the corpus callosum. Correlation with further anomalies of the brain. AJNR 1988;9:493-501.

30. Barkovich AJ. *Contemporary Neuroimaging, Pediatric Neuroimaging*. 2nd ed. New York: Raven Press; 1995:321-437.

31. Barkovich AJ. *Contemporary Neuroimaging, Pediatric Neuroimaging*. New York: Raven Press; 1990; 1:341-342.

32. Barkovich AJ. Neuroimaging of pediatric brain tumors. In: Berger MS, ed. Pediatric Neuro-oncology. In: Winn HR, Mayberg MR, eds. *Neurosurgery Clinics of North America*. Philadelphia, PA: WB Saunders; 1992:739-770.

33. Barkovich AJ, Maroldo TV. Magnetic resonance imaging of normal and abnormal brain development. Top Magn Reson Imaging. 1993;5:96-122.

34. Barros-Nunes P, Rivas F. Autosomal recessive congenital stenosis of aqueduct of Sylvius. Genet Couns 1993;4:19-23.

35. Barsky SH, Rosen S, Geer DE, et al. The nature and evolution of port-wine stains: a computer-assisted study. J Invest Dermatol 1980;74:154-157.

36. Baum JL, Feingold M. Ocular aspects of Goldenhar's syndrome. Am J Ophthalmol 1973;75:250-257.

37. Baum JL. Goldenhar's syndrome. Arch Ophthalmol 1992;110:750.

38. Baumgartner JE, Edwards MSB. Pineal tumors. In: Berger MS, ed. Pediatric Neuro-oncology. Philadelphia, PA: WB Saunders; 1992:853-862.

39. Beck RW, Greenberg HS. Post-decompression optic neuropathy. J Neurosurg 1985;63:196-199.

40. Beck RW, Hanno R. The phakomatoses. Int Ophthalmol Clin 1985;25:97.

41. Bell WO, Charney EB, Bruce DA, et al. Symptomatic Arnold-Chiari malformation: review of experience with 22 cases. J Neurosurg 1987;66:812-818.

42. Belman A. Neurologic complications of Lyme disease in children. Int Pediatr 1992;7:136-143.

43. Bender BL, Yunis EJ. The pathology of tuberous sclerosis. Pathol Annu 1982;17:339-382.

44. Berger L, Gauthier S, Leblanc R. Akinetic mutism and parkinsonism associated with obstructive hydrocephalus. Can J Neuro Sci 1985; 12:255-258.

45. Berger MS, Keles GE, Geyer JR. Cerebral hemispheric tumors of childhood. In: Berger MS, ed. *Pediatric Neuro-oncology, Neurosurgery Clinics of North America*. Philadelphia, PA: WB Saunders; 1992:839-852.

46. Bianchi-Marzoli S, Righi C, Broncato R, et al. Pseudotumor cerebri in men: the need for cerebral angiography. Presented as a poster at the North American Neuro-ophthalmology Society, Durango, Colorado, February 27–March 3, 1994.

47. Biglan AW. Ophthalmologic complications of meningomyelocele: a longitudinal study. Trans Am Ophthalmol Soc 1990;88:389-462.

48. Bilaniuk LT, Zimmerman RA, Littman P, et al. Computed tomography of brain stem gliomas in children. Radiology 1980;134:89-95.

49. Bixenman WW, Laguna JF. Acquired esotropia as initial manifestation of Arnold-Chiari malformation. J Pediatr Ophthalmol Strabismus 1987;24:83-86.

50. Bloom HJG. Intracranial tumors: response and resistance to therapeutic endeavors. Int J Radiat Oncol Biol Phys 1982;8:1083-1113.

51. Boesel CP, Paulsen GW, Kosnik EJ, Earle KM. Brain hamartomas and tumors associated with tuberous sclerosis. Neurosurgery 1979;4:410-417.

52. Bolande RP. Neurofibromatosis—The quintessential neurocristopathy: pathogenetic concepts and relationships. Adv Neurol 1981;29:67-75.

53. Bonnet P, Dechaume J, Blanc E. L'anevrysme cirsoide de la retine (Aneuryme recemeux): Ses relations avec l'aneurysme cirsoide de la face et avec l'anevrysme cirsoide du cerveau. J Med Lyon 1937;18:165-178.

54. Bouzas EA, Mastorakos G, Chrousos GP, et al. Lisch nodules in Cushing's disease. Arch Ophthalmol 1993;111:439-440.

55. Bouzas EA, Freidlin V, Parry DM, et al. Lens opacities in neurofibromatosis 2: further significant correlations. Br J Ophthalmol 1993;77:354-357.

56. Branco G, Goulao A, Ferro JM. MRI in aqueduct compression and obstructive hydrocephalus due to an ecstatic basilar artery. Neuroradiology 1993; 35:447-448.

57. Brock S, Dyke CG. Venous and arteriovenous angiomas of the brain: a clinical and roentgenographic study of eight cases. Bull Neurol Inst NY 1932;2:247-293.

58. Brodsky MC, Glasier CM. Optic nerve hypoplasia: clinical significance of associated central nervous system abnormalities on magnetic resonance imaging. Arch Ophthalmol 1993;111:66-74.

59. Brodsky MC, Harper RA, Keppen LD, et al. Anophthalmia in Delleman syndrome. Am J Med Genet 1990;37:157-158.

60. Brodsky MC, Hoyt WF, Higashida RT, et al. Bonnet-Dechaume-Blanc syndrome with large facial angioma. Arch Ophthalmol 1987;105:854-855.

61. Brodsky MC, Hoyt WF, Hoyt CS, et al. Atypical retinochoroidal coloboma in patients with dysplastic optic discs and transsphenoidal encephalocele: report of five cases. Arch Ophthalmol 1995; 113:624–628.

62. Brodsky MC. The "pseudo-CSF" signal of orbital optic glioma on magnetic resonance imaging: a signature of neurofibromatosis. Surv Ophthalmol 1993;38:213-218.

63. Brodsky MC. Morning glory disc anomaly or optic disc coloboma? Arch Ophthalmol 1994;112:153.

64. Buchanan TAS, Harper DG, Hoyt WF. Bilateral proptosis, dilatation of conjunctival veins and papilledema: a neuro-ophthalmological syndrome caused by arteriovenous malformation of the torcular herophili. Br J Ophthalmol 1982;66:186-189.

65. Buchhalter JR, Dichter MA. Migraine/epilepsy syndrome mimicking shunt malfunction in a child with shunted hydrocephalus. J Child Neurol 1990;5:69-71. Letter.

66. Bullard DE, Crockard A, McDonald WI. Spontaneous cerebrospinal fluid rhinorrhea associated with dysplastic optic discs and a basal encephalocele. J Neurosurg 1981;54:807-810.

67. Burch JV, Leveille AS, Morse PH. Ichthyosis hystrix (epidermal nevus syndrome) and Coat's disease. Am J Ophthalmol 1980;89:25-30.

68. Burke JP, West NFJ, Strachan IM. Congenital nystagmus, anisomyopia, and hemimegalencephaly in the Klippel-Trenauney-Weber syndrome. J Ophthalmol Strabismus 1991;28:41-44.

69. Burns AJ, Kaplan LC, Mulliken JB. Is there an association between hemangioma and syndromes with dysmorphic features? Pediatrics 1991; 88:1527.

70. Butler IJ. Cerebrovascular disorders of childhood. J Child Neurol 1993;8:197-200. Editorial.

71. Byrne JV, Kendall BE, Kingsley DPE, et al. Lesions of the brain stem: assessment by magnetic resonance imaging. Neuroradiology 1989;31:129-133.

72. Calogero JA, Alexander E. Unilateral amaurosis in a hydrocephalic child with an obstructed shunt. Case report. J Neurosurg 1971;34:236-240.

73. Canbaz B, Akar Z, Yilmazlar S, et al. Warburg syndrome. Neurol Res 1994;16:145-147.

74. Caprioli J, Lesser RL. Basal encephalocele and morning glory syndrome. Br J Ophthalmol 1983; 67:349-351.

75. Carney SH, Brodsky MC, Good WV, et al. Aicardi syndrome: more than meets the eye. Surv Ophthalmol 1993;37:419-424.

76. Cavanagh EC, Hart BL, Rose D. Association of linear sebaceous nevus syndrome and unilateral megalencephaly. AJNR 1993;14:405-408.

77. Cedzich C, Schramm J, Wenzel D. Reversible visual loss after shunt malfunction. Acta Neurochir Wien 1990;105:121-123.

78. Celli P, Ferrante L, Palma L, et al. Cerebral arteriovenous malformations in children. Clinical features and outcome of treatment in children and in adults. Surg Neurol 1984;22:43.

79. Charles SJ, Moore AT, Yates JRW, et al. Lisch nodules in neurofibromatosis type 2. Arch Ophthalmol 1989;107:1571.

80. Chiba Y, Takagi H, Nakajimi F, et al. Cerebrospinal fluid edema: a rare complication of shunt operations for hydrocephalus. J Neurosurg 1982; 57:697-700.

81. Chuang SH, Fitz CR, Chilton SJ, et al. Schizencephaly: spectrum of CT findings in association with septo-optic dysplasia. Radiology 1984;153: 118. Abstract.

82. Cibis GW, Tripathi RC, Tripathi BJ. Glaucoma in Sturge-Weber syndrome. Ophthalmology 1984;91: 1061-1071.

83. Cibis GW, Whittaker CK, Wood WE. Intraocular extension of optic nerve meningioma in a case of neurofibromatosis. Arch Ophthalmol 1985;103: 404-406.

84. Clark AC, Nelson LB, Simon JW, et al. Acute acquired comitant esotropia. Br J Ophthalmol. 1989; 73:636-638.

85. Cobbs WH, Schatz NJ, Savino PJ. Midbrain eye signs in hydrocephalus. Ann Neurol 1978;4:172.

86. Cogan DG, Wray SH. Internuclear ophthalmoplegia as an early sign of brain stem tumors. Neurology 1970;20:629.

87. Cogan DG. Convergence nystagmus. Arch Ophthalmol 1959;62:295-299.

88. Cohen ME, Duffner PK. *Brain Tumors in Children*. 2nd ed. New York: Raven Press; 1994.

89. Connolly MB, Jan JE, Cochrane DD. Rapid recovery from cortical visual impairment following correction of prolonged shunt malfunction in congenital hydrocephalus. Arch Neurol 1991;48:956-957.

90. Coppetto JR, Gahn NG. Bitemporal hemianopic scotoma. A complication of intraventricular catheter. Surg Neurol 1977;8:361-362.

91. Corbett JJ. Neuro-ophthalmologic complications of hydrocephalus and shunting procedures. Semin Neurol 1986;6:111-123.

92. Cotton MF, Reiley T, Robinson CC, et al. Acute aqueductal stenosis in a patient with Epstein-Barr virus infectious mononucleosis. Pediatr Infect Dis J 1994;13:224-227.

93. Coulon RA, Toll K. Intracranial ependymomas in children: a review of 43 cases. Childs Brain 1977; 3:154-168.

94. Coyle JT. Goldenhar's syndrome. Arch Ophthalmol 1991;109:916.

95. Crosley CJ, Binet EF. Sturge-Weber syndrome. Presentation as a focal seizure disorder without nevus flammeus. Clin Pediatrics 1978;17:606-609.

96. Cunliffe IA, Moffat DA, Hardy DG, Moore AT. Bilateral optic nerve sheath meningiomas in a patient with neurofibromatosis type 2. Br J Ophthalmol 1992;76:310-312.

97. Cushing H. Experiences with the cerebellar medulloblstoma: a critical review. Acta Pathol Microbiol Scand 1930;7:1-86.

98. Cusmai R, Curatolo P, Mangano S, et al. Hemimegalencephaly and neurofibromatosis. Neuropediatrics 1989;21:179-182.

99. Cusmai R, Curatolo P, Mangano S, et al. Hemimegalencephaly and neurofibromatosis. Neuropediatrics 1990;21:179-182.

100. Dagi LR, Chrousos GA, Cogan DC. Spasm of the near reflex associated with organic disease. Am J Ophthalmol 1987;103:582-585.

101. Davidson JE, McWilliam RC, Evans TJ, et al. Porencephaly and optic hypoplasia in neonatal thrombocytopenia. Arch Dis Child 1989;64:858-860.

102. Davis CH, Joglekar VM. Cerebellar astrocytomas in children and young adults. J Neurol Neurosurg Psychiatr 1981;44:820-828.

103. de Jong PTVM, Verkaart RJF, van de Vooren MJ, et al. Twin vessels in von Hippel-Lindau disease. Am J Ophthalmol 1988;105:165-169.

104. de Juan E, Green WR, Gupta PK, Baranano EC. Vitreous seeding by retinal astrocytic hamartoma in a patient with tuberous sclerosis. Retina 1984;4:100-102.

105. De-Santi MM, Magni A, Valletta EA, et al. Hydrocephalus, bronchiectasis, and ciliary aplasia. Arch Dis Child 1990;65:543-544.

106. Dearnaley DP, A'Hern RP, Whittaker S, et al. Pineal and CNS germ cell tumors: royal Marsden Hospital experience 1962-1987. Int J Radiat Oncol Biol Phys 1990;18:773-788.

107. Delleman JW, Oorthuys JEW. Orbital cyst in addition to congenital cerebral and focal dermal malformations. A new entity? Clin Genet 1981;19:191-198.

108. Destro M, D'Amico DJ, Gragoudas ES, et al. Retinal manifestations of neurofibromatosis: diagnosis and management. Arch Ophthalmol 1991;109:662-666.

109. Deutsch M. Medulloblastoma: staging and treatment outcome. Int J Radiat Oncol Biol Phys 1988;14:1103-1107.

110. Di-Rocco C. Is the slit ventricle syndrome always a slit ventricle syndrome? Childs Nerv Syst 1994;10:49-58.

111. Dias MS, McLone DG. Hydrocephalus in the child with dysraphism. Neurosurg Clin North Am 1993;4:715-726.

112. Diebler C, Dulac O. Cephalocoeles: clinical and neuroradiological appearance. Neuroradiology 1983;25:199-216.

113. DiMario FJ, Ramsby G, Greenstein R, et al. Neurofibromatosis type 1: magnetic resonance imaging findings. J Child Neurol 1993;8:32-39.

114. Dobyns WB, Pagon RA, Armstrong D, et al. Diagnostic criteria for Walker-Warburg syndrome. Am J Med Genet 1989;32:195-210.

115. Dosseter FM, Landau K, Hoyt WF. Optic disk glioma in neurofibromatosis type 2. Am J Ophthalmol 1989;108:602-603.

116. Dotan SA, Trobe JD, Gebarski SS. Visual loss in tuberous sclerosis. Neurology 1991;41(12):1915-1917.

117. Dowhan TP, Muci-Mendoza R, Aitken PA. Disappearing optociliary shunt vessels and neonatal hydrocephalus. J Clin Neuro-ophthalmol 1988;8:1-8.

118. Dropcho EJ, Wisoff JH, Walker RW, et al. Supratentorial malignant gliomas in childhood: a review of fifty cases. Ann Neurol 1987;22:355-364.

119. Dyste GN, Menezes AH, VanGilder JC. Symptomatic Chiari malformations. An analysis of presentation, management, and long term outcome. J Neurosurg 1989;71:159-168.

120. Eckman PB, Fountain EM. Unilateral proptosis: association with arteriovenous malformations involving the Galenic system. Arch Neurol 1974;31:350-351.

121. Edwards MSB, Hudgins RJ, Wilson CB, et al. Pineal region tumors in children. J Neurosurg 1988;68:689-697.

122. Effron L, Zakov ZN, Tomsak RL. Neovascular glaucoma as a complication of the Wyburn-Mason syndrome. J Clin Neuro-ophthalmology 1985;5:95-98.

123. Ellenbogen RG, Winston KR, Kupsky WJ. Tumors of the choroid plexus in children. Neurosurgery 1989;25:327-335.

124. Epstein F, Wisoff JH. Intrinsic brain stem tumors in childhood: Surgical indications. J Neuro-oncol 1988;6:309-317.

125. Ernestus RI, Wilcked O, Schroder R. Supratentorial ependymomas in childhood: clinicopathological findings and prognosis. Acta Neurochir 1991;111:96-102.

126. Ersahin Y, Mutluer S, Guzelbag E. Intracranial hydatic cysts in children. Neurosurgery 1993;33:219-225.

127. Espinosa JA, Giroux M, Johnson K, et al. Abducens palsy following shunting for hydrocephalus. Can J Neurol Sci 1993;20:123-125.

128. Evans AE, Jenkin RDT, Sposto R, et al. The treatment of medulloblastoma. J Neurosurg 1990;72:572-582.

129. Faillace WJ, Canady AI. Cerebrospinal fluid shunt malfunction signaled by new or recurrent seizures. Childs Nerv Syst 1990;6:37-40.

130. Farwell JR, Flannery JT. Pinealomas and germinomas in children. J Neuro-oncol 1989;7:13-19.

131. Felix I, Becker LE. Intracranial germ cell tumors in children: an immunohistochemical and electron microscopic study. Pediatrics Neuroscience 1991;16:156-162.

132. Feuerstein RC, Mims LC. Linear nevus sebaceous with convulsions and mental retardation. AJDC 1963;104:675-679.

133. Fielder A. Ophthalmic complications of spina bifida and hydrocephalus. Eye 1991;5 (pt 3):vii. Editorial.

134. Figueroa RE, Gammal TE, Brooks BS, et al. MR findings on primitive neuroectodermal tumors. J Comput Assist Tomogr 1989;13:773-778.

135. Fitz C. Magnetic resonance imaging of pediatric brain tumors. Top Magn Reson Imaging 1993;5:174-189.

136. Fivenson DP, Lucky AW, Iannoccone S. Sjogren-Larsson syndrome associated with the Dandy-Walker malformation: report of a case. Pediatrics Dermatol 1989;6:312-315.

137. Foltz EL, Blanks JP. Symptomatic low intracranial pressure in shunted hydrocephalus. J Neurosurg 1988;68:401-408.

138. Fox AJ. Angiography for third nerve palsy in children. J Clin Neuro-ophthalmology 1989;9:37-38.

139. Friedman HS, Oakes WJ, Bigner SH, et al. Medulloblastoma tumor: biological and clinical perspectives. J Neuro-oncol 1991;11:1-15.

140. Fryer AE, Chalmers A, Connor JM, et al. Evidence that the gene for tuberous sclerosis is on chromosome 9. Lancet 1987;1:659.

141. Gaffney CC, Sloane JP, Bradley NJ, et al. Primitive neuroectodermal tumours of the cerebrum. J Neuro-oncol 1985;3:23-33.

142. Galetta SL, Smith JL. Chronic isolated sixth nerve palsies. Arch Neurol 1989;46:79-82.

143. Garcia DM, Latifi HR, Simpson JR, et al. Astrocytomas of the cerebellum in children. J Neurosurg 1989;71:661-664.

144. Garg BP. Colpocephaly: an error of morphogenesis? Arch Neurol 1982;39:243-246.

145. Gass JDM. Cavernous hemangioma of the retina: a neuro-oculo-cutaneous syndrome. Am J Ophthalmol 1971;71:799-814.

146. Gass JDM. *Stereoscopic Atlas of Diffuse Macular Disease: Diagnosis and Treatment.* 3rd ed. St. Louis, MO: CV Mosby; 1990;2:640-648.

147. Gass JDM. *Stereoscopic Atlas of Macular Diseases: Diagnosis and Treatment.* 3rd ed. St. Louis, MO: CV Mosby; 1987:420-421.

148. Gaston H. Ophthalmic complications of spina bifida and hydrocephalus. Eye 1991;5(pt 3):279-290.

149. Gatti RA, Berkel I, Boder E, et al. Localization of an ataxia-telangiectasia gene to chromosome 11q22-23. Nature 1988;336:577.

150. Gelabert-Gonzalez M, Bollar-Zabala A, Prieto-Gonzalez A, et al. Neurofibromatosis and stenosis of the aqueduct of Sylvius. A magnetic resonance assessment. Rev Med Univ Navarra 1990;34:17-19.

151. Geyer JR. Infant brain tumors. In: Berger MS, ed. *Pediatric Neuro-oncology, Neurosurgery Clinics of North America.* Philadelphia, PA: WB Saunders; 1992:781-791.

152. Ghose S. Optic nerve changes in hydrocephalus. Trans Ophthalmol Soc UK. 1983;103(pt 2):217-220.

153. Gilbert JN, Jones KL, Rorke LB, et al. Central nervous system anomalies associated with meningomyelocele, hydrocephalus, and the Arnold-Chiari malformation: reappraisal of theories regarding the pathogenesis of posterior neural tube closure defects. Neurosurgery 1986;18:559-564.

154. Gilles FH, Sobel E, Leviton A, et al. Epidemiology of seizures in children with brain tumors. The childhood brain tumor consortium. J Neuro-oncol 1992;12:53-68.

155. Gingold SI, Winfield JA. Oscillopsia and primary cerebellar ectopia: case report and review of the literature. Neurosurgery 1991;29:932-936.

156. Glanzmann C, Seelentag W. Radiotherapy for tumours of the pineal region and suprasellar germinomas. Radiother Oncol 1989;16:31-40.

157. Glauser TA, Packer RJ. Cognitive deficits in long-term survivors of childhood brain tumors. Childs Nerv Syst 1991;7:2-12.

158. Goldberg MF, Custis PH. Retinal and other manifestations of incontinentia pigmenti (Bloch-Sulzberger syndrome). Ophthalmology 1993;100:1645-1654.

159. Goldwein JR, Galser TA, Packer RJ, et al. Recurrent intracranial ependymomas in children. Cancer 1990;66:557-563.

160. Goldwein JW, Leahy JM, Packer RJ, et al. Intracranial ependymomas in children. Int J Radiat Oncol Biol Phys 1990;19:1497-1502.

161. Gomez MR. Diagnostic criteria. In: Gomez MR, ed. *Tuberous Sclerosis.* 2nd ed. New York: Raven Press; 1985:63-74.

162. Good WV, Brodsky MC, Edwards MS, et al. Bilateral retinal hamartomas in neurofibromatosis type 2. Br J Ophthalmol 1991;75:190.

163. Good WV, Hoyt CS. Optic nerve shadow enlargement in the Klippel-Trenauney-Weber syndrome. J Pediatrics Ophthalmol Strabismus 1989;26:288-290.

164. Good WV, Jan JE, DeSa L, et al. Cortical visual impairment in children. Surv Ophthalmlol 1994;38:351-364.

165. Gorlin RJ, Pindborg JJ, Cogen MM. Oculoauriculovertebral spectrum. In: *Syndromes of the Head and Neck.* 3rd ed. New York: McGraw-Hill; 1989:641-649.

166. Guy JR, Friedman WF, Mickle JP. Bilateral trochlear nerve paresis in hydrocephalus. J Clin Neuro-ophthalmol 1989;9:105-111.

167. Hager BC, Dyme IZ, Guertin SR, et al. Linear sebaceous nevus syndrome: megalencephaly and heterotopic gray matter. Pediatrics Neurol 1991;7:45-49.

168. Halbach VV, Higashida RT, Hieshima GB. Treatment of intracranial aneurysm by balloon embolization therapy. Semin Intervention Radiol 1987;4:261-268.

169. Hamed LM, Fang E, Fanous M, et al. The prevalence of neurological dysfunction in children with strabismus who have superior oblique overaction. Ophthalmology 1993;100:1483-1487.

170. Hamed LM, Maria BL, Quisling RG, et al. Alternating skew on lateral gaze: neuroanatomic pathway and relationship to superior oblique overaction. Ophthalmology 1993;100:281-286.

171. Hamed LM. Alternating skew on lateral gaze simulating bilateral superior oblique overaction. Binocular Vision Q 1992;7:83-88.

172. Hamed LM. Superior oblique overaction: some nosologic considerations. Am Orthopt J 1993;43:82-86.

173. Hardwig P, Robertson DM. von Hippel-Lindau disease: a familial, often lethal, multisystem phakomatosis. Ophthalmology 1984;91:263-270.

174. Healey EA, Barnes PD, Jupsky WJ, et al. The prognostic significance of postoperative residual tumor in ependymoma. Neurosurgery 1991;28: 666-671.

175. Hered RW. Tuberous sclerosis. Arch Ophthalmol 1992;110:410.

176. Herskowitz J, Rosman P, Wheeler CB. Colpocephaly: Clinical, radiologic, and pathogenetic aspects. Neurology 1985;35:1594-1598.

177. Hertle RW, Quinn GE, Katowitz JA. Ocular and adnexal findings in patients with facial microsomias. Ophthalmology 1992;99:114-119.

178. Hogg D, Gorin MB, Heinzmann C. Nucleotide sequences for the C-DNA of the bovine Beta-B2 crystalline and assignment of the orthologous human locus to chromosome 22. Current Eye Res 1987;6:1335-1342.

179. Hogg JE, Schoenberg DS. Paralysis of divergence in an adult with aqueductal stenosis. Arch Neurol 1979;36:511-512.

180. Holschneider AM, Bliesener JA, Abel M. Brain stem dysfunction in Arnold-Chiari II syndrome. Z Kinderchir 1990;45:67-71.

181. Horowitz ME, Mulhern RK, Kun LE, et al. Brain tumors in the very young child. Cancer 1988;61: 428-434.

182. Hoyt CS, Billson FA. Buphthalmos in neurofibromatosis: Is it an expression of regional giantism? J Pediatrics Ophthalmol Strabismus 1977;14:228-234.

183. Hoyt WF: Congenital homonymous hemianopia. Neuro-ophthalmology Jpn 1985;2:252-260.

184. Humphreys RP. Vascular malformations of the brain. In: Check WR, ed. *Pediatric Neurosurgery: Surgery of the Pediatric Nervous System.* Philadelphia, PA: WB Saunders; pp. 1994:524-532.

185. Huson SM, Harper PS, Hourihan MD, et al. Cerebellar haemangioblastoma and von Hippel-Lindau disease. Brain 1986;109:1297-1310.

186. Imes RK, Hoyt WF. Magnetic resonance imaging signs of optic nerve gliomas in neurofibromatosis 1. Am J Ophthalmol 1991;111:729-734.

187. Iteiskanen O, Vilkki J. Intracranial arterial aneurysms in children and adolescents. Acta Neurochir 1981;59:55-63.

188. Iwach AG, Hoskins HD, Hetherington A, Shaffer RN. Analysis of surgical and medical management of glaucoma in Sturge-Weber syndrome. Ophthalmology 1990;97:904-909.

189. Jackson IT, Carbonnel A, Potparic Z. Orbitotemporal neurofibromatosis: classification and treatment. Plast Reconst Surg 1993;92:1-11.

190. James HE, Nowak TP. Clinical course and diagnosis of migraine headaches in hydrocephalic children. Pediatr Neurosurg 1992;17:310-316. Discussion.

191. Janotka H, Huczynska B, Szczudrawa J. Buphthalmos without glaucoma in Recklinghausen's neurofibromatosis. Klin Monatsbl Augenheilkd 1972;161:301-305.

192. Jenkin RDT, Boesel C, Ertel I, et al. Brain stem tumors in childhood: A prospective randomized trial of irradiation with and without adjuvant CCNU, VCR, and prednisone. J Neurosurg 1987;66:277-285.

193. Jennings MT, Gelman R, Hochberg F. Intracranial germ cell tumors: natural history and pathogenesis. J Neurosurg 1985;63:155-167.

194. Jereb B, Zupancic N, Petric J. Intracranial germinomas: report of seven cases. Pediatrics Hematol Oncol 1990;7:183-188.

195. Jesberg DO, Spencer WH, Hoyt WF. Incipient lesions of von Hippel-Lindau disease. Arch Ophthalmol 1968;80:632-640.

196. Jordan RM, Kendall JW, McClung M, Kammer H. Concentration of human chorionic gonadotropin in the cerebrospinal fluid of patients with germinal cell hypothalamic tumors. Pediatrics 1980;65:121-124.

197. Kaiser-Kupfer MI, Freidlin V, Datiles MB, et al. The association of posterior capsular lens opacities with bilateral acoustic neuromas in patients with neurofibromatosis type 2. Arch Ophthalmol 1989; 107:541-544.

198. Kandt RS, Steingold S, Wall S, et al. The majority of tuberous sclerosis (TSC) families show no evidence for linkage to purported linked foci, but 1 family sublocalizes TSC on chromosome 9. Ann Neurol 1992;32:457. Abstract.

199. Kandt RS. Tuberous sclerosis: the next step. J Child Neurol 1993;8:107-111.

200. Kanter WR, Eldridge R, Fabricant R, et al. Central neurofibromatosis with bilateral acoustic neuroma: genetic, clinical and biochemical distinctions from peripheral neurofibromatosis. Neurology 1980;30: 851-859.

201. Karch SB, Urich H. Occipital encephalocele: a morphological study. J Neurol Sci 1972;15:89-112.

202. Kashii S, Solomon SK, Moser FG, et al. Progressive visual field defects in patients with intracranial arteriovenous malformations. Am J Ophthalmol 1990;109:556-562.

203. Katz B, Wiley CA, Lee VW. Optic nerve hypoplasia and the syndrome of nevus sebaceous of Jadassohn. Ophthalmology 1987;94:1570-1576.

203a. Katz DM, Trobe JD, Muraszko, KM, Dauser RC. Shunt failure without ventriculomegaly proclaimed by ophthalmic findings. J Neurosurg 1994;81:721-725.

204. Kaye LD, Rothner Ad, Beauchamp GR, et al. Ocular findings associated with neurofibromatosis type 2. Ophthalmology 1992;99:1424-1429.

205. Keane JR: Pretectal pseudobobbing. Five patients with "V"-pattern convergence nystagmus. Arch Neurol 1985;42:592-594.

206. Kodsi SR, Bloom KE, Egbert JE, et al. Ocular and systemic manifestations of encephalocraniocutaneous lipomatosis. Am J Ophthalmol 1994;118:77-82.

207. Kojima N, Tamaki N, Hosoda K, Matsumoto S. Visual field defects in hydrocephalus. No-To-Shinkei. 1985;37(3):229-236.

208. Kroll AS, Reiken PD, Robb RM, Albert DM. Vitreous hemorrhage complicating retinal astrocytic hamartoma. Surv Ophthalmol 1981;26:31-38.

209. Kuban KC, Teele RL, Wallman J. Septo-optic-dys-plasia-schizencephaly. Radiographic and clinical features. Pediatrics Radiology 1989;19:145-150.

210. Kun LE, Kovnar EH, Sanford RA: Ependymomas in children. Pediatrics Neuroscience 1988;14:57-63.

211. Kupersmith MJ, Vargas M, Hoyt WF, Berenstein A. Optic tract atrophy with cerebral arteriovenous malformations. Direct and transsynaptic degeneration. Neurology 1994;44:80-83.

212. Lamas E, Lobato RD, Esparza J, Escudero L. Dural posterior fossa AVM producing raised sagittal sinus pressure. J Neurosurg 1977;46:804-810.

213. Lambert HM, Sipperley JO, Shore JW, et al. Linear sebaceous nevus syndrome. Ophthalmology 1987;94:278-283.

214. Landau K, Yasargil GM. Ocular fundus in neurofibromatosis type 2. Br J Ophthalmol 1993;77:646-649.

215. Landau K, Dossetor FM, Hoyt WF, et al. Retinal hamartoma in neurofibromatosis 2. Arch Ophthalmol 1990;108:328-329.

216. Landau K; Gloor BP. Therapy-resistant papilledema in achondroplasia. J Neuro-ophthalmol 1994;14(1):24-28.

217. Lannering B, Marky I, Lundberg A, et al. Long-term sequelae after pediatric brain tumors: their effect on disability and quality of life. Med Pediatr Oncol 1990;18:304-310.

218. Larson DA, Wara WM, Edwards MSB. Management of childhood cerebellar astrocytoma. Int J Radiat Oncol Biol Phys 1989;18:971-973.

219. Lee A, Goldberg MF, Gillard JH, et al. Intracranial assessment of incontinentia pigmenti using magnetic resonance techniques. Arch Pediatrics 1995. In press.

220. Legido A, Packer RJ, Sutton LN, et al. Suprasellar germinomas in childhood. Cancer 1989;63:340-344.

221. Leigh RJ, Mapstone T, Weymann C. Eye movements in children with the Dandy-Walker syndrome. Neuro-ophthalmology 1992;12:285-288.

222. Lennerstrand G, Gallo JE. Neuro-ophthalmological evaluation of patients with myelomeningocele and Arnold-Chiari malformations. Dev Med Child Neurol 1990;32:415-422.

223. Lennerstrand G, Gallo JE, Samuelsson L. Neuro-ophthalmological findings in relation to CNS lesions in patients with myelomeningocele. Dev Med Child Neurol 1990;32(5):423-431.

224. Lerone M, Pessagno A, Taccone A, Poggi G, Romeo G, Silengo MC. Oculocerebral syndrome with hypopigmentation (Cross syndrome): report of a new case. Clin Genet 1992;41:87-89.

225. Lewis RA, Gerson LP, Axelson KA, et al. von Recklinghausen neurofibromatosis. II: incidence of optic gliomata. Ophthalmology 1984;91:929.

226. Lewis RA, Riccardi VM: von Recklinhausen neurofibromatosis: incidence of iris hamartomata. Ophthalmology 1981;88:348.

227. Listernick R, Charrow J, Greenwald MJ, Esterly NB. Optic gliomas in children with neurofibromatosis type I. J Pediatr 1989;114:788.

227a. Listernick R, Charrow J, Greenwald M, Mets M. Natural history of optic pathway tumors in children with neurofibromatosis type 1: a longitudinal study. J Pediatr 1994;125:63-66.

228. Loggers HE, Oosterwijk JC, Overweg-Plandsoen WCG, et al. Encephalocraniocutaneous lipomatosis and oculocerebrocutaneous syndrome. Ophthalmic Ped Genet 1992;13:171-177.

229. Lopponen H, Sorri M, Serlo W, von-Wendt L. ENG findings of shunt-treated hydrocephalus in children. Int J Pediatr Otorhinolaryngol 1992;23:35-44.

230. Lowenstein DH, Koch TK, Edwards MS: Cerebral ptosis with contralateral arteriovenous malformation: A report of two cases. Ann Neurol 1987;21:404-407.

231. Lubs M-LE, Bauer M, Formas ME, Djokic B. Iris hamartomas in the diagnosis of neurofibromatosis-1. Int Pediatr1990;5:261.

232. Lubs M-LE, Bauer M, Formas ME, Djokic B. Lisch nodules in neurofibromatosis type I. N Engl J Med 1991;324:1264.

233. Luessenhop AJ. Natural history of cerebral arteriovenous malformations. In: Wilson CB, Stein BM, eds. *Intracranial Arteriovenous Malformations.* Baltimore, MD: Williams & Wilkins; 1984:13-23.

234. Lunsford LD, Kondziolka D, Flickinger JC, et al. Stereotactic radiosurgery for arteriovenous malformations of the brain. J Neurosurg 1991;75:512.

235. Lyons MK, Kelly PJ. Posterior fossa ependymomas: report of 30 cases and review of the literature. Neurosurgery 1991;28:659-665.

236. Maher ER, Yates JRW, Harries R, et al. Clinical features and natural history of von Hippel-Lindau disease. Q J Med 1990;66:233.

237. Maitland CG, Abiko S, Hoyt WF, et al. Chiasmal apoplexy: report of four cases. J Neurosurg 1982;56:118-122.

238. Malik S, Cohen BH, Robinson J, et al. Progressive vision loss: a rare manifestation of familial cavernous angiomas. Arch Neurol 1992;49:170-173.

239. Malzone WF, Gonyea EF. Exophthalmos with intracerebral arteriovenous malformations. Neurology 1973;23:534-538.

240. Manor RS, Bar-Ziv J, Tadmor R, et al. Pineal germinoma with unilateral blindness. Seeding of germinoma cells in optic nerve sheath. J Clin Neuro-ophthalmol 1990;10:239-243.

241. Mansour AM, Wang F, Henkind P, et al. Ocular findings in the facioauriculovertebral sequence (Goldenhar-Gorlin syndrome). Am J Ophthalmol 1985;100:555-559.

242. Margolis S, Aleksic S, Charles N, et al. Retinal and optic nerve findings in the Goldenhar-Gorlin syndrome. Ophthalmology 1984;91:1327.
243. Maria BL, Rehder KK, Eskin TA, et al. Brain stem glioma. I: pathology, clinical features and therapy. J Child Neurol 1993;8:112-128.
244. Martinez-Lage JF, Poza M, Costa TR. Bilateral temporal arachnoid cysts in neurofibromatosis. J Child Neurol 1993;8:383-385.
245. Martyn LJ, Knox DL. Glial hamartoma of the retina in generalized neurofibromatosis, von Recklinghausen's disease. Br J Ophthalmol 1972;56:487-491.
246. Matsubara O, Tanaka M, Ida T, Okeda R. Hemimegalencephaly with hemihypertrophy (Klippel-Trenauney-Weber syndrome). Virchows Arch A Pathol Anat Histopathol 1983;400:155-162.
247. Matzkin DC, Slamovits TL, Jenis I, et al. Disc swelling: A tall tale? Surv Ophthalmol 1992;37:130-136.
248. Mautner VF, Tatagiba M, Guthoff R, et al. Neurofibromatosis-2 in the pediatric age group. Neurosurgery 1993;33:92-96.
249. McLone DG, Knepper PA. The cause of Chiari II malformation: a unified theory. Pediatrics Neuroscience 1989;15:1-12.
250. Mealey J Jr, Dzenitis AJ, Hockey AA. The prognosis of encephaloceles. J Neurosurg 1970;32:209-218.
251. Mercuri S, Russo A, Palma L. Hemispheric supratentorial astrocytomas in children. Long-term results in 29 cases. J Neurosurg 1981;55:170-173.
252. Meyers SP, Kemp SS, Tarr RW. MR imaging features of medulloblastomas. Am J Roentgenol 1992;158:859-865.
253. Miller JH. Radiological evaluation of sellar lesions. Crit Rev Diagn Imaging 1981;16:311-347.
254. Miller NR. Solitary oculomotor nerve palsy in childhood. Am J Ophthalmol 1977;83:106-111.
255. Miller NR. *Walsh and Hoyt's Clinical Neuro-ophthalmology.* 4th ed. Baltimore, MD: Williams & Wilkins; 1988;3:1747-1765.
256. Miller NR. *Walsh and Hoyt's Clinical Neuro-ophthalmology.* Baltimore, MD: Williams & Wilkins; 1982;1:197.
257. Miller NR. *Walsh and Hoyt's Clinical Neuro-ophthalmology.* Baltimore, MD: Williams & Wilkins; 1991;3:1516.
258. Miyamoto S, Kikuchi H, Karasawa J, et al. Study of the posterior circulation in Moyamoya disease. Part 2: visual disturbances and surgical treatment. J Neurosurg 1986;65:454-460.
259. Moadel K, Yannuzzi LA, Ho AC, Uresaker A. Retinal vascular occlusive disease in a child with neurofibromatosis. Arch Ophthalmol 1994;112: 1021-1023.
260. Mohandessan MM, Romano PE. Neuroparalytic keratitis in Goldenhar-Gorlin sydnrome. Am J Ophthalmol 1978;85:111.
261. Mohr JP. Neurological manifestations and factors related to therapeutic decisions. In: Wilson CB, Stein BM, eds. *Intracranial Arteriovenous Malformations.* Baltimore, MD: Williams & Wilkins; 1984:1-11.
262. Morgan SA, Emsellem HA, Sandler JR. Absence of the septum pellucidum: overlapping clinical syndromes. Arch Neurol 1985;42:769-770.
263. Mori K, Murata T, Hasimoto N, et al. Clinical analysis of arteriovenous malformations in children. Childs Brain 1980;6:13.
264. Mossman SS, Bronstein AM, Gresty MA, Kendall B, Rudge P. Convergence nystagmus associated with Arnold-Chiari malformation. Arch Neurol 1990;47:357-359.
265. Murphy MJ, Risk WS, VanGilder JC. Intracranial dermoid cyst in Goldenhar syndrome. J Neurosurg 1980;53:408-410.
266. Naidich TP, Altman NR, Barffman BH, et al. Cephaloceles and related malformations. AJNR 1992;13:655-690.
267. National Institutes of Health Consensus Development Conference. Neurofibromatosis: Conference Statement. Arch Neurol 1988;45:575-578.
268. Neumann HPH, Berger DP, Sigmund G, et al. Pheochromocytomas, multiple endocrine neoplasia type 2, and von Hippel-Lindau disease. N Engl J Med 1993;329:1531-1538.
269. Neumann HPH, Eggert HR, Scheremet R, et al. Central nervous system lesions in von Hippel-Lindau syndrome. J Neurol Neurosurg Psychol 1992;55:898-901.
270. Neumann HPH, Wiestler OD. Clustering of features of von Hippel-Lindau syndrome: evidence for a complex gene locus. Lancet 1991;337:1052.
271. Newman NJ. Bilateral visual loss and disc edema in a 15-year-old girl. Surv Ophthalmol 1994; 38:365-370. Clinical Conference.
272. Newman SA. Ophthalmic features of craniosynostosis. Neurosurg Clin North Am 1991;2:587-610.
273. Nishizaki T, Tamaki N, Nishida Y, et al. Bilateral internuclear ophthalmoplegia due to hydrocephalus: a case report. Neurosurgery 1985;17:822-825.
274. Nowak TP, James HE. Migraine headaches in hydrocephalic children: a diagnostic dilemma. Childs Nerv Syst 1989;5:310-314.
275. O'Connor PS, Smith JL. Optic nerve variant in the Klippel-Trenauney-Weber syndrome. Ann Ophthalmol 1978;10:131-134.
276. Oakes WJ. The natural history of patients with the Sturge-Weber syndrome. Pediatrics Neurosurg 1992;18:287-290.
277. Obringer AC, Meadows AT, Zackai EH. The diagnosis of neurofibromatosis-1 in the child under the age of 6 years. AJDC 1989;143:717-719.
278. Ogata H, Oka K, Mitsudome A. Hydrocephalus due to acute aqueductal stenosis following mumps

infection: report of a case and review of the literature. Brain Dev 1992;14:417-419.

279. Oka K, Kumate S, Kibe M, et al. Aqueductal stenosis due to mesencephalic venous malformation: case report. Surg Neurol 1993;40:230-235.

280. Okuno T, Prensky AL, Gado M. The Moyamoya syndrome associated with irradiation of optic glioma in children: report of two cases and review of the literature. Pediatrics Neurol 1985;1:311-316.

281. Ondra SL, Troupp H, George ED, Schwab K. The natural history of symptomatic arteriovenous malformations of the brain: a 24-year follow-up assessment. J Neurosurg 1990;73:387-391.

282. Orcutt JC, Bunt AH. Anomalous optic disc in a patient with a Dandy-Walker cyst. J Clin Neuro-ophthalmology 1986;2:42-43.

283. Osenbach RK, Menezes AH. Diagnosis and management of the Dandy-Walker malformation: 30 years of experience. Pediatrics Neurosurg 1992;18:179-189.

284. Osher RH, Corbett JJ, Schatz NJ, et al. Neuro-ophthalmological complications of enlargement of the third ventricle. Br J Ophthalmol 1978;62:536-542.

285. Packer RJ, Nicholson HS, Vezine LG, Johnson DL. Brain stem gliomas. In: Berger MS, ed. *Pediatric Neuro-oncology, Neurosurgery Clinics of North America.* Philadelphia, PA: WB Saunders; 1992:863-879.

286. Pappas CTE, Rekate HL. Cervicomedullary junction decompression in a case of Marshall-Smith syndrome. J Neurosurg 1991;75:317-319.

287. Pascual-Castroviejo I, Roche MC, Fernandez VM, et al. Incontinentia pigmenti: MR demonstration of brain changes. AJNR 1994;15:1521-1527.

288. Pascual-Castroviejo I, Velez A, Pascual-Pascual SI, et al. Dandy-Walker malformation: analysis of 38 cases. Childs Nerv Syst 1991;7:88-97.

289. Passo M, Shults WT, Talbot T, Palmer EA. Acquired esotropia. A manifestation of Chiari I malformation. J Clin Neuro-ophthalmol 1984;4:151-154.

290. Pearson-Webb MA, Kaiser-Kupfer MI, Eldridge R. Eye findings in bilateral acoustic (central) neurofibromatosis: association with presenile lens opacities and cataracts but absence of Lisch nodules. N Engl J Med 1986;315:1553-1554.

291. Peerless SJ, Nemoto S, Drake CG. Giant intracranial aneurysms in children and adolescents. In: Edwards MSB, Hoffman HH, eds. *Cerebrovascular Disease in Children and Adolescents.* Baltimore, MD: Williams & Wilkins; 1988:255-273.

292. Phadke JG, Hern J, Blaiklock CT. Downbeat nystagmus—A false localizing sign due to communicating hydrocephalus. J Neurol Neurosurg Psychiatr 1981;44:459.

293. Pollack IF. Brain tumors in children. N Engl J Med 1994;331:1500-1507.

294. Pollack IF, Pang D, Albright AL. The long-term outcome in children with late-onset aqueductal

stenosis resulting from benign intrinsic tectal tumors. J Neurosurg 1994;80:681-688.

295. Price DB, Inglese CM, Jacobs J, et al. Pediatric AIDS. Neuroradiologic and neurodevelopmental findings. Pediatrics Radiology 1988;18:445-448.

296. Rabinowicz IM. Visual function in children with hydrocephalus. Trans Ophthalmol Soc UK 1974;94:353-366.

297. Radkowski MA, Naidich TP, Tomita T, et al. Neonatal brain tumors: CT and MR findings. J Comput Assist Tomogr 1988;12:10-20.

298. Ragge NK, Falk RE, Cohen WE, Murphree AL. Images of Lisch nodules across the spectrum. Eye 1993;7:95-101.

299. Ragge NK. Clinical and genetic patterns in neurofibromatosis 1 and 2. Br J Ophthalmol 1993;77:662-672.

300. Ragge NK; Hoyt WF. Midbrain myasthenia: fatigable ptosis, 'lid twitch' sign, and ophthalmoparesis from a dorsal midbrain glioma. Neurology 1992;42:917-919.

301. Rathbun JE, Hoyt WF, Beard C. Surgical management of orbitofrontal varix in Klippel-Trenauney-Weber syndrome. Am J Ophthalmol 1970;70:109-112.

302. Riaz G, Selhorst JB, Hennessey JJ. Meningeal lesions mimicking migraine. Neuro-ophthalmology 1991;11:41-48.

303. Riccardi VM, Eichner JE, eds. *Neurofibromatosis: Phenotype, Natural History, and Pathogenesis.* Baltimore, MD: Johns Hopkins University Press; 1986.

304. Riccardi VM: Neurofibromatosis: past, present, and future. N Engl J Med 1991;324:1283.

305. Riccardi VM: von Recklinhausen neurofibromatosis. N Engl J Med 1981;305:1617.

306. Richards SC, Bachynski BN. Ophthalmic manifestations of neurofibromatosis type 2. Int Pediatrics 1990;5:270.

307. Richkind KE, Boder E, Teplitz RL. Fetal proteins in ataxia-telangiectasia. JAMA 1982;248:1346.

308. Riela AR, Roach S. Etiology of stroke in children. J Child Neurol 1993;8:201-220.

309. Roach ES, Smith M, Huttenlocher P, et al. Diagnostic criteria-tuberous sclerosis. J Child Neurol 1992;7:221-224.

310. Robertson IJ, Leggate JR, Miller JD, et al. Aqueduct stenosis—presentation and prognosis. Br J Neurosurg 1990;4:101-106.

311. Roche JL, Choux M, Czorny A, et al. Intracranial arterial aneurysm in children. A cooperative study. Apropos of 43 cases. Neurochirurgie 1988;34:243-251.

312. Rollnick BR, Kaye CI, Nagatoshi K, et al. Oculovertebral dysplasia and variants: phenotypic characteristics of 294 patients. Am J Med Genet 1987;26:361-375.

313. Rosenfeld SI, Smith ME. Ocular findings in incontinentia pigmenti. Ophthalmology 1985;92:543-546.

314. Rouleau GA, Wertelecki W, Haines JL, et al. Genetic linkage of bilateral acoustic neurofibromatosis to a DNA marker on chromosome 22. Nature 1987;329:246.

315. Rozot P, Berrod JP, Bracard S, et al. Stase papillaire et fistule durale. J Fr Ophtalmol 1991;14:13-19.

316. Ruggieri V, Caraballo R, Fejerman N. Intracranial tumors and West syndrome. Pediatrics Neurol 1989;5:327-329.

317. Rutka JT, Hoffman HJ, Drake JM, Humphreys RP. Suprasellar and sellar tumors in childhood and adolescence. In: Berger MS, ed. *Pediatric Neurooncology.* Philadelphia, PA: WB Saunders; 1992:803-820.

318. Rydh M, Malm M, Jernbeck J, et al. Ectatic blood vessels in port-wine stains lack innervation: possible role in pathogenesis. Plast Reconstr Surg 1991;87:419-421.

319. Sainte-Rose C, LaCombe J, Peirre-Kahn A, et al. Intracranial venous sinus hypertension: cause or consequence of hydrocephalus in infants? J Neurosurg 1984;60:727-736.

320. Sandhu A, Kendall B. Computed tomography in management of medulloblastomas. Neuroradiology 1987;29:444-452.

321. Sardanelli F, Barodi RC, Ottonello C, et al. Cranial MRI in Ataxia-Telangiectasia. Neuroradiology 1995;37:77-82.

322. Sarkari NBS, Bickerstaff ER. Relapses and remissions in brain stem tumors. Br Med J 1969;2:21-23.

323. Sarwar M, Schafer M: Brain malformation in linear nevus sebaceous syndrome: an MR study. J Comput Assist Tomogr 1988;12:338-340.

324. Sarwar M. The septum pellucidum: normal and abnormal. Am J Neuroradiol 1989;10:989-1005.

325. Sato Y, Waziri M, Smith W, et al. Hippel-Lindau disease: MR imaging. Radiology 1988;166:241-246.

326. Saylor WR, Saylor DC. The vascular lesions of neurofibromatosis. 1974;25:510-519.

327. Schatz H, Chang LF, Ober RR, et al. Central retinal vein occlusion associated with arteriovenous malformation. Ophthalmology 1993;100:24-30.

328. Schijman E, Blumenthal L, Sevilla M, Landoni O. Neuro-ophthalmic complications of intracranial catheters. Neurosurgery 1994;34:769-770. Letter.

329. Schneider JH, Raffel C, McComb JG. Benign cerebellar astrocytomas of childhood. Neurosurgery 1992;30:58-63.

330. Schrander-Stumpel CTRM, De Die-Smulders CEM, Hennekam RCM, et al. Oculoauriculovertebral spectrum and cerebral anomalies. J Med Genet 1992;29:326-331.

331. Sclafani AP, DeDio RM, Hendrix RA. The Chiari-I malformation. Ear Nose Throat J 1991;70:208-212.

332. Seiff SR, Brodsky MC, MacDonald G, et al. Orbital optic glioma in neurofibromatosis: magnetic resonance diagnosis of perineural arachnoidal gliomatosis. Arch Ophthalmol 1987;105:1689.

333. Seizinger BR, Rouleau GA, Ozeluis LJ, et al. von Hippel-Lindau disease maps to the region of chromosome 3 associated with renal cell carcinoma. Nature 1988;332:268.

334. Sergeyev AS. On the mutation rate of neurofibromatosis. Hum Genet 1975;28:129-138.

335. Serville F, Benit P, Saugier P, et al. Prenatal exclusion of X-linked hydrocephalus-stenosis of the aqueduct of Sylvius sequence using closely linked DNA markers. Prenat Diagn 1993;13:435-439.

336. Serville F, Lyonnet S, Pelet A, et al. X-linked hydrocephalus: clinical heterogeneity at a single gene locus. Eur J Pediatr 1992;151:515-518.

337. Shami MJ, Benedict WL, Myers M. Early manifestation of retinal hamartomas in tuberous sclerosis. Am J Ophthalmol 1993;115:539-540.

338. Shapiro F. Osteopetrosis. Current clinical considerations. Clin Orthop 1993;294:34-44.

339. Shields JA, Decker WL, Sanborn GE. Presumed acquired retinal hemangiomas. Ophthalmology 1983;90:1292-1300.

340. Shults WT, Hamby S, Corbett JJ, et al. Neuro-ophthalmic complications of intracranial catheters. Neurosurgery 1993;33:135-138.

341. Slavin ML, Rosenthal AD. Chiasmal compression caused by a catheter in the suprasellar cistern. Am J Ophthalmol 1988;105:560-561.

342. Smirniotopoulos JG, Murphy FM. The phakomatoses. AJNR 1992;13:725-746.

343. Smith JL, Walsh TJ, Shipley T. Cortical blindness in congenital hydrocephalus. Am J Ophthalmol 1966;62:251-257.

344. Smith NM, Carli MM, Hanieh A, et al. Gangliogliomas in childhood. Childs Nerv Syst 1992; 8:258-262.

345. Smoller BR, Rosen S. Port-wine stains: A disease of altered neuromodulation of blood vessels? Arch Dermatol 1986;122:177.

346. Sorensen SA, Mulvihill JJ, Nielsen A. Long-term follow-up of von Recklinghause neurofibromatosis. N Engl J Med 1986;314:1010-1015.

347. Spooner JW, Baloh RW. Arnold-Chiari malformation. Improvement in eye movements after surgical treatment. Brain 1981;104:51-60.

348. Spoor TC, Kennerdell JS, Maroon JC, et al. Pneumosinus dilatans, Klippel-Trenauney-Weber syndrome, and progressive visual loss. Ann Ophthalmol 1981;13:105-111.

349. Spoto GP, Press GA, Hesselink JR, Solomon M. Intracranial ependymoma and subependymoma: MR manifestations. AJNR 1990;11:83-91.

350. Stanley P, Senac MO Jr, Segal HD. Intraspinal seeding from intracranial tumors in children. Am J Roentgenol 1985;144:157-161.

351. Staudenmaier C, Buncic JR. Periodic alternating gaze deviation with dissociated secondary face turn. Arch Ophthalmol 1983;101:202-205.

352. Stovner LJ, Kruszewski P, Shen JM. Sinus arrhythmia and pupil size in Chiari I malformation: evidence of autonomic dysfunction. Funct Neurol 1993;8:251-257.

353. Straube A, Witt TN. Oculo-bulbar myasthenic symptoms as the sole sign of tumour involving or compressing the brain stem. J Neurol 1990;237:369-371.

354. Sullivan TJ, Clarke MP, Morin JD. The ocular manifestations of the Sturge-Weber syndrome. J Pediatr Ophthalmol Strabismus 1992;29:349-356.

355. Sutton LN, Packer RJ, Rorke LB, et al. Cerebral gangliogliomas during childhood. Neurosurgery 1983;13:124-128.

356. Swash M. Disorders of ocular movement in hydrocephalus. Proc R Soc Med 1976;69:480-484.

357. Szenasy J, Slowik F. Prognosis of benign cerebellar astrocytomas in children. Childs Brain 1983;10:39-47.

358. Tampiere D, Moumdjian R, Melanson D, Ethier R. Intracerebral gangliogliomas in patients with partial complex seizures: CT and MR imaging findings. Am J Neuroradiol 1991;12:749-755.

359. Taylor D. *Pediatric Ophthalmology.* Boston, MA: Blackwell Scientific; 1990:583-589.

360. Terry A, Patrinely JR, Anderson RL, Smithwick W. Orbital meningoencephalocele manifesting as a conjunctival mass. Am J Ophthalmol 1993;115:46-49.

361. Theron J, Newton TH, Hoyt WF. Unilateral retinocephalic vascular malformations. Neuroradiology 1974;7:185-196.

362. Tien RD, Barkovich AJ, Edwards MSB. MR imaging of pineal tumors. AJNR 1990;155:143-151.

363. To KW, Rabinowitz SM, Friedman AH, et al. Neurofibromatosis and neural crest neoplasms: primary acquired melanosis and malignant melanoma of the conjunctiva. Surv Ophthalmol 1989;33:373-379.

364. Tomita T, McLone DG, Yasue M. Cerebral primitive neuroectodermal tumors in childhood. J Neuro-ooncol 1988;6:233-243.

365. Tonsgard JH, Oesterle CS. The ophthalmologic presentation of NF-2 in childhood. J Pediatr Ophthalmol Strabismus 1993;30:327-330.

366. Troost BT, Mark LE, Maroon JC. Resolution of classic migraine after removal of an occipital lobe AVM. Ann Neurol 1979;5:199-201.

367. Troost BT, Martinez J, Abel LA, et al. Upbeat nystagmus and internuclear ophthalmoplegia with brain stem glioma. Arch Neurol 1980;37:453-456.

368. Troost BT, Newton TH. Occipital lobe arteriovenous malformations. Arch Ophthalmol 1975;93:250-265.

369. Tychsen L, Hoyt WF. Occipital lobe dysplasia. Magnetic resonance findings in two cases of isolated congenital hemianopia. Arch Ophthalmol 1985;103:680-682.

370. Tzekov C, Cherninkova S, Gudeva T. Neuroophthalmological symptoms in children treated for internal hydrocephalus. Pediatr Neurosurg 1992;17:317-320.

371. Undjian S, Marinov M, Georgiev K. Long-term follow-up after surgical treatment of cerebellar astrocytomas in 100 children. Childs Nerv Syst 1989;5:99-101.

372. Undjian S, Marinov M. Intracranial ependymomas in children. Childs Nerv Syst 1990;6:131-134.

373. Van Allen M, Kalousek D, Chernoff D, et al. Evidence for multisite closure of the neural tube defects in humans. Am J Med Genet 1993;47:723-743.

374. Van de Hoeve T. Eye disease in tuberous sclerosis of the brain. Trans Ophthalmol Soc UK 1923;43:534-541.

375. van-Dorp DB, Kwee ML. Tuberous sclerosis. Diagnostic problems in a family. Ophthalmic Paediatr Genet 1990;11:95-101.

376. Volpe JJ. Intraventricular hemorrhage in the premature infant—Current concepts. Part I. Ann Neurol 1989;25:3-11.

377. Volpe JJ. Intraventricular hemorrhage in the premature infant—Current concepts. Part II. Ann Neurol 1989;25:109-116.

378. Volpe JJ. *Neurology of the Newborn.* 2nd ed. Philadelphia, PA: WB Saunders; 1987:311-361.

379. Vrabec TR, Sergott RC, Savino PJ, Bosley TM. Intermittent obstructive hydrocephalus in the Arnold-Chiari malformation. Ann Neurol 1989;26:401-404.

380. Walton DS. In discussion: Iwach AG, et al. Analysis of surgical and medical management of glaucoma in Sturge-Weber syndrome. Ophthalmology 1990;97:909.

381. Waner M, Orton S, Flock S. The treatment of port-wine stains: a long term study. Plast Reconstr Surg 1995. In press.

382. Watkins L, Hayward R, Andar U, Harkness W. The diagnosis of blocked cerebrospinal fluid shunts: a prospective study of referral to a paediatric neurosurgical unit. Childs Nerv Syst 1994;10:87-90.

383. Weber PC, Cass SP. Neurotologic manifestations of Chiari 1 malformation. Otolaryngol Head Neck Surg 1993;109:853-860.

384. Weinberg S, Bennett H, Weinstock I. CNS manifestations of sarcoidosis in children. Clin Pediatrics 1983;22:447-481.

385. Weiner A. A case of neurofibromatosis with buphthalmos. Arch Ophthalmol 1925:481.

386. Weleber RG, Zonana J. Iris hamartomas (Lisch nodules) in a case of segmental neurofibromatosis. Am J Ophthalmol 1983;96:740-743.

387. Wende-Fischer R, Ehrenheim C, Heyer R; et al. In spinal symptoms remember toxoplasmosis. Monatsschr Kinderheilkd 1993;141:789-791.

388. Wertelecki W, Rouleau GA, Superneau DW, et al. Neurofibromatosis 2: clinical and DNA linkage studies of a large kindred. N Engl J Med 1988;319:278.

389. Westerhof W, Delleman JW, Wolters E, Dijkstra P. Neurofibromatosis and hypertelorism. Arch Dermatol 1984;120:1579-1581.

390. Williams J, Brodsky MC, Griebel M, et al. Septo-optic dysplasia: the clinical insignificance of an absent septum pellucidum. Dev Med Child Neurol 1993;35:490-501.

391. Williams R, Taylor D. Tuberous sclerosis. Surv Ophthalmol 1985;30:143-154.

392. Williams AS, Hoyt CS. Acute comitant esotropia in children with brain tumors. Arch Ophthalmol 1989;107:376-378.

393. Williamson TH, Garner A, Moore AT. Structure of Lisch nodules in neurofibromatosis type 1. Ophthalmic Paediatr Genet 1991;12:11-17.

394. Wilson GN: Cranial defects in the Goldenhar syndrome. Am J Med Genet 1983;14:435-443.

395. Wilson RD, Traverse L, Hall JG, et al. Oculocerebrocutaneous syndrome. Am J Ophthalmol 1985; 99:142-148.

396. Wolin MJ, Saunders RA: Aneurysmal oculomotor nerve palsy in an 11-year-old boy. J Clin Neuro-ophthalmology 1992;12:178-180.

397. Woody RC, Reynolds JD. Association of bilateral internuclear ophthalmoplegia and myelomeningocoele with Arnold-Chiari malformation type II. J Clin Neuro-ophthalmology 1985;5:124-126.

398. Wyburn-Mason R. Arteriovenous malformation of the mid-brain and retina, facial nerve, and mental changes. Brain 1943;66:163-203.

399. Yang SY, Wang ML, Xue QC. Cerebral cysticercosis. Surg Neurol 1990;34:286-293.

400. Yasue M, Tanaka H, Nakajima M, et al. Germ cell tumors of the basal ganglia and thalamus. Pediatrics Neurosurg 1993;19:121-126.

401. Yee RD, Baloh RW, Honrubia V. Episodic vertical oscillopsia and downbeat nystagmus in a Chiari malformation. Arch Ophthalmol 1984;102:723-725.

402. Yokota A, Matsukado Y, Fuwa I, et al. Anterior basal encephalocele of the neonatal period. Neurosurgery 1986;19:468-478.

403. Zammarchi E, Calzolari C, Pignotti MS, Pezzati P, Lignana E, Cama A. Unusual presentation of the immotile cilia syndrome in two children. Acta Paediatr 1993;82:312-313.

404. Zaret CR, Behrens MM, Eggers HM. Congenital ocular motor apraxia and brain stem tumors. Arch Ophthalmol 1980;98:328.

405. Zerah M, Garcia-Monaco R, Rodesch G, et al. Hydrodynamics in vein of Galen malformations. Childs Nerv Syst 1992;8:111-117. Discussion 117.

406. Zimmerman CF, Roach ES, Troost BT. Seesaw nystagmus associated with Chiari malformation. Arch Neurol 1986;43:299-300.

Index